THIRD EDITION

COMPREHENSIVE WOUND MANAGEMENT

THIRD EDITION

COMPREHENSIVE WOUND MANAGEMENT

Glenn L. Irion, PhD, PT, CWS
Retired Professor of Physical Therapy

Jennifer A. Gardner, PT, DPT, MHA, CWS
Clinical Wound Care Specialist

Rose M. Pignataro, PT, DPT, PhD, CWS, CHES
Physical Therapy Program
Emory & Henry College
Emory, Virginia

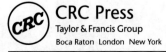

CRC Press
Taylor & Francis Group
Boca Raton London New York

CRC Press is an imprint of the
Taylor & Francis Group, an **informa** business

First Published in 2024 by SLACK Incorporated

Published 2024 by CRC Press
2385 NW Executive Center Drive, Suite 320, Boca Raton FL 33431

and by CRC Press
4 Park Square, Milton Park, Abingdon, Oxon, OX14 4RN

CRC Press is an imprint of Taylor & Francis Group, an informa business

Library of Congress Control Number: 2023943592

ISBN: 9781630915216 (hbk)
ISBN: 9781003523291 (ebk)

DOI: 10.1201/9781003523291

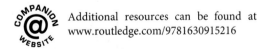

Additional resources can be found at
www.routledge.com/9781630915216

DEDICATION

This textbook is dedicated to my children, Lindsay, Kyle, Christina, Phillip, and Connor, and my wife Jean.
I also dedicate this book to the many patients who inspired me to create a Third Edition
that might better help others improve the lives of their patients.

—Glenn L. Irion, PhD, PT, CWS

I am dedicating this book to my wonderful husband, Wes Harbison, and our daughters, Delaney and Pyper.
I would also like to dedicate this book to my parents who have always supported me through all my endeavors.

—Jennifer A. Gardner, PT, DPT, MHA, CWS

I dedicate this work to my husband, Jack Murry Jr, and parents, Rose and Anthony Pignataro,
in appreciation for their love and support. I am grateful for a career enriched with colleagues, patients, and
students who have provided opportunities for continued personal and professional growth.
"Whatever you do, do all to the glory of God"—1 Corinthians 10:13

—Rose M. Pignataro, PT, DPT, PhD, CWS, CHES

CONTENTS

Comprehensive Wound Management, Third Edition, includes ancillary materials specifically available for faculty use. Please visit www.routledge.com/9781630915216 to obtain access.

ACKNOWLEDGMENTS

The authors wish to acknowledge the individuals who contributed to the production of the Third Edition. The book has been improved by the photos of patients, students, and colleagues who gladly allowed their images to be used to augment the text of the book. The assistance of those at SLACK Incorporated, including Tony Schiavo and Jennifer Cahill, is greatly appreciated.

ABOUT THE AUTHORS

Glenn L. Irion, PhD, PT, CWS, is a retired Certified Wound Specialist through the American Academy of Wound Management and Professor of Physical Therapy. He has taught integumentary and cardiovascular and pulmonary physical therapy and basic science for more than 30 years at the University of Central Arkansas and University of South Alabama and retired recently from Emory & Henry College. His clinical practice has included wound management, cardiopulmonary rehabilitation, and intensive care unit in both hospital and outpatient settings. He received a PhD in physiology at Temple University School of Medicine and furthered his research skills at the Medical College of Virginia (Virginia Commonwealth University) and the University of Cincinnati/Cincinnati Children's Hospital. He is the author of more than 50 research articles and co-editor with his wife Jean of *Women's Health in Physical Therapy.*

Jennifer A. Gardner, PT, DPT, MHA, CWS, has been a physical therapist since 1997 and a Certified Wound Specialist through the American Academy of Wound Management since 2001. She is the Clinical Director for Reapplix and its product, 3C Patch. Prior to joining the industry side of wound care, Dr. Gardner managed a wound care center, working with a multidisciplinary team of surgeons and nurses. In addition, she is an adjunct professor at Stockton University in Galloway, New Jersey, teaching integumentary to doctoral physical therapy students. Dr. Gardner is also one of the founding members of the American Physical Therapy Association Integumentary Specialty Council. She received her master's in physical therapy from Ithaca College and her doctorate in physical therapy from Temple University as well as her master's in health care administration from Walden University.

Rose M. Pignataro, PT, DPT, PhD, CWS, CHES, is a Certified Wound Specialist through the American Academy of Wound Management and Certified Health Education Specialist through the National Commission for Health Education Credentialing. She has been a physical therapist since 1990, with a clinical background in wound prevention and management, cardiopulmonary physical therapy, adult rehabilitation, and home health. Dr. Pignataro has been teaching integumentary physical therapy since 1999. She received a bachelor's degree in physical therapy from Hunter College: City University of New York, a master's degree in health science education and a doctorate of physical therapy from Stony Brook University, and a PhD in public health from West Virginia University. Dr. Pignataro is currently a member of the faculty and the Assistant Chair at Emory & Henry College Department of Physical Therapy. She also serves on the education committee for the American Physical Therapy Academy of Clinical Electrophysiology and Wound Management.

PREFACE

The text has been reorganized for the Third Edition. Two authors have been added to provide their unique experiences in industry, outpatient, and home health wound management. Although the text is no longer divided into units, the flow is largely similar to the previous editions. The first few chapters cover basic science; followed by examination of the patient and wound, common wound types, wound management techniques, and atypical types of wounds; and finishes with administrative concerns.

Although the text is written from the perspective of a physical therapist, the information is still applicable to the practice of a nurse, physician, physician assistant, occupational therapist, and other health care providers whose practice involves wound management.

An emphasis is on preparing students in professional programs with a multitude of descriptions, tables, and figures to successfully complete their programs and board examinations. However, the textbook is also written in sufficient detail to assist clinicians in a change in clinical practice emphasis or to aid in the preparation for a certification in wound management.

In this edition, common wound types now have their own chapters to increase the ease in finding a specific topic. Infection control and pain management have been moved into the basic sciences and scar management, and adjuncts have been combined into a single chapter.

As noted in the prefaces of the previous editions, we encourage the reader to use a systematic approach to managing the patient/client with a wound rather than treating a wound. The ability to change the management course across an episode of care in response to how the patient/client changes is the hallmark of a true wound management specialist.

Our flow from basic science to history taking, physical examination, and discussing the types of wounds and their treatments is summarized in the plan of care chapter, which we hope will be used to provide management that improves the quality of the lives of the patients/clients seen by the readers of this book.

—*Glenn L. Irion, PhD, PT, CWS*

Anatomy and Physiology of Skin

OBJECTIVES

- Describe the functions of the skin.
- Describe the types of cells in the epidermis.
- Discuss the maturation of epidermal cells as they migrate outwardly.
- Contrast the structure and functions of the papillary and reticular dermis.
- Describe the sensory organs of the skin, including their locations and stimuli.
- Describe the appendages of the skin and their role in regenerating the epidermis after injury.
- Describe basic pathological changes of the skin.

Working knowledge of the skin's anatomical and physiological processes is necessary to proceed with discussions of wound healing. Developing a diagnosis and a prognosis; selecting appropriate outcomes in consultation with the patient or caregiver; and developing an optimal plan of care, taking into account individual facets of the person's life and life span, rely on this knowledge.

Visual assessment of the skin may sometimes reveal the first indication of underlying pathology. For example, cyanosis, or bluish discoloration of the skin, may indicate insufficient oxygen supply due to cardiovascular or pulmonary impairments. Temporary dryness and loss of skin turgor can signal dehydration. Redness and warmth can be a sign of inflammation. Examination of accessory skin appendages, such as hair growth and nail growth, can provide information about a patient's nutritional status. When conducting a patient examination, health care practitioners should include a visual assessment of all exposed skin, especially areas of the body that patients cannot easily see, such as the low back, thighs, and posterior cervical region.

Irion GL, Gardner JA, Pignataro RM.
Comprehensive Wound Management, Third Edition (pp 1-18).
© 2024 Taylor and Francis Group.

The skin is the largest organ of the body. Depending on height and weight, skin is approximately 2 meters squared (m^2) and weighs about 4 kg. By adulthood, the human body contains an estimated 300 million skin cells. Despite its seemingly simple appearance and role as a protective cover for the body's internal components, skin integrity involves several diverse physiological processes, and regional differences exist to maintain that integrity. Although the ability to tolerate external stresses changes as we age, the skin structure allows it to be flexible and resilient, permitting movement and resisting trauma.

Skin acts as a physical barrier against microorganisms, trauma, ultraviolet light, and body fluid loss to the environment. Tight intercellular junctions, surface oils, and lipids create a waterproof barrier, allowing the body to maintain appropriate electrolyte and protein concentrations. Although it is not a perfect barrier, intact skin is generally successful at protecting underlying tissues. The skin surface's acidic nature with a pH of slightly below 5 eliminates many bacteria and maintains normal skin flora. Generally, bacteria on the skin are maintained at a low number of nonpathogenic species, but some patients will develop frequent skin abscesses due to their individual characteristics. Alterations in skin pH due to alkaline water, soaps, certain topical agents such as alcohol or acetone, and cosmetics may, in turn, alter the skin flora. Agents that strip away sebum and the protective layer of fatty acids at the surface of the skin also increase the risk of tissue breakdown and infection.

Skin also has a role in calcium metabolism through the effect of sunlight on the activation of vitamin D. Vitamin D plays a vital role in maintaining healthy bones and teeth by regulating the amount of calcium and phosphorous absorbed from the small intestine during digestion and reabsorption of calcium from the renal tubules. Vitamin D also supports immunity and is essential for the proper functioning of the nervous system and the cardiovascular and pulmonary systems. The amount of sunlight or ultraviolet exposure needed to synthesize sufficient amounts of vitamin D depends on multiple factors, including a person's skin pigment, geographic location, and time of day of exposure (ie, the position of the sun and strength of radiation), as well as the amount of skin surface area being exposed. Due to the associated dangers of excessive ultraviolet radiation, the use of vitamin D supplements is often advised.

Training in movement science, anatomy, physiology, and pathophysiology assists in risk assessment, prevention of skin injury, and direct wound management. This enables clinicians to screen for factors that contribute to delayed wound closure, including multisystem impact, ability to engage in effective self-care, identification of infection, and pain management. Historically, physical therapists were involved in wound management as a component of rehabilitation for injured soldiers during World War I. Today, rehabilitation specialists continue to play a vital role in the interprofessional wound management team. The involvement of rehabilitation specialists is particularly important when movement impairments affect the patient's risk of wounds and delayed closure, or the presence of an integumentary impairment increases the risk of movement dysfunction. Depending on their practice settings, rehabilitation professionals may encounter various acute wounds, including surgical incisions, traumatic lacerations, puncture wounds, abrasions, and burns. Chronic wounds are also commonly encountered in patients receiving rehabilitation services.

Wounds can interfere with various daily activities, such as work, education, leisure pursuits, self-care, and social participation. In addition to direct management of the wound site, rehabilitation clinicians can assist in pain management, functional mobility, and promoting role participation. Additionally, clinicians may be trained to work with patients to restore a sense of self-efficacy by identifying alternative means of participating in their own wound management and prevention.

GROSS ANATOMY OF THE INTEGUMENT

The interrelationship between the integumentary and other body systems is a major consideration of rehabilitation professionals. Musculoskeletal and neurologic impairments can place excessive stresses on the skin as well as on recovery from skin injuries. Abnormal movement, or lack of movement, can increase the risk of wound formation and delayed healing. Similarly, open wounds, delayed healing, and scar tissue formation can have a negative impact on strength, flexibility, and functional mobility.

The integumentary system is the largest organ in the human body and plays a critical role in homeostasis. The integument consists of the skin and its appendages. Skin may be described as having 3 layers—the epidermis, dermis, and hypodermis (also known as *subcutaneous tissue*). The thickness of the skin inclusive of the dermis and epidermis varies from 0.5 millimeters (mm) to 4 mm depending on the site. For example, the skin on the back, palms, and soles is the thickest. Tissues such as the eyelid or the bridge of the nose that do not have subcutaneous fat are substantially thinner and pliable, supporting subtle movements needed for facial expressions. The skin on the palms and soles of the feet is the thickest, protecting skin from friction and shear during gait and other weight-bearing activities. Variability in the thickness of the fatty hypodermis affects variability in skin thickness as a whole.

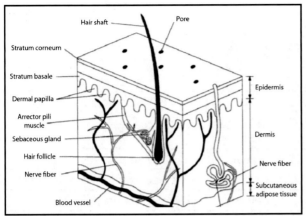

Figure 1-1. Components of the skin, including accessory structures of the epidermis. Note how deeply the hair follicles and sweat glands extend into the dermis.

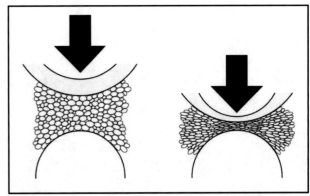

Figure 1-2. The cushioning effect of subcutaneous fat. Pressure and shearing forces between the skin and bony prominences are dissipated by deformation of subcutaneous fat before damage to the skin and subcutaneous tissues would otherwise occur.

Grossly, we can see only the epidermis in intact skin and some of the appendages. The appendages include hair, nails, sweat glands, and sebaceous glands. The epidermis consists of stratified squamous epithelium. The dermis consists of fibrous, dense irregular connective tissue (Figure 1-1). The hypodermis is composed of fatty, loose areolar connective tissue that allows movement and deformation of the skin around the underlying tissues (Figure 1-2). Beneath the hypodermis, fascia separates the skin from other structures, including major blood vessels (other than superficial veins) and nerves, muscle, tendon, ligaments, and bone. The ability of the fatty hypodermis to deform and distribute pressure and other mechanical forces reduces the potential for injury to the skin above it and the other tissues below it. Loss of body fat with malnutrition places the skin at greater risk of injury, especially with prolonged static positioning. However, excessive subcutaneous fat can cause the overlying skin to become taut and nondeformable, placing the skin at risk.

The dermis and epidermis have different embryologic origins. The epidermis and skin appendages are nearly all derived from the surface ectoderm, whereas the dermis develops from the mesoderm. Most of the epidermis cells are keratinocytes, named for the production of the keratin filaments that develop within them. Melanocytes that provide pigment to the skin and Merkel cells that provide some of the sensory input from the skin migrate to the epidermis from the neural crest during development. The other cell of the epidermis, Langerhans cells, are monocytes in origin and migrate to the epidermis, acting as resident macrophages.

HISTOLOGY OF SKIN

Due to regional differences in skin structure, we often divide skin into thick and thin skin. Thick skin is often described as *glabrous*, meaning smooth or hairless. Thick skin is restricted to the palms and soles, where the skin is subjected to tangential/shearing forces during normal activities such as ambulation and manipulation of objects in the hand. Skin elsewhere on the body is considered to be thin skin and develops hair. Much of this hair is short, thin, and less noticeable than scalp hair. However, it may become longer and coarser on the body's stereotypical locations throughout the life span, particularly during puberty. In thin skin, the epidermis is 70 nm to 150 nm thick, whereas thick skin ranges from 1 mm to 1.5 mm in thickness and consists of a cellular layer not found in thin skin.

The junction between the epidermis and dermis, the dermoepidermal border, is very complex and vascular, whereas the remainder of the dermis is much less vascular. The epidermis is completely avascular. The dermis composes most of the skin's thickness (1.5 mm to 4 mm depending on location). The upper layer of the dermis consists of capillary networks, and the lower layer contains larger blood vessels, lymphatics, and nerves that branch through the skin. The health of the avascular epidermis depends on the diffusion of nutrients from the network of capillaries in the dermis beneath it.

The dermis also contains 3 to 4 million sweat glands. Depending on environmental and bodily temperatures, sweat production volumes can range from 100 milliliters (mL)/day to 2 L within 1 hour. The capillary network of the superficial dermis and sweat glands aid thermoregulation. Vasodilation and perspiration promote heat dissipation, whereas vasoconstriction can help conserve heat during exposure to cold. Sebaceous glands within the dermis secrete oil or sebum to lubricate the skin and help maintain its waterproof barrier.

TABLE 1-1
Layers of Epidermis

DEPTH	LAYER	CHARACTERISTICS
Deepest ↓ Most superficial	Stratum basale	Regenerative layer; receives nutrition by diffusion from papillary dermis
	Stratum spinosum	Development of keratin filaments
	Stratum granulosum	Development of lipid granules assisting in waterproofing
	Stratum lucidum	Present only in thick skin of palms and soles; obscures pigmentation
	Stratum corneum	Devitalized flattened cells remain in layer for ~14 days

The dermis and epidermis interface has somewhat regular alternating peaks and valleys/corrugations producing what might be envisioned as a 3-dimensional jigsaw puzzle. These topographical features aid in maintaining the integrity of the dermoepidermal border. The 3-dimensional ridges are called *rete ridges* or *rete pegs* and provide massive surface area to allow both adhesion and nutrition for the epidermis.

The upper part of the dermis contributes to the rete pegs and is highly vascularized. This upper layer is called the *papillary dermis*. Papillary is a general term used to describe tissues with protrusions. The papillary dermis consists of a looser connective tissue composed of type I and III collagen. Interspersed elastic fibers and fibroblasts are also found in this layer, but its dense capillary network is the major feature.

The lower part of the dermis is not involved in rete pegs. It is composed of dense irregular connective tissue, which provides substantial strength. This part is called the *reticular dermis*, referring to its "netlike" fibrous construction. Fibers within the reticular dermis are generated from molecules produced in the dermis by fibroblasts. This network of very thick collagen bundles provides tensile strength to the skin while maintaining the ability to deform sufficiently to allow movement. In addition to fibroblasts, other cells found in the dermis include macrophages, mast cells, plasma cells, and lymphocytes. The vascularity and immune cells allow inflammation to occur in the dermis. Although inflammation of the dermis can often be seen through the epidermis, the lack of vasculature does not allow inflammation to occur in the epidermis itself. The epidermis has limited ability to stretch with inflammation. In contrast, the dermis can swell substantially, leading to blistering and exfoliation of the epidermis during severe dermis inflammation, including allergic reactions and infection.

Epidermal Histology

The epidermis is composed of stratified epithelial cells called *keratinocytes* that develop with the basement membrane at the dermoepidermal border. These cells migrate outwardly in a stereotypical fashion, producing apparent layers with different characteristics seen with light microscopy. Cellular migration consists of an orderly progression of mitosis, differentiation, maturation, keratinization, loss of organelles, cell death, and shedding as the cells progress outwardly. This process typically requires 14 days for new epithelial cells to migrate from the basal layer to the outermost layer and another 14 days for cells to be shed. The shedding process is termed *desquamation*.

Epidermal Layers

In thin skin, 4 layers of the epidermis are described in Table 1-1 and depicted in Figure 1-3. In thick skin, these 4 layers are thicker, and an additional epidermal layer is present that largely obscures any pigmentation of the soles and palms. The basal layer (stratum basale or germinativum) is a single layer of keratinocytes resting on the basement membrane. Mitosis constantly occurs, replacing cells that migrate outwardly. These cells approximate a columnar to cuboid shape that will become progressively flatter as they migrate superficially. In partial-thickness wounds, new keratinocytes produced within the stratum basale promote re-epithelialization and wound closure.

Progressing outwardly, the next layer is the stratum spinosum. The name of this layer refers to the histologic appearance of the cells under the microscope. During slide preparation, cells within the stratum spinosum shrink, accentuating the keratin fibers developing in them and producing an obvious histologic distinction from the

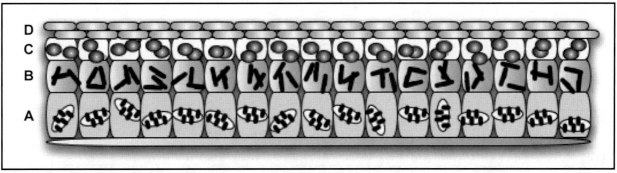

Figure 1-3. Cells and layers of the epidermis. The epidermis consists of 4 layers: (A) stratum basale, (B) stratum spinosum, (C) stratum granulosum, and (D) stratum corneum. See text for details about each layer. Each stratum consists of several layers of cells. Figure is simplified for clarity.

stratum basale. This "prickly" or spiny appearance is the source of another term for this layer—*prickle cells*. The stratum spinosum is several cells thick; cells become flatter as they migrate outwardly. Each cell is attached to adjacent cells by desmosomes, providing greater structural integrity of the epidermis. Keratohyalin granules appearing in the stratum spinosum contain a protein called *filaggrin* that cross-links with keratin. Several autoimmune diseases damage proteins of the desmosomes that bind adjacent epidermal cells, compromising skin integrity.

Superficial to the stratum spinosum is another 3- to 5-cell layer characterized by the development of granules that will eventually release a fatty substance that helps waterproof the epidermis. This layer is called the *stratum granulosum*. Due to lysosomes' activity, cells within the stratum granulosum have become nearly flat and have lost most of their organelles, including the nucleus. In thick skin, the next layer moving outward from the base to the surface is the *stratum lucidum*. The stratum lucidum consists of a few flattened cells without nuclei and organelles. This layer contributes to the thick skin's resistance to shearing forces from walking or using hand tools. The stratum lucidum received its name because it is transparent to light and contains 3 to 5 layers of clear keratinocytes.

The outermost layer of both thick and thin skin is the *stratum corneum*. The process of producing keratin-rich tissue is called *cornification* (coming from the term for horn). The term for cells of the outermost layer of the epidermis is *corneocyte*. The cells are extremely flat and take on a role similar to shingles on a roof. Cells are stacked in such a way that interlocking occurs in all 3 dimensions. Lipid released from granules developed in the stratum granulosum aids in the waterproofing function of the skin. Excessive handwashing removes the lipid component and reduces the passive barrier function of the epidermis, which can lead to skin cracking, especially in cold, dry weather. The thickness of the stratum corneum varies tremendously but is very thick in the thick skin and

is very thin in areas where the skin is thin such as eyelids. Desmosomes between cells break down as the stratum corneum cells migrate outwardly, resulting in desquamation. Much of house dust consists of desquamated epidermal cells. These particles from skin or hair from animals contribute to animal dander allergies and feed dust mites that also cause allergic reactions.

Cell Envelope

The cell envelope is a structure unique to keratinocytes. The cell envelope develops beneath the cell membrane as cells mature and migrate superficially through the epidermis. The envelope is constructed of several cross-linked proteins. These proteins are first detectable in the stratum spinosum. The envelope forms in the stratum granulosum and is complete in the stratum corneum. The enzymes required to synthesize the cell envelope develop as the cell matures. Involucrum, a component of the cell envelope, begins production in the basal layer and appears to be responsible for migration from the basal layer as the cell envelope is developed. Involucrum is also increased markedly in psoriasis, implicating cell envelope proteins' role in the abnormal migration of keratinocytes in this disorder.

Lipids

Lipids within the epidermis form the permeability barrier between adjacent keratinocytes. A distinct layering of lipid is observable in the stratum corneum. Sources of lipid within the stratum corneum include sebaceous glands, cell membranes, and lamellar granules. Lamellar granules develop in the stratum spinosum and are extruded in the stratum granulosum. In patients who lack essential fatty acids (discussed in Chapter 4), decreased amounts of lipids within the epidermis result in dry, scaly skin and increased skin permeability.

TABLE 1-2
Growth Factors

GROWTH FACTOR	FUNCTION
EGF	Stimulates growth of epidermis cells
FGF	Stimulates endothelial growth/angiogenesis; promotes fibroblast proliferation; promotes granulation; stimulates chemotaxis of epithelial cells
KGF	Specific form of FGF responsible for keratinocyte growth
PDGF	Stimulates growth of mesenchymal cells in context of wound healing
TGFα	Member of EGF family; binds to same receptor as EGF
TGFβ	Involved in skin aging; blocks conversion of dermal fibroblasts into fat cells, increasing wrinkling of skin
VEGF	Member of PDGF family; involved in angiogenesis; triggers angiogenesis with hypoxia via hypoxia-inducible factor

Growth Factors Affecting the Epidermis

Several growth factors affect the skin, including epidermal growth factor (EGF), acidic and basic fibroblast growth factor, insulin, insulin-like growth factor-1 (IGF-1), interleukin 2, colony-stimulating factors, nerve growth factor, platelet-derived growth factor (PDGF), and transforming growth factor-beta (TGFβ). These growth factors have multiple sites of action. Receptors for EGF and TGFβ are found on basal keratinocytes, sweat duct cells, hair follicles, sheath cells, basal sebocytes, vascular smooth muscle cells, and arrector pili muscle cells. Growth factors EGF and fibroblast growth factor increase fibroblast number; TGFβ has been linked to angiogenesis and fibroplasia; and PDGF has been linked to chemotaxis, DNA synthesis, collagen deposition, and wound contraction.

Experimentally, PDGF normalizes wound repair in diabetic animals but is also suspected to be involved in atherosclerosis and neoplasia. Signals for release of growth factors include phospholipase C/protein kinase C, which is activated by bradykinin, histamine, thrombin, EGF, and PDGF. Phospholipase C/protein kinase C is implicated in both proliferation and differentiation of skin cells, the release of prostaglandins, and increased gene expression. Another signaling mechanism, tyrosine kinase, has been associated with TGFβ, insulin, and basic fibroblast growth factor to promote the proliferation of skin cells. Prostaglandins and leukotrienes are associated with inflammation, which, as discussed later, is an important component of normal healing. However, prolonged inflammation can impede healing.

Normal skin appearance and function depend on a balance between cellular proliferation and differentiation. Scaling, plaques, and other disorders may result from an imbalance of these 2 processes. Production of normal layering of the epidermis requires both a sequence of timely production by mitotically active keratinocytes and subsequent differentiation of postmitotic cells. In addition to the skin's appearance, impaired wound healing and skin cancer may result from an imbalance between proliferation and differentiation. IGF-1 is an important regulator of proliferation and differentiation. Both epidermal keratinocytes and dermal fibroblasts possess specific receptors for IGF-1. Binding of IGF-1 to specific receptors located in keratinocytes and dermal fibroblasts leads to the proliferation of these cells. Lack of IGF-1 leads to thin, weak skin, whereas excessive quantities of IGF-1 may produce a range of effects from thickening to neoplasia. Excessive IGF-1 also inhibits the differentiation of keratinocytes required for normal layering of the epidermis. Alterations in the balance of different growth factors have been linked to several disorders, including psoriasis with interleukins 17 and 22 and scleroderma with interleukin 17B, interleukin 17E, and a subtype with interleukin 17F. The characteristics of several known growth factors are described in Table 1-2.

Keratinocytes

Within the stratum basale, keratinocytes contain large quantities of mitochondria and ribosomes to support the demands of reproduction and generation of filaments and granules. Tonofilaments, or intermediate filaments, of keratin proteins are found in all epithelial cells. The skin has approximately 50 types of keratin. Differences in the texture

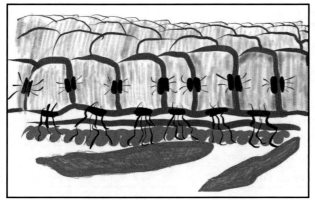

Figure 1-4. Attachments of keratinocytes to each other by desmosomes and to the basement membrane by hemidesmosomes.

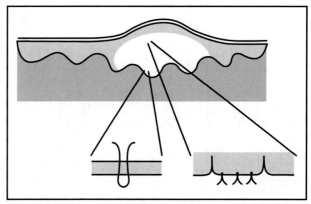

Figure 1-5. Formation of blisters. Fluid accumulation due to inflammation causes rupture of hemidesmosomes and the separation of epidermis from dermis.

of stratum corneum, hair, and nails are mainly due to variations in the types of keratin within them. Desmosomes link adjacent keratinocytes within the stratum basale and stratum spinosum, connecting tonofilaments within adjacent cells. Desmosomes provide tight, complex intercellular junctions by connecting adjacent cells. The desmosome is a complex structure consisting of anchoring points of keratin filaments within plaques on their own membranes and the anchoring points on plaques within those of adjacent cells through a large number of proteins connecting the plaques of adjacent cells. These complex adhesive bonds provide the skin with tensile strength.

Basal cells attach to the epidermal basement membrane through hemidesmosomes. Hemidesmosomes have a single attachment plaque that attaches basal cells to the epidermal basement membrane. Desmosomes have 2 attachments that bind adjacent keratinocytes to one another. Desmosomes and hemidesmosomes are depicted in Figure 1-4. Dermal cells attach to adjacent cells through desmosomes with attachment plaques with the adjoining cells and fibers running through them. The dermal cells produce the basal membrane, which allows anchoring filaments constructed of multiple proteins to attach cells firmly. Whereas the basement membrane's epidermal surface is lined with epidermal cells, the dermal side is lined with extracellular matrix and fibers provide attachment.

Blistering

The presence of proteoglycans and fibers allows the dermis to swell considerably without injury. However, when the dermis swells, the hemidesmosomes connecting the dermis and epidermis can become damaged. Inflammation of the dermis by a superficial injury such as a mild burn causes leakage of fluid between the dermis and epidermis. Accumulation of fluid stretches the epidermal attachments to their breaking points, lifting it into blisters.

If tension within the blisters exceeds the tissue tolerance, blisters can rupture and expose the dermis to potential contaminants with the possibility of infection.

Additionally, several autoimmune diseases specifically damage either desmosomes or hemidesmosomes, allowing fluid to accumulate either within the epidermis (intraepidermal blisters) or between the dermis and epidermis (subepidermal blisters). Blisters can form either by inflammation or fluid accumulation, causing hemidesmosomes to break. Alternatively, blisters may form due to hemidesmosomes' breakage, which allows fluid to accumulate between layers. Diagnostic testing and history would be necessary to distinguish which mechanism caused the formation of blisters. Blister formation is depicted in Figure 1-5.

Melanocytes

Melanin produces the pigmentation of skin, hair, and other structures of the body. Melanosomes are packets of melanin produced by melanocytes and distributed to surrounding keratinocytes over dendrites similar to those of neurons. Melanocytes are derived from the neural crest and share much histology with neurons. During embryonic development, melanocytes migrate from the neural crest to the epidermis, hair follicles, eyes, ear, and meninges. Each melanocyte provides melanin to approximately 30 adjacent keratinocytes. The activity of melanocytes, rather than their number, is generally the determinant of pigmentation. The amount of melanin produced varies from person to person based on race and genetic makeup. Ultraviolet light and adrenocorticotrophic hormone and a similar hormone, melanocyte-stimulating hormone, determine the production of melanin. It also changes in older adults, with irregular deposition of melanin leading to senile lentigo, or "age spots."

Two types of melanin are produced in humans. Although both are produced from tyrosine, a genetic variation

TABLE 1-3
Cells of Epidermis and Dermis

CELL	LOCATION	CHARACTERISTICS
Keratinocyte	Throughout epidermis	Flatten and lose organelles while migrating toward surface
Melanocyte	Stratum basale	3% of epidermal cells; produce melanosomes; melanosomes distributed to adjacent keratinocytes
Langerhans cell	Midepidermis	Resident macrophage; present antigen to immune cells
Fibroblast	Dermis	Produce ground substance and fibers

causes people with red hair to produce only pheomelanin. Pheomelanin (named for the chemical difference between it and eumelanin) is responsible for the redder color of lips and similar tissues, and a genetic variant produces a redder hair coloration and ruddier complexion. Pheomelanin does not produce as much protection against sunlight. Ultraviolet light does not cause a darker pigmentation of pheomelanin. Skin dominated by pheomelanin is more likely to be sunburned and develop skin cancers. People with other hair colors produce both types of melanin. Eumelanin (true melanin) is either brown or black. The black subtype of eumelanin produces a darker pigmentation than the brown.

Melanin content can also be affected by a noncontagious condition called *vitiligo*. Although its exact cause is unknown, people with vitiligo have skin areas that lose their pigment when melanocytes are destroyed. Wound care professionals should be aware that people with vitiligo also experience higher rates of certain autoimmune diseases, such as pernicious anemia, Addison's disease, myasthenia gravis, and systemic lupus erythematosus. In addition, with vitiligo, where patches of skin lack pigmentation, and in albinism, melanin is made in such small quantities that a person is at high risk of skin cancer and damage to the retina.

Langerhans Cells

The resident monocyte-derived cells of the epidermis are named Langerhans cells. These cells are produced in red bone marrow and migrate from the blood as monocytes. Langerhans cells are also found in the dermis, lymph system, and thymus. These cells are classified as dendritic cells as opposed to macrophages. Although both macrophages and dendritic cells phagocytose, dendritic cells have a greater role in presenting antigens to T cells. Langerhans cells patrol tissue and engulf unusual cells. Then, surface antigens of these cells and other immune-reactive antigens, such as plant oils and proteins associated with mycobacterium tuberculosis, are presented to T cells

to activate a targeted immune response. These cells occupy the stratum spinosum and stratum granulosum. Although Langerhans cells have the effect of a pre-emptive strike against pathogens, they can also cause numerous nuisance responses such as reactions to poison ivy and chemicals found on clothing. A type of cancer called *Langerhans cell histiocytosis* is a rare neoplasm of childhood. Langerhans cells are also involved in transmitting some viruses such as human immunodeficiency virus, herpes simplex, and human papillomavirus by transferring the virus to helper T cells. Cells of the epidermal and dermal layers are summarized in Table 1-3.

Dermal Structure

The dermis is a form of dense connective tissue. Two types of dense connective tissue are dense regular and dense irregular. Dense regular tissues, such as tendons and ligaments, have great tensile strength but little ability to accommodate deforming forces. In contrast, the dense irregular connective tissue of the dermis provides a compromise of tensile strength and the ability to deform and return to its resting shape when the force is removed. This balance between tensile strength and accommodation is due to a greater amount of ground substance and a less regular fiber alignment. The dermis must also allow neural and vascular structures to run through it and still provide enough tensile strength to prevent damage to vascular and neural structures. The ground substance of the dermis performs several roles—maintaining appropriate hydration, providing turgor and resilience to deformation, and strengthening fibers. The macromolecules within the ground substance can attract large numbers of water molecules and act as a buffer for water. Glycosaminoglycans create a water-holding gel. These molecules consist of large chains of sugar molecules with negative charges that retain water molecules and sodium ions. Proteoglycans are even larger molecules that link glycosaminoglycans to a protein backbone with an appearance similar to a bottlebrush.

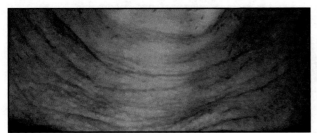

Figure 1-6. Tenting of skin secondary to aging. Loss of hypodermis, skin dehydration, and thinning of the dermal/epidermal junction allow wrinkling of the skin to occur when tension is removed at rest.

This structural arrangement gives ground substance a springy quality that allows the skin to deform and recoil. This property is termed *turgor*. Turgor is dependent on the amount of water. In a dehydrated state, turgor is low, and the release of the deforming force does not produce a brisk recoil but instead produces tenting when the skin is pinched. Tenting is common in aging skin, particularly that of the neck and elbows, as shown in Figure 1-6. Excessive hydration in edema allows free water to move in the skin, and deforming forces produce pitting, leading to the term *pitting edema*, as depicted in Figure 1-7.

Dermal Layers

The dermis consists of 2 major layers with important functional differences and 3 basic components as depicted in Figure 1-8. Fibroblasts are the principal cells of the dermis. Although they are not tremendously numerous or active cells in stable skin, fibroblasts secrete important macromolecules during the healing process. Fibers, especially collagen and elastic fibers, are common in the dermis and are described in the following section.

Papillary Layer

The papillary dermis (pars papillaris), or uppermost layer, is thin and molded against the epidermal ridges/grooves. It consists of smaller, more loosely distributed collagen fibers than the deeper reticular dermis. In contrast to the reticular dermis, which lies beneath, the fibers within the papillary layer consist mainly of type III and IV collagen. The major feature of the papillary dermis layer is the network of blood and lymphatic vessels, which are organized into plexuses. The papillary layer and its plexuses are important in regulating heat loss and providing nutrition to the stratum basale. Increased blood flow through the papillary dermis results in greater loss of heat to the environment.

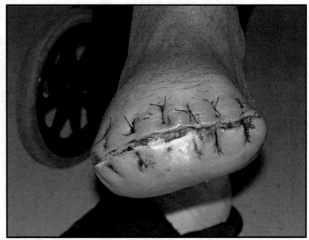

Figure 1-7. Pitting edema caused by inflammation causes tension on sutures and gapping between the sutures.

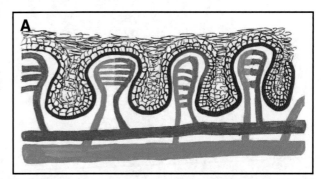

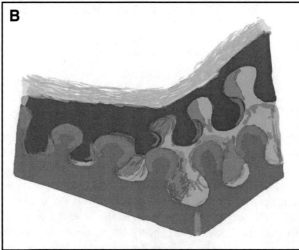

Figure 1-8. Structure of dermis. (A) Papillary plexus shown within the papillary dermis. Vasodilation allows heat to be dissipated through the skin. (B) Rete pegs form 3-dimensional jigsaw puzzle–like projections between the dermis and epidermis to increase adhesion between the layers.

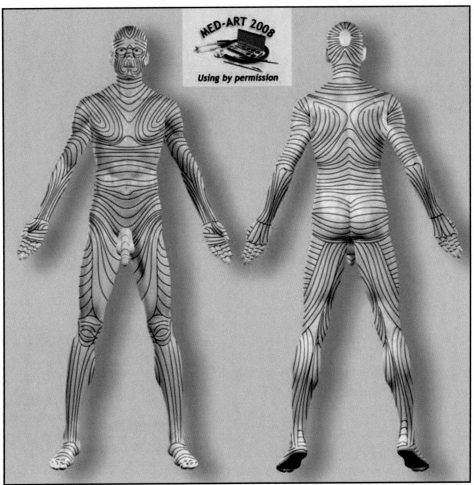

Figure 1-9. Langer's lines. These indicate lines of natural tension in the skin. A wound along these lines has little stress on it, whereas a wound running perpendicular to these lines will experience stress along its edges. (Reproduced with permission from Davide Brunelli, MD.)

Reticular Layer

The reticular layer of the dermis has a much greater thickness than the papillary layer and is relatively acellular and avascular compared with other tissues. It is characterized by denser fibers and less gel than the papillary layer. It also contains an abundance of type I collagen fibers arranged in a meshlike, preferential directional organization. This organization of the reticular fibers gives rise to the structures known as Langer's lines, forming a grainlike nature to the skin. Langer's lines are important in performing body composition analysis with skinfold calipers. A proper skinfold results only when the skin is pinched such that Langer's lines run perpendicular to the calipers. They are also important in understanding the preferential direction of skin contraction following injury. If possible, incisions for surgery are made parallel to Langer's lines to reduce the resulting scar's width. The general directions of Langer's lines are depicted in Figure 1-9.

Fibers of the Dermis

Fibrillar proteins found in the dermis include collagen, fibrillin, elastin, and fibronectin. Collagen is a large family of aggregated protein shaped into strings, fibers, and cables. The type of collagens and other fibers present in tissue largely determines the tissue's properties. The collagen in dermis provides tensile strength. In addition, the multidirectional arrangement of collagen fibers within the dermis produces some of the elasticity of the skin. Patterns of fiber deposition in the skin produce more tension in some directions than in others, resulting in the preferential directions of skin stress mapped as Langer's lines. When tension is removed from the skin, the collagen fibers recoil, allowing the tissue to resume its resting shape.

Fibroblasts synthesize collagen, which is synthesized as polypeptides and released into the extracellular space around the fibroblast. Hydroxylation of proline and lysine by vitamin C is necessary for full function. Vitamin C deficiency produces the condition of scurvy, in which collagen fibers are weakened. The triple helix of procollagen is formed within the fibroblast's endoplasmic reticulum cell and released into the extracellular space by exocytosis. Within the extracellular space, procollagen is converted to tropocollagen, capable of aggregating with other molecules to form collagen fibrils. Collagen fibrils assemble themselves into fibers, and the fibers aggregate into bundles producing the strength of collagen fibers. The thickness of collagen fibers increases in proportion to the stress placed on them. Judiciously applied stresses to collagen will increase the strength of connective tissue. However, excessive stresses, in terms of either too much intensity or frequency, damages connective tissue, as seen in pressure injuries.

Type I collagen is the most common type forming fibrils with tremendous tensile strength, meaning that it resists efforts to elongate it. A natural undulation along collagen fibers allows some lengthening of the tissue and recoil when the force is removed. Further stretch is resisted until fibers become permanently lengthened, and additional lengthening then results in the structure's tearing. The biomechanics of skin is discussed later in the chapter. Different collagen types may form fibrils such as type I in the dermis or sheets or mesh. Type III collagen forms reticular fibers, which create a netlike structure around the dermis that provides spaces for blood vessels and nerves to pass in and out of it. Type IV collagen is found in the basement membrane between the dermis and epidermis and in granulation tissue developed in wounded skin. The formation of collagen fibers is depicted in Figure 1-10.

Elastic fibers provide an additional elasticity to the dermis. Elastic fibers are composed of the proteins fibrillin and elastin. Fibrillin is a critical component of elastic fibers. In Marfan syndrome, a defect in fibrillin leads to defective elastic tissues. The elastic fibers in the dermis attach to collagen fibers and provide a better recoil to resting conditions when deforming forces are removed from the skin.

Dermal Vasculature

Skin vasculature consists of a deep plexus in the reticular dermis and a superficial plexus within the papillary dermis. The papillary dermis is very vascular, and the reticular dermis conveys both the vessels that feed the papillary dermis and plexuses responsible for thermoregulation. The largest vessels that bring blood flow in and back out of the skin are located in the subcutaneous connective tissue. Additional networks of vessels surround each sweat and sebaceous gland. Connections between the deep plexus of the reticular dermis and the superficial plexus of the papillary dermis are physiologically controlled as part of thermoregulation. In a warm environment, more blood

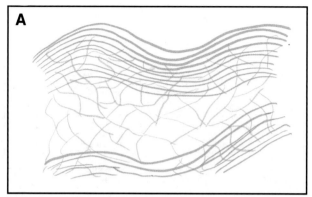

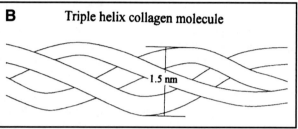

Figure 1-10. (A) Three-dimensional depiction of the undulating structure of a collagen bundle. Note the elastic fibers connecting adjacent collagen bundles. (B) Triple-strand structure of individual collagen fibers. Collagen fibers coalesce into multiple strands that become thicker along lines of stress in the skin.

flow is diverted to the papillary dermis to dissipate heat. In a cold environment, the blood flow of the superficial plexus can be diverted to the deep plexus to conserve heat. Lymphatic vessels are located in deep and superficial plexuses and follow venous vessels in the skin. The lymphatics are capable of managing about 10 times the normal leakage of fluid from skin vessels. When the lymphatic vessels fail to return fluid and proteins from the skin, swelling and fibrosis characteristic of lymphedema occurs.

Sensory Receptors

Skin is richly supplied by sensory structures capable of detecting very small changes in some areas, such as the fingertips. In addition to sensory nerves, autonomic motor nerves innervate sweat glands, blood vessels, and the arrector pili muscles that cause hair to become perpendicular to the skin's surface (ie, "goose bumps"). Extensive neural plexuses are found in the superficial reticular dermis associated with sensory receptors.

Pacinian corpuscles are encapsulated, lamellar end organs reminiscent of onion bulbs. They are located deep in the reticular dermis and hypodermis. Pacinian corpuscles fire with deformation and the release of deformation but not with sustained pressure. These characteristics make

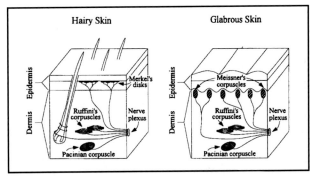

Figure 1-11. Sensory receptors in the skin.

the Pacinian corpuscle useful for detecting vibration and grasping and releasing objects by the hand.

Meissner corpuscles are encapsulated receptors with a pine cone appearance located in the papillary dermis of hairless skin. Like Pacinian corpuscles, Meissner corpuscles respond to the initial deformation and the release of deformation but not to sustained pressure. They have small receptive fields and are densely concentrated on thick, hairless skin, especially the fingertips. Meissner corpuscles allow the detection of shape and texture of objects, making them ideal for discriminatory touch, such as reading Braille. In skin with hair, Meissner corpuscles are not present, but the function is provided by hair receptors. Light touch with the bending and unbending of hair is determined by these receptors but not sustained bending.

Ruffini endings are spindle-shaped receptors located in the mid-dermis that adapt slowly to deformation, allowing them to detect sustained stretch and pressure.

Merkel cells are located within the epidermis and are separate from their associated nerves, whereas other named sensory receptors of the skin are specialized endings of neurons. Merkel cells are abundant in the fingertips and are slowly adapting, which allows them to detect sustained deformation from pressure and static touch. Information from Merkel cell receptors allows 2-point discrimination.

Free nerve endings are the most abundant nerve endings in the skin, sending plantlike roots throughout the dermis and penetrating the epidermis. These free nerve endings respond to multiple modalities, including temperature, mechanical, and noxious stimuli. Sensory receptors and their locations within the skin are depicted in Figure 1-11 and summarized in Table 1-4.

Accessory Structures

The skin has several accessory structures that are distributed differently throughout the body. Sweat glands, hair follicles, and associated sebaceous glands and nails are described in the following sections.

Sweat Glands

Two types of sweat glands are described in humans—eccrine and apocrine sweat glands. The vast majority are eccrine glands located throughout the body. Eccrine glands are responsible for heat loss by sweating and consist of a coiled tubule deep in the dermis, extending into the hypodermis with a relatively straight excretory duct. Eccrine glands develop as invaginations of the epidermis and are lined with epidermal cells. When wounding with loss of epidermal tissue occurs, sweat glands function as valuable sources of new epidermal cells along with hair follicles. During moderate exercise in reasonable temperature and humidity, the coiled nature of the deep portion of the sweat gland provides ample length to reabsorb ions from the fluid filtered into the gland from the blood, producing hypotonic sweat. With hypotonic sweat, electrolyte replacement is not necessary. Reabsorption of sodium and chloride is regulated by aldosterone, which prevents excessive loss of electrolytes. Sweat rate is determined by local skin temperature and general body temperature by thermoregulatory mechanisms controlled by the hypothalamus and executed by cholinergic sympathetic nerves, as opposed to the adrenergic sympathetic innervation of other tissues. Because of this difference, increased serum catecholamine levels due to mental stress do not increase sweating from eccrine glands. With heavier exercise in hotter temperatures and greater relative humidity, the secretory rate of eccrine sweat glands may become too great to reabsorb sufficient electrolytes, requiring replacement of both water and electrolytes. In cystic fibrosis, the inability to reabsorb chloride ions from sweat glands can lead to salt drying on the skin's surface and necessitates electrolyte replacement. The location of eccrine sweat glands is depicted in Figure 1-1.

Apocrine sweat glands are innervated by adrenergic sympathetic nerves and are associated with increased sweating during mental stress. Molecules believed to be pheromones are released along with sweat from these glands. Apocrine glands are located in areas associated with coarser body hair development with puberty, including the axilla, scrotum, labia majora, perineum, and around the anus and areola. Apocrine sweat glands can be the source of difficult-to-manage infections called *hidradenitis suppurativa*, which is discussed in Chapter 18 with other skin infections that lead to open wounds.

Pilosebaceous Units

The combination of the hair follicle, arrector pili muscle, and oil-secreting sebaceous gland is known as the *pilosebaceous unit* (see Figure 1-1). The arrector pili attaches to the hair and, in response to cold or other stresses that activate the sympathetic nervous system, it contracts, moving

TABLE 1-4
Sensory Receptors of the Skin

RECEPTOR	LOCATION	CHARACTERISTICS
Merkel disk	Base of epidermis	Slow adapting; respond to static stimuli—2-point discrimination, shapes
Meissner's corpuscle	Papillary dermis	Rapidly adapting; respond to vibration, texture
Ruffini endings	Deep dermis, joints	Slowly adapting; respond to movement
Pacinian corpuscles	Deep dermis	Rapidly adapting; respond to vibration, grasp/release

the hair from its normal oblique orientation with the skin's surface to a position close to perpendicular. Contraction is associated with bulging at the skin's surface, often referred to as *gooseflesh* or *goose bumps.*

The ducts of sebaceous glands empty into hair follicles obliquely, with the gland itself positioned between the hair follicle and the arrector pili muscle. Sebaceous glands are located throughout the body except in thick skin (palm and sole). These glands produce an oily secretion called *sebum,* which consists of decomposed cells of the glands themselves. Androgens increase sebum production. With the onset of puberty, sebaceous glands undergo such increased activity that sebum often obstructs the glands, leading to acne. Derivatives of vitamin A decrease the production of sebaceous glands and may be used to treat acne.

Hair follicles also develop from invaginations of the epidermis. Like sweat glands, hair follicles can be a source of new epidermal cells following an injury. The depth of the hair follicle changes during the life cycle of hair. The hair follicles, about 5 million, are developed by about 22 weeks of gestation. Therefore, hair follicles' density decreases during development as the skin increases in area, but the number of follicles does not change. A disproportionate number are located on the head, with about 1 million. The scalp alone has 100,000 hair follicles.

Hair follicles consist of a root sheath derived from the epidermis and an outer connective tissue component derived from dermal tissue. The epithelial component of the root sheath is then divided into an internal and external root sheath. The external root sheath performs a role similar to that of the stratum basale and stratum spinosum of the epidermis, constantly producing new cells to lengthen the hair during the hair cycle's growth phase. The internal root sheath takes on the stratum granulosum and stratum corneum roles and secures the hair within the follicle through the production of additional layering of cells. The widened base of the internal root sheath forms a bulb that does not allow an actively growing hair to be removed easily from the follicle. Similar to the epidermis, the desmosomes joining adjacent cells disintegrate as the cells

forming the hair flatten and become physically locked by their shape rather than desmosomes. This serves to push the hair outwardly from the bulb and lengthen the hair. The hair sheath ends below the opening of the sebaceous gland; therefore, the oily sebum is deposited onto the hair shaft itself as it pushes forward at a rate of about 0.3 mm to 0.4 mm/day.

Both hair growth and sebum production are increased with testosterone. Similar to keratinocytes of the epidermis, melanosomes are deposited in hair cells before they flatten and become keratinized cell remnants. The keratin of hair and nails is different from the epidermis, giving each of these somewhat different properties. The developing hair shaft produces 3 distinct layers—the medulla, cortex, and cuticle. Pigment is contained in the cortex and medulla. The types of melanin and thickness of the hairs determine its coloration. Thicker hair will appear darker, and thinner hair appears blond. A greater proportion of black melanin produces darker hair, a greater proportion of brown melanin produces brown hair, and a greater pheomelanin content creates redder hair. Loss of melanization with age or disease produces gray to white hair.

Hairs grow cyclically with different periods on the body, resulting in varying lengths of hair. For example, scalp hair may achieve lengths over 1 meter, and facial hair may grow to a much greater length than hairs elsewhere, such as eyelashes. The hair cycle consists of 3 stages called *anagen, catagen,* and *telogen.* During anagen, hair follicle cells actively produce new cells and push the hair outwardly as the follicle extends more deeply into the dermis. Depending on the location and individual, anagen may last from 2 to 6 years. Any previous hair shafts still present in the follicle, termed *club hairs,* are pushed out of the follicle during this process and shed. At any given time, most hairs (about 85%) are in the anagen phase. During the catagen phase, lengthening of the hair shaft ceases, and the outer sheath becomes attached to the hair shaft to produce the club hair. Under normal conditions, about 1% of hairs are in the catagen phase.

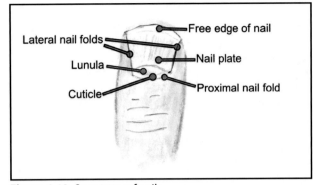

Figure 1-12. Structures of nails.

Melanin incorporation ceases with apoptosis of the follicular melanocytes. Over approximately 2 weeks, the follicle itself shrinks to about one-sixth of its maximum length and becomes remote from the dermal blood supply. This process occurs over approximately 2 weeks. The hair shaft appears to continue to move outwardly due to the shrinkage of the follicle. The telogen phase occurs for about 15% of hairs at any time. Follicles become dormant for about 100 days on the scalp and even longer elsewhere. The club hair is fully formed during the telogen phase and has a solid spherical mass forming a root. This tends to keep the hair in place within the follicle until the anagen phase begins anew. Anagen restarts the cycle, pushing the club hair out of the shaft as the new hair develops. Some hairs are growing in areas of dense hair follicles as other hairs are shed, resulting in a relatively constant hair density. With male-pattern baldness, aging, malnutrition, and ischemic disease, the skin will display gradual hair loss due to the inability of new hair growth to compensate for the loss.

Given that the hair follicle cells are among the most rapidly dividing of the body, cancer chemotherapeutic agents that impair cell division also result in hair loss. Hair follicles are also sensitive to radiation that may be used to treat cancer. This may cause localized hair loss in exposed areas.

Nails

Modified stratum corneum cells produce nails consisting of a more rigid formulation of keratin fibrils. Nails do not desquamate like stratum corneum. Instead, they develop into a semitransparent nail plate of compacted, interlocked keratinized squamous cell remnants continually pushed outwardly from a germinal layer. Only part of the nail is visible beyond the skin. The undersurface of the nail, the nail bed, consists of regenerative stratum basale epidermal cells with an underlying dermal layer attached firmly to the periosteum below, creating the finger/toe pulp (Figure 1-12). Ridges, rather than rete pegs, serve to increase the epidermal cells' attachment to the dermal

portion of the nail bed. These ridges allow the migration of the nail plate distally over the nail bed.

Keratinized cells are pushed outwardly in a wedge shape from the white, half-moon–shaped proximal area of the nail called the *lunula*. The nail matrix is the thickened area under the nail plate's proximal area, where new cells are added to push the nail bed outwardly in a wedgelike progression. The lunula is the visible part of the nail over the matrix. The most proximal portion of the nail matrix generates the most superficial portion of the nail bed, whereas the most distal portion of the matrix generates the deepest-part layers of the nail bed. The proximal nail fold and lateral nail groove are skin covering the nail's proximal end and sides, protecting the underlying tissue. These areas can become infected, particularly with poorly executed nail trimming. The term *paronychia* is used to describe infection around the nails through this tissue. A growth of epidermal cells, the cuticle, extends beyond the fold and groove onto the nail's surface to further protect this junction.

Nails generally are convex medially to laterally but have minimal curvature from proximal to distal, resulting in a cylindrical shape. The rate of nail growth is proportional to the distal phalanx's length, with the result that fingernails grow much more rapidly than toenails. Fingernails grow about 3 mm/month and toenails about 1 mm/month. Nails that are not periodically clipped can become very long and curve under the toes. Injuries and diseases often produce changes in nails. Chronic anemia can produce spoon-shaped, concave nails. The formation of spherical nail shape with substantial proximal to distal curvature is termed *clubbing* and occurs in disorders such as coronary artery disease, lung cancer, Eisenmenger's syndrome, and cystic fibrosis but can be a normal variant (Figure 1-13). Other types of nail changes are associated with a large number of diseases.

Toenails can become very thick, especially with poorly controlled diabetes mellitus, and require grinding to decrease their thickness (Figure 1-14). Otherwise, pressure from the toe box of a person's overlying shoes can damage the nail beds. Chronic trauma leads to the production of keratohyalin granules and increased keratinization and thickening of nails. Severe trauma may lead to permanent nail loss, and less severe injury can lead to continuous nail dystrophy. Splinter hemorrhages are visible as the nail grows outwardly, carrying coagulated blood with it. A fingernail will require 6 months to grow out completely, and a toenail may require 1 to 1.5 years to do so. A severely injured nail may cease growing. With nail bed recovery, a new nail may push out the old nail, similar to a club hair being pushed out by a new hair. The granular layer produced in traumatized nail beds prevents normal adherence of the nail to the nail bed, resulting in layering, separation, and premature loss of the nails' upper surface. Psoriasis frequently produces pitting of the nails. Banding, splitting,

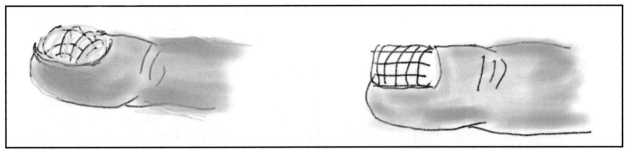

Figure 1-13. Change in nail structure characteristic of clubbing. The normal nail is cylindrical with curvature laterally only. The clubbed nail is spherical with curvature both laterally and proximal to distal as noted with the wire frame depiction.

and dystrophy accompany many diseases. Thick, yellow fungal-infected nails occur commonly with the combination of arterial disease and diabetes mellitus, as shown in Figure 1-14.

SKIN PATHOLOGY

Several terms must be introduced to allow the description of skin disease. Some of these terms apply to small lesions and others to larger versions of the same appearance. Some skin lesions are flat, some are raised, and some are fluid vs solid filled. After introducing these terms, some basic skin disorders will be described. Management of wounds related to these skin diseases will be discussed in the chapters on wound management.

Premature desquamation and migration through the epidermis are associated with several skin disorders. Accelerated maturation of keratinocytes leads to the accumulation of cells of the outermost layer, producing scaling, which is characteristic of diseases such as psoriasis. Scaling, in general, occurs when the stratum corneum accumulates more rapidly than it is shed. Scales may be slightly to more obviously raised and can have normal, brown, or whitish/silvery coloration that produces the classic appearance of psoriasis. Scales are dry and flaky compared with crusts from liquid debris dried on the skin's surface.

Macules, patches, papules, plaques, vesicles, bullae, cysts, pustules, wheals, hives, and scaling are terms used to identify the skin pathology. A *macule* is a flat area, and by strict definition, it is neither raised nor depressed and often has a different coloration. Macules can have markedly irregular shapes, and the color is typically tanner than the surrounding skin. White, brown, and reddish are most common. By strict definition, a macule is 5 mm or less. Common freckles are an example of a macule. A similar area that exceeds 5 mm is termed a *patch*.

Small, solid, elevated lesions are termed *papules*. Again, the definition limits the size to 5 mm in diameter. Papules may have a flat, pointed, or rounded top. The

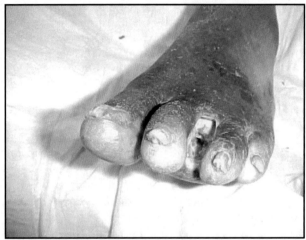

Figure 1-14. Changes in nails consistent with diabetic neuropathy.

presence of papules is not specific but can occur in several dermatologic conditions, particularly acne, fungal infections, and lichen planus. Fungal infections are among the most common dermatological conditions encountered in clinical practice, particularly among vulnerable individuals, such as older adults, people who are immunocompromised, newborns and young children, and people with circulatory conditions or diabetes. Topical fungal infections affect approximately 20% to 25% of the global population. Although these conditions are contagious, they can be prevented or reduced by proper hygiene and decreasing the skin's exposure to moisture. Risk factors include occlusive footwear and communal facilities, such as showers or locker rooms. Proper cleansing of objects and surfaces, such as bath mats and towels, is essential in reducing transmission risk. The most common types of superficial fungal infections of the skin are known as *tinea* and are further classified by location (eg, *tinea capitis*, which affects the scalp; *tinea pedis*, or "athlete's foot"; *tinea cruris*, or "jock itch"; and *tinea unguis*, also known as *onychomycosis*, fungal infections involving the nails).

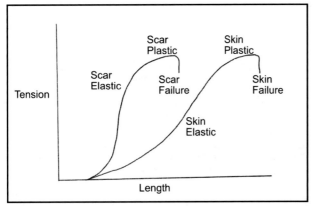

Figure 1-15. Length-tension relationship of scar tissue and normal skin. Note the 5 regions. In the first region, lengthening occurs with little stress. The next three phases (see text) exhibit a linear relationship between lengthening and stress. With further stress (plastic region), fibers are damaged and elasticity lost. Also note the greater extensibility of skin for a given stress.

A raised, solid area greater than 5 mm in diameter is a *plaque*. Plaques are more plateaulike, with some variation in height along the plaque. Plaques may combine other features such as *scaling*, particularly in psoriasis.

Fluid-filled lesions have additional names. A small blister, up to a few millimeters, is a *vesicle*. Vesicles are associated with several skin disorders, especially the lesions of herpes simplex virus. Larger blisters are *bullae* (bulla is singular). Bullae are associated with immune disorders that damage desmosomes or hemidesmosomes and allow fluid to accumulate within the skin. Bullae may also be seen with moderately severe burn injuries. If a vesicle is filled with purulent material from an infection, it is more appropriately termed a *pustule*. A fluid- to semisolid-filled, encapsulated lesion is given the term *cyst*. The capsule around purulent material often develops as the immune system attacks but does not prevail against bacteria. Cysts occur in cystic acne and other blockages of follicular ducts. Larger "boils" are more appropriately termed a *furuncle* and a coalescence of furuncles, particularly in the lower cervical/upper thoracic region, a *carbuncle*. Raised, firm, swollen skin created by an allergic or anaphylactic response is termed a *wheal* but is also known by the lay term of *hives*.

BIOMECHANICS OF SKIN

Skin is much more elastic than the dense connective tissue of bone, ligament, and tendon. Some of these differences in elasticity are due to tissue components, and some are due to the arrangements of these components within the tissues. Tendons are very stiff and barely elongate when forces are applied. Tendon stiffness is primarily due to the parallel arrangement of very thick bundles of collagen.

However, as discussed previously, the tendon has different proportions of glycosaminoglycans than elastic cartilage or skin. In addition to its elastic nature, normal skin has tensile and viscous properties. Much of this elasticity comes from viscous elements; therefore, skin is described as having a viscoelastic property.

In a simple model, collagen fibers may be ascribed the role of providing tensile strength (ie, the ability to resist lengthening). However, collagen fibers are both coiled and undulating. As stretch is applied to collagen fibers, they become straightened. Several elastic fibers attach to each other and other collagen bundles at several points along each bundle of collagen fibers. Further stretch straightens the alignment of collagen and elastic fibers. The 3-dimensional interaction of collagen fibers and the attachment of elastic fibers made of elastin allow the skin to recoil when an applied tension is released.

Ground substance, made of glycosaminoglycans and water, also provides some elasticity to the skin. Dehydration of the skin, as occurs with aging, diminishes skin turgor and allows the skin's fibers to become lax. This laxity is manifested as *tenting*, seen when the skin is pinched but does not recoil when this force is released. The response of a material to an applied force is graphically represented as a stress-strain curve (Figure 1-15). The force applied to the tissue represents the stress (dependent variable plotted on the y-axis); the length of the tissue represents the strain as the independent variable plotted on the x-axis. Therefore, the stress-strain curve represents a measurement of force across the tissue as its length is changed.

The stress-strain curve of connective tissue can be divided into 5 regions and subdivided into 2 major regions. In the elastic region, no permanent change in tissue length occurs with stretch (see Figure 1-15). The elastic region is subdivided into 3 phases. The compliant phase (toe region) represents taking up of slack within individual fibers. During the compliant phase, very little change in force across the tissue occurs with lengthening. The second phase, the transition phase, has a greater slope, producing more but still relatively little force as it is lengthened. However, in the third phase, the linear phase, the stress-strain relationship's slope becomes linear due to the lattice of fibers becoming aligned with the force across it.

The plastic region represents a permanent change in tissue length once a certain length is achieved. This point at which the plastic region is reached is termed the *yield point* because the material yields to the force applied, and tension actually produces increasing length. Within the plastic region, attachments between fibers are destroyed at the microscopic level, changing the fibers' 3-dimensional lattice. The release of stretch leaves the tissue in an elongated and weakened state. In the second yield region, individual fibers unravel further, yielding to the applied force up to the point of failure, manifested as tearing of the tissue.

Loss of collagen and elastic fibers and dehydration cause skin to become less extensible and weaker (more brittle) with age. Skin tears, especially with the imprudent use of adhesives, and multiple ecchymoses (bruises) become frequent in older patients. On the other hand, the prudent application of external forces can aid functional skin repair during the maturation phase of healing. Scar management is discussed extensively in Chapter 13.

BIOMECHANICS OF SCAR TISSUE

Scar tissue differs from normal skin in several ways. The collagen within scars is a different type, and the ground substance has different proportions of the component molecules. In scar tissue, collagen is primarily type IV, which is stiffer than type I. In normal skin, hyaluronic acid, chondroitin sulfate, and dermatan sulfate represent, respectively, about 42%, 5%, and 54% of the glycosaminoglycans. Hyaluronic acid decreases dramatically in scar tissue, and chondroitin sulfate increases to proportions similar to those of tendon and bone. Because of these changes, scar tissue is much stiffer than normal skin. Because all the skin is contiguous, its entire mass acts as a reservoir of elasticity. Therefore, flexing the fingers tightens the skin on the hand's dorsum as well as that on the forearm. The effect of finger flexion is much greater on the hand, but even the skin covering the opposite hand or foot has some of its elastic reservoir taken away. With small injuries, this loss of elastic reservoir can go un-noticed and may be compensated over time. However, when a large proportion of the skin is injured, as in a burn, we see the loss of range of motion at the joint involved in the burn and diminishing fashion in adjacent joints. A burn that causes extensive scarring at the elbow leads to profound loss of range of motion at the elbow and decreases the range of motion at the wrist, hand, and shoulder. A more extensive burn could limit the range of motion at the neck as well. Interventions directed toward maintaining range of motion following burn injuries are covered in Chapter 14.

SUMMARY

Skin consists of 2 primary layers and a subcutaneous fat layer. The epidermis consists primarily of keratinocytes and waterproofs the skin. Distinct layers of cells support the function of the epidermis as the cells mature and migrate toward the surface. Langerhans cells provide an immune function, and melanocytes protect the skin from ultraviolet radiation. The dermis consists of a papillary layer that attaches to and nourishes the epidermis and a reticular layer. The dermis consists of fibroblasts within a sea of collagen, elastic fibers, and ground substance. Both the fibers' structure within the dermis and their arrangement provide tensile strength and elasticity of the dermis. Excessive stretch applied to the skin results in tearing. Tearing occurs much more readily in the skin of older adults. Subcutaneous fat provides thermal insulation and cushions bony prominences. Emaciated individuals are at a much higher risk of pressure injuries because of the lack of soft tissue between the bony prominences and skin.

QUESTIONS

1. What is the history of physical therapy in the management of wounds?
2. How does skin interact with the other 3 systems—cardiovascular and pulmonary, neuromuscular, and musculoskeletal—in health and disease?
3. How does skin protect the body from infection passively and actively?
4. What are the pros and cons of the skin flora?
5. What can happen when the environment of the skin flora is altered (heat, moisture, etc)?
6. How does skin contribute to thermoregulation?
7. What happens to skin's role with autonomic dysfunction and burns?
8. How does skin temperature provide a window on the function of the vascular system?
9. How does injury/disease of the nervous system affect skin integrity?
   a. Sensory
   b. Motor
   c. Autonomic
10. What is meant by a reservoir of elasticity, and how can the reservoir be emptied?
11. What are the basic functions of the 3 layers associated with the skin?
    a. Epidermis
    b. Dermis
    c. Hypodermis/subcutaneous fat
12. Name the 3 major cells of the epidermis and their roles.
    a. Keratinocyte
    b. Langerhans cell
    c. Melanocyte

13. Name the 5 layers of epidermis and their functions.
    a. Stratum basale
    b. Stratum spinosum
    c. Stratum granulosum
    d. Stratum corneum
    e. Stratum lucidum
14. Describe the locations and roles of the accessory structures of skin.
    a. Hair follicles
    b. Sebaceous glands
    c. Sweat glands
    d. Nails
15. What lines each of the accessory structures, and how does that assist in wound healing?
16. What are the changes we commonly see in nails with aging and disease?
17. Name the 2 layers of the dermis and their roles in dermal function.
18. Contrast the blood supply of the 2 layers of dermis.
19. What are the components of the ground substance?
20. What are the different types of fibers found in the dermis, and what are their properties?
21. What is the significance of Langer's lines?
22. What are the 2 basic mechanisms leading to the formation of blisters?
23. What contributes to the biomechanics properties of healthy skin?
24. How are the biomechanics of scar tissue different than healthy skin?
25. What are the typical changes seen in aging skin?

BIBLIOGRAPHY

Canty EG, Kadler KE. Procollagen trafficking, processing and fibrillogenesis. *J Cell Sci.* 2005;118:1341-1353. doi:10.1242/jcs.01731

Ekman AK, Bivik Eding C, Rundquist I, Enerbäck C. IL-17 and IL-22 promote keratinocyte stemness in the germinative compartment in psoriasis. *J Invest Dermatol.* 2019;139(7):1564-1573.e8. doi:10.1016/j.jid.2019.01.014

Lambers H, Piessens S, Bloem A, Pronk H, Finkel P. Natural skin surface pH is on average below 5, which is beneficial for its resident flora. *Int J Cosmet Sci.* 2006;28(5):359-370. doi:10.1111/j.1467-2494.2006.00344.x

Ovalle WK, Nahirney PC. *Netter's Essential Histology.* 2nd ed. Saunders; 2013.

Robak E, Gerlicz-Kowalczuk Z, Dziankowska-Bartkowiak B, Wozniacka A, Bogaczewicz J. Serum concentrations of IL-17A, IL-17B, IL-17E and IL-17F in patients with systemic sclerosis. *Arch Med Sci.* 2019;15(3):706-712. doi:10.5114/aoms.2019.84738

Stevens A, Lowe J. *Human Histology.* 4th ed. Mosby; 2014.

Watt FM. Involucrin and other markers of keratinocyte terminal differentiation. *J Invest Dermatol.* 1983;81(1 Suppl):100s-103s.

2

Normal Healing

OBJECTIVES

- Identify the important aspects associated with the 4 phases of normal wound healing, including wound closure and ultimate healing.
- List the phases of normal wound healing and their time frames.
- List the 6 processes occurring in a healing wound.
- Describe events of the inflammatory (lag) phase, including hemostasis and roles of immune cells.
- Describe the events of granulation tissue formation.
- Describe the need for coordination of granulation tissue formation and re-epithelialization.
- Describe the events of the remodeling phases and factors determining wound strength.
- Contrast the injury and healing of superficial, partial-thickness, and full-thickness wounds with subcutaneous tissue involvement.
- Discuss the roles of oxygen in wound healing.
- Describe features distinguishing fetal wound healing from adult wound healing.

Irion GL., Gardner JA, Pignataro RM.
Comprehensive Wound Management, Third Edition (pp 19-30).
© 2024 Taylor and Francis Group.

Cutaneous wounds generally heal well with little intervention. The purpose of this chapter is to describe the events of well-executed wound healing as a prelude to issues that can delay or halt normal healing. Some tissues are capable of regeneration, whereas others must heal through repair with granulation tissue, which does not replace the defect with normal tissue but fills the defect and closes the skin.

NORMAL TISSUE HEALING

Depending on the extent of the injury, a simple regeneration of the epidermis may be sufficient. Deeper injuries may lead to defects extending beyond the skin, potentially to bone. These injuries involve tissues that cannot be regenerated and must be filled with new tissue to bridge the defect. Most of the wounds that will be seen by those reading this will involve full-thickness injuries and often subcutaneous injury.

Following a full-thickness injury, a programmed sequence of events unfolds, generating granulation tissue, which will eventually mature into a scar covered with regenerated epidermis. The clinician may either facilitate or disturb this repair with interventions. In this chapter, a description of these events is given. In subsequent chapters, the ways we can facilitate and avoid interfering with the processes are described.

REGENERATION VS REPAIR

The restoration of tissue to the same condition prior to the injury, consisting of the same cells and extracellular matrix, is *regeneration*. Only the epidermal covering of a wound can be fully regenerated. If a partial depth of dermis is damaged, epidermal regeneration including accessory structures is expected, and restoration of the thickness of the dermis can occur by the production of extracellular matrix by surviving fibroblasts, although tissue pigmentation may be changed. However, in full-thickness and subcutaneous wounds, accessory structures destroyed in the injury cannot be regenerated and will be absent in a scar. Hair, sebaceous glands, and sweat glands will be missing and lead to some degree of cosmetic and functional changes. Pigmentation and contour of the skin may also be significantly changed. In full-thickness injuries, regeneration of the epidermis from the edges of the wound can provide coverage but will not restore skin function. The depths of tissue injury are depicted in Figure 2-1.

The intermediate tissue that develops once the wounded area is cleared of debris is termed *granulation tissue*. It consists of fibroblasts that produce a provisional

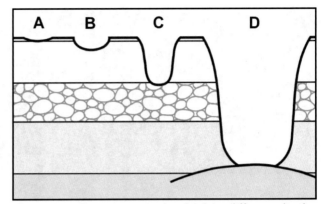

Figure 2-1. Skin structures involved in different depths. (A) Superficial, (B) partial thickness, (C) full thickness, and (D) full thickness with subcutaneous involvement.

extracellular matrix and angioblasts that build temporary vasculature to support the repair process. Although fibroblasts and angioblasts present during the process of repair are also normally found in the dermis, they leave the area when repair is complete, resulting in a tissue with different characteristics that simply serves to fill the void caused by the injury; therefore, only repair, not regeneration, of the dermis occurs. Granulation tissue only occurs in full-thickness injuries without any remaining viable dermis. Its eventual contraction leads to the loss of skin elasticity.

TYPES OF WOUND HEALING

Superficial thickness wounds are caused by shearing, friction, and mild burn (first degree). Healing occurs by regeneration of epithelial cells on the wound surface due to the loss of contact inhibition and migration of epidermal cells across the surface. Because no defect in skin continuity occurs, this type of healing does not cause scars, and accessory structures remain intact (see Figure 2-1A). However, a serious deep injury can sometimes be identified incorrectly as a superficial wound due to the death of tissue starting deeply below the seemingly intact epidermis. In many cases of pressure and shear injury, necrotic tissue may be hidden below an injured but still intact epidermis. Erosion through the remaining thickness of the skin (iceberg/volcano analogy; see Figure 2-1D) may lead to expulsion of necrotic tissue creating a large void. An example of a superficial wound with a small area of a partial-thickness wound caused by abrasion is shown in Figure 2-2.

Partial-thickness wounds (see Figure 2-1B) heal in a way similar to superficial thickness wounds. Damage to the dermis occurs, but accessory structures are spared. Depending on the cause, dry, necrotic tissue known as *eschar* may form on the wound, particularly with burn

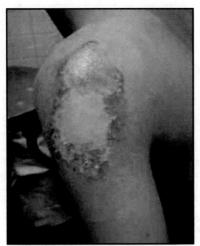

Figure 2-2. Photo of a superficial and partial-thickness wound.

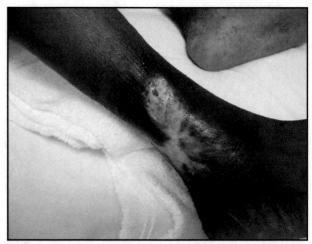

Figure 2-3. Partial-thickness wound adjacent to previously closed wounds.

injuries. Partial-thickness wounds can have similar causes as superficial wounds but generally with greater intensity or prolongation of insult. A partial-thickness wound adjacent to a previously closed wound is shown in Figure 2-3.

Full-thickness wounds (see Figure 2-1C) and wounds with subcutaneous involvement (see Figure 2-1D) may be closed by the following processes: primary intention, delayed primary intention (also known as *tertiary intention*), or secondary intention. Although inflammation is associated with vascular tissues, even superficial injuries may generate some inflammation without tissue necrosis due to the release of chemical messengers that promote inflammation. Chemicals diffusing from damaged epidermis into the vascularized tissue below produce the apparent inflammation. The processes used for wound closure are described in the following sections. An example of a full-thickness wound with subcutaneous involvement is shown in Figure 2-4.

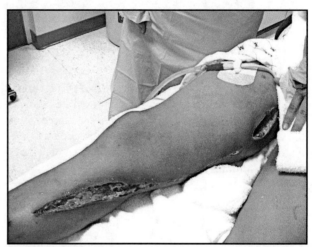

Figure 2-4. Full-thickness wound with subcutaneous involvement from harvesting the greater saphenous vein for coronary artery bypass grafting.

Primary Intention

Primary closure can be accomplished by suturing, stapling, or the use of adhesives. This type of closure (Figure 2-5) is reserved for surgical or traumatic wounds with clean, smooth edges and negligible subcutaneous tissue loss. Attempts to close wounds that do not have these characteristics increase the risk of infection or may cause cosmetic problems. Primary closure results in faster healing and less scarring than secondary or delayed primary closure due to the minimal amount of granulation tissue that must be generated. Epithelialization begins within the first 24 hours if the edges of the wound are approximated and may be complete within 48 to 72 hours.

Delayed Primary (Tertiary) Intention

In this type of healing, sutures or staples are employed at a later date, often after multiple days of irrigation and drainage of an abscess or osteomyelitis and the generation of some granulation tissue. This type of closure is chosen when contamination, tissue loss, or risk of infection is present. The wound is left open but covered with a suitable dressing material until closing it becomes prudent. Dead space of the wound is filled with suitable materials to prevent premature closure of the wound. Closing a wound that is likely to harbor harmful bacteria may lead to sepsis or death. Therefore, such wounds are initially allowed to stay open as they would with secondary intention. However, with tertiary intention, the wound is not allowed to fill completely with granulation tissue and re-epithelialize. Instead, when the wound is deemed clean and stable and

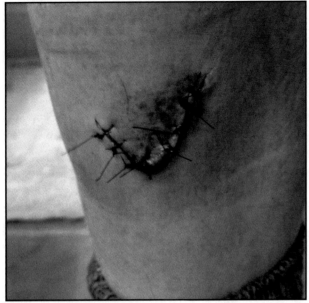

Figure 2-5. Use of primary intention to secure a laceration on the anterior leg.

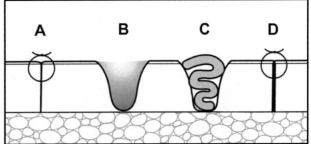

Figure 2-6. Comparison of (A) primary, (B) secondary, and (C and D) tertiary intention. C depicts packing of the wound to be closed later. D depicts the wound in C closed with sutures. Note the clean edges and minimal granulation tissue of primary healing. Secondary healing is characterized by the production of granulation tissue and wound contraction. Delayed primary healing may be associated with some amount of granulation tissue and contraction depending on the amount of tissue lost to necrosis.

therefore unlikely to pose a significant risk of infection, it is closed with sutures or staples as it would be with primary intention. In some cases, sutures are placed across the wound, but the edges are not approximated until later. As the ends of the wound granulate in, sutures are tied off until the wound is closed.

Secondary Intention

Healing by secondary intention refers to allowing wounds to close on their own, as opposed to closing them directly. In secondary intention, wounds fill completely with granulation tissue, contract, and are covered by regeneration of the epidermis. Wound contraction reduces the amount of granulation tissue required to close the defect but in doing so removes some of the reservoir of elasticity from the skin. Ideally, wound filling, resurfacing, and contraction are coordinated, resulting in a cosmetically and functionally acceptable scar. Secondary intention is used for wounds with tissue loss, irregular edges, tissue necrosis, high microbial count, or the presence of other debris such as depicted in Figure 2-4. The events of healing by secondary intention and necessary components are described in the following section. The 3 types of closure are summarized in Figure 2-6.

Events of Healing by Secondary Intention

Healing by secondary intention generally involves addressing the cause of the wound as well as the degradation and removal of necrotic tissue. This may include the

need for hemostasis and possibly an immune response against infectious agents. Both hemostasis and an inflammatory response are required to stop bleeding associated with wounding, restoring blood flow to the injured area, and removal of substantial quantities of necrotic tissue. Therefore, additional and time-consuming steps are involved in removing the cause of tissue injury as well as the necrotic tissue. This complex process introduces the opportunity for several problems to arise, which are discussed in the next chapter. Healing by secondary intention will be described initially for uncomplicated healing following a traumatic injury, rather than infectious etiology. Thus, hemostasis will be considered as the first step in healing, followed by a period of inflammation, proliferation, and remodeling or maturation of the scar. The process also involves several growth factors to promote proliferation and molecules such as matrix metalloproteinases (MMPs) to rid the area of debris to allow normal healing. The timeline for healing by secondary intention is depicted in Figure 2-7.

Hemostasis

Shortly upon injury to vascularized tissue, hemostasis is initiated. This can be stimulated by either the exposure of collagen to platelets or the release of tissue factor from injured tissue. Platelets adhere to the site of an injured blood vessel, activating the platelet. Adenosine diphosphate released by platelets binds to specific receptors on additional platelets, recruiting them to the site of injury and causing them to change shape and bind to each other (*aggregation*). Platelet activation results in a positive feedback mechanism that rapidly produces a platelet plug and stimulates the coagulation cascade to reinforce the platelet plug with fibrin. In normal hemostasis, the platelet plug stops bleeding and allows regeneration of the injured blood vessel, followed by degradation of the fibrin and restoration of blood flow to the area of injury. In addition to adhesion and recruitment of additional platelets, activation of platelets leads to the release of platelet-derived growth factor (PDGF) and activates inflammation.

Inflammation

A number of mechanisms can be responsible for the activation of inflammation. Neutrophils are the first cells attracted to an area of injury. They can perform phagocytosis of a large number of bacteria and control bacterial proliferation until more specific components of the immune system arrive. Neutrophils respond to molecules on some bacteria by phagocytosis. They release molecules that damage and kill bacteria nonspecifically and can also damage surrounding normal tissue. Neutrophils can also phagocytose damaged and dead cells and debris. Macrophages arriving later play a large role in removing dead cells, debris, and remaining bacteria. The removal of debris becomes important in allowing the production of granulation tissue to produce a scar. Other, more specific immune cells may arrive later, after macrophages present antigen to specific helper and killer T cells and plasma cells produce antibodies for antigens present on bacteria. Complement proteins binding to components of bacterial cells may also produce much of the inflammation.

Mast cells reside in connective tissue and can be stimulated to degranulate by injury and events of the inflammatory process. Histamine is a major component of mast cell granules and produces much of the vasodilation associated with inflammation.

Matrix Metalloproteinases

MMP enzymes aid in the degradation of necrotic tissue to clear the site of injury in preparation for repair. Different MMP species are designated MMP1, MMP2, and so on as they are discovered. MMPs are released during the inflammatory response, degrading extracellular matrix proteins, including different types of collagen, elastin, laminin, fibronectin, and aggrecan. Degradation of extracellular matrix also triggers the release of growth factors that assist in choreographing the neovascularization and production of a new tissue matrix.

A braking mechanism on MMPs is provided by tissue inhibitors of metalloproteinases (TIMPs). The 4 types are designated as TIMP-1, TIMP-2, TIMP-3, and TIMP-4. These molecules bind the zinc molecule of MMPs to inactivate them. As the source of inflammation is cleared from the wound, genetic expression of MMP genes is diminished and TIMP expression is increased, thereby allowing the building of a permanent matrix. In Chapter 3, the continued expression of MMP genes as a contributor of chronic wounds is discussed.

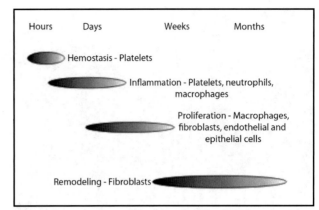

Figure 2-7. Timeline of the phases of healing by secondary intention.

Proliferative Phase

The proliferative phase consists of granulation tissue formation, regeneration of an epidermal covering (re-epithelialization), and wound contraction. Granulation tissue is created by the 2 coordinated processes of angiogenesis (formation of new blood vessels) by angioblasts and the deposition of a provisional extracellular matrix and type IV collagen by fibroblasts.

Temporary blood vessels are generated from existing blood vessels due to several factors. Vascular endothelial growth factor (VEGF) and low tissue oxygen are major factors in the process. A provisional extracellular matrix is produced by the excretion of type IV collagen and fibronectin by fibroblasts attracted to the site of injury. A clean surface such as fascia or periosteum aids the development of granulation. Failure to provide a clean surface for the provisional matrix leads to very slow healing.

Epidermal regeneration occurs along the surface due to the loss of contact inhibition. Proliferating epidermal cells either move across the edge of the injured area or spread from sweat glands, hair follicles, and sebaceous glands until contact with other epidermal cells occurs. Under normal circumstances, re-epithelialization is limited to granulation tissue that has reached the previous surface level of the skin, providing normal contour to the wound. Granulation tissue can be seen in both Figures 2-4 and 2-8. In both photographs, granulation tissue is intermingled with necrotic tissue. The granulation tissue in Figure 2-8 is very healthy, but the tissue in Figure 2-4 is stringy and has an unhealthy appearance due to infection of this surgical site. Good-quality granulation tissue with re-epithelialized edges can be seen in Figure 2-8. Events of proliferation are depicted in Figure 2-9.

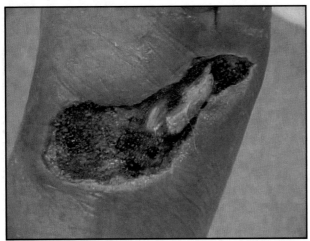

Figure 2-8. Granulation tissue and re-epithelialized edges from a wound receiving negative pressure wound therapy. Note the exposed tendon within the wound bed.

Contraction

In concert with filling and covering of the skin defect, myofibroblasts with contractile elements and adhesion to surrounding tissue pull the edges of the wound toward each other. Contraction occurs more readily in directions that correspond to lines used by surgeons in planning incisions. The best known of these lines are Langer's lines, which are often drawn perpendicular to the line of pull of underlying muscles. For example, a horizontal wound on the abdomen will close more rapidly than a vertical wound. Over the course of contraction, a circular wound will appear to close more in one plane and become elliptical and then linear before closing. The pulling of contracting scars on surrounding skin can be seen in Figures 2-10A to 2-10D.

Remodeling

Over the course of several months and up to 2 years, a closed wound will continue to remodel or mature. Initial fibroplasia involves random orientation of collagen bundles and reduced strength. Over this maturation period, collagen bundles are degraded and rebuilt. Those aligned with stress become reinforced and are not degraded. Early in the maturation process, following wound closure, blood vessels built in the granulation tissue are degraded as oxygen demand falls and the tissue becomes hyperperfused. Closed wounds are expected to be slightly red and swollen but lose the erythema and swelling over the course of several days to a few weeks due to the regression of blood vessels. An example of a maturing scar is shown in Figure 2-5. Note that this scar has not yet achieved normal pigmentation. Migration of melanocytes into the new epidermis is evident by the uneven transition of pigmentation from the surrounding skin across the scar. Over the course of multiple weeks to months, pigmentation is expected to normalize.

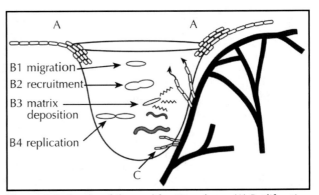

Figure 2-9. Events of the proliferative phase. (A) Proliferation and migration of epithelial cells from wound margins. (B) Proliferation of fibroblasts and production of collagen fibers. (C) Proliferation of angioblasts and angiogenesis.

Healing

A wound is considered healed when function and appearance become optimized. A closed wound must mature and regain its strength to be considered healed. Health care professionals working with wounds need to recognize the difference between a closed and healed wound. A wound that is simply closed may lack sufficient strength and function to withstand stresses placed on the skin and reopen or become *dehiscent* (term for reopening of a surgically closed wound). Some areas of the body are well known for poor healing due to the stresses placed on the skin. This concept is addressed further in the next chapter.

OPERATIVE REPAIR

If possible, direct closure of an acute wound is preferable to prevent contamination and chronic inflammation. Indications for direct closure include lacerations with minimal tissue loss, surgical wounds, and other incisions. Regardless of the cause of the wound, for direct closure to be the method of choice, the wound must be clean and likely to heal. Prior to direct closure, the site must be irrigated and debrided of any foreign material or necrotic tissue. A surgeon may choose delayed primary closure (tertiary closure) if significant undermining or contamination is present. Should direct closure be chosen, deep sutures are placed in the depth of the wound to decrease stress on the skin's surface and remove any dead space. Subcutaneous dead space is a major risk factor for infection as this space fills with fluid (blood or serum) that can nourish the bacteria and shield them from the immune system.

Surgical staples or adhesives (glue) may be used in the place of sutures. Staples are primarily used for the scalp and linear incisions. Sutures are preferred with nonlinear wounds. A number of techniques are available to

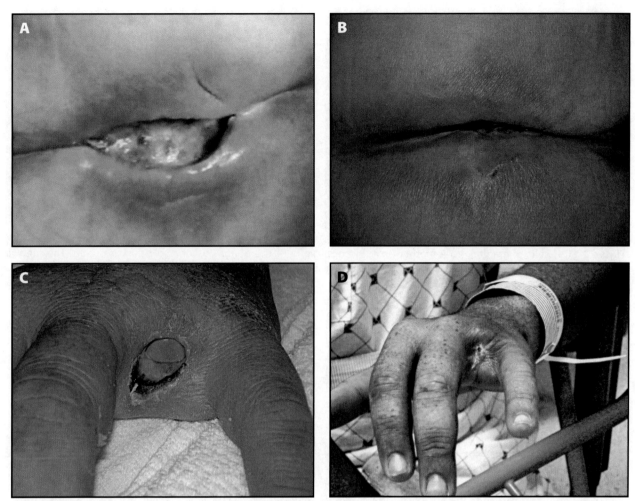

Figure 2-10. Examples of wound contraction. (A) Wound created by excision of rectal carcinoma. (B) The same wound following granulation, re-epithelialization, and contraction. (C) Wound caused by amputation of the fourth finger of the left hand due to ischemic necrosis. (D) The same wound following granulation, epithelialization, and wound contraction. In both B and D, note the tension placed on the surrounding skin by the contraction and the uneven nature of the contraction.

plastic surgeons to close even complicated wounds with minimum evidence of scarring. In some cases, however, primary closure is not sufficient, and grafts are required.

Grafts

In the event that a wound is too large to close optimally, tissue may be transplanted from one part of the body to another. Types of grafts used in plastic surgery include skin grafts, which have no blood supply, and flaps, which are transplanted with a blood supply. Grafts can also be defined by their sources. An *autograft* is taken from another part of the patient's body. Although rejection will not occur, significant shortening and scarring can occur. *Allografts* are skin from another person. They may not be permanent. Autografts or transplants from an identical twin (*syngeneic transplant*) will last, although tissue will turn over just as normal skin does over time. Allografts

can provide temporary coverage necessary for preventing infection and fluid loss, but allografts may transmit infectious agents, particularly viral diseases, or undergo rejection. This type of graft becomes useful for large burn injuries, skin loss secondary to trauma, or necrotizing fasciitis. *Xenografts* come from species other than humans. Xenografts are temporary until they are replaced by the patient's own skin. Porcine skin has been used extensively but can also transmit disease and may not be accepted by some patients for religious reasons. Fish skin has recently been proposed as a form of xenograft.

Skin Grafts

Skin grafts are indicated for wounds that are not expected to close spontaneously in a reasonable time frame, provided the patient has suitable graft donor sites with sufficient vascularity to take at the graft recipient

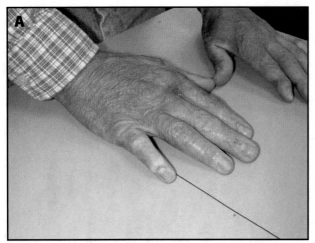 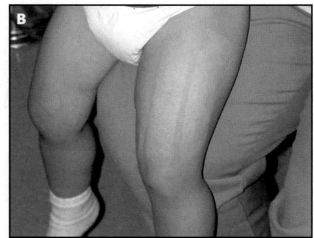

Figure 2-11. Results of grafting. (A) A meshed split-thickness graft. (B) The donor site for a split-thickness graft. The site will re-epithelialize and regain thickness, allowing repeated harvesting from this site. (Reproduced with permission from Arkansas Children's Hospital, Little Rock, Arkansas.)

site. Skin grafts are only indicated if the site has no need for subcutaneous tissue to act as padding. Additional considerations include aesthetics of the healed graft site. Either split-thickness or full-thickness grafts may be used depending on the area to be covered. The advantage of a split-thickness skin graft is its ability to cover a larger area due to meshing, which allows coverage of a surface area approximately 3 times as large as the donor area. Additionally, the area may be reharvested multiple times.

A meshed split-thickness graft also has the advantage of allowing fluid to escape rather than accumulate under the graft and prevent adherence. The stretching of the meshed graft has the important effect of converting a single large defect in the skin into multiple small wounds that can close by re-epithelialization more rapidly than a single large wound of the same cumulative surface area. As the donor site heals by re-epithelialization, it can be reharvested after 10 to 14 days to provide a graft for another area of the body (Figure 2-11). Drawbacks of split-thickness grafts include cosmetic problems and diminished function on flexor surfaces. Certain areas of the body such as the face, hands, and flexor surfaces may require a full-thickness graft. Full-thickness grafts have sufficient strength to function on flexor surfaces such as the anterior elbow, axilla, and posterior knee and are much more cosmetically acceptable than the residual diamond effect left in a healed meshed split-thickness skin graft. However, full-thickness skin grafts can only cover one-third of the area that a split-thickness graft can, and the available surface area for taking full-thickness grafts may be limited. Cultured skin is another way of covering a wound. A small piece of skin is harvested from the patient and grown under optimal conditions in a laboratory setting. After several weeks, a piece of skin originally only a few square centimeters may reach a size approaching a square meter. Precautions following successful grafting include the risk of infection, protecting the graft from the effect of shear for 7 to 14 days, and the need for lubrication.

Flaps

In certain cases, flaps are preferable to grafts. Benefits of a flap include better-quality skin cover, sensation more likely to remain intact, the provision of padding, the ability to cover exposed anatomical structures and prostheses, the ability to maintain blood supply, cosmesis, and the possibility of functional restoration. Flaps are classified based on the type of tissue grafted and the anatomical relationship between the donor and graft site of the flap. The tissue type may include skin and subcutaneous tissue, muscle with or without overlying skin, or bone with or without original overlying tissue. The anatomical relationship between the donor and graft site may be classified as local, in which the tissue harvested is adjacent to the defect to be filled; distant, in which the harvested tissue is attached temporarily to its original site until vascularization occurs at the new location; or a free flap, which has been removed from its donor site, but blood vessels are anastomosed to blood vessels in the new location.

Skin Flaps

Although the purpose of using a skin flap rather than a skin graft is the presence of intact blood vessels, blood supply to the skin flap can be unpredictable. If blood vessels are identifiable within the flap, the preference is for a flap with an axial, arterial supply running the length of the flap. An axial supply can provide a larger flap than a flap with horizontal blood supply.

Muscle Flaps

This type of flap can be done without overlying skin, but if overlying skin is not used, then it must be covered with a split-thickness skin graft. As with the skin flap, an axial blood supply is preferred with perforating blood vessels to revascularize skin. In contrast to skin flaps, muscle flaps provide padding. Good blood supply decreases the risk of infection or failure of the graft to take.

Free Flaps

To perform a free flap, the surgeon must be able to identify vessels to anastomose in both the flap and recipient site. If this vessel anastomosis can be done, the free flap provides well-vascularized tissue to a site that does not have a good local blood flow. In addition, a skilled surgeon may be able to anastomose a nerve. Other specialized flaps exist, and the reader is directed toward texts covering these flaps.

Micrografting

Another recent development is an extension of split-thickness grafting called *micrografting*. Skin cells are spaced over a clean granulation bed with a device that allows the spreading of cells to eventually coalesce into intact skin. Different techniques range from small pinch grafts to techniques that could be compared to spray-painting skin cells on the bed of granulation.

Skin Substitutes

Skin substitutes are often marketed as a temporary covering that allows the recipient to eventually replace the applied product with their own skin. A large number of skin substitutes have been developed. Older types are based on dermal-derived and epidermal/dermal-derived processes. Historically, cells harvested from neonatal foreskins have been used to avoid rejection. The material is grown in culture without immune markers or accessory structures of the skin. Products may combine human keratinocytes, fibroblasts, and other components such as nonhuman collagen. Extracellular matrix, cytokines, and growth factors that are normally found in human skin are purported to stimulate healing.

Newer forms of skin substitutes continue to be developed along with guidelines of which products may be the most suitable for different applications. Recently developed products include portions of placental membranes. Both growth factors and mesenchymal stem cell availability are suggested as mechanisms for the use of placental membranes. Products may contain an amniotic membrane, chorionic membrane, or both. Frozen and freeze-dried products are available. Fish skin is now also available as a temporary skin substitute. Fish skin is promoted as being safer than mammalian tissues that must be processed to destroy any potential infectious agents.

Skin substitutes do not always take and may need to be reapplied, especially in cases of arterial disease or excessive edema of the application site. Even with good results, additional applications may be required to promote full closure.

SUMMARY

Normal wound healing differs with the depth of injury. Simple partial-thickness wounds heal by re-epithelialization, whereas full-thickness wounds may heal by either primary intention or secondary intention. Primary intention refers to surgical closure of clean, narrow wounds. Delayed primary or healing by third intention is used after a wound is sufficiently clean and narrow to be closed later. Healing by secondary intention requires a coordination of hemostasis, inflammation, re-epithelialization, production of granulation tissue, wound contraction, and remodeling of the scar tissue. In some cases, none of these processes will produce a satisfactory result, and grafts, flaps, or skin substitutes are used to allow healing. Types of healing are summarized in Figure 2-12, and the progression through normal healing is summarized in Figure 2-13. A summary of the actions of cells involved in normal healing is provided in Table 2-1.

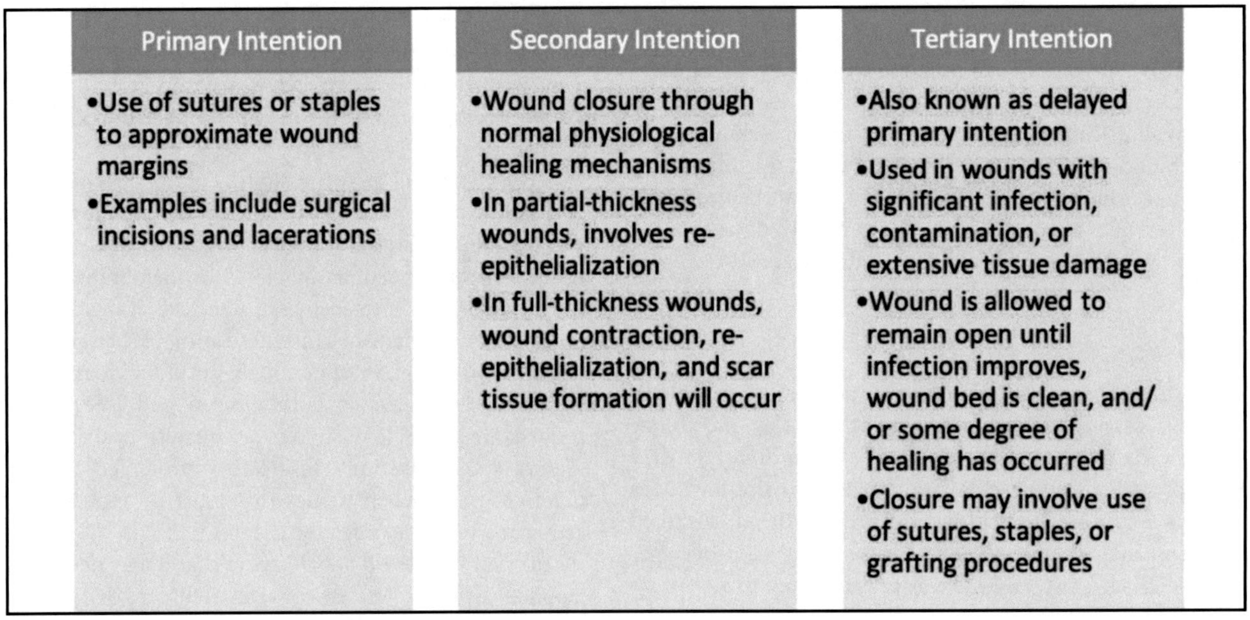

Primary Intention	Secondary Intention	Tertiary Intention
•Use of sutures or staples to approximate wound margins •Examples include surgical incisions and lacerations	•Wound closure through normal physiological healing mechanisms •In partial-thickness wounds, involves re-epithelialization •In full-thickness wounds, wound contraction, re-epithelialization, and scar tissue formation will occur	•Also known as delayed primary intention •Used in wounds with significant infection, contamination, or extensive tissue damage •Wound is allowed to remain open until infection improves, wound bed is clean, and/or some degree of healing has occurred •Closure may involve use of sutures, staples, or grafting procedures

Figure 2-12. Types of wound healing.

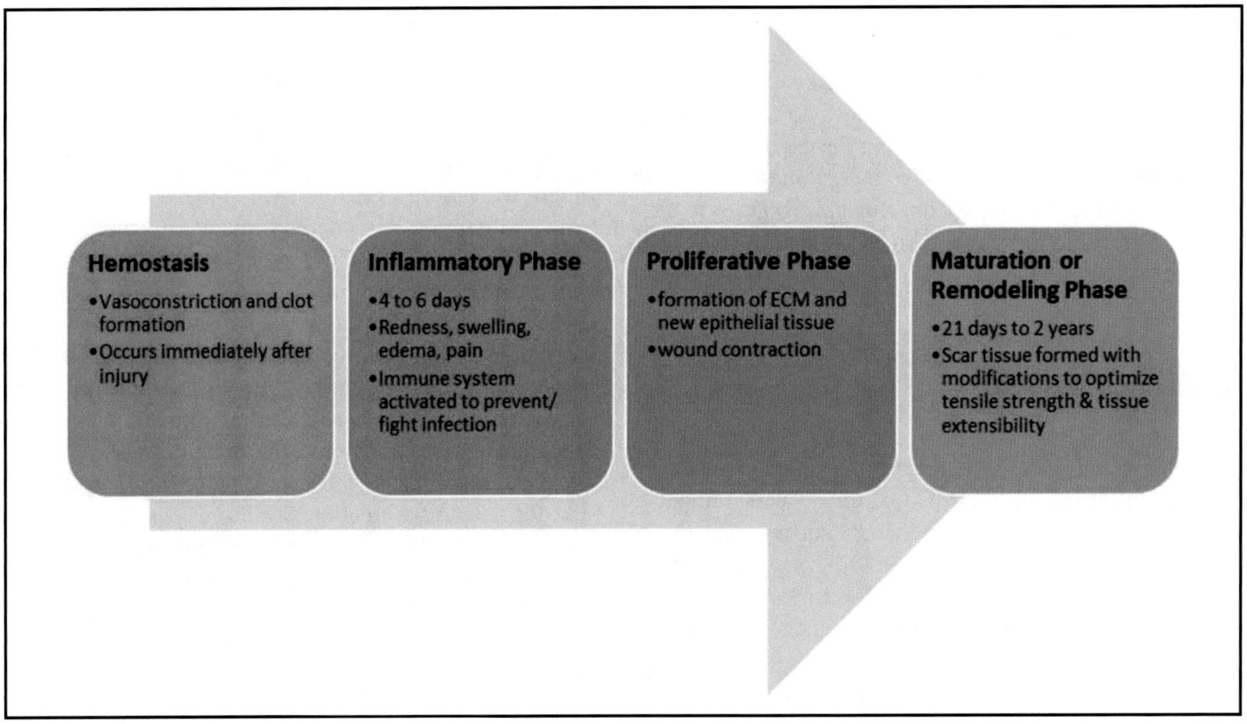

Hemostasis
•Vasoconstriction and clot formation
•Occurs immediately after injury

Inflammatory Phase
•4 to 6 days
•Redness, swelling, edema, pain
•Immune system activated to prevent/fight infection

Proliferative Phase
•formation of ECM and new epithelial tissue
•wound contraction

Maturation or Remodeling Phase
•21 days to 2 years
•Scar tissue formed with modifications to optimize tensile strength & tissue extensibility

Figure 2-13. Wound healing cascade.

TABLE 2-1
Cells Essential for Integumentary Repair/Wound Healing

Platelets	Responsible for hemostasis through clotting and fibrin release
Mast cells	Release histamine during the inflammatory stage
	Histamine increases vascular permeability; assists arrival of cells needed to fight infection and begin tissue repair
PMNs	Polymorphonuclear leukocytes, white blood cells that transform into neutrophils and mast cells during the inflammatory stage
Neutrophils	White blood cells (PMNs) that fight infection through phagocytosis and release of antimicrobials
Monocytes	Largest type of white blood cell; responsible for innate immunity; help fight known pathogens
Macrophages	Type of white blood cell responsible for phagocytosis of debris and large pathogens/bacteria present at the wound site; help activate stem cells to assist in angiogenesis
Fibroblasts	Most prominent cell during the proliferative phase; release vascular endothelial growth factor and promote angiogenesis; deposit collagen—help form extracellular matrix (ECM)
Myofibroblasts	Derived from fibroblasts; assist in wound contraction during the proliferative phase; manufacture glycoproteins and proteoglycans to help form ECM
Keratinocytes	Generate new epithelial layer after granulation tissue is formed

QUESTIONS

1. What are the differences among the following?
   a. Healing
   b. Wound closure
   c. Regeneration
   d. Scarring
2. How does healing of a superficial wound occur?
3. What stops epithelial cell migration?
4. Why does erythema often occur in a superficial wound?
5. What do we expect in terms of recovery from superficial wounds?
6. What are the potential sources of epidermal cells for healing a partial-thickness wound?
7. Why does blistering or coagulation occur in a partial-thickness wound?
8. What do we expect in terms of the range of recovery from partial-thickness wounds?
9. How do we distinguish a deep partial-thickness wound from a superficial partial-thickness wound?
10. What potential sources of epidermal cells are still available with a full-thickness or deeper wound?
11. How do we distinguish a full-thickness wound from a deep partial-thickness wound?
12. What is the result of a full-thickness wound?

13. What is closure by primary intention, and what mechanisms are commonly used?
14. When is primary intention contraindicated?
15. What is closure by secondary intention?
16. What characteristics of wounds are indications for secondary intention?
17. What is closure by tertiary intention/delayed primary?
18. What characteristics of wounds are indications for tertiary intention?
19. What types of physical therapy interventions help promote wound closure by the following?
    a. Primary intention
    b. Secondary intention
    c. Tertiary intention
20. What are the contributions of the processes of secondary intention?
    a. Hemostasis
    b. Inflammation
    c. Granulation
    d. Re-epithelialization
    e. Contraction
21. What are the timelines for the following?
    a. Hemostasis
    b. Inflammation
    c. Proliferation
    d. Remodeling

22. What are the pros and cons of scab formation?
23. What are the roles and timelines of neutrophils vs macrophages?
24. Why are MMPs needed? What happens if they persist?
25. How can we determine whether the inflammatory response is appropriate?
26. What are the 2 primary cells responsible for creating granulation tissue?
27. What are the contributions of angioblasts?
28. What are the contributions of fibroblasts?
29. What is the appearance of healthy granulation tissue?
30. What is the appearance of healthy re-epithelialization?
31. What cells produce wound contraction?
32. How do Langer's lines relate to wound contraction?
33. Describe the progression of normal full-thickness wound closure.
34. Describe the progression of normal subcutaneous wound closure.
35. What is the importance of having healthy fascia, periosteum, and allografts?
36. What is the ideal environment for the production of granulation tissue?
37. What is the ideal environment for re-epithelialization?
38. What is the appearance of a closed wound?
39. How strong is a closed wound?
40. What is the appearance of a mature scar?
41. How strong is a mature scar?
42. What are the purposes of skin grafts?
43. What are the sources of skin grafts?
44. What happens to the donor site of an autograft?
    a. Full thickness
    b. Split thickness
45. What is the purpose of meshing a split-thickness graft?
46. Why are flaps used instead of skin grafts?
47. What is the difference between free flaps and other flaps?
48. What is the purpose of using skin substitutes, allografts, and xenografts?

BIBLIOGRAPHY

Borena BM, Martens A, Broeckx SY, et al. Regenerative skin wound healing in mammals: state-of-the-art on growth factor and stem sell based treatments. *Cell Physiol Biochem.* 2015;36(1):1-23. doi:10.1159/000374049

Broughton G 2nd, Janis JE, Attinger CE. The basic science of wound healing. *Plast Reconstr Surg.* 2006;117(7 Suppl):12S-34S. doi:10.1097/01.prs.0000225430.42531.c2

Broughton G 2nd, Janis JE, Attinger CE. Wound healing: an overview. *Plast Reconstr Surg.* 2006;117(7 Suppl):1e-S-32e-S.

Bush JA, Ferguson MWJ, Mason T, McGrouther DA. Skin tension or skin compression? Small circular wounds are likely to shrink, not gape. *J Plast Reconstr Aesthet Surg.* 2008;61(5):529-534.

Guo S, DiPietro LA. Factors affecting wound healing. *J Dent Res.* 2010;89(3):219-229. doi:10.1177/0022034509359125

Keylock KT, Vieira VJ, Wallig MA, DiPietro LA, Schrementi M, Woods JA. Exercise accelerates cutaneous wound healing and decreases wound inflammation in aged mice. *Am J Physiol Regul Integr Comp Physiol.* 2008;294(1):R179-R184.

Larouche J, Sheoran S, Maruyama K, Martino MM. Immune regulation of skin wound healing: mechanisms and novel therapeutic targets. *Adv Wound Care (New Rochelle).* 2018;7(7):209-231. doi:10.1089/wound.2017.0761

Liu T, Yang F, Li Z, Yi C, Bai X. A prospective pilot study to evaluate wound outcomes and levels of serum C-reactive protein and interleukin-6 in the wound fluid of patients with trauma-related chronic wounds. *Ostomy Wound Manage.* 2014;60(6):30-37.

Pang C, Ibrahim A, Bulstrode NW, Ferretti P. An overview of the therapeutic potential of regenerative medicine in cutaneous wound healing. *Int Wound J.* 2017;14(3):450-459. doi:10.1111/iwj.12735

Pence BD, DiPietro LA, Woods JA. Exercise speeds cutaneous wound healing in high-fat diet-induced obese mice. *Med Sci Sports Exerc.* 2012;44(10):1846-1854.

Sheehan P, Jones P, Caselli A, Giurini JM, Veves A. Percent change in wound area of diabetic foot ulcers over a 4-week period is a robust predictor of complete healing in a 12-week prospective trial. *Diabetes Care.* 2003;26(6):1879-1882.

Abnormal Healing

OBJECTIVES

- Use the patient history and physical exam to identify factors that may slow healing as modifiable or unavoidable.
- Address modifiable and unavoidable factors in the plan of care.
- Distinguish infection from inflammation.
- Identify and control problems with moisture and edges of wounds.

Normal healing was addressed in the previous chapter. Normal healing of an acute wound follows a predictable trajectory. An abnormal healing trajectory may consist of not showing any signs of healing within 3 days, failure to decrease in size in 4 weeks, or failure to close in 6 to 12 weeks. Commonly, acute wounds are handled without any extraordinary measures and are not referred for specific wound management. Referrals in outpatient settings will come from wounds that are not following the normal trajectory or wounds that are established as chronic wounds that are now being addressed by another provider or through

direct access. The size of the wound is immaterial in terms of the requirement for wound management beyond simple cleaning and dressing changes. The quality of the wound is the issue driving the referral, and restoring the quality of the wound is paramount in re-establishing a normalized wound healing trajectory. Chronicity of a wound, high risk of infection, and poor quality of the wound bed and surrounding skin lead to referrals for wound management. The ability to identify impediments to wound healing guides the selection of treatment interventions.

Irion GL, Gardner JA, Pignataro RM.
Comprehensive Wound Management, Third Edition (pp 31-44).
© 2024 Taylor and Francis Group.

CHRONIC WOUNDS

Epidemiological data reflecting the prevalence and incidence of chronic wounds are unreliable due to the lack of uniform surveillance. Globally, the lifetime prevalence of chronic wounds is estimated to be 1% to 2% of the entire population. Compromised healing places a burden on the individual as well as society. In the United States alone, among Medicare beneficiaries, 8.2 million people had at least one type of wound or related infection. The estimated cost of care ranged from $28.1 billion to $96.8 billion. The economic impact is likely much larger because these data only reflect care rendered to Medicare beneficiaries. Escalating costs are expected to continue based on the aging of the population and increased burden of associated chronic conditions, such as peripheral arterial disease, obesity, sedentary lifestyle, and diabetes. Chronic wounds are generally characterized by failure to achieve wound closure within a 3-month period. Delayed healing is often related to the wound etiology and comorbid conditions that interfere with normal healing processes. Impediments to healing might include circulatory and/or metabolic impairments, as well as physiological changes associated with aging. Long-standing wounds create additional health risks, such as infection, pain, reduced mobility, social isolation, and psychological issues such as depression. Wounds may also interfere with patients' usual roles within their families, occupations, and community.

In normal healing, the hemostatic and vasodilatory responses are expected to be completed within 3 days and then progress into inflammation. Inflammation should then prepare the wounded area for proliferation. Depending on the extent of damage and bioburden, an inflammatory response should subside within 3 weeks. Then, depending on the extent of tissue injury, the proliferative phase should be complete and progress to remodeling in 1 to 6 weeks. Additional factors, such as injury from radiation therapy, may increase the time required for wound closure, but a progression should be evident. The failure to move through the vascular response to inflammation and inflammation into proliferation will be the typical scenarios in abnormal wound healing. If a wound proceeds to proliferation, only very unusual events would prevent the remodeling phase.

Chronic inflammation will have signs of repeated trauma such as hemosiderin staining, ecchymoses, and induration/fibrosis of the surrounding skin that can be readily determined visually and by palpation. Hemosiderin staining is characterized by a dark red to rusty discoloration of the skin, typically consistent with venous insufficiency. In people with darker skin pigments, hemosiderin staining can appear as dark brown to violet. The discoloration occurs when red blood cells break down, leaving behind components of hemoglobin, causing the hemosiderin stain. Within the bed of a chronic wound, one might see persistent, wet, necrotic tissue; a darker red to dusky color of the wound bed; stringy easily bleeding/friable granulation tissue; and maceration of the wound edges and surrounding skin. Biochemical changes characteristic of chronic inflammation are not visible. Due to the inability to remove the cause of inflammation, genetic expression of chemical mediators of inflammation such as matrix metalloproteinases is increased, and the expression of chemicals needed for proliferation is downregulated.[1] In addition to the persistence of inflammation, macrophages fail to change their role from degradation to support of growth. The switch from inflammatory cytokines initially while degradation of necrosis occurs to anti-inflammatory cytokines characteristic of proliferation fails to occur as well as a reduction in tissue inhibitors of matrix metalloproteinases. Table 3-1 depicts the biochemical background of acute compared with chronic wounds. Normal quantities of growth factors apparent in the acute wound are not seen due to increased degradation in the chronic wound as well as stimulation of fibrosis. Photographs of wounds with chronic inflammation are shown in Figure 3-1.

In addition to excessive inflammation, the inability to mount a sufficient inflammatory response to tissue injury can slow healing. Lack of inflammation occurs primarily in ischemic conditions but also with immunosuppression, including cancer chemotherapy, treatment for autoimmune disorders, and prevention of transplant rejection. Wounds demonstrating lack of inflammation have a less red and more pink wound bed and may have desiccated necrotic tissue in the wound.

FACTORS AFFECTING HEALING

The failure to progress to proliferation and closure can usually be attributed to a cascade/vicious cycle of repeated tissue injury, ischemia, and elevated bioburden. As usual in the case of a vicious cycle, intervention must be directed to stop it. Precipitating factors must be identified to adequately determine the most appropriate intervention.

Repeated Tissue Injury

Two common types of wounds are characterized by repeated tissue injury. Pressure injuries result from excessive, unrelieved passive force placed on tissues in cases with a lack of sensation, physical ability, or cognitive status to relieve the pressure. Neuropathic ulcers/diabetic foot ulcers result from repeated, excessive shearing and pressure forces placed on the foot during the gait cycle. A person with altered gait biomechanics, altered foot shape and

TABLE 3-1
Environment of Acute vs Chronic Wound

COMPONENT	ACUTE	CHRONIC
Neutrophils	Arrive early and stop	Continued activity
Macrophages	Transition to noninflammatory	Continued inflammatory
Inflammation	Ramps up and down	Persistent, low level
Cytokines	Low	High
Anti-inflammatory cytokines	High	Low
Growth factor turnover	Slow	High
MMP	Low	High
TIMP	Normal	Low
Granulation tissue	Increasing	Slow, stop and start, poor quality
Fibrosis	Minimal to none	High

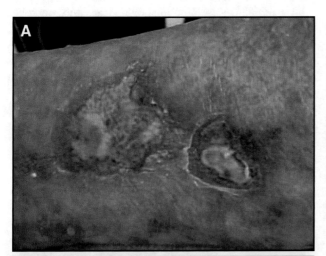

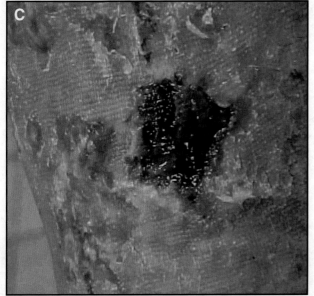

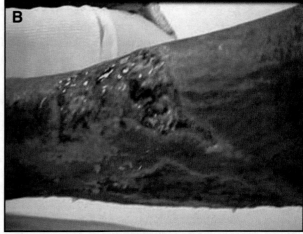

Figure 3-1. Chronic inflammation. (A) Failure to debride necrotic tissue has maintained inflammation. (B) Inflammation caused by untreated venous disease. (C) Close-up of skin affected by venous disease.

compliance, and dry skin and the lack of sensory awareness to address the problem is at high risk of developing such ulcers. Additionally, failure to protect a wound or poor wound management perpetuates the vicious cycle of injury, ischemia, and bioburden. Issues related to poor wound management are addressed under iatrogenic causes later in this chapter. Venous hypertension can also be considered a form of constant tissue injury. Ischemia exacerbates repeated tissue injury due to the inability of the tissue to repair itself, and infection diverts resources away from the tissue subjected to repeated tissue injury.

Ischemia

Ischemia is the lack of adequate blood flow to meet tissue needs, generally manifesting as a lack of oxygen. Chronic wounds tend to have lower transcutaneous oxygen levels (5 to 20 mm Hg) compared with healthy tissue (30 to 50 mm Hg). In addition to circulatory impairments, blood flow may be insufficient due to the need to compensate for other types of hypoxia, the lack of delivery of nutrients or removal of waste due to impairments of other systems, and the loss of regulation of interstitial fluid volume. Demand for oxygen is also greater in healing tissues due to increased cellular metabolism. Three major types of hypoxia are hypoxic, anemic, and ischemic. Hypoxic hypoxia, also known as *hypoxemia*, refers to low partial pressure of oxygen in the blood due to respiratory disorders. Anemia refers to diminished capacity of a volume of blood to carry oxygen. Thus, greater blood flow is required to supply tissues with oxygen in the face of respiratory disease and anemia. A fourth type of hypoxia, histotoxic, refers to poisoning of the enzymes responsible for using oxygen to regenerate adenosine triphosphate, such as cyanide poisoning, and will not be addressed further.

In the case of hypoxic hypoxia, gas exchange in the alveoli is compromised, resulting in a diminished partial pressure of oxygen in the blood. Because of this, oxygen content per volume of blood is reduced, and more blood flow is required by tissues to meet oxygen demands. Moreover, low partial pressure of oxygen in the blood reduces the distance that oxygen can diffuse from capillaries into tissues. One of the benefits of hyperbaric oxygen is that increasing partial pressure of oxygen in the blood can drive oxygen a greater distance from capillaries. Anemic hypoxia, or more simply anemia, decreases the amount of oxygen that a volume of blood can carry for a given partial pressure of oxygen due to either a diminished quantity or quality of hemoglobin in the red blood cell. The net result of either hypoxemia or anemia is a reduced content of oxygen for a volume of blood, thereby requiring more blood flow to deliver the same amount of oxygen.

Anemia and hypoxemia exacerbate the effect of ischemia, and infection diverts resources from ischemic tissues. Ischemia can also alter the wound flora with increased potential for infection, especially with anaerobic bacteria. Moreover, ischemia suppresses the immune response to bacteria. During the inflammatory phase, oxygen supply is crucial for collagen synthesis and proper functioning of polymorphonuclear leukocytes to fight infection. Additionally, insufficient circulation can impair the removal of debris and pathogens, predisposing the individual to chronic infection.

Elevated Bioburden

Elevated bioburden can result in either systemic infection in which cytokine release may impair healing or local infection. Local infection/bioburden, as noted earlier, diverts resources from wound healing. Both circumstances lead to a prolonged inflammatory response as neutrophils and macrophages become unable to clear either microbes or necrotic tissue. Infection lowers the resilience of the tissue, allowing ischemia and trauma to cause further necrosis. Additional immune compromise can result from insufficient responses of the liver and spleen to infection and digestive system disease and other forms of malnutrition.

CAUSES OF SLOW HEALING

Causes of slow healing can be divided into systemic causes affecting the entire body, local causes affecting the immediate environment of the wound, and iatrogenic causes resulting from issues with medical therapy and how the wound is managed.

Systemic Factors

Malnutrition can be caused by several diseases or conditions (Chapter 4). Briefly, the choice of food and the inability to prepare, digest, absorb, or distribute nutrients deprive the wound of needed materials for health or repair. Frequent comorbidities seen in patients with chronic wounds (eg, diabetes mellitus, heart failure, and respiratory disease) have a similar effect as malnutrition. Wounded tissue is deprived of nutrients, including oxygen and glucose, by these diseases. Immunodeficiencies, including diabetes, excessive tobacco, and alcohol intake, and inherited decreased response to specific microbes increase the risks of elevated bioburden discussed earlier. Burn injuries and cancer depress immunity, as do aging, immobility, and frailty, creating a generalized catabolic state.

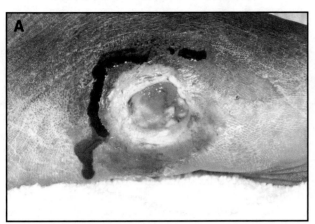 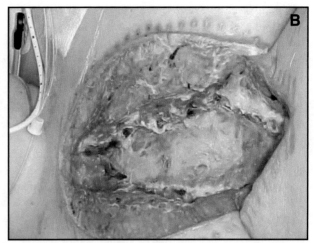

Figure 3-2. Lack of inflammation. (A) Despite the presence of a wound, the patient fails to mount a normal inflammatory response. (B) Lack of inflammation in a wound with desiccated necrotic tissue.

Local Factors

Factors that affect the local environment include peripheral arterial disease, neuropathy, local infection/critical colonization, chronic or suppressed inflammation, and either excessive or inadequate moisture in the wound bed. Additionally, changes in the edges of the wound can slow healing because new epidermal cells in full-thickness and deeper wounds must originate from the edges. Callused, excessively wet or dry edges, and edges that roll over—a condition termed *epibole*—impair the ability to re-epithelialize a wound.

Iatrogenic Factors

Iatrogenic factors include treatments for other disorders or improper wound care. Medical treatments for cancer, as well as radiation, impair the ability to generate the cells necessary for prompt wound healing. Drugs used for autoimmune disorders include corticosteroids, which produce a catabolic effect and impair immunity. Both older antirheumatic drugs and newer biological drugs used for forms of arthritis, psoriasis, and inflammatory bowel disease suppress aspects of the immune system, resulting in slower wound healing. The use of inappropriate dressings or noncompliance with wound care recommendations can also affect the patient's ability to heal.

Addressing Causes of Slow Healing

Optimizing wound healing often requires vigilance to maintain the "Goldilocks" principle of wound management. Constant management of the wound bed is required to ensure that the moisture is just right; the temperature is just right; and the quality of the surrounding skin, edges, and wound bed is just right. Debridement and dressing choices, in addition to the use of adjunctive therapies, must be addressed continuously as characteristics of the wound change. Stated to fit the principle, one must keep checking which bowl of porridge is best.

LACK OF INFLAMMATION

Options to correct lack of inflammation include providing a dressing that maintains moisture and temperature as well as changing the dressing at appropriate intervals. Dressings are covered in detail in Chapter 16. Both the interval of dressing and the type of dressing may need to be altered during an episode of care. Aggressive debridement of necrotic tissue may allow healing of a wound that lacks a sufficient inflammatory response to degrade necrotic tissue by itself. If the wound is supplied by an insufficient arterial system, referral to a vascular surgeon may be necessary to restore adequate blood flow to allow healing. Photographs of wounds showing an insufficient inflammatory response are shown in Figures 3-2A and 3-2B.

INFECTION

Infection is commonly assumed to be the cause of slow healing, and certainly addressing infection is an important step to restore a normal healing trajectory. Thus, infection is an easy target, but it is often incorrect and allows the actual cause of slow healing to be missed. Worse, treating incorrectly is not harmless; it can harm both the wound and the patient. Patients may have severe responses to antibiotics such as anaphylaxis and other immune responses as well as renal and inner ear damage from some antibiotics. The failure to restore healing with one antibiotic may result in treatment with several antibiotics and lead to *Clostridium difficile* infection.

Signs of Infection

Before infection is treated to restore healing, one should assess whether a wound is likely to be infected. The acronym IFEE (Induration, Fever, Erythema, and Edema) may be used in the examination process. *Induration* is a hardening of the surrounding skin that is caused by edema and fibrosis. Fibrosis is associated with chronic wounds. *Fever* represents an increased temperature of the wound. *Erythema* extending well beyond the edges of the wound, whether due to excessive inflammation or to cellulitis (infection spreading through the interstitial space), is also indicative of infection. Lastly, *edema* is also an indicator. Although IFEE itself does not guarantee infection, other pieces of the clinical picture, especially stringy, bleeding, degrading tissue and purulence, assist in the diagnosis. The term *friable* is used to describe the deterioration observed in an infected wound with stringy, bleeding, degrading tissue. Green drainage accompanied by a fruity odor is suggestive of *Pseudomonas aeruginosa* infection.

Although purulence is an indication of infection, someone with limited experience with wounds may confuse drainage of solubilized necrotic tissue with pus. Pus consists of thick, commonly yellow, drainage containing dead bacteria and spent neutrophils. Clearer, thinner yellow drainage is common in wounds that are breaking down necrotic tissue on their own (autolytic debridement). Infection control is covered extensively in Chapter 5. Photographs of wounds with signs of wound infection are shown in Figure 3-3.

Symptoms of systemic infection include loss of appetite, nausea, elevated body temperature, chills, and malaise. Sometimes, the only outward sign of infection and the presence of biofilms is the wound's failure to heal. In addition, the longer a wound takes to close, the greater the chances of infection; chronic wounds are particularly susceptible to infections involving anaerobic bacteria, which tend to thrive in an oxygen-deficient environment. A mixture of aerobic and anaerobic bacteria can increase the risk of bone infection, or osteomyelitis, and bacteremia, particularly in deeper, full-thickness wounds. Bacteremia is when pathogens enter the bloodstream and can travel to other areas, possibly resulting in sepsis. During sepsis, bacteria overwhelm the body's immune system, triggering a massive inflammatory reaction that can threaten organs and body systems. Sepsis can be life-threatening.

SUBCUTANEOUS DEFECTS

Subcutaneous defects include sinuses, tunneling/tracts, undermining, and pocketing. These defects are depicted in Figure 3-4. Mechanical stresses that produce ulcers, such as unrelieved pressure in an immobile person over a bony prominence and shearing forces placed on the plantar surface of an insensate foot, produce undermining. Undermining can be described as a clifflike wound edge that has been "mined under" with an arc of tissue missing below a seemingly intact skin surface corresponding to the direction that stress was placed on the tissue. For example, undermining at the upper edge of a sacral pressure injury is common.

Sinuses represent the remnants of an abscess that has generally been incised, drained, and irrigated before referral for wound management. A pocket is a specific type of undermining that can be missed unless one checks under the wound's edges. Pockets cannot be seen as well as ordinary undermining due to their relative lack of depth. Any time a wound displays characteristics of infection, even if it appears to be closing, one must probe under the edges as demonstrated in Figures 3-4A and 3-4B. Even seemingly intact skin may be covering necrotic tissue and even infection. Discoloration below intact skin that has been subjected to damaging stresses must be monitored for heat, bogginess, and leakage of liquefied tissue.

A sinus tract implies a linear erosion of tissue emanating from the abscess or sinus. Pus is commonly found within tunnels. Probing for tunnels requires some skill and patience so that all of them can be found because more than one tunnel can emanate from an abscess, and they can branch off each other. The same defect may be simply called *tunneling*. Tunnels are produced by bacteria capable of digesting tissue along the path of least resistance between the skin and fascia. When a tight area of fascia is reached, erosion may then occur through the skin and produce a second opening with a tunnel or sinus tract between them. Subcutaneous defects must be debrided thoroughly and packed open to allow them to fill from the bottom/edges and not allow them to close over a void and become infected again in the future. Consequences of abnormal healing are depicted in Figures 3-5A and 3-5B.

WOUND EDGES

Optimal healing requires optimal moisture and clean, healthy, adherent, re-epithelializing edges that allow the filling of the bottom and sides coordinated with an advancing epithelial edge. Problems with edges include moisture, callus, and epibole. Desiccated edges can occur along with desiccation of the wound bed, particularly with peripheral arterial disease. If the injury site does not have enough

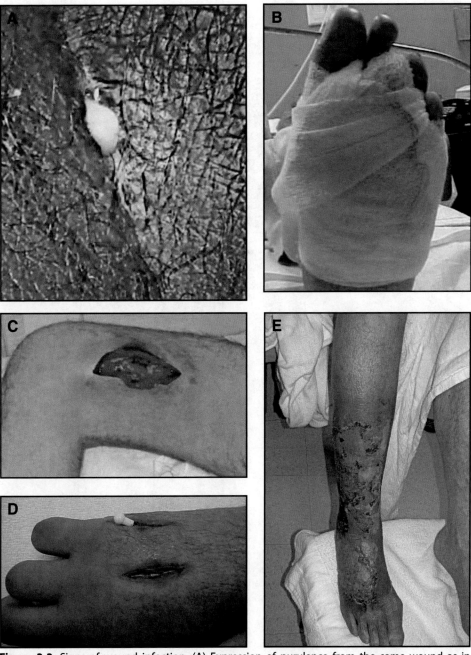

Figure 3-3. Signs of wound infection. (A) Expression of purulence from the same wound as in Figure 3-4D. (B) Drainage from the wound indicative of *Pseudomonas aeruginosa*. Both blood and green drainage can be seen on dressing (serosanginous drainage with greenish tint). (C) Four classic signs of inflammation are demonstrated—induration (hardness), fever (heat), edema, and erythema. Induration and fever are detectable with palpation. The original width of the wound was the width of a scalpel blade used to drain the abscess. The edema has produced the gapping shown here. In addition, the presence of stringy yellow slough in the wound, black eschar in the wound and on some of the edges, and hemosiderin in the surrounding skin are indicative of infection. This wound and similar wounds are generally accompanied by rapid and seemingly sudden swelling and pain, and in some cases, the expression of purulence. In other cases, purulence is not released until surgical incision and drainage. (D) Failure of the wound to close in a timely manner and continued edema in metacarpal fracture fixation. Pin was removed from the fourth metacarpal due to infection. (E) Classic signs of infection of the right leg and foot with induration, fever, erythema, and edema. Tissue necrosis is present without purulence. Crepitus is present with palpation due to the anaerobic bacteria releasing gases contributing to this case of necrotizing fasciitis.

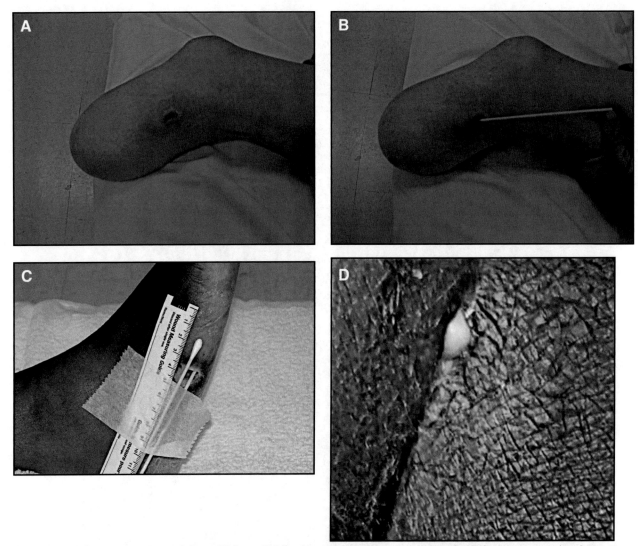

Figure 3-4. Subcutaneous tissue defects. (A) Superficially, this wound appears to be closed. (B) The same wound with a cotton-tipped applicator inserted 1.5 cm into a tunnel caused by infection of a wound produced by prosthesis injury. (C) Undermining of the same wound shown in Figure 3-2A. This wound has 1.8 cm of undermining detected by careful palpation and probing of the wound. (D) Example of a wound with a very small opening (1-mm diameter) with a subcutaneous defect 1 cm around the opening and 4 mm deep. This wound continued to produce purulent drainage until the subcutaneous defect filled with granulation tissue. Special effort was needed to prevent re-epithelialization until the subcutaneous defect was filled to the surface.

moisture, wound desiccation can occur. Lack of moisture also reduces the number of growth factors, and a dry wound bed or scab can create a mechanical impediment to cellular proliferation. Dry wound beds will be slow to granulate, and migration of epidermal cells across the wound edge will also be delayed. Failure to protect the wound with an appropriate dressing to maintain moisture or the use of a dressing that is too absorbent for the amount of drainage may also desiccate a wound. Desiccation may be improved by either debridement to remove old tissue and/or the addition of moisture to the wound. In cases of arterial disease, revascularization surgery may be necessary. Desiccation is shown in Figure 3-6.

Excessive moisture produces maceration of the surrounding skin. This condition can occur in normal skin that is left in water too long. Skin loses color, swells, and may appear fissured. Venous disease produces tremendous amounts of fluid that become difficult to manage and lead to maceration. Excessive drainage from other types of wounds can occur. Maceration is generally the result of inappropriate dressing selection and changing intervals and failure to address the underlying problem such as venous hypertension or failure to debride necrotic tissue and treat infection adequately. In addition to wound exudate, perspiration and/or incontinence can contribute to excessive moisture at the wound site and introduce

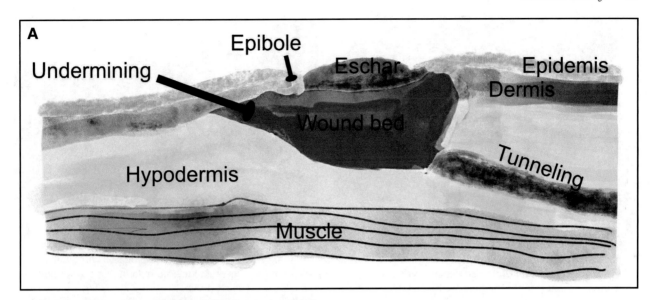

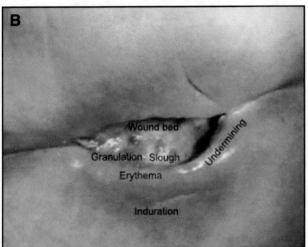

Figure 3-5. Problems with wound healing. (A) Undermining, tunneling, epibole, and eschar are depicted. (B) Undermining, epibole, erythema, and induration are labeled on a photo of a wound.

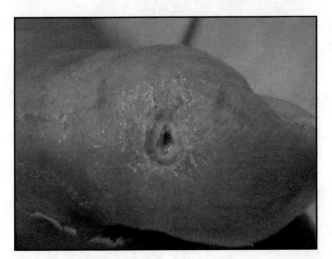

Figure 3-6. Desiccated wound secondary to diabetic neuropathy. Lack of moisture and callus formation produce a dry wound bed that will be slow to heal without intervention.

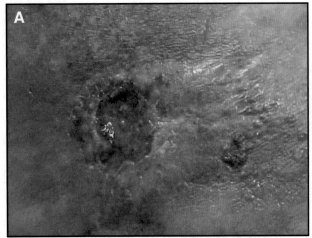

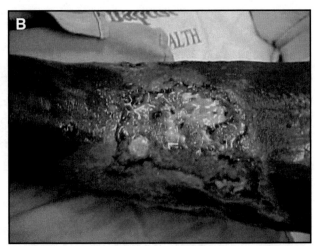

Figure 3-7. Maceration. (A) Excessive drainage allowed to accumulate on skin has injured the surrounding skin with swelling and loss of pigmentation. (B) Untreated venous hypertension leading to copious serous drainage accumulating on the surrounding skin. In this example, heavily pigmented skin has lost its color from moisture damage to skin.

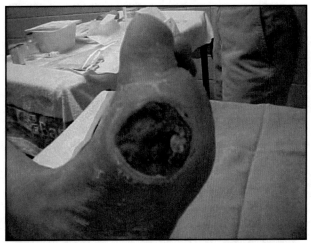

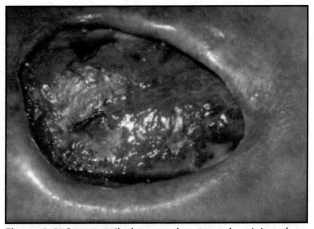

Figure 3-9. Severe epibole secondary to undermining along the entire perimeter of a wound.

Figure 3-8. Wound on same foot as in Figure 3-6 displays a number of issues related to slow healing. Epibole is seen on the lateral wound edge, and thick callus is seen around most of the wound bed, indicative of diminished arterial supply and likely wound infection.

pathogens. Maceration leads to wound chronicity due to impairment of re-epithelialization. Maceration is shown in Figure 3-7.

Callus is a normal response of skin to excessive shearing forces. Callus is very common on the plantar surface of neuropathic feet. Often, the edges of neuropathic ulcers have heavily callused edges (see Figures 3-6 and 3-8). Callus must be debrided and the edges beveled with a scalpel in addition to off-loading the foot. Callus is likely to re-form, and repeated debridement of the edges may be required to provide a clean edge to allow re-epithelialization.

Epibole is the rolling under of a wound's edge. Epibole is a frequent occurrence in chronic wounds (Figure 3-9). When edges roll under as seen in Figure 3-9, contact inhibition of epithelial cells occurs, and migration occurs slowly or not at all. Epibole may be corrected by either burning the edge with a silver nitrate stick (Figure 3-10) or surgical excision of the edge. Debridement of underlying necrotic tissue should also be performed. Epibole can also accompany the formation of hypergranulation as described later in this chapter.

SUBCUTANEOUS HEMATOMA

Injury to tissue beneath intact skin can result in bleeding. Without ulceration of the skin, the clinician cannot determine whether the tissue remains viable. In

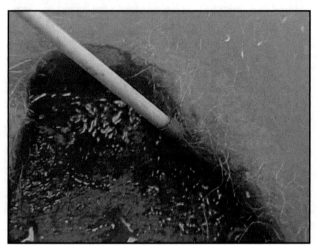

Figure 3-10. Silver nitrate stick, which may be used to burn rolled-over edges to aid epithelialization in a wound slow by epibole.

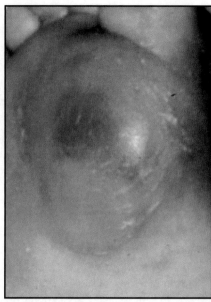

Figure 3-11. Subcutaneous hematoma of the forefoot. The clinician cannot determine the extent of the subcutaneous necrosis (if any) in this case.

such cases, the area of injury must be inspected daily for what is termed *fluctuance*, meaning the wound is unstable. If the area remains firm, has a normal temperature, and does not have any drainage, it should be considered stable and allowed to heal. If the area becomes boggy, warm, and expresses liquefied or semisolid material, the area of injury is considered unstable and needs debridement. An example of a subcutaneous hematoma is shown in Figure 3-11.

HYPERGRANULATION

The formation of granulation tissue that rises above the normal skin contour is termed *hypergranulation*. Under normal circumstances, granulation tissue becomes covered by the advancing epithelial edge as it rises to the level of the wound's edge; however, in some instances, granulation tissue becomes stimulated to grow above the wound's edge. Potential causes of hypergranulation include rough handling of wound edges that damages the advancing epidermal cells, such as whirlpools, wet-to-dry dressings, and maceration. Epibole may also lead to hypergranulation. Other causes need to be considered, particularly if the granulation tissue has a "fungating" appearance with tremendous variation in the height of the granulation, which is suggestive of carcinoma. Carcinoma should be suspected in cases in which the wound has been chronic for many years. An example of hypergranulation is shown in Figure 3-12.

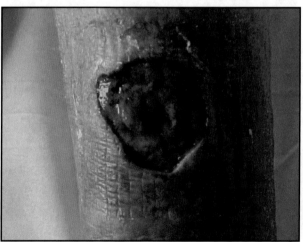

Figure 3-12. Hypergranulation of a leg wound. Note maceration of the surrounding skin and granulation exceeding the height of the surrounding skin. Injury to the surrounding skin or carcinoma are potential causes.

OVER-REPAIR

Forms of over-repair include hypertrophic, keloid, and burn scars. Scar management is addressed specifically in Chapter 17. These scars have the 3 "R's" in common. They are red, raised, and rigid, but vary in other characteristics and are caused by overproduction of different growth factors. Specific solutions for keloid and burn scars are under development. The 3 names are frequently used interchangeably but have specific differences.

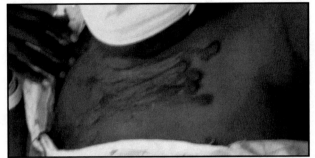

Figure 3-13. Keloid scar on the chest. Note the raised nature and the extension of keloid beyond the original sternotomy incision.

Keloid

This type of scarring has a genetic component and occurs in the skin of people of sub-Saharan African origin and, to a lesser extent, people of Asian, Latin American, or Mediterranean descent. Control of collagen deposition is largely lost, allowing scarring to extend well beyond the edges of the wound, as seen in Figure 3-13. This photograph demonstrates a midsternal vertical incision that has scarred well beyond its origin. These scars are more persistent and tend to regrow and spread with excision when compared to hypertrophic scars.

Hypertrophic Scars

Although hypertrophic scars are red, raised, and rigid, they are limited to the area of the injury, and they tend to regress with time. Most of these become significantly flatter and become white. Examples of both raised and red hypertrophic scars and regressed hypertrophic scars are visible in Figure 3-14.

Burn Scars

Burn scars are frequently referred to as keloids and hypertrophic scars but have characteristics that easily distinguish them. Proliferative scarring from burns occurs after apparent healing and may occur up to 2 years after injury. Grafting and compression garments are commonly used to reduce the extent of this scarring. Bridging of areas of skin such as the mouth, nose, and eyes is common. Bridging causes tension on the surrounding skin, producing both cosmetic and functional problems. Multiple plastic surgery procedures can be used to regain improved cosmesis and more normalized movement.

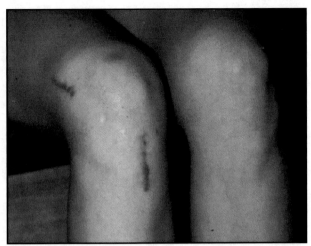

Figure 3-14. Hypertrophic scarring produced by hardware removal several months following anterior cruciate repair. Note the presence of faint white resolved hypertrophic scars from the original surgical procedure.

UNDERHEALING

Many people consider a closed wound to be healed. However, closure alone does not restore normal skin function. The term *healed* should be reserved for skin that has regained its function despite any scarring. Skin should have regained its thickness and contours. In some areas of the body, mechanical stresses may prevent sufficient regeneration of dermis to restore skin function. These areas may require grafting. Superficial tendons and large bony prominences that increase the stress on the skin are particularly susceptible to underhealing. The transition from the distal leg to the foot with the large dorsiflexor tendons is particularly problematic (Figure 3-15).

NEUROPATHY

Normal healing requires innervation. Either nerve injury or nerve disease slows wound healing. Experimentally, the removal of nerve growth factor or its replacement is correlated with wound healing. Slow healing is common in both neuropathic ulcers of the plantar foot and pressure injuries of those with spinal cord injuries. A typical neuropathic ulcer with surrounding callus is shown in Figure 3-16.

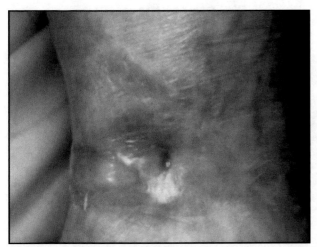

Figure 3-15. Underhealing. Failure of the skin to regain normal thickness before closure secondary to forces of large tendons beneath the skin of the distal leg/dorsum of foot.

HOME REMEDIES

Culturally based home remedies are common. These can be a major source of nonhealing and frustration. Soaking feet and placing neuropathic feet in front of a fireplace or other sources of heat can damage the feet as well as slow healing. Home remedies may include Epsom salt soaks, raw eggs, WD-40 (The WD-40 Company), Windex (SC Johnson), and allowing dogs to lick wounds. Although many animals lick their wounds and heal normally, bacteria in dogs' mouths may be harmful to wounds. Honey, aloe, turmeric, garlic, and peroxide may not be harmful, but the use of home remedies should be discussed with the patient and documented. Substances such as PRID (Hyland's Naturals) and Boil-Ease (Prestige Consumer Healthcare) are available over the counter, and patients may self-treat abscesses with these. These may prove ineffective and lead to a severe abscess requiring substantial intervention.

SUMMARY

Abnormal wound healing has multiple causes that require intervention to prevent chronicity of wounds or to put chronic wounds back onto a trajectory of healing. Chronic wounds have specific biochemical characteristics such as the upregulation of matrix metalloproteinases, which impair healing. A cascade or vicious cycle of 3 factors is commonly responsible for poor healing—repeated tissue injury, ischemia, and bioburden. Breaking this vicious cycle is imperative to restore healing trajectory. Systemic, local, and iatrogenic causes should be identified. To the degree possible, these causes should be eliminated

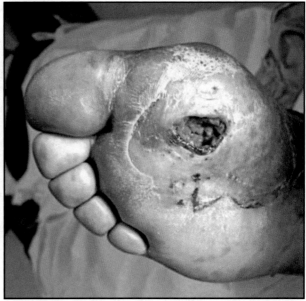

Figure 3-16. Appearance of a neuropathic foot secondary to diabetes. Note the thick callus caused by abnormal shearing forces on the sole during ambulation.

or mitigated. The need for drugs that suppress the immune system complicates healing. Cancer and cancer chemotherapy and radiation therapy may also be problems. Poor wound management practices such as excess trauma and failure to maintain a moist wound bed and prevent excess moisture on the skin must be corrected. Subcutaneous defects can hide infection and must be addressed. Callus and epibole removal were also addressed in the chapter.

QUESTIONS

1. How is abnormal healing defined?
2. Which should be a greater concern—the size of the wound or its healing trajectory?
3. What is responsible for the vast majority of wounds with abnormal healing for which patients are referred to physical therapy?
4. What are the signs of chronic inflammation?
5. What are the signs of lack of inflammation?
6. What are the most common causes of slow wound healing?
7. What are the most common iatrogenic causes of slow wound healing?
8. What are typical causes of chronic inflammation?
9. What is the simplest means of ameliorating chronic inflammation available to a physical therapist?
10. What can be done by a physical therapist to address lack of inflammatory response?

11. What do most laypeople and many health care providers think causes all cases of slow healing?

12. What can happen if we treat all wounds as if they are infected?

13. What are the elements of the IFEE acronym for an infected wound?

14. What additional aspects beyond the IFEE acronym can point to infection?

15. What specifically indicates infection with *Pseudomonas*?

16. What should a physical therapist do when infection is highly suspected but no purulence can be visualized in the wound bed?

17. What type of dressing should be used if a wound is determined to be infected or is highly suspicious?

18. Define the following subcutaneous defects.
    a. Sinus
    b. Sinus tract/tunnel
    c. Undermining
    d. Pocketing

19. Why is exploration of subcutaneous defects important?

20. What is a subcutaneous hematoma, and what does it signify?

21. What must we do in cases of subcutaneous hematomas?

22. How can inadequate moisture be managed?

23. Is callus good or bad? Why? What can be done to correct it?

24. What is epibole? What causes it? Why are we concerned about it?

25. How is epibole managed?

26. What causes hypergranulation? What is the major concern when it is encountered?

27. Distinguish among the 3 types of over-repair.
    a. Keloid
    b. Hypertrophic scars
    c. Burn scars

REFERENCE

1. Mulholland EJ, Dunne N, McCarthy HO. MicroRNA as therapeutic targets for chronic wound healing. *Mol Ther Nucleic Acids.* 2017;8:46-55.

BIBLIOGRAPHY

Alison WE, Phillips LG, Linares HA, et al. The effect of denervation on soft-tissue infection pathophysiology. *Plast Reconstr Surg.* 1992;90(6):1031-1035.

Bayat A, Bock O, Mrowietz U, Ollier WE, Ferguson MW. Genetic susceptibility to keloid disease and hypertrophic scarring: transforming growth factor beta1 common polymorphisms and plasma levels. *Plast Reconstr Surg.* 2003;111(2):535-543.

Bohn GA, Schultz GS, Liden BA, et al. Proactive and early aggressive wound management: a shift in strategy developed by a consensus panel examining the current science, prevention, and management of acute and chronic wounds. *Wounds.* 2017;29(11):S37-S42.

Cohen PR. The lunula. *J Am Acad Dermatol.* 1996;34(6):943-953.

Fleckman P. Anatomy and physiology of the nail. *Dermatol Clin.* 1985;3(3):373-381.

Himel HN. Wound healing: focus on the chronic wound. *Wounds.* 1995;7 Suppl A(5):70A-77A.

Hui P-S, Pu LL, Kucukceleki A, et al. The effect of denervation on leukocyte function in soft tissue infection. *Surgery.* 1999;126(5):933-938.

Ladwig GP, Robson MC, Liu R, Kuhn MA, Muir DF, Schultz GS. Ratios of activated matrix metalloproteinase-9 to tissue inhibitor of matrix metalloproteinase-1 in wound fluids are inversely correlated with healing of pressure ulcers. *Wound Repair Regen.* 2002;10(1):26-37.

Matsuda H, Koyama H, Sato H, et al. Role of nerve growth factor in cutaneous wound healing: accelerating effects in normal and healing-impaired diabetic mice. *J Exp Med.* 1998;187(3):297-306.

McCarthy DJ. Anatomic considerations of the human nail. *Clin Podiatr Med Surg.* 1995;12(2):163-181.

McCauley RL, Chopra V, Li YY, Herndon DN, Robson MC. Altered cytokine production in black patients with keloids. *J Clin Immunol.* 1992;12(4):300-308.

Polo M, Ko F, Busiollo F, Cruise CW, Krizek TJ, Robson MC. Cytokine production in patients with hypertrophic burn scars. *J Burn Care Rehabil.* 1997;18(6):477-482.

Robson MC. Wound infection. A failure of wound healing caused by an imbalance of bacteria. *Surg Clin North Am.* 1997;77(3):637-650.

Robson MC, Mannari, RJ, Smith PD, Payne WG. Maintenance of wound bacterial balance. *Am J Surg.* 1999;178(5):399-402.

Sheehan P, Jones P, Caselli A, Giurini JM, Veves A. Percent change in wound area of diabetic foot ulcers over a 4-week period is a robust predictor of complete healing in a 12-week prospective trial. *Diabetes Care.* 2003;26(6):1879-1882.

Souza BR, Cardoso JF, Amadeu TP, Desmoulière A, Costa AMA. Sympathetic denervation accelerates wound contraction but delays reepithelialization in rats. *Wound Repair Regen.* 2005;13(5):498-505.

Trengove NJ, Stacey MC, MacAuley S, et al. Analysis of the acute and chronic wound environments: the role of proteases and their inhibitors. *Wound Repair Regen.* 1999;7(6):442-452.

Wang J, Jiao H, Stewart TL, Shankowsky HA, Scott PG, Tredget EE. Improvement in postburn hypertrophic scar after treatment with IFN-alpha2b is associated with decreased fibrocytes. *J Interferon Cytokine Res.* 2007;27(11):921-930.

Winter GD, Scales JT. Effect of air drying and dressings on the surface of a wound. *Nature.* 1963;197:91-92.

Yang L, Scott PG, Dodd C, et al. Identification of fibrocytes in postburn hypertrophic scar. *Wound Repair Regen.* 2005;13(4):398-404.

Yang L, Scott PG, Giuffre J, Shankowsky HA, Ghahary A, Tredget EE. Peripheral blood fibrocytes from burn patients: identification and quantification of fibrocytes in adherent cells cultured from peripheral blood mononuclear cells. *Lab Invest.* 2002;82(9):1183-1192.

Nutrition, Medications, and Substance Use

Wound healing requires adequate nutrition. Both calorie expenditure and protein usage are increased substantially. Malnutrition can lead to increased risk of integumentary damage and delayed healing. In addition, nutritional deficiencies increase the risk of wound development, especially pressure injuries. The term *malnutrition* encompasses both overconsumption of calories and underconsumption of food and essential nutrients. Therefore, people who are overweight or obese can be malnourished due to a lack of essential nutrients despite excess caloric intake. In individuals with chronic wounds, caloric demand can increase by 50%, and the need for protein intake can increase by

Irion GL, Gardner JA, Pignataro RM.
Comprehensive Wound Management, Third Edition (pp 45-56).
© 2024 Taylor and Francis Group.

250%. Drainage from wounds contributes to the loss of fluid, protein, and other nutrients. Venous ulcers, burns, and large wounds that cover a significant surface area tend to produce more drainage, and greater surveillance for fluid and nutrient loss is required.

Proper tissue repair relies on the proper supply of calories, protein, vitamins, and minerals. This is especially relevant in wounds that occur in older adults or individuals with existing comorbidities. Malnutrition can occur at any point in the chain of events between selecting foods to distributing nutrients through circulation. Preparation of food, consumption, digestion, and absorption by the digestive system also play a role in nutrition.

NUTRIENTS

Nutrients include protein as a source of amino acids; carbohydrates as a source of energy; fats as a source of energy and fat-soluble vitamins A, D, E, and K; water-soluble vitamins B and C; minerals, including iron, copper, and zinc; and water.

Calories

The amount of energy that can be derived from food has historically been quantified in calories. A calorie is defined as the amount of energy necessary to increase the temperature of 1 g water by 1°C. This unit is quite small relative to what can be obtained from food, so the term *kilocalorie* (kcal) is used instead. Calorie spelled with an uppercase C may be used to indicate a kilocalorie (the amount of energy necessary to raise the temperature of 1 kg of water by 1°C). Therefore, nutritional information is provided as kcal or Calories. Regardless of the source, energy to regenerate adenosine triphosphate from chemical bonds of ingested foods is required. Calories can be obtained from carbohydrates, protein, and fat. Fat is the most efficient source of calories. Other metabolic products such as ketones and lactic acid can be salvaged as sources of calories.

Protein

Protein is a critical building block of structures in the body, particularly of fat-free body mass. Proteins are used to create many of the chemical signals, components of the immune system, and the plasma proteins that allow water to remain within blood vessels despite the hydrostatic pressure within them. Protein can also be used as a source of energy. Consequences of protein deficiency extend through all 4 phases of healing. During hemostasis and the inflammatory phase, protein is required for production and proper functioning of platelets, polymorphonucleocytes, and macrophages. Due to immune dysfunction, rates of infection increase in people who are malnourished. During the proliferative phase, insufficient protein intake can impede the formation of new blood vessels as well as synthesis of collagen and proteoglycans in the extracellular matrix. Wound contraction will also be impaired.

Proteins are chains of amino acids. The amino acids are harvested from proteins by the digestive system, providing cells with the opportunity to assemble necessary proteins from amino acids present in the bloodstream.

Amino acids are composed of nitrogen in addition to carbon, hydrogen, and oxygen atoms. Nitrogen atoms are removed as ammonia (NH_3) to provide molecules that can be used to provide energy through oxidative metabolism. Ammonia is converted to the less toxic urea and excreted from the body primarily in the urine. Severe liver dysfunction as in cirrhosis results in rising ammonia and hepatic encephalopathy.

Protein nutrition is complicated in renal disease. Protein is lost in the urine in nephrotic syndrome, and ingestion may need to be supplemented. Patients with renal insufficiency or renal failure may be required to limit protein consumption as part of their therapy. Consultation with a dietitian may be necessary to ensure that the patient receives sufficient amounts of essential amino acids without further injury to the kidneys.

Dispensable vs Indispensable Amino Acids

Amino acids may be divided into the groups of dispensable and indispensable. Dispensable amino acids can be synthesized from other amino acids. Indispensable amino acids cannot be synthesized by rearranging the molecules of dispensable amino acids. Meat sources contain indispensable amino acids; diets that exclude meat must be adjusted or supplemented to provide all the necessary amino acids.

Of the 20 amino acids, 9 are indispensable and must be obtained from the diet—isoleucine, leucine, lysine, threonine, tryptophan, methionine, histidine, valine, and phenylalanine. If a specific amino acid must not be ingested (eg, phenylalanine in phenylketonuria), other amino acids (in this example, tyrosine) can become nondispensable. Six amino acids are dispensable and can be synthesized from other amino acids—alanine, aspartic acid, glutamic acid, serine, selenocysteine, and asparagine. Newborns cannot synthesize histidine and arginine and must ingest these. In a stressed state, some dispensable amino acids may also become indispensable amino acids. This list includes arginine, cysteine, glutamine, glycine, proline, and tyrosine.

Arginine is a precursor to proline, the major component of collagen. Arginine also increases the release of insulin-like growth factor, is a precursor to nitric oxide synthesis necessary for vascular function, increases nitrogen balance, and acts as a precursor to polyamines. Lack of polyamine production decreases cell migration, which is necessary for wound repair.

Glutamine is the most abundant amino acid. It is a source of energy for rapidly proliferating cells, including fibroblasts, lymphocytes, epithelial cells, and macrophages. Serum glutamine concentration is decreased following sepsis, trauma, major surgery, and burns. Patients in a stressed state (eg, major burns) recover better with diets higher in glutamine. Glutamine supplementation increases wound-breaking strength, improves nitrogen balance, and increases immune response.

Micronutrients

Micronutrients consist of components other than protein and calories. These include vitamins, minerals, and water.

Vitamins

Vitamins were originally described as the presumed fat-soluble factor (vitamin A) and water-soluble factor (vitamin B) necessary for health. Following the discovery of different components of water-soluble vitamins, the terminology was altered. The B vitamins may be termed by a subscript following the B or given their own names. For example, vitamin B12 is also termed *cyanocobalamin*. The discovery of more vitamins follows the same lettering from C, D, E, and then skipping to vitamin K. Historically, all of the letters from A to K have been used, but F, G, H, I, and J have been abandoned because of the discovery of the actual nature of the substance so named. K also stands for coagulation, spelled in German with a K. In addition to B, water-soluble vitamins also include C. Excessive quantities of water-soluble vitamins are excreted in the urine and cannot be stored for long periods of time. In contrast, fat-soluble vitamins can be stored in fatty tissue and released as their concentration in the blood falls. However, excessive consumption of fat-soluble vitamins can produce toxicity. The fat-soluble vitamins are A, D, E, and K. These vitamins can be supplemented specifically for individuals who digest fat poorly, particularly many people with cystic fibrosis.

Vitamin A (retinol) is stored in the liver and obtained in the diet as beta-carotene from plants and retinol esters from animals. Retinoic acid binds to receptors to affect gene expression. Vitamin A acts as a morphogen to regulate epidermal development and is harmful to unborn babies. Pregnant women must avoid exposure to the high doses of vitamin A and its analogs (eg, Retin-A [tretinoin], which is used for treating skin disorders such as acne). Retinol suppresses the maturation of keratinocytes. Excess retinol causes thinning and drying of the skin. Deficiency of vitamin A causes hyperkeratosis and metaplasia of glands of the epidermis. Retinol and chemicals of similar structure are used therapeutically to treat acne through the suppression of oil production by sebaceous glands. Deficiency of vitamin A has been shown to delay wound healing as well as increase susceptibility to infection, presumably because of a requirement of vitamin A by the immune system.

The B vitamins are necessary for energy metabolism and synthesis of DNA. Deficiency of niacin produces pellagra, a condition characterized by hyperkeratotic eruptions of sun-exposed skin and damage to other organs. Deficiency of vitamin B6 (pyridoxine) or essential fatty acids causes scaling. Both riboflavin and thiamine are required for collagen synthesis, but no links have been shown between deficiencies of these vitamins and impairment of wound healing.

Vitamin C is essential for collagen development. Vitamin C deficiency (scurvy) causes diminished tensile strength of connective tissues and slows wound healing but does not prevent wound healing. Vitamin C deficiency can also lead to higher infection risk. Vitamin C deficiency in Western civilization is rare, and supratherapeutic doses of vitamin C have not been demonstrated to enhance healing of either acute or chronic wounds.

Vitamin D is related to calcium metabolism. Sunlight reaching the skin converts vitamin D into its more active form. Vitamin D deficiency may result from a lack of exposure to sunlight, including the use of high SPF sunscreen. Those with more darkly pigmented skin are also at risk of vitamin D deficiency.

Vitamin E has been attributed with antioxidant properties and is thought to have a protective effect on the skin by reducing sun and other types of damage. It is frequently used as an additive to over-the-counter skin products with a suggestion of improved skin integrity. However, vitamin E has also been shown to decrease wound healing, possibly by interference with collagen synthesis, and vitamin E has not been demonstrated to be important to wound repair.

Vitamin K is responsible for producing the active form of several of the coagulation factors in the blood (II [prothrombin], VII, IX, X, protein C, protein S, and protein Z). Vitamin K deficiency increases coagulation time and leads to excessive bleeding with trauma. Warfarin (Coumadin) is a drug used to interfere with the recycling of vitamin K, leading to its depletion, which, in turn, decreases the risk of excessive coagulation therapeutically. This drug is used by individuals at risk for myocardial infarction and stroke and in other conditions that may stimulate coagulation, such as heart valve replacement and atrial fibrillation. Patients using warfarin or other anticoagulation medications may bleed excessively during debridement. History taking should include questions about the patient's use of anticoagulants, vitamin K deficiency, or other conditions leading to excessive bleeding.

Minerals

Several minerals are required in low concentrations for healthy skin. Although copper, manganese, and iron appear to be necessary for tissue regeneration, they have not been directly related to impaired wound healing other than the role of iron as a component of hemoglobin. Selenium is part of an enzyme system (glutathione) that reduces oxidative damage by free radicals. Zinc is a part of many metalloenzyme systems, notably DNA and RNA polymerase. Zinc deficiency leads to dermatitis and slow healing. However, supplemental zinc has not been shown to aid wound healing in those without demonstrable zinc deficiency, and excessive zinc may slow healing as well as have deleterious effects on immune function and copper metabolism. Unna's boots applied directly over venous insufficiency ulcers have been demonstrated to slow healing, which may be attributable to the zinc oxide in the material. Copper is also essential to the production of collagen, as well as elastin and melanin. Copper is present in the enzymes that produce cross-linking of collagen, elastin, and keratin. Supplementation of selenium, copper, and zinc may be critical for patients with major burns due to their roles in antioxidant mechanisms.

Water

Although not often considered as a nutrient, adequate hydration is necessary for normal wound healing. Water represents a large fraction of body weight dependent on lean body mass. Water represents about two-thirds of body mass. This number is higher in lean individuals and may approach 75%. In individuals with obesity, the percentage of body weight may be substantially lower than 60%. A general guideline for water consumption is 30 mL water/day/kg body weight. In general, water ingestion is encouraged because excess water can be excreted in the urine without harm to the patient, but dehydration can lead to significant electrolyte disturbances. Although excessive water consumption is difficult to achieve, extreme consumption can lead to water intoxication with cerebral swelling as the most serious consequence. Because intact skin acts as a barrier for water loss, large open wounds, especially burns, can require greater consumption of water. Heavily draining wounds, vomiting, diarrhea, and the use of specialty beds that cause evaporation of fluid from wounds will require increased water consumption. However, all patients should not be encouraged to drink water; those with congestive heart failure, pulmonary edema, or other disease characterized by water retention may have input/output of fluid monitored carefully. In such cases, any water intake restrictions should be communicated clearly to all health care providers and visitors to ensure adherence.

MALNUTRITION

A person not meeting dietary needs may be classified as at risk or malnourished. Nutritional screening is used to determine whether a given person is at risk for malnutrition; further testing is needed to determine if malnutrition exists and what interventions are required.

Dietary needs may be divided into 3 basic categories: energy quantified by the number of calories consumed; protein to regenerate necessary enzymes and other structures; and cofactors necessary for metabolism, notably vitamins and trace minerals. Nutrition of the skin requires a healthy vascular supply through the dermis, which provides a rich supply to the papillary dermis. Blood flow through the papillary dermis provides nourishment to the metabolically active stratum basale where new cells of the epidermis are generated. Diffusion of nutrients occurs from the papillary dermis to stratum basale to support its metabolic needs. In addition, these plexuses are involved in thermoregulation. However, the blood supply to the relatively acellular reticular dermis is rather low due to its low metabolic rate.

Nutrition is frequently poor in ill or injured individuals with an estimated 30% to 55% rate of malnutrition in the hospital patient population. Impaired nutritional intake, lower dietary protein intake, impaired ability to feed oneself, and recent weight loss have been shown to be independent predictors of pressure injury development. Moreover, these factors are likely to occur in combination in many individuals. Even individuals receiving nutritional support may develop hospital-induced malnutrition. Patients on total parenteral nutrition for extended periods will have difficulty receiving nutrients that cannot be adequately supplied through this means. Malnutrition is a major risk factor for pressure injuries and delayed wound healing.

In adults who have access to adequate food, hypoalbuminemia is generally a result of an acute insult such as surgery or illness. Protein malnutrition may have a rapid onset and may be difficult to detect. Any given individual may experience several deficiencies in the diet, whether due to a lack of food in general, disease of the digestive system, or a lack of nutrients.

According to epidemiological data, approximately 16% of community-dwelling seniors living in the United States may experience malnutrition. This prevalence is even higher among older adults who are hospitalized (35% to 65%) or residing in institutions (30% to 60%). As people age, reasons for malnutrition include sensory decline, leading to decreased taste and appetite, and physical impairments

TABLE 4-1
Risk Factors for Malnutrition

- Report of poor intake by patient, family, or caregivers
- Weight less than 80% of ideal body weight (see calculation in Ideal Body Weight section)
- Loss of greater than 10% of usual body weight within last 6 months
- Alcohol use disorder
- Advanced age
- Impaired cognitive status
- Malabsorption syndromes
- Renal failure or nephrotic syndrome
- Heavily draining wounds
- Multiple trauma
- Edema not attributable to congestive heart failure or venous disease

TABLE 4-2
Types of Malnutrition Proposed by the Academy of Nutrition and Dietetics/American Society for Parenteral and Enteral Nutrition

TYPE	CHARACTERISTICS
Malnutrition in the context of social or environmental circumstances (starvation-related malnutrition)	Pure starvation due to financial or social reasons or anorexia nervosa
Malnutrition in the context of chronic illness	Organ failure, sarcopenic obesity (osteoarthritis), cachexia (cancer, rheumatoid arthritis)
Malnutrition in the context of acute illness or injury	Major infection, burns, trauma, brain injury
Data source: White et al, 2012.	

such as edentulism (tooth loss), xerostomia (dry mouth), trouble chewing, and dysphagia (difficulty swallowing). Older adults with mobility issues may also have difficulty with food shopping and meal preparation. Retirement or unintentional unemployment sometimes results in limited income, and a lack of financial resources may reduce access to healthy foods. Other issues to consider include depression and social isolation, which can decrease motivation for self-care.

METHODS USED TO ASSESS NUTRITION

Nutritional status has historically been assessed by a combination of anthropometric and biochemical data. Within the past several years, the accuracy of this assessment has come into question, and newer means of evaluation have been proposed. The Academy of Nutrition and Dietetics/American Society for Parenteral and Enteral Nutrition have proposed new criteria for a diagnosis of malnutrition. Several patient characteristics are known risk factors for undernutrition or malnutrition. These factors are listed in Table 4-1.

Three types of malnutrition have been described as shown in Table 4-2. Pure chronic starvation without inflammation occurs in anorexia. A second type is chronic disease that imposes sustained inflammation of a mild to moderate degree. The second type occurs with disease characterized by catabolic cytokines. Such diseases include

rheumatoid arthritis, osteoarthritis, and some types of cancer that produce cachexia. In rheumatoid arthritis and several types of cancer, both sarcopenia (loss of lean body mass) and decreased body weight occur. Osteoarthritis is an example of sarcopenic obesity in which loss of muscle mass is accompanied by increased storage of fat. The third type of malnutrition is acute disease or injury with marked inflammatory response. This is seen with major infection, burns, and trauma. Although the third type may frequently be the issue in wound management, many patients with wounds may be in the second category and, sometimes, the first. Managing a large pressure injury with systemic infection in a patient already in a catabolic state will require significant nutritional support.

The newest means of assessing nutrition is based on the elements of Table 4-1, which specifically include 6 clinical characteristics: energy intake, weight loss, body fat, muscle mass, fluid accumulation, and grip strength. Energy intake relative to need (body size, activity level, illness/trauma) is discussed specifically later in this chapter. Criteria proposed for malnutrition based on energy intake are shown in Table 4-3.

Weight loss criteria are also provided in Table 4-3. Note that the percentage weight loss criteria are given for several different time frames in weeks and months. Generally, we are interested in involuntary weight loss. However, deliberate weight loss can also be a risk for malnutrition depending on how it was achieved. No specific measurement is given for either body fat or muscle mass. Judgment of what is considered normal distribution of fat is utilized. Loss of periorbital fat, triceps, and ribs are specifically mentioned

TABLE 4-3

Components of Assessment for Malnutrition Proposed by the Academy of Nutrition and Dietetics/ American Society for Parenteral and Enteral Nutrition

CHARACTERISTIC	ACUTE ILLNESS/ INJURY MODERATE	ACUTE ILLNESS/ INJURY SEVERE	CHRONIC ILLNESS MODERATE	CHRONIC ILLNESS SEVERE	STARVATION MODERATE	STARVATION SEVERE
Energy intake	<75% for >7 days	≤50% for ≥5 days	<75% for ≥1 month	<75% for ≥1 month	<75% for ≥3 months	≤50% for ≥1 month
Weight loss	1% to 2% in 1 week; 5% in 1 month; 7.5% in 3 months	>2% in 1 week; >5% in 1 month; >7.5% in 3 months	5% in 1 month; 7.5% in 3 months; 10% in 6 months; 20% in 1 year	>5% in 1 month; 7.5% in 3 months; >10% in 6 months; >20% in 1 year	5% in 1 month; 7.5% in 3 months; 10% in 6 months; 20% in 1 year	>5% in 1 month; >7.5% in 3 months; >10% in 6 months; >20% in 1 year
Loss of body fat	Orbital, triceps, ribs	Orbital, triceps, ribs	Orbital, triceps, ribs	Orbital, triceps, ribs	Orbital, triceps, ribs	Orbital, triceps, ribs
Loss of muscle mass	Wasting at temples, clavicles, guttering of hands, etc	Wasting at temples, clavicles, guttering of hands, etc	Wasting at temples, clavicles, guttering of hands, etc	Wasting at temples, clavicles, guttering of hands, etc	Wasting at temples, clavicles, guttering of hands, etc	Wasting at temples, clavicles, guttering of hands, etc
Fluid accumulation	Generalized or dependent Extremities, scrotal/vulvar, ascites	Generalized or dependent Extremities, scrotal/vulvar, ascites	Generalized or dependent Extremities, scrotal/vulvar, ascites	Generalized or dependent Extremities, scrotal/vulvar, ascites	Generalized or dependent Extremities, scrotal/vulvar, ascites	Generalized or dependent Extremities, scrotal/vulvar, ascites
Reduced grip strength	N/A	Measurably reduced	N/A	Measurably reduced	N/A	Measurably reduced

Data source: White et al, 2012.

in the guideline because these produce obvious changes in the patient's appearance. Similarly, wasting of the temporal muscles, muscles attached to the clavicle, scapula, and knee, cause bony prominences to become so prominent that muscle loss becomes obvious by sight.

Fluid accumulation due to loss of albumin results in dependent edema. Based on whether the person is ambulatory or bedbound, the distribution of edema will vary. Dependent edema for a bedbound person maintained in a Fowler's position in a hospital bed may manifest as scrotal or vulvar edema. Ascites, fluid accumulation in the abdomen, may also occur, particularly with liver disease. Clinicians must also be aware that fluid accumulation can mask loss of body mass. Concurrent muscle wasting, body fat loss, and fluid accumulation may allow body mass changes to go un-noticed if only routine weight checks are used to assess nutritional status.

No specific guidelines are given for hand grip other than reductions when compared with published norms. Hand grip does correlate with loss of muscle mass, but one needs to be aware of the context of a given individual's grip strength. A relatively slender person or a person who was rather robust prior to the assessment may skew results of this single test, and, therefore, the larger picture of nutritional status needs to be taken as a whole. The Academy of Nutrition and Dietetics/American Society for Parenteral and Enteral Nutrition guidelines require at least 2 indicators for a diagnosis of malnutrition.

Anthropometric

Anthropometric assessment methods typically use body measurements such as height and weight. Based on normative data, one estimates whether a patient's mass is sufficient for height. Ideal body weight (IBW) is commonly used as a basis for comparison. A patient's body weight is compared with normative data to determine the percentage of IBW. A person who is malnourished would likely have a body weight less than 100% IBW, although an overweight person can be malnourished and may be in a catabolic state despite adequate caloric intake.

Ideal Body Weight

IBW may be computed in several ways. A commonly used set of equations is as follows. For men, the equation is 106 pounds for the first 5 ft plus 6 pounds for each additional inch above 5 ft of height (106# for 5' + 6# per inch). For women, the equation is 100 pounds for the first 5 ft and 5 pounds for each additional inch (100# for 5' + 5# per inch). Adjustments are made for body types by subtracting 10% for a small frame and adding 10% for a large frame.

For example, a 6'1" man has an IBW of $106 + 6 \times 13 = 184$ pounds, and a 5'3" woman has an IBW of $100 + 5 \times 3 = 115$ pounds. Computing percent of IBW provides an index of risk of either malnutrition or overnutrition. Overnutrition is also an important risk factor due to the relationships among obesity, type 2 diabetes mellitus, and atherosclerosis. Percent IBW is computed by dividing current body weight (CBW) by IBW as follows: percent IBW = CBW/IBW × 100. Normal is between 90% and 110% IBW. A value of 80% to 90% is underweight, and a value of 79% or less is considered malnutrition.

Other anthropometric considerations are body mass index (BMI), waist circumference, and hip-to-weight ratio. BMI is computed as mass in kilograms divided by the square of height in meters (BMI = mass [kg]/height [m^2]). To convert from pounds and inches, multiply the number of pounds by 703 and divide by the square of height in inches ($[180 \times 703/742] = 23$). A value between 19 and 25 for BMI is considered healthy. A value of 25 to 30 is considered overweight; 30 to 40 is considered obese. Greater than 40 is considered clinically significantly obese (morbid obesity). Guidelines for bariatric surgery restrict gastric bypass to those with a BMI greater than 50 or greater than 40 if the body weight is associated with significant morbidity such as refractory hypertension. A value of BMI less than 19 is considered underweight. Although BMI may give misleading results for people with large muscle mass, it is a quick and reliable means for the general population. A waist circumference greater than 40 inches for men and 35 inches for women is indicative of metabolic syndrome and a risk factor for cardiovascular disease. Greater than 43.5 inches for women and greater than 47 inches for men is very high risk. The waist-to-hip ratio is an indicator of where fat is deposited in the body. A high waist-to-hip ratio (greater than 0.95 for men and greater than 0.86 for women) represents the apple shape of metabolic syndrome and greater risk of cardiovascular disease than a low ratio, which is represented as the pear shape. Although weight loss for obese patients is generally encouraged to improve overall health, weight loss while a person has a significant wound is discouraged. Gastric bypass surgery is discussed further in Chapter 19.

Biochemical

Several lab tests have historically been used to assess whether nutritional needs are being met adequately. Three tests are related directly to protein: albumin, transthyretin/prealbumin, and nitrogen balance. Other tests used to assess nutrition include blood work such as hematocrit, hemoglobin concentration, and white blood cell count.

Nitrogen Balance

Under normal circumstances, the amount of nitrogen entering the body in the form of protein is equal to the amount of nitrogen excreted in the urine as urea. A positive nitrogen balance indicates accumulation of nitrogenous compounds in the body as would occur with an increase in fat-free mass. If a person does not take in enough calories, proteins already in the body in addition to those taken in from the diet can be broken into amino acids and deaminated for regenerating adenosine triphosphate, which results in greater excretion of nitrogen through the urine than nitrogen intake.

Like a bank account, a positive nitrogen balance means that the patient is accumulating nitrogen in the form of protein such as building or rebuilding muscle mass. When a patient must consume protein to meet energy needs, more nitrogen goes out in the urine than comes into the body by ingestion of protein, and the patient has a negative nitrogen balance. Ideally, protein intake during wound healing should result in a positive nitrogen balance.

Albumin and Transthyretin (Formerly Known as Prealbumin)

Albumin has long been considered the gold standard for assessing protein malnutrition. A normal value of albumin is 3.5 to 5.0 g/dL. Moderate depletion is a value between 3.2 and 3.5 g/dL, and severe hypoalbuminemia is defined as a value less than 2.8 g/dL. Recent evidence suggests that albumin is a poor predictor of nutritional status. Instead, depletion of albumin, transthyretin, and other proteins produced by the liver indicates systemic inflammation. During systemic inflammation, chemical mediators of inflammation restrict the production of protein by the liver. Serum albumin is positively correlated with hemoglobin and red blood cell count and negatively associated with C-reactive protein (CRP), an indicator of systemic inflammation, but not correlated with caloric intake. Greater albumin does serve as a predictor of faster healing rates. A rise in albumin and a fall in CRP occur as the status of the wound improves during treatment. A fall in albumin and a rise in CRP occur in deteriorating wounds. A decrease in albumin can still be used to address nutritional needs. Falling albumin is indicative of an inflammatory, catabolic state and suggests a need for nutritional supplementation. However, treating the underlying inflammation is needed to restore proteins produced by the liver.

Evaluation of albumin is particularly important for the person with a chronic wound due to the potential for albumin and other plasma proteins to be lost in wound exudate. The problem with low albumin is compounded by its effect on fluid distribution. Albumin loss leads to edema, which, in turn, causes decreased diffusion of nutrients through the interstitial space. However, in acute protein malnutrition, albumin may not have fallen yet and would not be indicative of an inadequate intake. The half-life of albumin is 20 days, and large stores of albumin are available; thus, malnutrition may be well along before a fall in albumin can be measured.

For an indicator of short-term protein intake, transthyretin can be measured. This protein transports thyroxin and retinol in the blood. The name *prealbumin* had previously been used, but this word was misleading because it has nothing to do with albumin. The name prealbumin has more historical significance, having been given because it showed up before albumin on gel electrophoresis. Mild, moderate, and severe depletion are defined as less than 17 g/dL, less than 12 g/dL, and less than 7 g/dL of transthyretin, respectively. In acute protein malnutrition, a decline in transthyretin will occur prior to a decline in albumin because of the shorter half-life. Hemoglobin, hematocrit, and blood cell counts may also be used as indicators of nutritional status.

COMPUTING NUTRITIONAL REQUIREMENTS

Both total calories and protein intake need to be computed to meet an individual's nutritional needs. If possible, a thorough assessment by a licensed clinical dietitian should be performed. A simple guideline is to provide 30 to 35 calories/kg to maintain CBW and 40 to 45 calories/kg to promote anabolism. For a more precise determination of the nutritional requirements, the Harris-Benedict equation is frequently used. The equation for basal energy expenditure (BEE) for men is as follows: BEE (kcal) = 66 + (13.7 × mass in kg) + (5 × height in cm) − (6.8 × age in years). For women, the equation is BEE (kcal) = 665 + (9.6 × mass in kg) + (1.8 × height in kg) − (4.7 × age in years). To calculate total daily expenditure, one must take into account the patient's activity (activity factor) and severity of injury (injury factor). The BEE is adjusted to derive total daily expenditure as BEE × AF × IF, where AF is activity factor, which ranges from 1.2 for bed rest to 2.0 for an extremely active person, and IF is injury factor, which ranges from 1.2 for minor surgery to 2.5 for extreme thermal injury. Using the conversions of 2.54 cm/inch and 2.2 pounds/kg, the following examples are given: (1) 160-pound male, 73 inches tall, 40 years old, low activity: 30 to 35 kcal/kg × 160 pounds/2.2 kg/pounds = 2182-2545 kcal/day or using the Harris Benedict formula = (66 + 996.4 + 927.1 − 272) × 1.5 (AF) = 2576 kcal/day and (2) 120-pound female, 63 inches tall, 38 years old, extremely active: 30 to 35 kcal/kg × 120 pounds/2.2 kg/pounds = 1636 to 1909 kcal/day or using the Harris Benedict formula = (665 + 523.6 + 288.0 − 178.6) × 2 (AF) = 2596 kcal/day.

Required protein intake is computed as 0.8 to 2.0 g protein/kg. The effectiveness of this intake can be monitored by calculating nitrogen balance.

Assessing the diet is not just an issue for undernourished individuals. Anyone with an injury will have increased nutritional needs. Although weight reduction is an important long-term goal to maintain overall health, the person with a wound should not be placed on a weight reduction diet until they are no longer at risk for developing a wound or having slow wound healing. Therefore, adjusting the diet to promote weight loss should not be a goal during wound healing. An individual with obesity needs a positive nitrogen balance, sufficient calories, and trace elements to promote wound healing. Tools available for nutritional screening include the Malnutrition Universal Screening Tool (MUST) (https://www.bapen.org.uk/pdfs/must/must_full.pdf) for community use; the Nutrition Risk Screening (NRS-2002) (https://www.mdcalc.com/nutrition-risk-screening-2002-nrs-2002) for hospital use; the Nestle Mini Nutritional Assessment (MNA; https://www.mna-elderly.com/sites/default/files/2021-10/mna-mini-english.pdf) for community, especially for older adults; and the Nestle Self-MNA (https://www.mna-elderly.com/sites/default/files/2021-10/Self-MNA-English-Imperial.pdf), which can be performed by either a patient or caregiver.

INTERVENTIONS

Several options are available depending on calorie and protein needs, the degree of malnutrition, and any comorbidities that will influence the processing of nutrients. A licensed dietitian should be the first resource for assessment and recommendations for nutritional interventions. The most conservative approach is addressing the selection and preparation of food. Although this seems simple on the surface, culture, personal preference, financial, and other resources can impact the ability to obtain, store, and prepare food. Options for patients with food insecurity include 211, which can be accessed by phone at 2-1-1 or on the internet by www.211.org. Patients can also be referred to a local food bank. A website for locating food banks is www.feedingamerica.org/find-your-local-foodbank.

A second line is the provision of supplements. Supplements may be provided in a hospital setting or can be purchased by the patient. Supplements do not always need to be name brand preparations but can include the selection of more nutrient-dense food.

In some cases, supplements are not enough, or digestive system issues require feedings either into the gastrointestinal system (enteral nutrition) or directly into the bloodstream (parenteral nutrition).

DIETARY INTERVENTIONS

Depending on several factors, notably the ability to ingest adequate calories and protein, the diet may need to be manipulated by the clinician. The least invasive dietary intervention sufficient for some patients is to increase food intake by increasing intake of nutrient-dense foods such as cheese, nuts, peanut butter, eggs, ice cream, and milkshakes. A further step is the use of commercial supplements such as Sustacal (Mead Johnson) and Ensure (Ross Products). More extreme and invasive interventions include enteral and parenteral feeding.

Formulations of specific ingredients thought to aid wound healing have been developed. A formulation of L-arginine, vitamins, sugar, protein, and minerals is available as Arginaid Extra (Nestle Health Science). Branched-chain amino acid formulations containing leucine, isoleucine, and valine, which are all indispensable amino acids, have been used for burn injuries, trauma, and sepsis. Beta-hydroxy beta-methylbutyrate, denoted as HMB, is a product of leucine that has been used to promote wound healing, especially burn injuries.

Feedings

Enteral feeding refers to the delivery of nutrients artificially to the gastrointestinal tract, usually utilizing a pump and a line placed into the gastrointestinal tract. For short-term feeding, a tube may be placed through the nose into the stomach (nasogastric tube). Long-term feeding requires a surgically placed tube either through the skin into the stomach or into the jejunum. A line placed into the stomach is called a PEG (percutaneous endoscopic gastrostomy) tube. A J tube is surgically placed into the jejunum to provide nutrients for the individual who cannot ingest a sufficient diet. The placement of the feeding tube will be determined by several factors, including the patient's tolerance. For example, a tube may be placed into the duodenum if the patient does not tolerate a nasogastric tube.

The introduction of nutrients directly to the bloodstream, bypassing the gastrointestinal tract, is termed *parenteral feeding*. Because nutrients are dissolved in water, the provision of adequate nutrition would cause fluid overload if the fluid were isotonic. Nutrients must be concentrated in parenteral feeding, resulting in hypertonic fluid that would damage a peripheral vein. For this reason, parenteral feeding must be delivered by a central venous line directly into the right atrium where the fluid can be immediately diluted by the entire cardiac output. Another problem with parenteral feeding is providing fat-soluble nutrients and lipids. In the short term, the provision of water-soluble nutrients can be adequate because of storage of fat and fat-soluble vitamins in adipose tissue. If needed, a short-term solution for feeding using a 5% dextrose (D5W) solution can be used. Over a longer time, lipids and fat-soluble vitamins will also need to be provided.

Medications

In general, pharmaceuticals provide a therapeutic effect by altering a physiologic process. In some cases, the effect is mostly limited to abnormal cells and bacteria, but many times, adverse effects on healthy cells and those necessary for wound healing must be weighed against their benefits. There are many pharmacological agents that can delay wound and tissue repair.

Anti-Inflammatories

Many disorders are treated with anti-inflammatory agents. These can range from baby aspirin used to prevent a second myocardial infarction to drugs that largely eliminate a component of the immune system such as tumor necrosis factor to treat an autoimmune disease like rheumatoid arthritis, psoriasis, ulcerative colitis, or Crohn's disease. Patients who have received an organ transplant may be taking multiple drugs that suppress the immune system. Reducing inflammation interferes with destroying bacteria and clearing debris from a wounded area and makes an individual more susceptible to infection.

Common anti-inflammatory drugs include aspirin and nonsteroidal anti-inflammatory medications. Nonsteroidal anti-inflammatory drugs frequently prescribed for pain relief include ibuprofen, naproxen, and selective cyclooxygenase-2 inhibitors (eg, celecoxib [Celebrex]). Cyclooxygenase-2 inhibitors work by suppressing prostaglandin E2 synthesis. Ordinarily, prostaglandin E2 helps initiate the healing cascade.

Corticosteroids

In addition to the anti-inflammatory effects, corticosteroids have a catabolic effect, breaking down protein structures and decreasing the immune response. Glucocorticosteroids can be used for several disorders, particularly autoimmune diseases and preventing transplant rejection. Prednisone is a commonly prescribed corticosteroid for autoimmune disorders. It is often used to manage pulmonary and rheumatological conditions. Systemic glucocorticosteroids can also suppress fibroblast activity. This can result in delayed or insufficient formation of granulation tissue as well as reduced wound contraction. Decreased collagen content in healing wounds also increases the risk of reinjury, such as wound dehiscence. In addition, prolonged use of systemic steroids can interfere with immune response, increasing the risk of chronic infection.

Disease-Modifying Antirheumatic Drugs

Other immunosuppressants and disease-modifying antirheumatic drugs used in the treatment of conditions such as rheumatoid arthritis, psoriasis, ankylosing spondylitis, and systemic lupus erythematosus include mycophenolate (Cellcept), azathioprine (Imuran), and cyclosporine (Neoral). New drugs that block the effects of tumor necrosis factor and various interleukins continue to be developed for autoimmune disease and increase the risk of infection.

Cancer Chemotherapy

Many cancer chemotherapeutic agents have their primary effects on rapidly reproducing cells. Although chemotherapy is intended to slow rates of cell division at the cancer site, unfortunately, these agents also cause slower cell division within injured tissues. Reduced rates of mitosis can lead to fewer fibroblasts, with decreased collagen synthesis, impairing formation of the extracellular matrix and new blood vessels. Chemotherapy also frequently results in immunosuppression with increased risk of chronic infection. An example of a chemotherapeutic drug that reduces cell division and immune response is methotrexate. In addition to cancer, this drug is used in the treatment of autoimmune conditions. Due to the adverse effects of chemotherapy on wound healing and susceptibility to infection, a patient's oncologist and infectious disease physician must coordinate their efforts to treat the cancer without unduly increasing the risk of sepsis.

Anticoagulants

Patients may be taking anticoagulants for several reasons. History of pulmonary embolism or recurrent clotting disorders and atrial fibrillation should make the clinician aware of the possibility of a patient using these medications. When a patient is taking these, one should be aware of the possibility of increased bleeding with tissue trauma including sharp debridement and dressing removal. Accumulation of blood in a wound, creating a hematoma, also increases the risk of infection. Patients may be taking warfarin, low-molecular-weight heparin, or unfractionated heparin if still an inpatient or one of the novel oral anticoagulants. Common novel oral anticoagulants include rivaroxaban (Xarelto), apixaban (Eliquis), and dabigatran (Pradaxa). In addition, aspirin functions as a nonsteroidal anti-inflammatory, multiplying its potential negative effects on wound repair. This is because medications that suppress the inflammatory response can cause delays in healing.

Antiplatelets

In some cases, antiplatelet drugs are used instead of anticoagulants. Patients with a history of stroke or myocardial infarction are likely to be taking these. These drugs work by decreasing the likelihood of platelets signaling each other to aggregate and release platelet-derived growth factor.

Anabolic Steroids

Oxandrolone is an anabolic steroid indicated for offsetting the effects of long-term corticosteroid use and recovery from burn injuries. As opposed to other anabolic steroids, it has a greater anabolic than androgenic effect and less hepatotoxicity.

BEHAVIORAL FACTORS THAT CAN IMPEDE WOUND HEALING

Alcohol Use

In addition to obtaining a full list of medications, rehabilitation professionals must screen patients and clients for behavioral factors that increase the risk of delayed healing. In acute wounds, intoxication at the time of injury has been associated with a greater likelihood of wound infection. Alcohol interferes with the regulation of proinflammatory cytokines and proper functioning of immune cells such as neutrophils and macrophages. It also suppresses angiogenesis, collagen production, formation of the extracellular matrix, and the release of growth factors. These impairments in fibroblast function also impede migration to keratinocytes during the proliferative phase. In addition, fibroblast dysfunction and increased production of matrix metalloproteinases reduce the tensile strength of healing wounds and elevate the risk of wound dehiscence. Hypoxia at or near the site of injury may also be an issue because circulatory compromise is more prevalent among people with chronic alcohol abuse. Reducing or eliminating chronic alcohol use can improve integumentary health by decreasing oxidative stress. This is also true for other types of tissue repair, including bone and muscle.

Tobacco Use

Tobacco use is another behavioral risk factor that interferes with wound healing and tissue repair. The long-term effects of tobacco use are widely acknowledged; increased incidence of cardiovascular and pulmonary disease has a negative impact on wound closure. However, the acute effects of tobacco use must also be considered.

Although dosage matters, tobacco can impede tissue repair because of nicotine and other harmful by-products. Nicotine is a powerful vasoconstrictor; it stimulates the release of epinephrine and causes decreased tissue perfusion. Diminished circulation at the wound site leads to a reduction in oxygen content, which impairs the normal inflammatory response and increases the risk of infection. Low oxygen tension promotes the colonization of bacteria. In addition, smoking is associated with an impaired immune response because of suppressed migration of lymphocytes, leading to fewer polymorphonuclear leukocytes and macrophages at the wound site. Lack of adequate blood flow also contributes to lower levels of platelet-derived growth factor and transforming growth factor beta. Nicotine also interferes with fibrinolysis, thereby increasing blood viscosity and predisposing tobacco users to abnormal clot formation. The use of cigarettes and other combustible forms of tobacco also causes an increase in blood concentrations of carbon monoxide, disrupting oxygen's ability to bind with hemoglobin. Another by-product of tobacco smoke is hydrogen cyanide, which impairs cellular oxygen metabolism. During the proliferative phase, smoking impairs fibroblast function, which decreases angiogenesis, impedes formation of the extracellular matrix, and slows re-epithelialization. It may also impair function of myofibroblasts, slowing rates of wound contraction in people who use tobacco. Fortunately, in terms of wound healing, the benefits of tobacco cessation happen almost immediately. Within 60 minutes, abstinence from smoking can restore normal levels of cutaneous blood flow and oxygenation levels. This is because both nicotine and carbon monoxide have relatively short half-lives (1 to 4 hours, respectively). Two weeks after quitting tobacco use, the number of polymorphonuclear leukocytes increases, and the likelihood of spontaneous platelet aggregation, or abnormal clot formation, decreases. Although each of these factors improves localized wound healing, patients and clients should be encouraged to maintain abstinence even after the wound has closed so that they also limit the long-term health risks associated with tobacco use.

SUMMARY

Wound healing requires sufficient nutrition to produce new tissue to fill and close defects. Both calories and protein are considered. The definition of malnutrition has changed with more emphasis on clinical characteristics rather than relying on chemistry. Changes in body weight, visual changes indicative of fat and muscle loss, and edema are used. The intake relative to the calculated need for calories and protein is still an important aspect of determining nutrition. Interventions proceed from changes in diet to supplementation to feeding either enterally or parenterally. Medications that impair wound healing and may increase risk of infection include anti-inflammatories, corticosteroids, cancer chemotherapeutics, anticoagulants, and antiplatelet drugs.

QUESTIONS

1. What are the 2 basic elements of nutrition regarding wound healing?
2. What is the importance of calorie consumption in wound healing?
3. What is the importance of protein consumption in wound healing?
4. What is the difference between dispensable and conditionally dispensable amino acids?
5. Which amino acid frequently needs supplementation?
6. What is the difference between albumin and prealbumin in terms of protein malnutrition?
7. What is the difference between positive and negative nitrogen balance?
8. What is the role of copper in wound healing?
9. What is the role of iron in wound healing?
10. What is the role of vitamin C in wound healing?
11. How does pancreatic insufficiency (eg, cystic fibrosis) affect nutrition?
12. Which vitamins need to be supplemented with pancreatic insufficiency?
13. Why is hydration particularly important in wound healing?
14. What disease complicates the issue of hydration?
15. What formula is used to determine adequate calorie intake?
16. Why are the activity and injury factors needed?
17. What is the effect of anti-inflammatory medications on healing?
18. What effects do different classes of cancer chemotherapy have on wound healing?

BIBLIOGRAPHY

Beitz JM. Pharmacologic impact (aka "Breaking Bad") of medications on wound healing and wound development: a literature-based overview. *Ostomy Wound Manage.* 2017;63(3):18-35.

Berger MM, Baines M, Raffoul W, et al. Trace element supplementation after major burns modulates antioxidant status and clinical course by way of increased tissue trace element concentrations. *Am J Clin Nutr.* 2007;85(5):1293-1300.

Boyce ST, Supp AP, Swope VB, Warden GD. Vitamin C regulates keratinocyte viability, epidermal barrier, and basement membrane in vitro, and reduces wound contraction after grafting of cultured skin substitutes. *J Invest Dermatol.* 2002;118(4):565-572.

Collins N, Friedrich L. Multivitamin supplements—magic bullet or waste of money? *Ostomy Wound Manage.* 2010;56(5):18-24.

Collins N, Friedrich L. Nutrition 411: changing the malnutrition paradigm. *Ostomy Wound Manage.* 2013;59(2):18-22.

Fraser C. The identification of barriers to pressure ulcer healing. *Wound Care Canada.* 2010;8(2):20-25.

Heintschel M, Heuberger R. The potential role of zinc supplementation on pressure injury healing in older adults: a review of the literature. *Wounds.* 2017;29(2):56-61.

Molnar JA, Underdown MJ, Clark WA. Nutrition and chronic wounds. *Adv Wound Care (New Rochelle).* 2014;3(11):663-681.

Shils ME, Olson JA, Shike M, Ross AC. *Modern Nutrition in Health and Disease.* Williams & Wilkins; 1999.

Sugino H, Hashimoto I, Tanaka Y, Ishida S, Abe Y, Nakanishi H. Relation between the serum albumin level and nutrition supply in patients with pressure ulcers: retrospective study in an acute care setting. *J Med Invest.* 2014;61(1-2):15-21.

Thomas DR. Specific nutritional factors in wound healing. *Adv Wound Care.* 1997;10(4):40-43.

White JV, Guenter P, Jensen G, Malone A, Schofield M; Academy of Nutrition and Dietetics Malnutrition Work Group; A.S.P.E.N. Malnutrition Task Force; A.S.P.E.N. Board of Directors. Consensus statement of the Academy of Nutrition and Dietetics/American Society for Parenteral and Enteral Nutrition: characteristics recommended for the identification and documentation of adult malnutrition (undernutrition). *J Acad Nutr Diet.* 2012;112(5):730-738. doi:10.1016/j.jand.2012.03.012

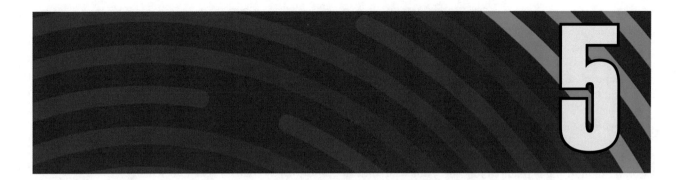

Infection Control

Infection control is a critical aspect of wound management. Infection is the most common cause of delayed healing in chronic wounds. Many patients will be referred for wound management due to infected wounds including surgical site infections and skin abscesses. In addition, an open wound or any breach in the skin provides an opportunity for infection. As discussed in Chapter 3, many times, infection is a cause of slow wound healing. During the inflammatory stage, an impaired immune response elevates the risk of infection due to the body's inability to control invading pathogens. Without an appropriate immune response, microbes present within the wound release endotoxins and cause higher concentrations of proinflammatory cytokines. By exacerbating and prolonging inflammation, wound infection contributes to delayed wound closure. Persistent activity of polymorphonucleocytes can also perpetuate tissue damage due to the release of free radicals and proteolytic enzymes. Both acute and chronic infections can be life-threatening if bacteria enter the bloodstream and cause systemic infection or sepsis.

Irion GL, Gardner JA, Pignataro RM.
Comprehensive Wound Management, Third Edition (pp 57-90).
© 2024 Taylor and Francis Group.

Therefore, detailed assessment, timely recognition, and early treatment are essential. Signs of local infection include an increase in wound exudate or fluid production, a change in color and consistency of wound exudate (ie, pus or purulent drainage), fragile granulation tissue with frequent bleeding, localized warmth and redness, and pain on palpation. Symptoms of systemic infection include loss of appetite, nausea, elevated body temperature, chills, and malaise. Sometimes, the only outward sign of infection and the presence of biofilms is the wound's failure to heal. Careful monitoring is required for older adults and others with existing factors that increase risk of infection, such as metabolic disease, long-term steroid use, prolonged antibiotic therapy, insufficient circulation, and immunocompromised patients. In addition, the longer a wound takes to close, the greater the chances of infection; chronic wounds are particularly susceptible to infections involving anaerobic bacteria that tend to thrive in an oxygen-deficient environment. However, wounds that are not infected and treated as such or treated for the wrong causative agent can also slow healing. This chapter discusses different states related to infection and methods for mitigating the risk of infection as well as increasing the likelihood of discovering the cause of infection.

SOURCES OF MICROBES

Microbes can originate from the environment or from patients themselves. Body fluids, feces, respiration, wound drainage, and spores from the environment are common infectious sources. These sources can be divided into endogenous and exogenous microbes.

Endogenous Microbes

Endogenous microbes are considered resident flora that are not pathogenic under normal circumstances. Alterations in host immunity, environmental conditions, or competition from other microbes can cause these microbes to become pathogenic. Most importantly, a breach in the skin, respiratory, urogenital, or digestive tracts can allow infection to occur. In addition, the patient's resident flora may be pathogenic to others. This person may be an asymptomatic carrier.

Protection from endogenous organisms includes skin preparation with antiseptics such as iodine/alcohol mixture before surgery, irrigation and lavage of open wounds, protection from fecal contamination, and use of either topical or systemic antimicrobial drugs. Prior to surgery, hair is clipped and not shaved. Shaving risks nicking the skin and driving bacteria into the damaged skin.

Exogenous Microbes

Exogenous microbes are introduced to the patient through the environment, other people, or organisms. Contamination of objects in a patient's room by touching or coughing by other people or using equipment that has previously been used on other patients can easily transmit exogenous microbes. Prevention of infection from exogenous microbes includes sterilization of invasive instruments, disinfection of surfaces and objects that come in contact with patients, hand hygiene, and use of personal protective equipment (PPE).

TERMS RELATED TO THE PRESENCE OF MICROBES

Several terms are used to describe states on a continuum between the presence of microbes and frank infection. The terminology continues to evolve. Recent discussion has focused on the use of the terms *critical colonization* and *local infection* for the same condition. For the purposes of this chapter, the terms are interchangeably.

Contamination

In terms of infection control, contamination refers to the unintended introduction of potentially infectious material. Due to bacteria that normally exist on the surface of the skin, all open wounds are automatically assumed to be contaminated. In healthy individuals, once bacteria enter the wound, polymorphonucleocytes work to fight the foreign invaders. However, if the immune system is compromised or the host's immunity becomes overwhelmed by pathogens, wound infection will occur. For the purposes of the discussion of infection control, contamination refers to a breach of infection control, allowing other surfaces, fluids, or aerosolized bacteria or fungus to come in contact with the wound. Infection control protocols are utilized to minimize any exposure, even though perfect sterile technique cannot guarantee that microbes will not come in contact with an open wound.

Colonization

Colonization can be defined as the presence of microbes without interaction between the host and the microbe. Thus, a stable population of microbes on a surface, including an open wound, characterizes colonization. Any chronic wound is expected to be colonized. With balanced colonization in which no one species of bacteria

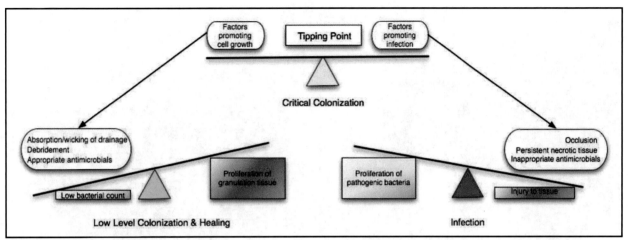

Figure 5-1. Relationship between cells of the wound bed and bacteria that define colonization, critical colonization, and infection. This diagram illustrates the principle of a tipping point in which conditions become favorable for granulation tissue formation at the expense of bacterial growth, or conditions become favorable for bacterial growth at the expense of the cells of the wound producing infection. An area near the tipping point represents critical colonization. Granulation cannot take place rapidly due to competition for resources between the cells of the wound and bacteria.

or fungus becomes dominant and the entire population remains in small numbers, no damage is done to the tissue and the tissue has sufficient resources for wounds to heal. However, if bacterial replication continues unchecked, the wound infection continuum progresses until critical colonization, or the number of bacteria needed to cause a local infection, occurs.

Critical Colonization/Local Infection

Critical colonization or local infection refers to a state in which the density of bacteria or fungus becomes so great that healing becomes slow or halts. Critical colonization can be considered a tipping point from which improving the environment leads to wound healing, but deterioration of the environment leads to frank (clinically evident) infection with damage to tissue, inflammation, and other signs of infection (described later). The concept of a tipping point is illustrated in Figure 5-1. An environment that is created by retaining necrotic tissue or using inappropriate antimicrobials can tip the wound toward infection, whereas absorption of drainage, debridement of necrotic tissue, and appropriate antimicrobials tip the environment toward a low bacterial count and healing.

Chronic infection often involves several different species of microbes. Therefore, whether an infection develops depends on both the total number of bacteria within the wound and individual and synergistic virulence. The overall health of the host must also be considered because comorbidities or multiple infections can contribute to a less effective immune response. The most common infectious agents found in chronic wounds include *Staphylococcus*, *Enterococcus*, *Pseudomonas*, *Proteus*, and *Bacteroides*.

Infection

Infection can be defined as a state in which microbes thrive at the expense of the host and produce localized necrosis.

CULTURING

Culturing is a technique of growing microbes obtained from a surface to determine the quantity and identity of microbes. Cultures may also be taken from the environment, inside a patient's nose or mouth, and other areas. Wound culturing involves a sample taken from tissue within the wound bed. The culture is taken by the use of a culturette, a long stick with an absorbent tip, commonly made of alginate. The culturette is moved across a medium in a petri dish and processed based on what is suspected to be present. The microbes are allowed to grow to estimate the quantity of microbes on the surface sampled. In addition, antibiotic discs can be placed on the medium to determine the sensitivity to antibiotics in an effort to direct medical treatment. Thus, one can have a quantitative culture to estimate the number of microbes and a qualitative culture.

A major emphasis on the quantitative culture is to determine whether the common cutoff threshold for infection of 100,000 organisms per gram is reached. However, more virulent organisms such as beta-hemolytic streptococci can cause infection at 10,000 organisms per gram.

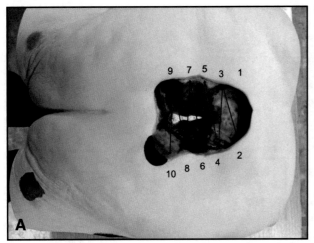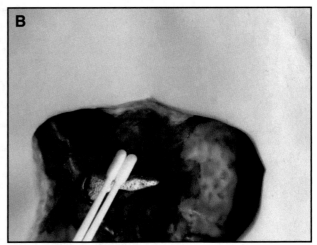

Figure 5-2. (A) Culturing using the Z technique. (B) Culturing using the Levine technique.

Swab Cultures

This type of culture sampling is performed by rolling the culturette from side to side in a zigzag pattern with 10 points (Figure 5-2A). The principle of this technique is to sample as much of the surface as possible. This technique should only be used after the wound bed is clean. Skin, eschar, and purulence are to be avoided. Despite this, only the surface is being sampled. What is actually of interest is the bacteria within the wound tissue itself, which is not what swabbing accomplishes. A culturette typically used is shown in Figure 5-2B.

Problems with swab cultures include failing to identify the organism and identifying the wrong organism. Failing to identify the organism that is causing the infection can lead to inadequate antimicrobial treatment. In many cases, antibiotics will be started before culture results are obtained. A broad-spectrum antibiotic may be able to control the infection, but using such antibiotics increases the risk of developing antibiotic resistance.

Identifying an organism that is not actually causing a problem with the wound can result from swabbing eschar, slough, purulence, or intact skin. Treatment with the wrong antibiotic may result in an inadequate treatment but can also cause further problems with healing. Killing the wrong bacteria can reduce the competition for the actual causative agent, making the infection worse. It may also create a facultative infection, allowing an otherwise innocuous bacterium to become virulent.

Levine Technique

An alternative technique that is more likely to contain bacteria from within the tissue is the Levine technique. This is accomplished by choosing a spot that has the most interest. The culturette is pressed into the wound bed and rotated over a 1-cm^2 area.

Alternative Techniques

Other options for obtaining material for culturing include tissue biopsy and aspiration of fluid from deep in a wound bed using a syringe. These types of culturing are generally reserved for physicians.

SIGNS OF INFECTION

Frank infection is a term implying that the signs of infection are unmistakable or clinically evident. Such signs include inflammation extending well beyond the wound margins, foul odor, and production of purulence and have very high specificity for infection. In addition, a trained clinician will look for damage to the wound bed as a sign of infection. Weak, bleeding granulation tissue that pulls apart easily is described as *friable* (Figure 5-3). Friable tissue with a progressive darkening of the red color, often referred to as "dusky," is also indicative of infection. Further subcutaneous tissue loss such as tunneling and lack of response to treatment are also indicators of infection. The clinician should also consider that the lack of response to treatment may simply mean the treatment was wrong and should look for additional indicators of infection. A combination of induration, erythema well beyond the margin of the wound, significant edema, and significantly greater temperature of the tissue surrounding the wound combined with foul odor and purulence should accompany slow healing to be considered infection. This combination of features comprises the acronym for infection of IFEE (Induration, Fever, Erythema, and Edema).

A series of studies based on emergency room patients discovered that quantitative cultures with 100,000 organisms per gram were predictive of infection, whereas cultures with 10,000 or fewer per gram predicted no infection. However, some bacteria such as beta-hemolytic streptococcus, the causative agent of strep throat, will produce infection at a lower concentration. This likelihood of infection occurring at a given quantity per gram is termed *virulence*. The relationship among infection, virulence, and quantity is also influenced by the immune system of the host. The relationships among these terms are often expressed in a pseudoequation as follows: infection = dose × virulence/host resistance. The virulence of beta-hemolytic streptococci is greater than other common bacteria.

When wounds are infected, grafts will not take, acute wounds will not heal, and they become chronic. Confirming infection and identifying the causative agent are discussed later in the chapter.

TERMS RELATED TO INFECTION CONTROL

The prevention of contamination and, thereby, infection is dependent on maintaining the cleanliness of anything being introduced into the body. Terms related to the cleanliness of materials and surfaces, including the surface of the wound, are defined in the following sections.

Sterile/Sterilized

A sterile object or field has no viable microbes, including spores. Anything that enters an acute wound should be sterile. An object that has been sterilized will have some type of packaging with a marker that indicates that the sterilization process has been completed. Tools used for sharp debridement, the same as those used for surgery, must be sterilized. A place created specifically for sterile objects to be kept sterile is called a *sterile field*. Only sterile materials are allowed to be placed in a sterile field or the field becomes contaminated and is no longer considered sterile. An autoclave is typically used for sterilizing instruments. The autoclave provides a very high temperature and pressure sufficient to kill any living microbes and degrade any spores. Objects that would be damaged by an autoclave can be sterilized by ethylene gas, X-rays, or gamma rays.

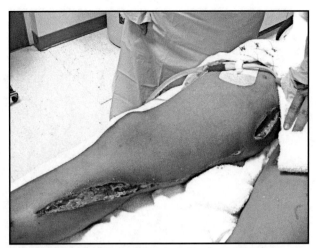

Figure 5-3. Friable tissue characteristic of wound infection.

Clean/Decontamination

Cleaning and *decontamination* are nonspecific terms to indicate an attempt at removing contaminants from a surface. This level of cleanliness does not guarantee complete elimination or any specific level of microbes. Decontamination is a term that could refer to either a living or inanimate surface.

Asepsis/Antiseptic

The deliberate removal of microbes from a living surface is called *asepsis*. The material used to accomplish this task is called an *antiseptic*. Antiseptics may kill all or nearly all microbes on a surface, but no indicators are available on a routine basis to determine the effectiveness. Skin over surgical sites is routinely treated with antiseptics such as iodine and alcohol mixture to reduce the risk of contaminating a surgical site.

Disinfect/Disinfectant

Disinfection is the deliberate removal of microbes from an inanimate surface using a disinfectant. Different levels of disinfection are accomplished with different agents. Labels clearly indicate whether the substance is appropriate for routine cleaning or high-level disinfection. High-level disinfectants are appropriate for objects such as scopes used for examining the gastrointestinal and respiratory tracts as well as hydrotherapy equipment. Lower-level, less toxic disinfectants are used for work surfaces, doorknobs, and handles and knobs on drawers and cabinets in work areas to minimize the spread of microbes that may have originated from a patient's body fluids.

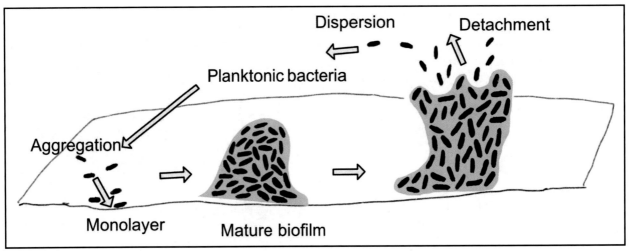

Figure 5-4. Life cycle of biofilm-producing bacteria.

BIOFILM

In some instances, bacteria form complex aggregate communities embedded in a self-secreted matrix called *biofilms*. These biofilms consist of intricate channels to facilitate gas exchange and the delivery of essential nutrients to the bacteria, diverting resources from the healing tissue of the host. Because of this, the presence of biofilms can contribute to localized wound hypoxia.

Biofilm is defined as a syntrophic consortium of microorganisms, meaning that the organisms with the biofilm respond to their environment and communicate through primitive processes to form a protective polymeric structure that protects the colony as a whole. Their elaborate structure makes biofilms more resistant to topical and systemic antimicrobials that may enable infection to spread to surrounding areas. Bacteria on the surface of the biofilm are at greater risk of injury from antibiotics, but the colony as a whole is able to survive and continue to proliferate. Plaque on teeth is considered a biofilm. Slimy surfaces on wounds are frequently referred to as "biofilm," but biofilm exists as a microscopic entity that cannot be seen with an unaided eye. Life cycles of biofilms are depicted in Figure 5-4. Biofilms are estimated to occur on more than 70% of chronic wounds and only 6% of acute wounds.

PLANKTONIC BACTERIA

Planktonic is the term used to describe bacteria that live and act independently. Under specific conditions, planktonic bacteria can aggregate and form a biofilm. As biofilm becomes more mature, planktonic bacteria can free themselves from the biofilm and spread to adjacent or distant sites to form a new biofilm. The life cycle of a biofilm can be described in 5 steps: (1) attachment of planktonic bacteria (or fungus) to a surface, (2) formation of a monolayer and initiation of a polysaccharide matrix, (3) microcolony with multiple layers, (4) mature biofilm in a characteristic mushroom configuration embedded in the polysaccharide film, and (5) detachment and release of planktonic bacteria to start a new cycle in either adjacent or distant sites. The ability to disrupt biofilm by debridement and other means is an important aspect of chronic wound management.

CONSEQUENCES OF WOUND INFECTION

Five major consequences of wound infection in order of severity can be described as follows:

1. Competition for resources slowing a wound that would otherwise heal. As described in Chapter 3, increased bioburden, ischemia, and repetitive trauma work together to increase the risk of infection.

2. Ability to evade host defenses and produce a biofilm that is difficult to eradicate. Biofilm production in bone is particularly difficult to manage and may require multiple weeks of antibiotic use, aggressive bone debridement, or amputation.

3. Injury to tissue producing friable wound bed tissue that becomes stringy and bleeds easily.

4. Enzymes from bacteria degrade tissue, allowing infection to spread along fascial planes.

5. Infection spread to blood and/or lymph resulting in systemic signs of infection, including fever, anorexia, malaise, and somnolence. Lymphadenitis and lymphangitis may occur. Bacteremia refers to the entry of these pathogens into the bloodstream and traveling to

other areas, possibly resulting in sepsis. During sepsis, bacteria overwhelm the body's immune system, triggering a massive inflammatory reaction that can threaten organs and body systems, potentially resulting in death (Table 5-1).

CAUSES OF INFECTION

A framework for considering how infection might occur includes impaired immunity, the individual's genetic component of immunity, engineering controls, work practices, and luck. Immunosuppression increases the risk of infection from both typical causes of infection and opportunistic infections that would not otherwise occur with a competent immune system. In addition, the immune system is inherited from contributions by each parent. Primary immunosuppression is caused by genetic deficiency of the immune system. A given individual may have an immune system that protects against most microbes but misses some or may miss large classes of microbes. Members of that individual's family may also have the same gaps in the immune system. Iatrogenic causes should also be considered. Corticosteroids, especially taken systemically for autoimmune diseases or prevention of organ transplant rejection, decrease inflammation and immune responses. Other drugs used to treat autoimmune diseases and cancer and to prevent transplant rejection also increase the risk of infection. Secondary immunosuppression results from diabetes mellitus, cancer, burns, AIDS, alcoholism, and drug abuse, among other causes.

Facultative infection refers to an infection that occurs due to an altered environment facilitating the ability of some microbes to thrive. Environment changes include temperature, moisture, pH, and reduced competition from other potential pathogens. For example, skin-on-skin contact due to obesity keeps skin warm and moist, thereby facilitating fungal infection of the skin. The use of multiple antibiotics in an effort to eradicate infection often results in *Clostridium difficile* infection because competition within the gut is reduced. Work practice and engineering controls discussed later have an effect on the environment of potential pathogens. An element of luck also plays a role in infection. A given person may be either fortunate or unfortunate to have exposure to certain microbes at a certain time. A fortunate person may have a severe injury to the skin but only be exposed to microbes that the immune system can handle, whereas an unfortunate person may happen to be exposed to a virulent organism at a susceptible moment despite the best engineering and practice controls.

TABLE 5-1 Host Defense Mechanisms		
CELL MEDIATED	HUMORAL	MOLECULAR
• T cell • Neutrophils • Macrophages	• Antibodies, especially IgA	• Defensins • Collectins

RECURRENT INFECTION

Some patients are seen intermittently with recurrent surgical site or skin and soft tissue infections. These patients may also be susceptible to urinary or vascular catheter infections. Factors that contribute to recurrent infections include primary immunosuppression and family history of susceptibility to particular microbes, especially community-acquired methicillin-resistant *Staphylococcus aureus* (MRSA). Others may be susceptible to recurrent infection due to secondary immunosuppression, especially due to diabetes mellitus. Facultative infection can also be recurrent due to obesity, lymphedema, and other conditions that make the skin a more favorable environment for bacterial growth. Any combination of primary and secondary immunosuppression and facultative infection may occur.

INFECTION CONTROL

Two major components of infection control are engineering controls and practice controls. Unfortunately, the development of technology, policies, and procedures to ensure the lowest possible risk to both patients and health care providers is frequently undermined by complacency. Human nature is such that when processes become burdensome, the purposes appear arbitrary, and when no bad outcomes occur when breaks in procedure occur, shortcuts are taken. Once down the road of making small violations of procedures without negative consequences, the seriousness of the violations become steadily greater until an incident occurs. Policies and procedures related to infection control, provision of better technology, and education must be constantly scrutinized and policed to avoid infection control disasters. Patients have died from infections at prestigious facilities due to failure to provide optimal infection control.

Engineering Controls

Engineering controls refer to the development and implementation of technology to minimize risk. This includes the development of protocols by which tasks are implemented. The development of sharps containers and PPE, as well as the development of policies of disinfecting surfaces, wearing PPE, and standard precautions, would qualify as engineering controls. Infection control officers at facilities are responsible for ensuring that the latest and best technologies and procedures are available and that staff are appropriately trained.

Practice Controls

Practice controls refer to how tasks are done, including how carefully the policies developed are actually carried out. Complacency is the greatest risk factor leading to the failure of practice controls. Shortcuts in technique can creep into practice due to complacency. For example, only putting gowns over forearms, not washing hands before eating, not changing gloves after touching the patient's body fluids, and touching objects without following up with hand hygiene can lead to infection. Complacency can be seen in practice control in seemingly benign ways such as using eyeglasses for eye protection, failing to pull face masks over the nose, not tying gowns so that they stay over the shoulders, or changing gloves without washing hands. Infection control officers are responsible for continuing education and policing the practices within institutions. Giving the same online multiple-choice exams and announced visits to practice areas on an annual basis are not considered best practice for institutional practice controls. Unannounced visits and updated methods of education should be employed.

Universal Precautions

The underlying principle of universal precautions is that the health care providers can become complacent due to the assumption that a patient does not have a communicable disease if an infection is not identified in a patient's history. Thus, we are to practice as if every patient has blood-borne pathogens. Universal precautions have since been superseded by standard precautions.

Standard Precautions

As with universal precautions, standard precautions refer to all patients, but more specific isolation requirements may also apply. Visitors as well as health care providers are expected to clean hands when entering and exiting a patient's room, cover the mouth and nose when coughing or sneezing, not apply makeup or lip balm, keep nails

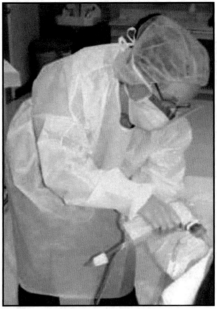

Figure 5-5. PPE—surgical cap, face shield, gown, and gloves.

short, use gloves and gowns when soiling is likely, and wear a mask with eye protection if splashing is likely.

PERSONAL PROTECTIVE EQUIPMENT

In the course of wound management, the clinician must be protected from accidental exposure to pathogens. In addition to pathogens involved in wounds, clinicians must be protected against the transmission of blood-borne pathogens such as hepatitis B virus, hepatitis C virus, and human immunodeficiency virus. Patients must also be protected against the transmission of pathogens from the clinician. Pathogenic organisms can be transmitted easily from one patient to a clinician's clothing to another patient. The Occupational Safety and Health Administration (OSHA) requires the protection of all workers from biohazards. Specific OSHA requirements are discussed at the end of this chapter. PPE consists of gloves, devices to protect mucous membranes such as masks and eye shields, and coverings for clothing and shoes. PPE is shown in Figure 5-5.

PPE is designated by facility policy and procedure and should be appropriate to the circumstances of the task and the person performing it. The least configuration of PPE is the use of exam gloves that are discarded between patients. Full PPE would cover the entire body and clothing and would therefore include a cap, face shield extending beyond the neck, gown extending beyond the knees, and boots extending above the bottom of the gown and gloves. Typically,

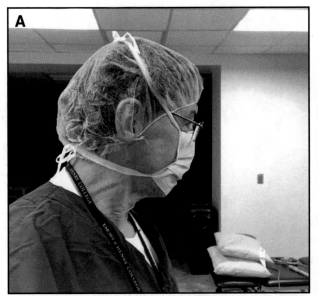

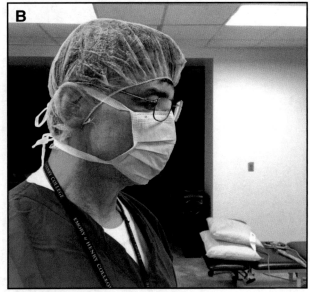

Figure 5-6. Donning of face mask. (A) Tying over the head. (B) Tying around the neck.

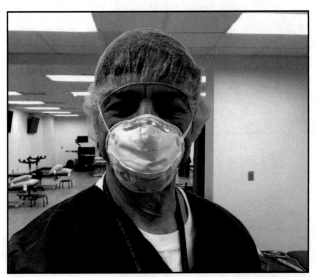

Figure 5-7. Donning an N95 mask.

shoe covers are used, which exposes pants below the knees and socks. Face masks and caps typically leave much of the neck, some of the forehead, and some of the side of the face uncovered. Splattering, splashing, or aerosolization can contaminate these areas. Policies must cover the possibility of decontaminating the skin or clothing in these cases.

Donning and Doffing

The act of putting equipment on—don or donning—and taking it off—doff or doffing—should follow a general plan of donning the item that needs to be cleanest last and doffing the most contaminated first. Another

consideration needs to be what is touched prior and after. Hand hygiene practices must be employed before donning PPE. Using this approach with typical PPE for potential splashing, a bouffant cap is donned first, preferably in front of a mirror so that all hair is captured. Initially placing the front of the cap below the eyebrows and pulling up should capture the hair in front. A tie-on face mask with a built-in eye shield is next. Typical masks are shown in Figure 5-6 and can be donned by securing the upper ties over the ears and the lower ties on the top of the head. This method pulls the sides of the mask tighter to the face, minimizing the risk of splashes entering the sides. Securing the lower ties around the neck can result in gapping of the sides of the mask. If a surgical type of cap is used instead of a bouffant cap (see Figures 5-6 and 5-7), the face mask may be donned before the cap.

After donning the cap and mask, shoe covers are donned. Shoe covers should be donned after donning equipment on the face to prevent contaminants on the shoes reaching the face. A clinician should be able to don shoe covers without the hands coming in contact with the shoes. The front and back edges of the shoe covers should be grasped such that the edges roll over and cover the fingers, thereby preventing contact with the shoes as shown in Figure 5-8. The front end of the shoe cover should be pulled over the forefoot securely before attempting to pull the back end over the heel. Pulling out all wrinkles and having the front tight over the toes maximizes the slack available at the heel end. If a clinician wears shoes much larger than a US size 12, extra-large shoe covers should be provided. Immediately following donning of the shoe covers, hand hygiene should be repeated.

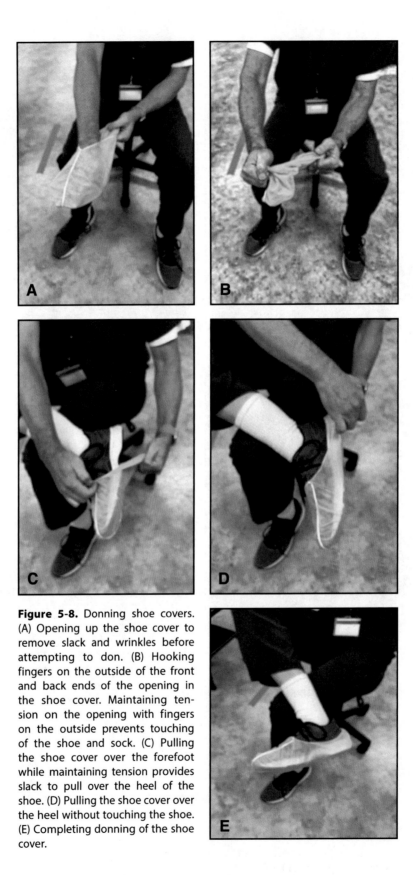

Figure 5-8. Donning shoe covers. (A) Opening up the shoe cover to remove slack and wrinkles before attempting to don. (B) Hooking fingers on the outside of the front and back ends of the opening in the shoe cover. Maintaining tension on the opening with fingers on the outside prevents touching of the shoe and sock. (C) Pulling the shoe cover over the forefoot while maintaining tension provides slack to pull over the heel of the shoe. (D) Pulling the shoe cover over the heel without touching the shoe. (E) Completing donning of the shoe cover.

Following hand hygiene, a gown is donned. Gowns can be either waterproof or splash resistant (Figure 5-9). Waterproof gowns (see Figure 5-9A) are made of plastic and do not allow evaporation of sweat. Long procedures in a warm room can lead to gowns adhering to sweating skin and to overheating. Splash-resistant gowns (see Figure 5-9B) are made of woven paper material and protect against simple, small splashes but will soak through if a stream of liquid hits them. Gowns may have either a head hole or ties for the neck. Another tie around the waist secures them. Ideally, the waist ties wrap around and can be torn loose from the front at the end of the procedure. The gown should have a mechanism such as thumb loops/holes to stop the sleeves from riding proximal to the glove and exposing any forearm (see Figure 5-9C). Many of the paper gowns only have an elastic band at the end of the sleeve that will not prevent the sleeve from riding up. A common practice with these is to tear thumb holes just above the elastic band at the end of the sleeve (see Figure 5-9D).

Gloves are donned last because these are most likely to contact the patient and the wound. For most procedures, clean exam gloves are sufficient because they only touch handles and dressing materials. Sterile gloves, for the most part, are a wasted resource. Studies comparing the infection rate using sterile gloves and exam gloves have found no difference in infection rates during emergency room procedures. Sterile gloves and gowns are used, however, when making direct contact with a patient's skin in burn rehabilitation due to the risk of spreading infection on burned skin.

When doffing PPE, gloves must be discarded first to avoid contamination, and gowns follow. Some clinicians are able to doff the gloves and gowns together. The removal of face protection precedes the removal of shoe covers to minimize any contamination from shoes onto the head. When doffing, only the inside or the back of the PPE is touched with the hands because any body fluids present on the PPE will only be on the front and outside.

Types of Masks

The mucus membranes of the eyes, nose, and mouth are potential sites for pathogen transmission. Aerosolization of fluid under pressure used to irrigate wounds, splashing of body fluids from open wounds, and spurting blood may result in contamination of mucus membranes. When any of these situations might occur, the clinician is expected to use protective eyewear and a mask. A combination face mask with an attached antifog eye shield provides better protection than separate eyewear and mask (Figure 5-10). Splashes may bounce off the face, under eyewear, and strike the eye. A full-face shield provides even greater

protection but can become uncomfortable and impede visibility due to fogging. Although almost all clinicians will never experience a facial splash, one cannot predict with complete confidence that fluid from any given wound will never splash. The cost of disposable masks and reusable goggles is small compared with the possible outcome of infectious material contacting the eyes, nose, or mouth.

Gloving

As a minimum, clean examination gloves should be worn both to protect the clinician from the patient's body fluids and to protect the patient's body fluid from contaminants on the clinician's hands not removed by handwashing. Donning sterile gloves requires special techniques, which are sometimes obvious from following package instructions, but not all manufacturers include instructions. The technique for donning sterile gloves is derived from 2 basic rules: (1) the inside of the gloves is considered unsterile, and (2) the outside of the gloves is considered sterile. Therefore, the hands may only make contact with the inside of the gloves, and only the outside of a glove is allowed to touch another glove. Furthermore, the inside of the package is sterile until touched by hands. Based on these rules, the clinician peels the package open and makes certain that all other needed packages are open before gloving and that the clinician's hands will not need to go outside of the sterile field.

The glove package is oriented so the words *right* and *left* or the letters *R* and *L* are upright. The inside package is folded so the part of it that becomes the outside of the wrapper can be grasped without touching the inside of the package. The inside package can then be pulled open using this folded-over part of the wrapper in the center. Avoid touching the inner surface of this wrapper, and pull hard enough to keep the wrapper open. The wrapper will re-close if not pulled far enough. The following sequence is based on the concepts discussed previously.

Reaching carefully, place the fingers of the nondominant hand into the glove in a scooping manner. With the dominant hand, pull on the inside surface of the glove, which is folded over to allow the glove to be grasped this way. Pull gently until the fingers are in, but do not try to pull the first glove completely onto the hand. Pulling hard enough that the fingers go entirely into the glove is likely to disturb the cuff and cause it to unfold and lose the handle for pulling the glove on correctly. Next, using the gloved nondominant hand, scoop underneath the fold in the cuff of the glove for the dominant hand so that the glove on the nondominant hand only makes contact with the outside of the glove on the dominant hand. The partially gloved nondominant hand is used to pull the glove entirely onto the dominant hand but only by touching the outside of the

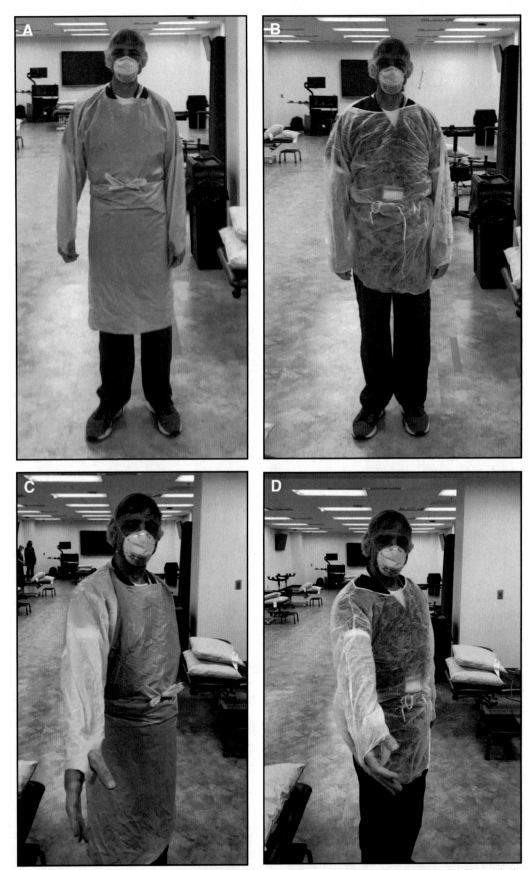

Figure 5-9. Gowns. (A) Waterproof. (B) Water resistant. (C) Thumbholes provided by manufacturer. (D) Thumbholes created in water-resistant gown by user.

2 gloves to each other. At this point, the dominant hand is completely gloved, and the nondominant hand is partially gloved. To finish gloving the nondominant hand, place the fingers of the gloved dominant hand inside the folded cuff of the other glove, and pull the glove all the way onto the nondominant hand, only touching the outside of the glove. The procedure for donning sterile surgical gloves is shown in Figure 5-11.

When gloves are removed, the outsides of the gloves should only touch the outside of the other glove, not the skin; carefully pull gloves off inside out so that the hands contact only the inside surface of the gloves. Wash your hands as soon as possible after gloves and another PPE are removed. Do not write notes, restock supplies, or anything else before washing your hands to avoid secondary contamination from the gloves onto other objects.

Latex Allergy

Latex has been a significant concern in wound management. Much of the PPE containing latex has been replaced with other materials. In particular, nitrile gloves have supplanted latex and vinyl in the clinic. Both the clinician and patient need to be considered. Due to the institution of universal precautions, a large number of both patients and clinicians have been exposed and sensitized to latex. Latex allergy is potentially fatal and must be taken seriously. An irritant dermatitis (type IV immune injury) is much more common than a type I allergic/anaphylactic reaction. About 7% to 12% of health care workers who are exposed to latex regularly have positive skin tests to proteins present in latex gloves. All patients with spina bifida are automatically treated as if they are latex sensitive, although the actual percentage is believed to be between 28% and 67%.

Moreover, clinicians must be familiar with objects other than gloves containing latex that may contaminate surfaces that contact the latex-sensitive person. For this reason, latex and nonlatex exam gloves should be kept apart, and hands should be washed after using latex gloves to avoid contaminating others with latex proteins. Powder-free gloves are less likely to expose individuals to latex proteins by minimizing airborne latex exposure. Other PPE may contain latex in elastic bands and other parts. Latex-free equivalents for these may be necessary. Employers are required to provide latex-free PPE to employees. Clinicians should also keep fingernails trimmed and remove jewelry to avoid an accumulation of latex molecules beneath them. Non–water-based skin care products should not be used under latex gloves because these may degrade the gloves. The Centers for Disease Control and Prevention recommends using these skin care products only at the end of patient care for the day.

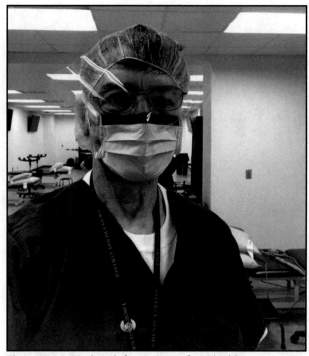

Figure 5-10. Mask with fog-resistant face shield.

ISOLATION

Isolation precautions are used to mitigate the risk of transmission of specific organisms. Contact precautions are common for patients with wounds. Gloves and gowns are the minimum requirements for contact. Airborne precautions are for organisms that linger in the air such as Mycoplasma tuberculosis and requires a special NIOSH-95 (N-95) mask that seals tightly on the face and is rated to prevent the entry of 95% of particles the size of a virus. Droplet precautions are for organisms that travel in droplets that settle within 3 feet (or 1 meter). Regular masks are required for this precaution.

ANTIMICROBIAL METHODS

Antimicrobial methods may be divided into physical and chemical methods. Certain types are more appropriate for sterilization and others for antisepsis or disinfection. Factors to be considered for any method include how long the process is applied; the temperature and pressure at which the process is applied; the quantity or concentration of heat or chemical; the nature of the item receiving the process; the type and quantity of microbe, including spores; and whether the items are contaminated with body fluids that may act as a protective layer for the microbe.

Physical methods include heat (both dry and moist), pressure combined with heat, cold, desiccation, radiation,

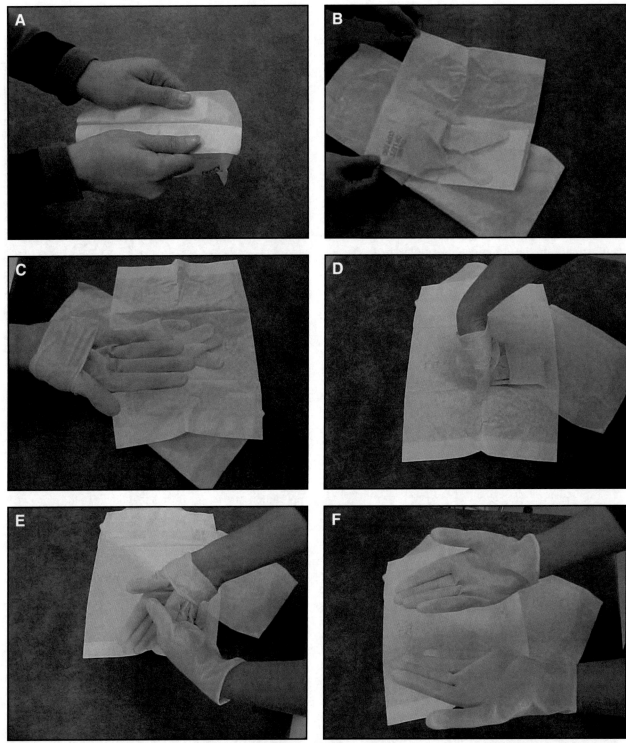

Figure 5-11. (A) Opening any sterile package should be done in this manner to avoid touching inside the package. (B) Opening package to reveal the first glove. (C) Donning first glove to leave cuff turned over. (D) Scooping second glove, touching on the outside of the second glove with the outside of the first glove. (E) Pulling down the cuff of the first glove with the second glove, touching only the outside of the first glove. (F) Completed gloving.

ultrasound, filtration, and hypertonicity. In general, physical methods are useful for sterilization, whereas chemicals are frequently used for antisepsis and disinfection. However, a combination of physical and chemical methods may be used for any of the 3 types of antimicrobial methods.

Physical Methods of Infection Control

Paper and gauze may be used to filter substances to decrease contamination with microbes. Paper is frequently used for face masks, and gauze is frequently placed as a covering over wounds. Paper and gauze need to be kept dry to be effective as filters. Wet gauze, in particular, can transmit microbes into a wound. Moist dressings are usually covered by a dry gauze or paper material to prevent the transmission of microbes from the air into the wounds. Additionally, HEPA (high-efficiency particulate air) filters are used to decrease microbes as well as allergens from the air. Ionizers may also be used to remove particulate material from the air; however, the ionized particles settle on surfaces and require dusting, vacuuming, or mopping to remove them.

Cold is primarily bacteriostatic rather than bactericidal. Cold reduces the rate of growth of microbes. Allowing temperature to increase to room temperature causes bacterial growth to resume and spores to germinate. Refreezing will simply slow the growth of a larger number of bacteria. Desiccation (drying) is frequently used in the preparation of foods and drugs. Desiccation combined with a vacuum is called *lyophilization*. Unfortunately, desiccation can also preserve microbes, especially spores. These microbes encased within desiccated body fluids may be found in a patient's environment, particularly on floors, dressings, clothing, and other items. Disturbing these may result in airborne dust that can be carried into wounds where a warm, moist, and frequently occluded environment may aid in the proliferation of the microbe. Hypertonicity is generally used for preserving food rather than wound management.

Disinfection

Three levels of disinfection are commonly described. High-level disinfection destroys all microorganisms and viruses. Intermediate-level disinfection destroys all microbes except spore-forming and some nonlipid and small viruses. The third type, low-level disinfection, provides little action against spore-forming bacteria, mycobacteria, and some fungi and small viruses. Some items, such as laundry, can be disinfected sufficiently by using very hot water. The effectiveness of chemical disinfection can be altered by the interaction of disinfectants and microbes. The concentration of the chemical, the pH,

and the presence of any body fluids on the items to be disinfected determine the effectiveness of chemical disinfectants; therefore, instructions need to be followed carefully. As discussed with sterilization, instruments and other items should be washed thoroughly before disinfection to remove proteinaceous material that may protect microbes from the disinfectant. High-level disinfection needs to be used when concern exists regarding spore-forming bacteria or viruses.

Chemicals for disinfection should be chosen for the specific situation. A large number of high-level disinfectants are available commercially. Their effectiveness is determined by the factors described previously, in particular, concentration, temperature, and the presence of body fluids. Surfaces should be scrubbed with detergent to remove body fluids. Surfactant and chelating agents in the detergent increase their effectiveness in removing proteinaceous contaminants. In addition, the disinfectant should be left on the surface for the prescribed time to be effective.

Disinfectants include several types of agents such as soaps/detergents, alcohols, heavy metals, oxidants, chlorine and iodine compounds, and other agents. Phenolics are used commercially in home disinfectants (eg, Lysol [Reckitt Benckiser]). Phenolics include carbolic acid, the disinfectant originally used by Lister, as well as phenol, xylenols, cresol, and orthophenylphenol. Similar to alcohols, these agents are effective tuberculocides and sporicides. In particular, chlorine compounds are used in hydrotherapy. Sodium hypochlorite, the active ingredient of laundry bleach, has a short half-life and is inactivated readily by organic material. Sustained-release forms of chlorine, such as Chlorazene (Ferno-Washington, Inc), are frequently used to disinfect water used for hydrotherapy in a whirlpool tank. Although they are indicated for skin preparation and hand scrubbing prior to surgery, sustained-release forms of iodine, such as povidone-iodine, have also been used to disinfect water used for hydrotherapy.

Antisepsis

Like disinfection, chemical antimicrobial methods are the mainstay of antisepsis. Chemicals used for antisepsis are called *antiseptics*. Physical means are generally not suitable for antisepsis due to the potential damage to skin or body tissues. Moreover, many chemicals that are highly effective for disinfection are too toxic to be used as antiseptics. Although antiseptics reduce the number of microbes on the body surface, microbes may still be harbored in hair follicles and the ostia of sweat and sebaceous glands. A reduction of approximately 95% is expected with proper technique. Soaps and detergents act as antiseptics by removing surface microbes. In addition, they damage cell membranes by dissolving phospholipids. As with disinfection, some degree of scrubbing is necessary with antiseptics to remove residues that could harbor bacteria beneath them. Chlorhexidine gluconate (Hibiclens, Molnlycke Health Care US, LLC) and hexachlorophene (Phisohex, Sanofi-aventis US) are commonly used as antiseptics for handwashing or topical bacterial infections. Both of these should be rinsed thoroughly from the skin. Hexachlorophene is neurotoxic if it is absorbed through the skin. These agents are used occasionally as whirlpool disinfectants, although they have questionable value at the dilutions used and may be ineffective against many organisms at their full strengths.

Ethyl and isopropyl alcohol in 70% solutions are effective disinfectants for bacteria and are tuberculocidal and sporicidal. Aerosolized ethyl alcohol foams and isopropyl alcohol gels are available for handwashing to rapidly reduce the counts of transient bacteria. Because these formulations appear to be more effective antiseptics than soap and water, some organizations have suggested these be used either in place of, or in addition to, handwashing with soap and water.

Iodine can be formulated as a slow-release polymer such as Betadine to produce a continual release of iodine on the skin surface or combined with alcohol (tincture of iodine). Alcohol and iodine solutions are used for antiseptic scrubs to reduce microbial counts further. Even with surgical scrubbing, microbial counts are still unacceptably high, requiring the use of sterile gloves. Iodine compounds are approved by the Food and Drug Administration for surface antisepsis as either a skin scrub or surgical prep but are not approved for use in open wounds. Iodine compounds have been shown clearly to interfere with the processes of wound healing. In addition, high concentrations of iodine can cause iodine burns, and absorption of antiseptics can lead to systemic iodine toxicity manifested as neuropathy or cardiovascular, renal, and hepatic toxicity.

Acids such as acetic acid and boric acid are effective against many common bacteria. Acetic acid is commonly used for treating wounds infected by *Pseudomonas aeruginosa*, and Dakin's solution (made of hypochlorite, or diluted bleach, and boric acid) is used to destroy *Staphylococcus* and *Streptococcus* species. Antiseptics are also used in sprays as air fresheners containing ingredients such as alcohol, triethylene glycol, and benzethonium chloride. Hydrogen peroxide is a commonly used, commercially available agent proposed to work as an oxidizing agent, particularly for anaerobes, and produces effervescence due to the reaction with tissue catalase, providing a mild debriding function. Although commercially available concentrations of hydrogen peroxide can interfere with the formation of granulation tissue when used repeatedly in chronic wounds, low levels of hydrogen peroxide released by macrophages and neutrophils during the inflammatory phase of healing help attract leukocytes to the area of injury. This assists with the release of matrix metalloproteinases and the suppression of tissue inhibitors of matrix metalloproteinases to facilitate the removal of necrotic tissue, debris, and wound contaminants. Hydrogen peroxide released by macrophages also stimulates endothelial cells and promotes the release of vascular endothelial growth factor to encourage angiogenesis.

Heavy metals, halogens, iodine, and bromine are bactericidal, virucidal, tuberculocidal, and sporicidal. Salts of heavy metals are available commercially as antiseptics. Mercury chloride is commonly used for first aid on acute wounds (Merthiolate, Mercurochrome), and silver nitrate has been used as an ophthalmic antiseptic for neonates. Silver nitrate left on the skin or open wounds is highly toxic. It causes severe drying and necrosis of tissue and is not recommended for use on open wounds.

In addition to chemical means of antisepsis, ultraviolet lamps have been approved. Like X-rays and gamma rays, ultraviolet produces severe genetic damage. The dose necessary for antisepsis is relatively small, requiring exposure for several seconds with minimal risk to growing tissue in the wound when used appropriately.

As discussed with iodine compounds, the use of antiseptics as topical agents for wounds is discouraged. No research has shown that the use of antiseptics on wounds reduces bacterial counts within them. Some antiseptics can be absorbed and cause toxicity, as noted earlier for iodine and hexachlorophene. The excessive use of antiseptics (and disinfectants) may lead to the development of resistant microbes. Other limitations on antiseptics are their ineffectiveness with high bacterial counts and the inactivation of antiseptics by excessive organic material, especially purulence.

Sterilization

Heat can be used for either sterilization or disinfection. However, heat is not suitable for many items and certainly not for antisepsis. To achieve sterilization, a combination of time and temperature is necessary. The heat required for sterilization is increased if items are contaminated with any body fluids that might form an insulating coat on the microbes. If instruments are contaminated with body fluids, thorough cleaning and chemical disinfection may be required before sterilization with heat. Dry heat is less effective on some types of microbes, especially on items contaminated with body fluids. Moist heat delivered as either steam or boiling is more effective at removing proteinaceous material from instruments. Of particular concern is the destruction of viruses that may withstand boiling. The combination of pressure and heat used in an autoclave is effective at destroying spores and viruses that may survive heat alone. Safe guidelines promoted in the literature include autoclaving for 20 minutes at 250°C and

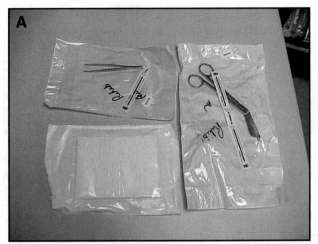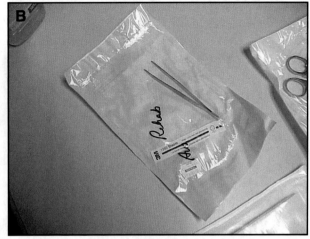

Figure 5-12. (A) Variety of sterile packages including sterilized forceps, scissors, and disposable towel. (B) Sterile packages. Note the indicator strip in the packages to insure sterilization has occurred.

15 psi, boiling for 30 minutes (longer at higher elevations), or dry heat (baking) for 1 hour at 356°C. Appropriate packaging, including pressure-sensitive tape, should be used for autoclaving. Photographs of autoclaved instruments are shown in Figure 5-12. Due to the heat and pressure of the autoclave, no sealed containers should be used. Items that cannot tolerate normal autoclave temperatures may be treated at a lower temperature for a longer time or may require chemical disinfection. Another approach for heat-sensitive items such as catheters is gas sterilization. Ethylene oxide is a chemical oxidizing agent that is highly effective but is also difficult to use. Radiation is another method used to sterilize items. X-rays or gamma rays (ionizing radiation) induce sufficient genetic damage to sterilize instruments as well as foods and drugs. Ultrasound is highly effective at removing adherent materials from the surface of metal. The cleansed materials may then be further disinfected and sterilized.

HANDWASHING

Although not completely effective in removing microbes from the skin, care needs to be taken during handwashing to minimize what is left on the skin of the clinician. Handwashing or the application of approved hand sanitizer is to be done before and after each patient. One must distinguish between handwashing, which is done to minimize the number of transient organisms on the hands, and scrubbing, which is done to minimize both transient and resident organisms present on the hands. Handwashing is a vigorous and brief rubbing of hand surfaces together with lathered hands, followed by rinsing with flowing water. Scrubbing is a specific sequence lasting up to 10 minutes using antiseptics before surgery is performed in an operating room. A surgical cap, mask, shoe covers, and sterile gown are required. Handwashing involves soap or detergent. Scrubbing is done with a combination of iodine and alcohol or other harsh antimicrobial agents.

For handwashing, disposable soap containers are preferred to refillable containers; bar soap should not be used due to potential contamination from other users. During handwashing, nothing should touch the hands and forearms other than soap, running water, and one's own hands and forearms. Because the average person only washes hands when they are obviously contaminated, the sink, its controls, and soap dispensers are generally heavily contaminated and should not be touched directly with the hands. One must also avoid being splashed at the sink due to the possibility of microbes being transmitted from the sink. Touchless controls for soap, water, and paper towels are all now commonly available. When touchless controls are not available, care must be taken to prevent contamination with *Pseudomonas* and other microbes from contact with the sink, handles, or faucet or from using solutions diluted with nonsterile water. If hands-free controls are not available, use clean paper towels to touch faucet controls. A scrub cannot be performed without knee or foot controls. A scrub must be followed by drying with a sterile towel, whereas clean paper towels are sufficient for handwashing. In obtaining paper towels, contact with the outside of the towel dispenser must be avoided. Proper handwashing techniques are depicted in Figure 5-13. The steps of proper handwashing are listed in Table 5-2.

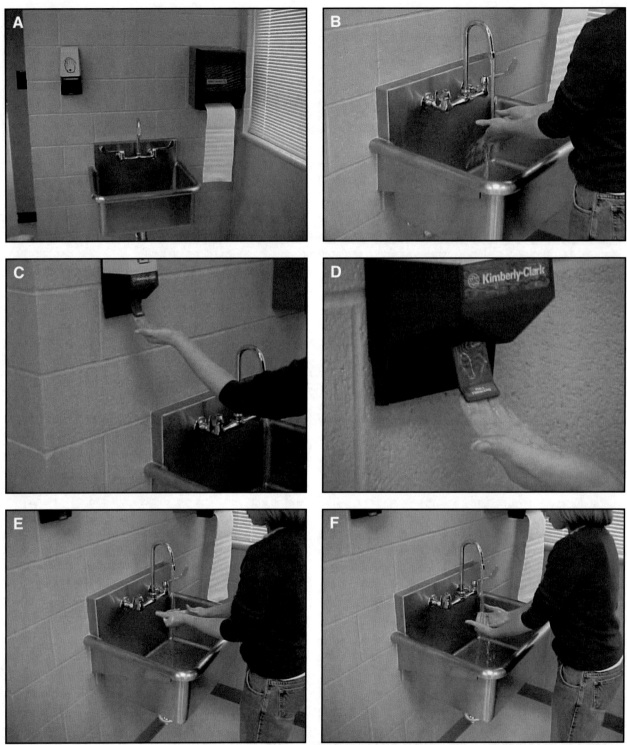

Figure 5-13. Handwashing. (A) Soap dispenser, sink, and paper towel dispenser. (B) Wetting hands. (C) Obtaining soap. (D) Close-up of nonrefillable soap dispenser. (E) Lathering. (F) Rinsing. *(continued)*

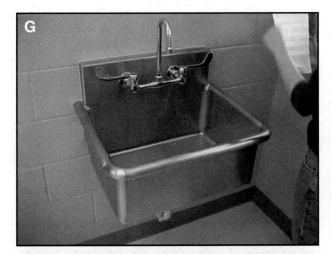

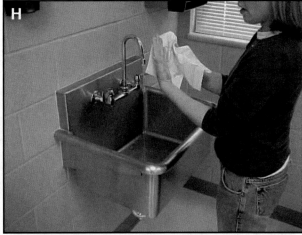

Figure 5-13 (continued). (G) Obtaining paper towel. (H) Drying hands. (I) Turning off faucet handles with paper towel.

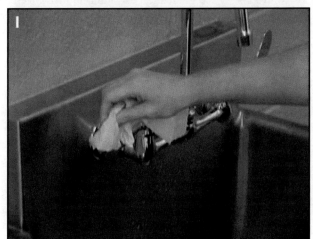

TABLE 5-2
Handwashing Technique

- Turn on the faucet with foot or knee control, or a clean paper towel.
- Operate soap control with foot control or use a clean paper towel.
- Wash thoroughly for 30 seconds.
- Rinse thoroughly under flowing water, but do not make contact with the faucet or sink; do not allow splashing from the bottom of the sink.
- If contact or splashing occurs, handwashing must be restarted.
- Allow water to run toward elbows; do not allow water from arm to run down to hands.
- Dry with clean paper towels, and then turn off water with paper towels.
- Use of automatic paper towel dispenser is preferred; avoid using crank-type dispenser.
- Disposable soap containers are preferred to refillable containers; bar soap should not be used.

Practical Issues Related to Handwashing

Several practical implications can be missed if not considered ahead of time. Cracking of skin can occur with frequent handwashing, especially in the winter. Periodic use of moisturizers must be employed to prevent cracking. Avoiding touching the faucet, sink, and paper towel controls can be difficult, particularly in older facilities that do not yet have touchless controls. Many older sinks are too small to use without accidental contact and splashing. A large, deep sink with a faucet that is far from the back of the sink, as shown in Figure 5-13, should be used whenever possible. Jewelry should not be worn when washing hands. It should be placed in a secure location and left off the wrists and hands for the duration of patient care. Long sleeves need to be rolled up or short sleeves worn so that cleaning of the forearms can be done effectively. Assuming that everyone else is compliant with hand hygiene is another common mistake. Assume that anything that can be touched with bare hands has been contaminated with the worst thing imaginable. In particular, avoid opening doors with freshly washed hands. Use the paper towel used for hand drying to open doors that open inwardly or use a shoulder or back to open doors that open outwardly.

TREATMENT OF LOCAL INFECTION

A large number of antimicrobial agents have been used on open wounds. However, most of these are antiseptics designed for preparation of the skin preoperatively and immediate use on acute wounds. They are not designed, indicated, or approved for use on chronic wounds. These agents are frequently misused or overused. Although they may be useful temporarily, they must be used prudently with the specific goal of preventing or treating infection. Because infection and eschar slow healing, these agents are used often in an illogical attempt to speed healing. Considering that these agents are toxic to bacteria, fungi, protozoa, and even many viruses, the clinician should also consider what these agents do to fibroblasts and epithelial cells. If the immediate goal is to rid the wound of unacceptable numbers of microbes, then a limited course may be prudent. One must keep in mind, however, that the concern is for organisms that have achieved a true tissue level, not merely bacteria colonizing the surface of a wound.

Moreover, many topical agents lack the penetration necessary to be effective when applied topically. Of the commonly used topical agents, silver sulfadiazine is sufficiently water soluble to be effective. Once a wound is debrided, clean, and stable, these topical antiseptic agents

will only retard wound healing. The Agency for Health Care Policy and Research (AHCPR) recommends a 2-week trial of topical antibiotics for clean ulcers that are not healing or are continuing to produce exudate after 2 to 4 weeks of optimal care. If an antibiotic is selected for topical use, the AHCPR recommends using an agent that is effective against gram-negative, gram-positive, and anaerobic organisms. Triple antibiotic (discussed later) and silver sulfadiazine are explicitly mentioned.

The AHCPR guidelines recommend against the use of topical antiseptics such as povidone-iodine, iodophor, sodium hypochlorite, Dakin's solution, hydrogen peroxide, and acetic acid in wound tissue. In these guidelines, systemic, rather than topical, antibiotic therapy is suggested for patients with bacteremia, sepsis, advancing cellulitis, or osteomyelitis. These guidelines also indicate that systemic antibiotics are not required for pressure injuries with only clinical signs of local infection. The American Diabetes Association recommends against the use of any topical antiseptics or antibiotics and recommends aggressive sharp debridement and systemic antibiotics. As discussed previously, povidone-iodine is a compound designed to produce sustained release of iodine. It is beneficial in reducing the risk of infection as a surgical preparation and temporary use on acute wounds. However, it is not recommended for use in chronic wounds. It may be used to prevent cross contamination of hydrotherapy equipment. At a concentration of 0.001%, it is noncytotoxic for fibroblasts. However, it is often used on gauze-packed wounds in concentrations much higher than this and has never received approval to be used in wounds but only for prepping skin for surgery or as a surgical hand scrub solution. Hypochlorite (household bleach) and the less cytotoxic chloramine (Chlorazene) are used routinely to prevent cross contamination of hydrotherapy equipment. Unless a patient has more than one wound in a whirlpool tank or other container, the use of these chlorine compounds is questionable.

Triple antibiotic is a solution of 3 antimicrobials: neomycin, polymyxin B, and gramicidin. It is useful topically temporarily for either a deep acute wound, such as a gunshot wound, or as a short topical course for a nonhealing chronic wound suspected to be infected. Silver sulfadiazine inhibits DNA synthesis of microbes and is a broad-spectrum antimicrobial with a cream formulation for topical application. It is especially useful for burns; it has a soothing effect and prevents gauze bandages from adhering to wounds. Although it may have adverse effects on fibroblasts and keratinocytes, it is highly effective in re-establishing bacterial balance. Therefore, it should be discontinued once bacterial balance is achieved. Silver sulfadiazine has also been implicated in Stevens-Johnson syndrome, an immune reaction that results in epidermal and mucosal blistering. This condition is potentially but rarely lethal. Stevens-Johnson syndrome has also been linked to several other antibiotics in addition to silver sulfadiazine. An alternative to silver sulfadiazine is sulfamylon (mafenide). Sulfamylon may be preferred for full-thickness burn injuries because it penetrates eschar better. However, silver sulfadiazine may be preferred with large percent body surface area wounds. Sulfamylon may cause electrolyte problems when applied to large surface area wounds. Patients need to be monitored and instructed to look for local reactions or more widespread allergic/anaphylactic reactions.

Cadexomer iodine is available in multiple forms—an ointment, sheet, or powder. It has been used in a variety of wounds, both acute and chronic, including venous, arterial, pressure injuries, and purulent wounds. It releases iodine gradually as the material absorbs exudate, and manufacturers claim that the release rate of iodine is not cytotoxic. In addition to absorption, it reduces odor and prevents maceration that might otherwise occur due to leakage of drainage onto the surrounding skin. Although it may be applied to cover the wound bed, it requires a secondary dressing over it. When the material changes color from brown to a yellow or gray color, it should be replaced. However, the nature of the ointment and its color also obscure the visibility of the wound bed and interfere with the assessment of drainage quantity and quality.

Mercurochrome has useful antimicrobial action on small, partially healed, superficial wounds or for a small number of applications to minor acute wounds. Neosporin is a combination of 3 antibacterial drugs (neomycin, polymyxin B, and bacitracin), is highly effective against most gram-negative and gram-positive bacteria found on skin, and is indicated for most minor acute wounds. Moreover, its petrolatum base allows moisture retention to prevent scab formation. Polysporin only contains 2 of the 3 antimicrobials present in Neosporin (missing neomycin). Sensitivity to neomycin is common. Because polysporin does not contain neomycin, it is a good alternative to Neosporin. It also has a petrolatum base, and it is commonly used on facial wounds, including burns. Polysporin is also available in a powder, which can be poured into open wounds.

Although hydrogen peroxide is a household staple for the treatment of minor acute wounds, it has little antimicrobial action compared with other available agents. It is sometimes used for its mechanical effect of effervescence. The enzyme catalase in blood converts H_2O_2 to H_2O and O_2, but this provides minor debridement value, which could be performed in other ways. Silver nitrate is very effective against gram-negative bacteria, especially in a single application following contamination, but it is more useful as a hemostatic agent. It is very caustic and will discolor the skin (black). Its caustic nature allows the skilled clinician to use it to burn off excessive granulation tissue or to open curled-over wound margins (epibole).

Dakin's solution is a combination of sodium hypochlorite and boric acid that is effective against *Staphylococcus* and *Streptococcus* species. Dakin's solution was an important development in treating acute wound infections and likely prevented a number of wartime amputations. However, it is frequently prescribed for use on chronic wounds that are not infected. It is highly cytotoxic unless diluted, and the AHCPR guidelines state explicitly that Dakin's solution should not be used on chronic wounds. Acetic acid, the active ingredient of vinegar, in a 0.25% solution is highly effective against *Pseudomonas* but is caustic and damages healthy tissue. The AHCPR guidelines also make specific mention of acetic acid in terms of harming healing tissue. Acetic acid may be useful for a short course of several days in wounds infected by *Pseudomonas aeruginosa*.

The development of nanocrystal technology has allowed silver to be incorporated into wound dressings of many types. Silver is a broad-spectrum antimicrobial. Dressings will be discussed further in Chapter 16. Polyhexamethylene biguanide can also be placed into dressings. In addition to its antimicrobial effects, it appears to be useful for managing biofilm-producing organisms. In general, a treatment strategy for local infection is silver sulfadiazine or silver dressings, cadexomer iodine, or polyhexamethylene biguanide. Dakin's solution for *Staphylococcus* or *Streptococcus* infection and acetic acid for *Pseudomonas* infections should be used sparingly and only for a few days. If Dakin's solution or acetic acid does not clear a local infection within a few days, an infectious disease consult should be considered. Povidone-iodine and hydrogen peroxide are considered worthless, and disinfectants such as chlorhexidine and quaternary ammonium are considered harmful and should never be placed on open wounds.

SYSTEMIC AGENTS

Many systemic antimicrobial drugs are available to treat infection. Entire texts are written to describe them. For chronic wounds, antibiotics are often not useful because systemic antibiotics do not reach therapeutic levels in chronic granulation tissue. However, these drugs become important in cases of acute wounds with advancing cellulitis. The purpose of this section of the chapter is to provide some background information for the clinician working with a patient for whom these drugs have been prescribed by a physician. As with any type of drug, antimicrobial agents have a therapeutic index (TI) that must be considered. TI is the ratio of the median toxic concentration (TD50) to the median effective concentration (ED50) (TI = TD50/ED50). Ideally, all antimicrobial drugs would have selective toxicity that would only harm bacteria (or protozoa or fungi), rather than the patient. Another consideration physicians have in prescribing antibiotics is that some antibacterial drugs are bacteriostatic, whereas others are bactericidal. Under most conditions, simply rendering bacterial replication difficult (bacteriostatic agents) is sufficient to allow the immune system to tip the wound away from infection and toward healing. However, certain conditions dictate using drugs that kill existing bacteria (bactericidal agents).

RESISTANT ORGANISMS

Inappropriate use and overuse of antibiotics have also increased the prevalence of antibiotic-resistant strains of bacteria, creating further challenges in the management of chronic wounds. MRSA is now a common problem. Prior to the use of penicillin, *S. aureus* bacteremia had a mortality of greater than 80%. Methicillin was developed to overcome the mechanism of penicillin resistance of strains of *S. aureus*. MRSA was reported in 1961 and now represents a large proportion of isolated *S. aureus*. Vancomycin has been the major antibiotic used against penicillin-resistant *S. aureus* since the 1950s. The proportion of *S. aureus* strains varies tremendously among locations. Once primarily nosocomial, community-acquired MRSA is now among the most common causes of skin and soft tissue infections. MRSA may be a resident microbe on the skin and inside the nose. Patients may develop recurrent skin abscesses and spread MRSA to others. Methicillin-resistant *Staphylococcus epidermidis* is considered to be less of a problem than MRSA, but it may become important in those with reduced immunity and implanted devices, including catheters.

Another important resistant organism is vancomycin-resistant *Enterococcus* (VRE). These bacteria (*Enterococcus faecalis* and other species) are spread easily by contact between health care providers and patients due to breakdown in standard precautions. VRE may be present in fecal matter and inadvertently spread to a patient's skin, where it may then be transmitted to a person or object coming in contact with the contaminated area.

Vancomycin-resistant *S. aureus* (VRSA) was reported in 2002, presumably due to the transfer of genes from VRE to *S. aureus*. Although it is somewhat resistant to vancomycin, it is still treatable by trimethoprim/sulfamethoxazole (Bactrim, Septra) and other antibiotics. The term *vancomycin-intermediate resistant* S. aureus is used for strains that require lower concentrations of vancomycin to inhibit growth than VRSA requires. By definition, the concentration of vancomycin needed to inhibit the growth of VRSA is 2 to 4 times that needed for vancomycin-intermediate resistant *S. aureus*.

Multidrug-resistant tuberculosis (MDR TB), although not directly involved in skin and soft tissue infections, has become an increasing problem. MDR TB may, however, be transmitted between patient and clinician. By definition, MDR TB is resistant to at least 2 of the primary antituberculosis drugs, particularly isoniazid and rifampicin. Extensively drug-resistant tuberculosis is resistant to isoniazid, rifampicin, fluoroquinolones, and at least one of the drugs used for cases resistant to these 3. For those with compromised immunity, especially those with human immunodeficiency virus infection, mortality is very high.

PROBING WOUNDS

Any open wounds suspected to be infected should be probed with a cotton-tipped applicator to inspect for the spread of the infection along fascial planes. In particular, wounds that are increasing in size or failing to respond to treatment may have subcutaneous defects such as tunneling or pockets that could be missed by only visual inspection. A mixture of aerobic and anaerobic bacteria can increase the risk of bone infection, or osteomyelitis, and bacteremia, particularly in deeper, full-thickness wounds. The ability to probe to the bone has a 50% sensitivity for osteomyelitis (50% of cases of osteomyelitis do not probe to bone) and 80% specificity (20% that probe to bone do not have osteomyelitis). Early detection of osteomyelitis might lead to earlier treatment and less likelihood of amputation.

ISSUES MAINTAINING STANDARD PRECAUTIONS

Compliance with standard precautions seems simple, but in actual practice can be difficult. PPE can be hot and uncomfortable. The trade-off of using waterproof gowns and water-resistant gowns should be considered. The likelihood of being hit with a stream of water is extremely low, whereas the risk of a waterproof gown raising body temperature to unacceptable levels can be great, particularly if worn in a room that already has an elevated temperature. A designated helper should be present when working with wounds that require the use of instruments. This person could be a technician, assistant, or student. The person must be reliable and trained in infection control procedures.

Additional packages of materials may need to be opened when gloves have already been donned and used. The designated person does not wear gloves and does not touch anything that has touched or will touch the patient. This individual can open drawers and cabinets, open packages, and retrieve supplies from outside the room such as additional towels. When gloves are donned, nothing other than things that touch the patient should be touched. Drawers and cabinets are to be closed when working with patients. If something is needed from a drawer or cabinet, work is stopped, and the cabinet or drawer is opened by someone with bare hands. Depending on the work, the handle or knob may need to be disinfected first. Never reach into a drawer or cabinet with the gloves that have been donned for patient care. If a helper is not available, gloves must be doffed and the hands sanitized before reaching into cabinets or drawers for supplies.

Nothing should be stored in open storage containers. Supplies must be behind closed doors. Work should be arranged such that the possibility of aerosolization or splashing does not reach any drawers or cabinets. For practical purposes, nothing should be stored in the same room as whirlpools.

Avoid touching the face. If itching occurs, try to ignore it; it will usually pass. If not, a helper or the arm portion of the sleeve may be used to pat over the mask or other PPE. Do not use a telephone or any other non–patient-related equipment until PPE is removed and hand hygiene is performed. In the case of an emergency, work is stopped when practical and PPE is doffed.

PERSONAL PROTECTIVE EQUIPMENT OUTSIDE PATIENT CARE SPACE

PPE is used for patients on isolation, whether because of the patient's infectious disease or because of their immunodeficiency. Facilities generally have a policy regarding the wearing of PPE in hallways. The assumption is that PPE has been worn due to isolation and the PPE has been contaminated by the patient. Once PPE is donned, one must avoid going back into a hallway. Therefore, having all the necessary equipment and supplies before entering a patient's room or room designated for wound care is paramount. Even in cases in which a designated wound care room exists, whether in a hospital, outpatient clinic, or a dedicated wound care facility, supplies and equipment should be checked frequently. Checking for materials should be minimally done at the beginning and end of the day and also after large quantities have been used for a patient. Having assistance and constant vigilance for supplies and equipment will reduce the need to leave the room during patient care.

CLEANING WORK SURFACES

High-level disinfectant should be used on all horizontal surfaces between patients. Horizontal surfaces include tabletops, stretchers, and bedside tables but also any handles or knobs to drawers or cabinets in the work area and any other surfaces where airborne material could settle. Disinfection should occur before the first patient is seen and after the last. High-level disinfection should be performed on vertical surfaces daily. Any soft surfaces that cannot be wiped adequately with disinfectant need to be covered with towels or other suitable materials that are then placed in a hamper located nearby with a foot control to minimize the risk of any transmission.

WHAT PERSONAL PROTECTIVE EQUIPMENT IS NEEDED?

The types of PPE needed will vary depending on what tasks are contemplated. If an unanticipated task is required, one simply starts the PPE donning procedure anew rather than lack appropriate protection.

- Gloves only: (1) the patient is not on contact precautions; (2) the intervention is simply inspection and redressing a stable wound, and one can be 100% certain that no fluids will leak from the wound; and (3) the intervention does not involve an open wound (eg, patient education, gait training, or exercise).
- Gloves and gown only: (1) no potential for splashing, splattering, or aerosolization, and (2) the patient is on contact precautions. Consider shoe covers if any risk of fluids dripping exists.
- Gloves, gowns, and mask only: (1) contact and droplet precautions; (2) wear an N-95 mask if airborne; and (3) no risk of splashing, splattering, or spurting.
- Gloves, gown, cap, mask, and shoe covers: procedures with any risk of splashing, splattering, spurting, or aerosolization. These include sharp debridement, pulsed lavage, whirlpools, and working with wounds with a history of severe bleeding.

STERILE TECHNIQUE

Most wound care does not need sterile technique. Colonized open wounds in patients with a reasonable level of immunity can be treated with clean technique. Clean exam gloves and PPE that are stored properly can be used. The use of clean gloves and PPE assumes that gloves have not been exposed to any splashing or aerosolization. For example, glove boxes should never be left in a room where whirlpool or pulsed lavage procedures are performed. Sterile instruments are used for debridement with clean gloves. Sterile gowns are used infrequently outside the operating room or burn unit. These gowns are considered sterile only down to the waist in the front. The forearms (up to the elbow) are considered sterile, but anywhere between the elbow and shoulder is not considered sterile. The logic behind the declaration of sterile and nonsterile areas along the upper extremity is due to the inability to see behind and the possibility of bumping an object. For these same reasons, one should never face the back of

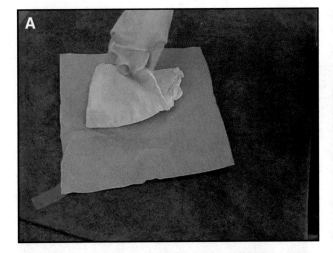

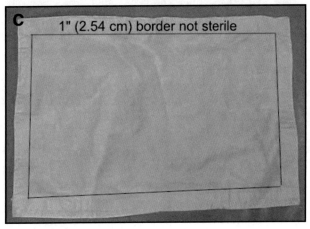

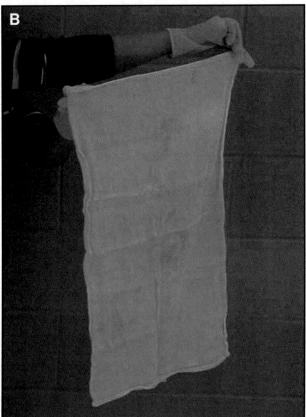

Figure 5-14. (A) Sterile towel. Removal of package by its corner. (B) Handling of sterile towel by 2 corners. By convention, none of the corners or edges within 1 inch are considered sterile. (C) One-inch border of sterile towel. This area is not considered to be part of the sterile field.

another person working with a sterile field; being back to back or front to front is acceptable. Communication with the other individuals, however, is the best way to prevent the contamination of others. Also, using the same simple rules, sterile gloved hands must be kept within prescribed sterile areas of the gown and not allowed to hang below the waist. When using sterile materials on a sterile, draped table, similar rules apply. Tables draped with a sterile field are considered sterile only on the top surface; sides are not.

Sterile technique is not an absolute term. Different levels exist for different procedures. In particular, surgery involving open bones comes the closest to sterile. Other surgical procedures in which skin is opened require sterile gloves and instruments and rules to prevent contaminating sterile fields. A sterile field is an area designated as being sterile. Only materials and instruments that will not be touched by anything other than the area involved in the procedure are allowed in the sterile field. Sterile towels (Figure 5-14) are commonly used to create a sterile field. In surgery, surrounding skin is prepared with antiseptic, and a sterile drape is placed over the surgical field.

For chronic wound procedures, antisepsis of surrounding skin and drapes are not necessary. Work spaces are disinfected and covered with a clean, dry towel or pillowcase. Towels are preferred for their absorption. Sterile towels can be used for a sterile field if a large workspace is needed. Frequently, however, packaging of equipment and supplies can be used as a sterile field. If a sterile towel is used, it must be removed first from the outer package. A marker indicating sterility should be present. The marker is usually on the tape used to seal the package. The outer package is removed, and the towel should be folded in such a way that a corner can be easily grasped without touching anywhere else on the towel. Before opening the package, a suitable site for placing the towel must be chosen. The towel is grasped by the corner and lifted straight up to avoid touching anything outside the package (see Figure 5-14A). When the towel is steady, an adjacent second corner is grasped (see Figure 5-14B), and the towel is swung into a horizontal position and allowed to settle on the work surface such that only the bottom of the sterile towel makes contact with the surface below it (see Figure 5-14C). When working with the sterile towel,

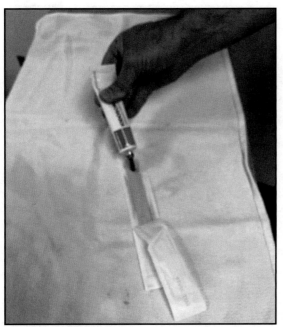

Figure 5-15. Squeezing sterile material from a tube onto an acceptable sterile field.

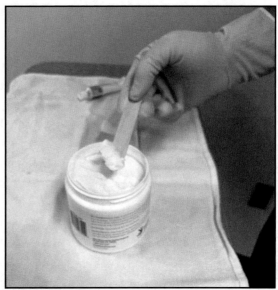

Figure 5-16. Dipping sterile material from a jar using a sterile tongue depressor.

a 1-inch (2.5-cm) border, as demonstrated on the towel in Figure 5-14C, is considered to be outside the sterile field. No sterile materials should touch within this border. The purpose of the border is to allow the towel to be picked up without sterile gloves.

Because wet materials can transmit bacteria, care must be taken to minimize wetting sterile fields. A basin of sterile saline or having an assistant wet materials as needed are options to avoid wetting a sterile field completely. Bandage rolls in plastic packages can have sterile saline added to them. Paper packages of gauze sponges that are wetted will soak through within the time of many procedures. Having a helper wet them just before using them can mitigate the issue. Nothing outside the sterile field should ever be touched when wearing gloves. If no helper is available, gloves can be doffed, hand hygiene performed, and wetting performed before donning new gloves. Similarly, materials in tubes, bottles, or jars should never be touched with gloved hands. Contents of tubes can be squeezed onto a sterile field such as tongue depressors (Figure 5-15) or cotton-tipped applicators either by a helper or before donning gloves. Ointments in jars can be scooped out with a tongue depressor in the same way. Double-dipping into jars is not permitted (Figure 5-16). A new tongue depressor or, if possible without contamination, the other end of the tongue depressor may be used. Having a helper alleviates the problem of having to retrieve more materials than anticipated. In addition to using sterile instruments for debridement, sterile dressings should be used. In the case of materials such as a packing strip that are used a bit at a time, the cap is taken off inside up, the measured length of

packing strip is cut with disinfected scissors, placed on a sterile field, and the cap replaced (Figure 5-17). Materials such as this should not be kept indefinitely or used for additional patients. All such materials are single-patient use only. They should be discarded when the episode of care ends or after several days. The cost of the material is much less than the cost of dealing with an un-necessary infection.

Packages of sterile instruments will be marked clearly. Instruments that have been autoclaved have a paper back and clear plastic front. As shown in Figure 5-12, an indicator with instructions printed will be inside the package. The black line seen in the photograph indicates adequate sterilization. Packages of dressing materials do not have an indicator but will have the words *sterile* or *sterilized* marked clearly on the package. Sterile gauze sponges may be individually packaged in paper, or a number of them may be packaged in a plastic tray with a paper top. All sterile packages have flaps above the seal on their ends. When opening sterile packages, especially paper packages, as much of the flap as possible should be grasped and pulled evenly, as shown in Figure 5-11, so the package does not tear. A torn package cannot be opened successfully without contaminating its contents.

When working with a sterile field, nothing should be held or passed over the field other than what will be placed in it. For example, if an object on the other side of a sterile field needs to be retrieved, walk around the sterile field. Instruct helpers not to pass open packages of sterile materials over the sterile field. The helper will pull the package open sufficiently to allow reaching the material without touching the outside of the package (Figure 5-18). The helper is only allowed to touch the outside of the package,

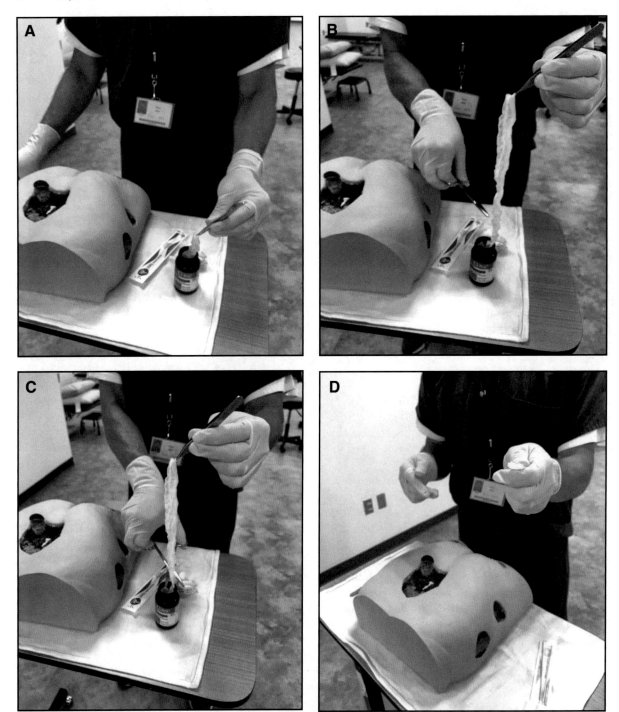

Figure 5-17. Removing the sterile packing strip from a bottle. A sufficient length is removed and cut instead of allowing the packing strip to drape over the edge of the bottle or touch the patient's surrounding skin. (A) Removing the packing strip with sterile forceps. (B) Pulling the length required of the packing strip without touching the sides of the bottle. (C) Using sterile scissors to cut the packing strip. (D) Most of the length is worked into the nondominant hand to avoid contaminating the strip.

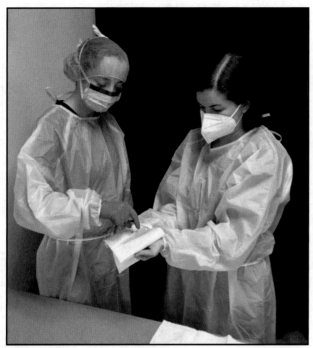

Figure 5-18. A nonsterile person passing sterile materials to a person already wearing gloves.

and the person performing wound care is only allowed to touch inside the package. The helper should walk around the sterile field to allow the material to be removed from the package.

If packages of sterile materials are used as a sterile field, the materials should never touch the edges of the package. For example, instruments from a plastic tray should be placed entirely inside the tray and not with their handles hanging over the edge (Figure 5-19). If gauze sponges inside a paper package are to be made wet, have a helper do it just as it is needed or carefully wet it just before donning gloves. Generally, people tend to tremendously overly wet gauze sponges and saturate the paper package, as shown in Figure 5-20.

Clean dressings, rather than sterile ones, may be used on pressure injuries and other chronic wounds as long as dressing procedures comply with institutional infection control guidelines. Clean dressings may also be used in the home setting. Disposal of contaminated dressings in the home should be done in a manner consistent with local regulations. In some areas, this may allow the disposal of all items in the regular trash or may require the use of biohazard containers. Recommended techniques for body substance isolation precautions are listed in Table 5-3.

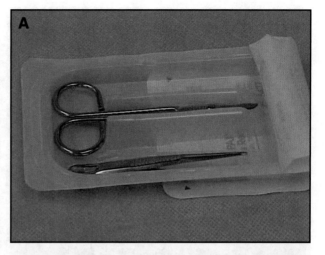

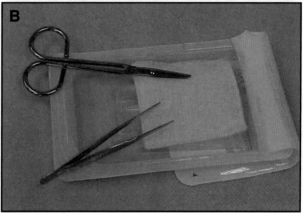

Figure 5-19. (A) Proper use of a package as a sterile field. Inside of the package is considered sterile and may be used as a sterile field. (B) Placing items on the edges of packages contaminates them.

WHIRLPOOLS

Equipment used for whirlpool therapy requires specialized care for infection control. The tank and turbine might be used for multiple patients daily. Pathogens potentially could be transmitted from one patient into the whirlpool tank or into the turbine and then to another patient. Areas of particular concern are the drain, the uppermost part of the tank, and the inside of the turbine where disinfection may prove difficult. A further concern is the possibility of aerosolization due to the agitation created by the turbine. Bacteria and other microbes present in the wound will be randomly distributed throughout the tank. Although this may remove pathogens from the wound, their distribution on the tank, within the tank, and onto any parts of the patient's body can become problematic. Pathogens from multiple wounds, intact skin, and the perineal area will be deposited in the tank, turbine, and elsewhere on the body, including the open wound. Therefore, the potential for a wound to become more contaminated instead of less

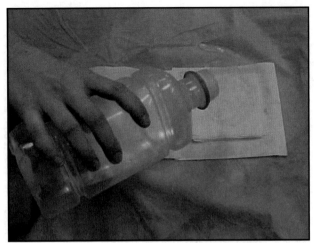

Figure 5-20. Excessive wetting of a sterile 4 × 4 leads to contamination due to soaking through the package.

exists. The movement of pathogens from one area on a patient to another is termed *cross contamination*. For infection control and other reasons to be discussed with wound debridement, whirlpool use is specifically discussed in the "Choosing Wisely" campaign of the American Physical Therapy Association (https://www.choosept.com/choosingwisely/default.aspx).

High-level disinfectants need to be rinsed thoroughly to avoid injury to the patient. Surfaces of whirlpool tubs usually receive high-level disinfection, but they are left open to airborne contamination, and contaminants may be present in tap water used to fill the whirlpool tub. When hydrotherapy is used, potential aerosolization of microbes onto other surfaces must be taken into account. In addition to keeping equipment and supplies covered, all horizontal surfaces in the treatment room must be disinfected between patients. After a patient is removed from a whirlpool, the submerged body part should be rinsed to remove contaminants, including disinfectants/antiseptics that were in the tank. Although sterile normal saline has been used routinely for irrigation, the infection rate is lower when wounds are irrigated with tap water than with normal saline provided a comparable decrease in bacterial count occurs.

Strategies for minimizing contamination and cross contamination consist of the addition of iodine or chlorine-releasing molecules such as povidone-iodine (Betadine) and chloramine T (Chlorazene). Whirlpool liners decrease the risk of contamination from patient to tank and tank to patient. However, they do not address contamination between the inside of the turbine and the patient, nor do they address cross contamination. Between patients, the tank and turbine must be cleaned and disinfected. A cleansing agent that removes proteinaceous residue must be used first to allow the disinfectant to reach the tank's surface. During this cleansing and disinfecting procedure, care must be taken to reach all surface areas that may contact the patient or the water that will be placed in the tank for the next patient. Difficult-to-reach areas include the drain, the rim, along the contours of the turbine, and a thermometer if it is present. Overlooked areas that may be missed include the upper part of the tank, the rim, and over the outside of the tank. Although the floor may become wet from doing so, these areas should be cleaned and disinfected. In addition to disinfection of the whirlpool tub, the inside and outside of the turbine must be disinfected. Running the turbine inside of a bucket of appropriate disinfectant for 10 minutes is usually recommended by manufacturers. Following cleaning and before the next patient uses the tank, high-level disinfectants must be rinsed from the tank thoroughly to avoid injury to the patient.

Spills onto the floor must be promptly cleaned and the floor disinfected. Patients at risk for respiratory infection may require a mask. Aerosolization and splashing may also occur during irrigation, especially pulsatile lavage. Masks should be worn by both the clinician and patient and splashing contained by a plastic sheet or a towel. In addition to keeping equipment and supplies covered, surfaces must be disinfected between patients.

OCCUPATIONAL SAFETY AND HEALTH ADMINISTRATION

Facilities are obligated to examine engineering controls periodically and maintain or replace them on a regular schedule. Critical work practice controls dictated by OSHA include a specific statement that all procedures involving blood or other potentially infectious materials are to be done to minimize splashing or spraying. OSHA also requires specific work practice controls. Eating, drinking, smoking, applying cosmetics or lip balm, and handling contact lenses are prohibited in work areas where exposure is likely to occur. Food and drink are not allowed to be kept in refrigerators, shelves, or other areas where blood or other potentially infectious materials are present. For conditions for which engineering and work practice controls cannot eliminate or minimize exposure, PPE is required by the OSHA regulations. For such conditions, employers are obligated to provide PPE at no cost to employees. According to OSHA, appropriate PPE may consist of gloves, gowns, laboratory coats, face shields or masks and eye protection, mouthpieces, resuscitation bags, pocket masks, or other ventilation devices. OSHA defines appropriate in such a way that the PPE does not permit blood or other potentially infectious materials to pass through to or reach the employee's work clothes, street clothes, undergarments, skin, eyes, mouth, or other mucous membranes. This statement is qualified by stating that blood and other potentially infectious material does not pass through the PPE under normal conditions of use and for the duration of time during which PPE is used. Employers are responsible for ensuring that employees use appropriate PPE except for extraordinary circumstances in which the PPE, in the opinion of the employee, might cause more harm than benefit. Under these circumstances, an analysis of the circumstances is to be undertaken to determine whether policy or procedure changes are necessary to prevent such problems from recurring. Employers are responsible for having PPE appropriate for any personnel requiring it, including any necessary sizes or accommodating allergies (eg, providing hypoallergenic gloves). Employers are also responsible for cleaning, laundering, disposal, repair, or replacement of PPE as needed to maintain its effectiveness at no cost to the employee. To prevent the spread of pathogens contaminating the PPE, all PPE must be removed and left within the work area. Facilities will typically place disposal containers within the appropriate work area rather than in common areas such as gyms or hallways, and durable PPE is left in a designated area within the work area and not carried out into common areas. OSHA states that after use, all PPE is to be placed in an appropriately designated area or container for storage, washing, decontamination, or disposal.

Employers are responsible for ensuring and maintaining clean and sanitary work sites. Because of variation in the type of activities and patient populations, appropriate written schedules for cleaning and methods of decontamination are to be determined and implemented based on characteristics of the work site, type of surface to be cleaned, type of soil present, and tasks or procedures being performed in the area. Regardless of the cleaning schedule, however, all equipment and environmental and working surfaces are to be cleaned and decontaminated after contact with blood or other potentially infectious materials. Contaminated work surfaces are to be decontaminated with an appropriate disinfectant after the completion of procedures. Decontamination is to be done immediately or as soon as feasible if surfaces are overtly contaminated or after any spill of blood or other potentially infectious materials.

Employers are obligated to offer the hepatitis B vaccine and vaccination series to all employees who have occupational exposure. Employers are also responsible for postexposure evaluation and follow-up to all employees who have had an exposure incident. Evaluations are to be made available at no cost to the employee, at a reasonable time and place, and performed by or under the supervision of a licensed physician or by or under the supervision of another licensed health care professional and provided according to recommendations of the US Public Health Service. All laboratory tests are to be conducted by an accredited laboratory at no cost to the employee.

OSHA regulations require that employers provide and ensure participation by all employees with occupational exposure in a training program at no cost to the employee and during working hours. Training is to be provided at the time of initial assignment to tasks where occupational exposure may take place and at least annually. Employers are also to provide additional training as needed if changes in tasks or how tasks are performed affect the employee's occupational exposure. The training program must at the minimum address the elements shown in Table 5-4.

WASTE DISPOSAL

Waste disposal is generally the last item that occurs following patient care, although some waste disposal may be necessary during procedures. In many facilities, clinicians may be observed to dispose of all waste in red biohazard containers. Noncontaminated waste placed in biohazard containers costs each facility thousands of dollars each year needlessly for special disposal. Careful consideration allows the clinician to be selective in the disposal of materials. The number of outer packages that are grossly contaminated during procedures can be minimized by handling only the contents or through the judicious use of sterile fields. Certainly, any grossly contaminated items and sharp instruments must be placed in appropriate biohazard containers. In contrast, packages that do not contact body fluids directly should be placed in regular waste containers. Contaminated dressings, gauze, gloves, and similar items should be placed in a red, marked biohazard bag. Waste containers are depicted in Figure 5-21. Personnel should never attempt to retrieve items that have been placed accidentally or deliberately in any waste containers, whether regular, biohazard, or sharps. In addition to trash, soiled reusable articles and

TABLE 5-4
OSHA Requirements for Employee Training

- Where the regulations can be accessed and an explanation of the regulations
- The epidemiology and symptoms of blood-borne diseases
- The modes of transmission of blood-borne pathogens
- The employer's exposure control plan
- Tasks and other activities that may involve exposure to blood and other potentially infectious materials
- Use and limitations of methods to prevent or reduce exposure, including appropriate engineering controls, work practices, and personal protective equipment
- Types, proper use, location, removal, handling, decontamination, and disposal of personal protective equipment
- The basis for selection of personal protective equipment
- Information on the hepatitis B vaccine and the appropriate actions to take and persons to contact in an emergency involving blood or other potentially infectious materials
- Methods for reporting any incident involving blood-borne pathogens and the medical follow-up that will be made available
- Information on the postexposure evaluation and follow-up that is required of the employer
- Signs, labels, and any color coding required for biohazardous materials
- An opportunity for interaction with the person conducting the training session

linen should be placed in containers that are securely sealed to prevent leaking. Double bagging is not necessary unless the outside of the bag is visibly soiled.

SHARPS CONTAINERS

Sharp instruments include needles, scalpel blades, forceps, and scissors. These objects can puncture plastic bags; therefore, they must be placed in puncture-resistant, rigid containers. Two types of containers may be used. A red, biohazard-marked container designed for disposable items is called a *sharps container*. They are equipped with a tamper-proof lid that allows objects to be placed in them but does not allow removal or overflow. Cotton-tipped applicators should also be placed in a sharps container (see Figure 5-21A). If they break after being placed in a plastic bag, a jagged edge can pierce a plastic bag and injure another person.

Regulations exist for both reusable and disposable sharps. For reusable sharp instruments, the regulations call for them to be placed immediately or as soon as possible after use in appropriate containers until properly reprocessed. By OSHA regulations, a container is considered appropriate if it is puncture resistant, it is labeled or color coded, and it is leakproof on the sides and bottom. Generally, these are metal containers with lids.

Single-use contaminated sharps are to be discarded immediately or as soon as feasible in closable, puncture-resistant, leakproof (sides and bottom), labeled or color-coded containers (see Figure 5-21B). Staff must be trained to identify the appropriate sharps container. Only disposable instruments are to be put in a designated sharps container. Items to be resterilized being placed into a sharps container is the equivalent of throwing them away. Untrained staff placing reusable instruments in sharps containers results in unwanted costs to replace lost instruments and a mystery as to where the instruments have gone.

OSHA calls for the placement of containers such that during use containers are easily accessible and located as close as is feasible to the immediate area where sharps are used. The containers are to be kept upright throughout use, replaced routinely, and are not allowed to be overfilled. Sharps containers must be closed immediately prior to removal or replacement to prevent spillage or protrusion of contents during handling, storage, or transport and placed in a secondary container that is closable and made to contain all contents and prevent leakage if leakage is possible. Secondary containers must also be labeled or color coded according to OSHA standards.

Reusable containers, typically used for reusable sharps, are not to be opened, emptied, or cleaned manually or in any other manner that would expose employees to the risk of percutaneous injury. Note that the requirement is for sharps containers to be puncture resistant. Protrusion of the contents through the walls of puncture-resistant containers will not occur under normal use. However, the mishandling of these containers could result in puncture. Also, note that the primary container is to be leakproof on the bottom and sides. These containers can leak if moved from an upright orientation or if overfilled. Personnel using or handling these containers should be trained to avoid spilling or puncturing the containers. Sharps containers and containers used to return sharp instruments for resterilization should be placed on carts and wheeled to their locations and never carried due to the risk of both spilling and potential injury from sharp edges.

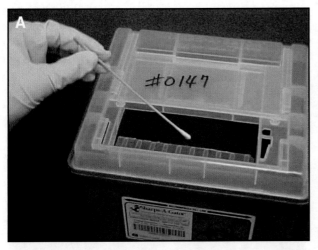
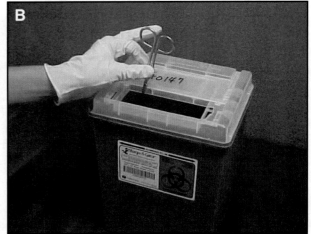
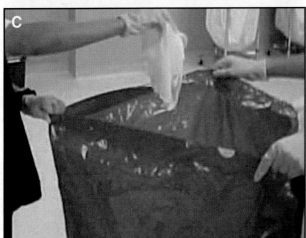
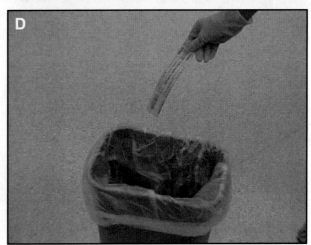
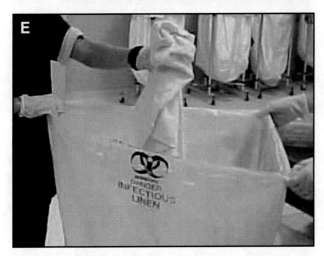

Figure 5-21. (A) Cotton-tipped applicators are placed in a sharps container due to the possibility of breaking and creating a sharp edge that could puncture a bag. (B) Disposable scissors being placed in an approved sharps container. (C) Typical biohazard disposal bag. (D) Items not grossly contaminated with body fluids are placed in a regular trash can. (E) Typical contaminated laundry bag.

BIOHAZARD VS ORDINARY TRASH RECEPTACLES

Contaminated waste is placed in containers that are readily recognized by any employees. Labels are to be fluorescent orange or orange-red or predominantly so, with lettering and symbols in a contrasting color and affixed as close as feasible to the container by string, wire, adhesive, or another method that prevents their loss or unintentional removal. Red bags or red containers may be substituted for labels (see Figure 5-21C).

Facilities should have policies in place regarding what is placed in biohazard containers. Facility policy must follow any local regulations regarding handling waste. In the past, biohazard bags placed inside residential-type trash cans have been filled indiscriminately with all sorts of trash, including wrappers that have never come close to being contaminated. A typical policy is to reserve biohazard bags for items dripping in blood or wound drainage with other items being placed in ordinary trash containers (see Figure 5-21D). This policy also means that the contents of ordinary trash containers should be treated as potentially infected. Nothing should ever be removed from any type of waste container.

LAUNDRY

OSHA regulations state that handling of contaminated laundry should be minimized, and it should be bagged or containerized at the location where it was used. To minimize handling, contaminated laundry is not to be sorted or rinsed in the location of use. Laundry bags should not be held close to the body or squeezed according to OSHA regulations. Once laundry is placed in a hamper and it is filled, the hamper should be rolled to the appropriate location rather than lifting bags out of the hamper. Contaminated laundry is to be placed and transported in bags or containers labeled or color coded appropriately. In cases in which standard precautions are used in the handling of all soiled laundry, any labeling or color coding that permits recognition by all employees is acceptable. As discussed with sharps containers and any other biohazard container, any time that soak through or leakage from the bag or container is likely, laundry is to be placed and transported in leakproof bags or containers.

Employers are also responsible for ensuring that employees who have contact with contaminated laundry wear protective gloves and other appropriate PPE. Towels or other linens used for wound care containing blood or wound drainage are placed in laundry containers based on facility policies. Laundry is assumed to be contaminated and is treated as such at some laundering facilities. OSHA regulations make a distinction between facilities that use universal precautions and those that do not. For facilities that use universal precautions, any sufficient labeling or color coding (see Figure 5-21E) is sufficient if it permits all employees to recognize the containers as contaminated. For facilities that do not use universal precautions, red bags or bags marked with the biohazard symbol are required. For such facilities, communication that the bags are not to be disposed is necessary. OSHA states that normal laundry cycles should be used according to the washer and detergent manufacturers' recommendations. Facility policies for laundry dripping with blood and wound drainage should be followed. Policies may include segregating and labeling bags containing contaminated laundry.

SUMMARY

Working with wounds creates the opportunity for wounds to be contaminated and for wounds to contaminate clinicians and others working in the facility, including those who empty waste containers or transport or clean laundry. Control of infection in wounds requires an understanding of the terms *colonization*, *infection* and *contamination*, *resident microbes*, and *transient microbes*. Acute wounds contaminated with any microbes are at risk for infection and, therefore, are treated harshly with aggressive debridement, irrigation, and application of topical antibiotics and, on occasion, systemic antibiotics. Chronic wounds are colonized by many species of microbes in a limited number. Contamination of an open wound presents the opportunity for a new microbe to grow out of control, causing infection. The terms *sterilization*, *antisepsis*, and *disinfection* were introduced. Sterilization removes all microbes and is necessary whenever invasive procedures or sharp debridement are performed. Routine wound care requires clean technique, but following general principles of sterile technique reduces the risk of contamination. Individuals with compromised immune systems require greater care to minimize the introduction of new microbes to the wound. OSHA standards require both work practice and engineering controls to minimize the risk of exposure to blood-borne pathogens and the use of PPE when these controls cannot eliminate the risk. PPE includes the protection of the eyes, nose, and mouth with face masks or face shields as appropriate; gloves at any time of exposure to body fluids; and gowns, caps, and shoe covers when appropriate. Universal precautions dictate assuming that any body fluids contain blood-borne pathogens. Both the employer and employee are obligated to follow OSHA regulations, as described previously. Annual review of OSHA regulations is required.

QUESTIONS

1. Distinguish among the following terms.
   a. Contaminated
   b. Colonized
   c. Critical colonization/local infection
   d. Infection
   e. Sterile/sterilization
   f. Clean/decontamination
   g. Asepsis/antiseptic
   h. Disinfect/disinfectant
   i. Biofilm

2. What are the typical causes of a wound changing from colonized to critically colonized?

3. What are the typical causes of a wound's environment becoming suitable for infection?

4. What are the typical interventions to return a wound's environment to promote healing?

5. List 5 consequences of wound infection.

6. List major causes of immunosuppression.

7. What is a facultative infection? What are common causes?

8. What is responsible for most cases of *C. difficile* infections?

9. What are common causes of postoperative infections?

10. Why are some people prone to recurrent infections?

11. Contrast exogenous and endogenous organisms.

12. How are exogenous and endogenous organisms controlled?

13. What options are available for identifying microbes?

14. What is the preferred culturing technique? Why?

15. What are the problems with using swab cultures?

16. What are the consequences of failure to find the correct organism?

17. What are the consequences of falsely finding the wrong organism?

18. Which surfaces need to be disinfected between patients?

19. What methods provide sterilization?

20. What are common pitfalls of handwashing?

21. What is the preferred method of hand hygiene? Why?

22. When is this method not preferred?

23. What are common antiseptics used in wound management?

24. How long should antiseptics be used on wounds?

25. What is the advantage of intravenous over oral antibiotics?

26. What is the advantage of intravenous and oral antibiotics over local antibiotics/antiseptics?

27. What is the purpose of probing a wound with respect to infection?

28. What is the major concern in terms of infection control in wound management?

29. What do the terms *engineering controls* and *practice controls* mean in terms of infection control?

30. What role does complacency play in terms of practice controls?

31. What are meant by *universal precautions* and *standard precautions*? Which term is considered to be the standard?

32. List common problems that break standard precautions.

33. Why is wearing PPE in the hallways considered to be a problem?

34. Under what conditions do you need to wear the following?
    a. Gloves only
    b. Gloves and gown
    c. Gloves, gown, and mask
    d. Gloves, gown, mask with eye shield, caps, and shoe covers

35. When are sterile gloves required instead of exam gloves?

36. Should instruments and dressings always be sterile?

37. What are the potential consequences of using hydrotherapy with regard to infection control?

38. Why do whirlpool tanks need to be scrubbed with abrasive cleaners?

39. Why do whirlpool tanks require high-level disinfection?

40. What is considered to be the weakest point of whirlpool disinfection?

41. Why do used cotton-tipped applicators go into a sharps container instead of a bag?

42. How are resterilizable instruments sent for processing?

BIBLIOGRAPHY

Ad Hoc Committee of the Committee on Trauma, Division of Medical Sciences, National Research Council. Report: postoperative wound infections: the influence of ultraviolet radiation of the operating room and the influence of other factors. *Ann Surg.* 1964;160(Suppl 2):11-192.

Berríos-Torres SI, Umscheid CA, Bratzler DW, et al. Centers for Disease Control and Prevention Guideline for the Prevention of Surgical Site Infection, 2017. *JAMA Surg.* 2017;152(8):784-791. doi:10.1001/jamasurg.2017.0904

Bill TJ, Ratliff CR, Donovan AM, Knox LK, Morgan RF, Rodeheaver GT. Quantitative swab culture versus tissue biopsy: a comparison in chronic wounds. *Ostomy Wound Manage.* 2001;47(1):34-37.

Bochner BS, Lichtenstein LM. Anaphylaxis. *N Engl J Med.* 1991;324(25):1785-1790.

Bohannon RW. Whirlpool versus whirlpool rinse for removal of bacteria from a venous stasis ulcer. *Phys Ther.* 1982;62(3):304-308.

Bucknall TE. The effect of local infection upon wound healing: an experimental study. *Br J Surg.* 1980;67(12):851-855.

Burton GRW, Engelkirk PG, Fader, RC. *Microbiology for the Health Sciences.* Lippincott-Raven Publishers; 1996.

Centers for Disease Control and Prevention. Guide to infection prevention in outpatient settings. https://www.cdc.gov/infectioncontrol/pdf/outpatient/guide.pdf

Cooper ML, Laxer JA, Hansbrough JF. The cytotoxic effects of commonly used topical antimicrobial agents on human fibroblasts and keratinocytes. *J Trauma.* 1991;31(6):775-782.

Cutting KF, White RJ. Criteria for identifying wound infection—revisited. *Ostomy Wound Manage.* 2005;51(1):28-34.

Demling RH, Waterhouse B. The increasing problem of wound bacterial burden and infection in acute and chronic soft-tissue wounds caused by methicillin-resistant Staphylococcus aureus. *J Burns Wound.* 2007;7:86-98.

Gardner SE, Frantz RA, Doebbeling BN. The validity of the clinical signs and symptoms used to identify localized chronic wound infection. *Wound Repair Regen.* 2001;9(3):178-86.

Grayson ML, Gibbons GW, Balogh K, Levin E, Karchmer AW. Probing to bone in infected pedal ulcers. A clinical sign of underlying osteomyelitis in diabetic patients. *JAMA.* 1995 ;273(9):721-723.

Greif R, Akca O, Horn E-P. Kurz A, Sessler DI. Supplemental perioperative oxygen to reduce the incidence of surgical-wound infection. *N Engl J Med.* 2000;342(3):161-167.

Hospital Infection Control Practices Advisory Committee. Guidelines for Isolation Precautions in Hospitals Hospital Infection Control Advisory Committee. http://wonder.cdc.gov/wonder/prevguid/p0000419/P0000419.asp#head002004000000000

Levine NS, Lindberg RB, Mason AD, Pruitt BA. The quantitative swab culture and smear: a quick, simple method for determining the number of viable aerobic bacteria on open wounds. *J Trauma.* 1976;16(2):89-94.

Lineaweaver W, Howard R, Soucy D, et al. Topical antimicrobial toxicity. *Arch Surg.* 1985;120(3):267-270.

Mertz PM, Oliveira-Gandia MF, Davis SC. The evaluation of a cadexomer iodine wound dressing on methicillin-resistant Staphylococcus aureus (MRSA) in acute wounds. *Dermatol Surg.* 1999;25(2):89-93.

Moscati RM, Mayrose J, Reardon RF, Janicke DM, Jehle DV. A multicenter comparison of tap water versus sterile saline for wound irrigation. *Acad Emerg Med.* 2007;14(5):404-409.

Moscati RM, Reardon RF, Lerner EB, Mayrose J. Wound irrigation with tap water. *Acad Emerg Med.* 1998;5(11):1076-1080.

Niederhuber SS, Stribley RF, Koepke GH. Reduction of skin bacterial load with use of the therapeutic whirlpool. *Phys Ther.* 1975;55(5):482-486.

OSHA Regulations (Standards 29 CFR). Bloodborne Pathogens. 1910.1030. https://www.osha.gov/laws-regs/regulations/standard-number/1910/1910.1030

Perelman VS, Francis GJ, Rutledge T, Foote J, Martino F, Dranitsaris G. Sterile versus nonsterile gloves for repair of uncomplicated lacerations in the emergency department: a randomized controlled trial. *Ann Emerg Med.* 2004;43(3):362-370.

Robson MC. Wound infection. A failure of wound healing caused by an imbalance of bacteria. *Surg Clin North Am.* 1997;77(3):637-650.

Robson MC, Duke WF, Krizek TJ. Rapid bacterial screening in the treatment of civilian wounds. *J Surg Res.* 1973;14(5):426-430.

Robson MC, Stenberg BD, Heggers JP. Wound healing alterations caused by infection. *Clin Plast Surg.* 1990;17(3):485-492.

Shankowsky HA, Callioux LS, Tredget EE. North American survey of hydrotherapy in modern burn care. *J Burn Care Rehabil.* 1994;15(2):143-146.

Siegel JD, Rhinehart E, Jackson M, Chiarello L, the Healthcare Infection Control Practices Advisory Committee. 2007 Guideline for Isolation Precautions: Preventing Transmission of Infectious Agents in Healthcare Settings. https://www.cdc.gov/infectioncontrol/pdf/guidelines/isolation-guidelines-H.pdf

Sussman GL, Beezhold DH. Allergy to latex rubber. *Ann Intern Med.* 1995;122(1):43-46.

Sussman GL, Liss GM, Deal K, et al. Incidence of latex sensitization among latex glove users. *J Allergy Clin Immunol.* 1998;101(2 Pt 1):171-178.

Ward RS, Saffle JR. Topical agents in burn and wound care. *Phys Ther.* 1995;75(6):526-538.

White RJ, Cutting KF. Critical colonization—the concept under scrutiny. *Ostomy Wound Manage.* 2006;52(11):50-56.

Zamora JL, Price MF, Chuang P, Gentry LO. Inhibition of povidone-iodine's bactericidal activity by common organic substances: an experimental study. *Surgery.* 1985;98(1):25-29.

Zhou LH, Nahm WK, Badiavas E, Yufit T, Falanga V. Slow release iodine preparation and wound healing: in vitro effects consistent with lack of in vivo toxicity in human chronic wounds. *Br J Dermatol.* 2002;146(3):365-374.

Pain Management

Irion GL, Gardner JA, Pignataro RM.
Comprehensive Wound Management, Third Edition (pp 91-99).
© 2024 Taylor and Francis Group.

OBJECTIVES

- List causes of pain and itch in wounds.
- Discuss physical therapy management of pain, including electrotherapy (transcutaneous electrical nerve stimulation, interferential current, and iontophoresis).
- Discuss the medical management of pain and the need to communicate with the patient's physician to optimize pain management.
- Discuss the relevance of newly occurring itch or pain.

Pain is another factor that can influence wound healing. Pain is the product of nociception and the pain matrix. In patients with normal sensation, acute and chronic wounds can induce pain that corresponds to the severity of the wound. However, pain can also occur without nociceptive input, and significant nociceptive input does not necessarily result in pain. In addition, patients with neurologic impairments, such as spinal cord injury and peripheral neuropathy, may lack awareness of pain, reducing their perception and protection from noxious stimuli that can damage the skin. Wound-related pain levels may also depend on certain aspects of treatment, such as choice of dressing, frequency of dressing changes, circulatory damage, or any underlying neuromuscular or musculoskeletal injuries. Therefore, pain associated with wound management may have multiple causes and, at the same time, may vary widely among patients, even those with identical pathology. Injury, infection, surgical management, and harsh treatments that lead to inflammation contribute to the potential for pain. For example, an abscess requiring incision and drainage, which is then packed and then needs to be unpacked for further debridement, is highly likely to result in a painful experience for the patient. However, components of the pain matrix may modulate the nociceptive input creating a situation that the patient might easily tolerate without any medical pain management, whereas another person receiving the upper limit of morphine may not be willing to participate in treatment. Expectation of pain, history of pain responses, fear avoidance, and lack of confidence in the health care provider are all possible modulators of nociceptive input.

A patient is unlikely to have complaints of pain without nociceptive input; therefore, the integrity of nociceptors plays a major role in pain. Superficial and partial-thickness wounds can involve less substantial tissue injury in comparison to full-thickness wounds, but when superficial and partial thickness wounds leave nociceptors intact, they can produce tremendous pain. Although aggressive debridement obviously incurs substantial risk of causing pain, one should be aware that dressing changes and even incidental tugging on devitalized structures that are still attached to innervated, sensitized tissues can also lead to pain.

INFLAMMATION

Inflammation can produce pain due to the swelling but also due to the release of chemical mediators that produce hyperalgesia, which is defined as an increased sensitivity to a given nociceptive input. Heat and redness observed around the wound should indicate the great likelihood of increased sensitivity. Acute wounds such as abscess incision and drainage can have substantial inflammation due to the combination of infection followed by surgical intervention. Chronic wounds may also be painful due to the constant activation of nociceptors, potentially leading to increased sensitivity. Moreover, wound chronicity may lead to allodynia, in which trivial sensory input is interpreted as a painful stimulus. Allodynia is often considered on a spectrum of heightened sensitivity with hyperalgesia.

PAINFUL AND PAINLESS WOUNDS

During the intake process, clinicians can start with some initial assumptions concerning the patient's pain burden while a full pain assessment is performed. Burns will always have painful areas. Full-thickness portions with nociceptors completely damaged will not provide nociceptive input, but the adjacent tissue with intact nociceptors may lead to exquisite pain. Arterial wounds are generally considered painful. Venous ulcers are generally considered less painful, but the quality of ischemic pain is also different. Ischemia produces chemical mediators sensitizing nociceptors, whereas venous disease produces more of a pressure

or bursting type of discomfort/pain. Pressure injuries can be painful along edges where nociceptors are intact. Ulcers produced by sickle cell disease, calciphylaxis, Behcet's syndrome, and malignancies can also be painful. Sickle cell ulcers, in particular, tend to be very sensitive to trauma of debridement and even dressing changes. Neuropathic wounds are typically not painful, but neuropathy itself can lead to neuropathic pain with sharp, brief, intermittent discomfort (dysesthesia) or periods of "pins and needles" (paresthesia).

PAIN ASSESSMENT

Adequate pain management helps promote patient comfort and better quality of life. When left untreated, pain can also have a negative impact on physiological processes of healing. Extreme and/or prolonged pain may perpetuate the inflammatory response and interfere with cellular proliferation. Research has also shown that the pain response stimulates the release of neuropeptides, such as substance P and neurokinin A, which trigger leukocytes to produce proinflammatory cytokines. Pain can also promote release of cortisol, an endogenous glucocorticoid that interferes with cellular proliferation. During the transition from proliferation to maturation, the pain response can also lead to increased tissue fibrosis. Additionally, patients with pain tend to limit their mobility to avoid further discomfort. This can lead to greater functional loss and impaired activities of daily living. Other aspects of a biopsychosocial approach to wound management must also be considered, such as the close association among pain, anxiety, and depression. For these reasons, wound assessment and a comprehensive plan of care must incorporate the need for appropriate pain management prior to interventions.

Several tools are available to assist in pain assessment. The simplest is the visual analog scale. A patient makes a mark on the scale along a horizontal line with the left end representing no pain and the right end representing the worst pain imaginable. The clinician then measures the distance across the scale with the left end being 0 and the right end being 10. An alternative is to simply ask the patient to give a number between 0 and 10, with 10 representing the maximum pain. In a written format, the patient can mark a visual analog scale (Figure 6-1) that can then be converted to a 0 to 10 scale. Verbal descriptors can also be used to convey pain quality (eg, sharp, dull, achy, pulsating, burning, etc). The short-form McGill Pain Questionnaire is a common tool (Figure 6-2). The Wong-Baker FACES Pain Rating Scale is one of several graphic representations that can be used to help people with limited verbal or reading ability to select a picture representing their present level of distress and is often used with children (Figure 6-3). Pain location can be documented using a body diagram.

No pain ━━━━━━━━━━━━━━━━━━━━━━━━━━━━━━ Worst pain imaginable

Directions: Indicate your pain in relation to the two extremes. Make a mark at the distance across that you think your pain is. A mark made in the middle of the line means your pain is half of the worst possible pain you could experience.

Figure 6-1. Visual analog scale used for patients to indicate the intensity of pain.

SHORT FORM McGILL PAIN QUESTIONNAIRE

Date: _____

Name: _____

Check the column to indicate the level of your
pain for each word, or leave blank if it does not
apply to you.

	Mild	Moderate	Severe
1. Throbbing	_____	_____	_____
2. Shooting	_____	_____	_____
3. Stabbing	_____	_____	_____
4. Sharp	_____	_____	_____
5. Cramping	_____	_____	_____
6. Gnawing	_____	_____	_____
7. Hot-burning	_____	_____	_____
8. Aching	_____	_____	_____
9. Heavy	_____	_____	_____
10. Tender	_____	_____	_____
11. Splitting	_____	_____	_____
12. Tiring-exhausting	_____	_____	_____
13. Sickening	_____	_____	_____
14. Fearful	_____	_____	_____
15. Cruel-punishing	_____	_____	_____

Indicate on this line how bad your pain is—at the left end of line means no pain at all, at right end means worst pain possible.

No Pain _____ Worst Possible Pain

S/33   A /12   VAS /10

Figure 6-2. Short Form from McGill Pain Questionnaire. (Reproduced with permission of author, Dr. Ron Melzack, for publication and distribution.)

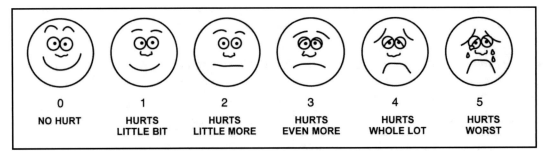

Figure 6-3. Wong-Baker FACES pain rating scale. Originally designed for children but can be used for individuals who cannot use a visual analog scale. Instructions are also available in a number of other languages. (Mosby; 2009. Used with permission. Copyright Mosby.)

TYPES OF PAIN ASSOCIATED WITH WOUNDS

While magnitude of pain is an important characteristic, the clinician should also seek information about quality, timing, and alleviating or exacerbating factors. The acronym PQRST is often used with pain assessment. What Provokes the pain, what is the Quality of the pain, does it Radiate, how Severe is it, and what are the Temporal characteristics of the pain? Does the patient experience background, breakthrough, or procedural pain (2 of these or all 3)? If the pain characteristics using PQRST do not fit the descriptions of background, breakthrough, and procedural pain as described in the following section, a more thorough investigation into the pain is required.

Subsequent pain assessment should use a consistent scale and continue to incorporate each of these dimensions when determining whether the level and pattern of discomfort experienced by the patient have changed. Additional attention should be given to nonverbal signs of distress, such as facial expressions and the patient's overall affect.

Background Pain

Pain associated with the underlying cause of the wound and occurring at rest can be described as background pain. The quality and radiation of background pain vary with the underlying cause. A throbbing or aching type of pain can occur with traumatic injuries and pressure injuries. Cramping type of pain is expected with arterial ulcers, and venous ulcers often have a bursting type of low to moderate pain. In addition, we need to consider operative pain from the trauma to surrounding tissue, inflammation secondary to the trauma, and packing or other procedures performed prior to referral.

Breakthrough Pain

Pain of a rapid onset that is severe, brief, and seems to occur "out of the blue" describes breakthrough pain. It is related to the underlying pathology and may be triggered by minor trauma such as dressing movement, dependency of a limb, or movement in general. It tends to be accompanied by wincing and verbal output.

Procedural Pain

Pain that occurs with interventions such as dressing changes, debridement, or removal of packing can be categorized as procedural pain. This type of pain is graded with the degree of trauma induced by the procedure and does not persist much beyond the event. The intensity can be severe depending on how sensitized the patient is prior to the intervention.

PAIN MANAGEMENT STRATEGIES

Following a thorough assessment of baseline pain, the patient, clinician, and care team must decide whether the pain associated with the selected intervention(s) will be tolerated or how the pain can be made tolerable. Surgical debridement under general anesthesia can be utilized for cases in which the pain will be too great and/or too much tissue needs to be removed. However, some patients are not candidates for general anesthesia. Another option is for a physician to prescribe either a local anesthetic or an analgesic for interventions. In particular, severe background pain with fear avoidance may require surgical intervention.

Before beginning any interventions, a series of questions should be asked. First, who is responsible for the patient's pain management? In an outpatient setting, a referring physician is generally available to consult. In a self-referral situation, another physician may need to be identified. In an acute care hospital, a given patient may have a number of physicians. More than one physician may believe that they are managing pain, or none of the physicians may be managing pain. Second, is pain management even necessary? In many cases, a patient is already on a pain management regimen, or in the case of many neuropathic ulcers, nociception is absent. Third, is medical management necessary? A wound may not be painful for a number of reasons. Gentler treatment and reassurance may be enough in many cases. Alternatives to prescription pain medications include the use of topical local anesthetics or non–prescription-strength nonsteroidal anti-inflammatory drugs. A confident and competent clinician is far less likely to evoke pain than one who cannot gain the confidence of the patient. Patients may ask, "Is this going to hurt?" The correct response can be yes, no, or maybe. Before attempting any interventions, even removing a dressing for the first time, the clinician simply does not know. One can try to be honest and state that it likely will be but that can sensitize a patient into perceiving pain that would not have occurred without the anticipation of pain. If a patient is told that pain will not occur and it does, the clinician loses credibility, and pain is more likely to be perceived. One potential answer to the question is simply, "Some patients say they feel better, and others find it a bit uncomfortable." This approach deliberately avoids the sensitizing words of "but" and "pain." This approach does not guarantee patient satisfaction, but clinicians should attempt anything that can minimize sensitization.

Pain management strategies are more likely to be effective if the type of pain is identified. Identifying and treating the cause of background pain can lessen any sensitization that would otherwise reduce a patient's tolerance for procedures. Reducing trauma by gentler interventions and better management of the wound environment and surrounding skin can lessen the severity of background pain. Unfortunately, treatment of the underlying cause of pain is not always possible. For example, off-loading pressure injuries or providing compression therapy for venous insufficiency ulcers may lessen background pain, but for patients experiencing pain due to ischemia or arterial ulcers, revascularization or some other form of medical management is generally needed to reduce background pain. Medical strategies for background pain are done in a stepwise strategy that starts with nonopioid analgesics. Nonsteroidal anti-inflammatory drugs can be augmented with tricyclic antidepressants, benzodiazepines, or anticonvulsants. If this strategy is insufficient, the next step involves opioid analgesics such as codeine or tramadol. The third step is hydrocodone or oxycodone, possibly combined with acetaminophen, in the forms of Vicodin, Lortab, or Norco.

Breakthrough pain can be very severe and can sensitize patients to procedural pain. Strategies for managing breakthrough pain include assurance and desensitization. Patients are assured that breakthrough pain is a normal phenomenon and brief, severe pain does not mean that any additional injury is occurring. Relaxation techniques, such as modulated breathing, can be used. Addressing movement patterns that jostle the wounded area, use of assistive devices, orthoses, positioning (especially dependency for venous ulcers), and aggravators such as coughing or constipation may improve breakthrough pain tremendously for some patients. In some cases, the same type of pharmacologic intervention as background pain may be necessary.

Management of background and breakthrough pain can mitigate procedural pain. Reducing background and breakthrough pain raises the threshold for pain during interventions. In addition, maintaining a moist wound bed and protecting the integrity of the surrounding skin reduce tissue injury and sensitivity to mechanical stimuli that could lead to pain. Avoiding adhesives by using nonadherent dressing materials and using silicone adhesives instead of stronger types can reduce wound trauma. When possible, address painful areas of the wound last to minimize sensitization.

INTERVENTIONS AVAILABLE FOR NONPHYSICIANS

Affective strategies can be effective in mitigating pain. The clinician's calming presence and air of competence and credibility reduce the likelihood of reaching a painful threshold, whereas waffling and insecure demeanor can sensitize patients to pain. Eliminating surprises by explaining interventions, setting expectations for the patient, and avoiding conflict and shaming gain the trust of the patient. Music that the patient finds pleasant and other diversions can also be helpful. Other possible interventions include electrotherapy, topical local anesthetics, and sedation.

PATIENT EDUCATION

Strategies commonly employed in outpatient spine clinics can also be used in the wound management arena for select patients. As seen in spine clinics, patients with wounds may also learn maladaptive responses to their wounds, resulting in amplification of pain through central sensitization and catastrophizing. Clinicians trained in dealing with central sensitization can assist patients to change any maladaptive perceptions and pain cognitions as well as restore normal movement patterns that may have been altered through kinesiophobia ("an excessive, irrational, and debilitating fear of physical movement and activity resulting from a feeling of vulnerability due to

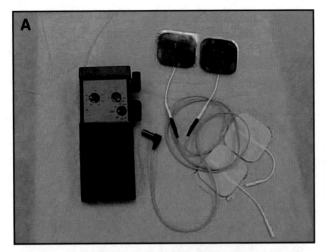
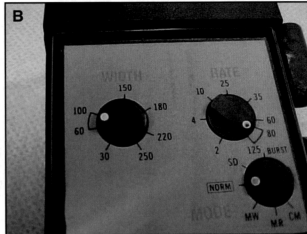
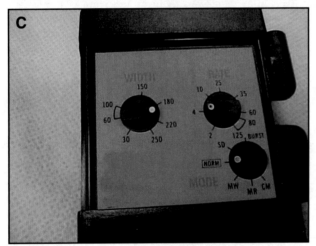
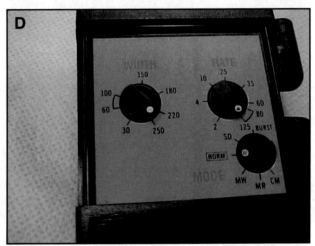

Figure 6-4. (A) Typical TENS unit. (B) Conventional TENS settings. (C) Low-frequency TENS settings. (D) Brief intense TENS settings.

painful injury or reinjury"[1]), fear avoidance, and catastrophizing. The fear-avoidance model is used to explain how a negative pain experience results in amplification of pain, in contrast to a more positive response to pain that leads to recovery. In this model, some people will develop a negative pain experience leading to a cycle of catastrophizing pain, pain-related fear, avoidance, and hypervigilance. This leads to disuse, depression, and disability, which produce an even more negative pain experience, further amplifying the negative perceptions. Patients may need to be trained in learning what movements are potentially harmful and guided through normal, nonharmful movements that may result in less perception of pain.

ELECTROTHERAPY

Electrotherapeutic interventions for reducing wound-related pain include transcutaneous electrical nerve stimulation (TENS) and interferential current (IFC). The brief intense mode of TENS can produce near anesthesia. A similar condition can be produced by IFC. Iontophoresis with lidocaine is another possibility to achieve a state similar to infiltration with lidocaine. Complications of using electrotherapy include maintaining a sterile/clean field without wires contaminating the field, the potential need for a physician's referral to use electrotherapy, and whether the patient is willing to use it.

Transcutaneous Electrical Nerve Stimulation

A typical TENS device is depicted in Figure 6-4A. Controls include intensity, frequency, and pulse width. Default settings for conventional TENS frequency and pulse width are typically marked on these controls as a means of modulating intensity, pulse width, or a combination of them. Modes of TENS that might be used include conventional, low frequency, and brief intense.

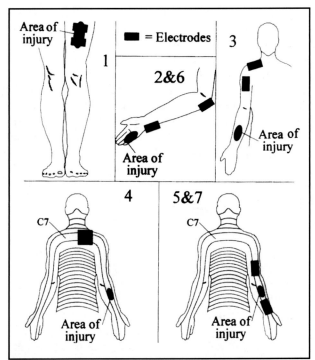

Figure 6-5. Rationales for TENS electrode placement. The 7 rationales include the following. (1) Directly over the site of injury or pathology, providing the skin is intact. (2) Over the trunk of the peripheral nerve innervating the area of injury or pathology. The nerve must be superficial (eg, peroneal or ulnar nerve). (3) Over the nerve plexus from which the nerve innervating the area of pain originates. In particular, the brachial plexus can be very useful for pain anywhere in the upper extremity. An electrode is placed over Erb's point (the area between the clavicle and trapezius where the brachial plexus is the most superficial). (4) Over the sensory nerve roots innervating the site of pain (using a dermatome chart). (5) Within the same dermatome as the site of pain (assuming affected nociceptors are entering the same dorsal root as the stimulated mechanoreceptive neurons). (6) Over the motor point of an injured or painful muscle. The motor point is the location at which one obtains a muscle contraction with the lowest current. Presumably this location is directly over the nerve of the muscle, which also contains sensory neurons of the muscle (Aα fibers). (7) Arranged so that the current will run between 2 electrodes through the area of pain.

Modes of Transcutaneous Electrical Nerve Stimulation

Conventional TENS may be used during or following a procedure. TENS could also potentially be used to manage background and breakthrough pain. As depicted in Figure 6-4B, conventional TENS uses a shorter pulse width and a high frequency or pulse rate. The intensity is set to a sensory level, which produces a tingling sensation. Conventional TENS is more likely to be used following rather than during procedures.

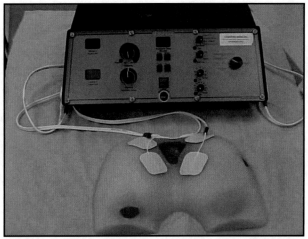

Figure 6-6. Setup for IFC treatment. Note the electrode placement pattern of 2 leads set perpendicular to each other.

Low-frequency TENS is depicted in Figure 6-4C. As the name implies, frequency is very low. Pulse width is at the upper end available. Intensity is set to produce a "pricking" sensation that some people may not tolerate. Low frequency is often claimed to be an acupuncturelike mode. It seems best suited for mitigating postprocedural pain.

Brief intense TENS is produced by gradually increasing both frequency and pulse width as tolerated by the patient (Figure 6-4D). Intensity may also be increased. Done well, brief intense TENS can produce anesthesia. However, some patients may be reluctant to try electrotherapy, and others may not tolerate the brief intense mode.

Multiple approaches for TENS electrode placement can be tried. The simplest is to place an electrode on each side of the wound as depicted in Figure 6-5. Other methods include placing the electrodes over the peripheral nerve serving the area, over the spinal nerve serving the area, and over the brachial plexus for upper extremity wounds.

Interferential Current

Setting up IFC is complicated by the need to cross the 2 alternating currents. Electrodes from one lead are set up perpendicular to the second lead such that the 2 currents produce constructive interference. This produces a sensation similar to conventional TENS, with the sensation of varying pulse rate and/or intensity within the area of tissue central to the placement of the electrodes. IFC setup is shown in Figure 6-6. By gradually increasing pulse width, frequency, and intensity, brief intenselike anesthesia may be created. Because of the number of wires involved, care in setting it up to avoid the wound and any sterile fields must be taken. Similar to TENS, some people may not tolerate the current.

MEDICAL MANAGEMENT

Potential medical pain management strategies include general anesthesia or local anesthesia using infiltration, localized block, and either epidural or spinal anesthesia. Due to costs of personnel, general anesthesia is reserved for surgical debridement. Infiltration of local anesthesia is accomplished by the use of a hypodermic needle and multiple small injections in different directions in the tissue involved. In most open wounds, infiltration of local anesthesia is difficult to perform and unrealistic. Nerve or plexus blocks are commonly used for orthopedic surgery but are cost prohibitive for the nonphysician. Local anesthetics are injected or slowly released from a device onto either a peripheral nerve or the brachial plexus.

Over-the-counter or prescription-strength nonsteroidal anti-inflammatory drugs are sometimes sufficient for some patients. Opioids can be given either orally or by an intravenous line. Oral medications will require a longer lead time before a procedure, whereas intravenous morphine or other opioids will be effective almost immediately. Regardless of setting, opioids increase the patient's risk of falls. In addition, outpatients using opioids should not be driving themselves to appointments. If a patient is using opioids, clinicians should determine that a patient is not driving a vehicle to outpatient appointments. Patient-controlled analgesia may already be in use before a referral, but it is unlikely to be provided for wound interventions by a nonphysician.

Benzodiazepines are commonly used as antianxiety drugs. Valium (diazepam), Xanax (alprazolam), Klonopin (clonazepam), Ativan (lorazepam), and Versed (midazolam) are common examples of anxiolytic medications. The reduction of anxiety can decrease the perception of pain. Both Ativan and Versed have the additional benefits of creating amnesia for the event and reduce agitation during procedures. For some patients, benzodiazepines may allow wound interventions to be performed that otherwise may not have been possible and, thereby, avoid surgery and general anesthesia.

Topical Anesthetics

Topical local anesthetics can be provided as a liquid, gel, or spray. Liquid is more difficult to localize because it will run downhill and may not stay in place long enough to be effective. Gels will stay in place much better. A third option is spray. Administration of local anesthetic to a wound may require a physician's order. In the outpatient setting, a patient may obtain their own ointment, gel, or spray and apply it ahead of time. Spray such as Hurricaine contains benzocaine. Both lidocaine and benzocaine are available in gel form. Orajel is a benzocaine-containing gel designed for oral use. Benzocaine and lidocaine are both available in cream form. Another cream is EMLA (eutectic mixture of local anesthetics), which is used for local anesthetics over vascular ports used for antibiotics and cancer chemotherapy at home. EMLA contains prilocaine and lidocaine.

Antipruritic Medications

Itching is physiologically similar to pain. Although itching can be beneficial in alerting one to potentially harmful chemicals or exoparasites, it can create a strong urge to scratch the skin. In some cases, people have created open wounds due to the intense desire to scratch. Patients can be taught to mechanically stimulate the skin in a less harmful manner, such as patting the skin instead of scratching. If this strategy is unsuccessful, medications can be prescribed. Five percent doxepin cream sold under the name Prudoxin, oral gabapentin (Neurontin), ondansetron (Zofran), or diphenhydramine (Benadryl) may be effective. Doxepin has many other uses as a serotonin-norepinephrine reuptake inhibitor. It is used as an antidepressant, anxiolytic, and antihistamine. Gabapentin is also used for chronic pain. Ondansetron is an antiemetic drug, and diphenhydramine is an antihistamine.

ONSET OF NEW PAIN OR ITCH

Itch frequently occurs during healing and can be considered a normal response when a wound is on a good healing trajectory. However, itch occurring when a wound is not healing well can be a sign of wound deterioration. New pain in a wound is generally a bad sign and likely due to infection. If pus, cellulitis, and other signs of infection are not obvious, the clinician should probe the wound for subcutaneous defects that might be harboring infection that are not visible from the wound's surface. If pain and new or worsening infection are observed, the patient's physician should be contacted as soon as practical. If systemic signs of infection (fever, malaise, somnolence, and anorexia) are present along with new pain and signs of new or worsening infection, the physician should be contacted immediately. If the physician cannot be contacted immediately, the patient should be transported to an emergency facility.

SUMMARY

Pain management is an important part of wound management. Patients should be evaluated for the sources of pain using the PQRST system to determine whether pain is background, breakthrough, procedural, or more than one. Both medical and nonmedical pain management can be used. Using a team approach, clinicians need to identify which team members are responsible for the patient's pain management and whether medical management is necessary. Because pain perception involves multiple physiological, mechanical, psychological, and emotional stimuli, affective strategies that reduce the sensitization to pain may also be useful. Knowing the type of pain management being used and the additional effects of the strategy impacts the plan of care. Intravenous opioids allow wound management to begin almost immediately, whereas oral opioids require up to 30 minutes to be effective and should be coordinated with wound interventions. Alternatives to medical management include electrotherapy and topical local anesthetics. One should ascertain whether a physician's order is required for topical anesthetic application. In an outpatient setting, patients may obtain over-the-counter local anesthetics and apply to the wound's edges themselves. Itch from a well-healing wound is a common but normal phenomenon. Pain or itch with a poor healing trajectory should raise the suspicion of new or worsening infection.

QUESTIONS

1. What causes patients to experience pain related to a wound?

2. What can be done in the context of physical therapy wound management to ameliorate pain?

3. What pain medications may be administered by a physical therapist? What limitations apply?

4. What precautions should be followed when a patient uses strong analgesics to control wound pain?

5. What may a patient use on their own to manage pain?

6. What alternatives to analgesics are available to manage pain?

7. What is the advantage of Ativan or Versed as an adjuvant to pain medications?

8. What is itch?

9. When does itch occur in the course of wound healing?

10. What options are available for dealing with itching?

11. What does a sudden change in pain and/or itch usually mean? What should you do to confirm your suspicion?

12. What should you do with new onset of pain in a wound?

REFERENCE

1. Kori S, Miller R, Todd D. Kinesiophobia: a new view of chronic pain behavior. *Pain Manag.* 1990;3(1):35-43.

BIBLIOGRAPHY

Bechert K, Abraham SE. Pain management and wound care. *J Am Col Certif Wound Spec.* 2009;1(2):65-71.

Broadbent E, Petrie KJ, Alley PG, Booth RJ. Psychological stress impairs early wound repair following surgery. *Psychosom Med.* 2003;65(5):865-869.

Buer N, Linton SJ. Fear-avoidance beliefs and catastrophizing: occurrence and risk factor in back pain and ADL in the general population. *Pain.* 2002;99(3):485-491. doi:10.1016/S0304-3959(02)00265-8

Ciccone CD. *Pharmacology in Rehabilitation.* 2nd ed. F.A. Davis; 1996.

Fischerauer SF, Talaei-Khoei M, Bexkens R, Ring DC, Oh LS, Vranceanu AM. What is the relationship of fear avoidance to physical function and pain intensity in injured athletes? *Clin Orthop Relat Res.* 2018;476(4):754-763. doi:10.1007/s11999.0000000000000085

Gatchel RJ, Mayer TG, Theodore BR. The pain disability questionnaire: relationship to one-year functional and psychosocial rehabilitation outcomes. *J Occup Rehabil.* 2006;16(1):75-94.

Gatchel RJ, Peng YB, Peters ML, Fuchs PN, Turk DC. The biopsychosocial approach to chronic pain: scientific advances and future directions. *Psychol Bull.* 2007;133(4):581-624.

Gatchel RJ, Robinson RC, Pulliam C, Maddrey AM. Biofeedback with pain patients: evidence for its effectiveness. *Semin Pain Med.* 2003;1(2):55-66.

Greaves MW. Recent advances in pathophysiology and current management of itch. *Ann Acad Med Singap.* 2007;36(9):788-792.

Hockenberry MJ, Wilson D, Winkelstein ML. *Wong's Essentials of Pediatric Nursing.* 7th ed. Mosby; 2004.

Katzung BG, ed. *Basic Clinical Pharmacology.* Appleton & Lange; 1998.

Krasner D. The chronic wound pain experience: a conceptual model. *Ostomy Wound Manage.* 1995;41(3):20-25.

Melzack R. The short-form McGill Pain Questionnaire. *Pain.* 1987;30(2):191-197. doi:10.1016/0304-3959(87)91074-8

Melzack R, Wall PD. Pain mechanisms: a new theory. *Science.* 1965;150(3699):971-979.

Peppin JF, Albrecht PJ, Argoff C, et al. Skin matters: a review of topical treatments for chronic pain. Part one: skin physiology and delivery systems. *Pain Ther.* 2015;4(1):17-32.

Price P, Fogh K, Glynn C, Krasner DL, Osterbrink J, Sibbald RG. Managing painful chronic wounds: the Wound Pain Management Model. *Int Wound J.* 2007;4(Suppl 1):4-15.

Reddy M, Kohr R, Queen D, Keast D, Sibbald RG. Practical treatment of wound pain and trauma: a patient-centered approach. An overview. *Ostomy Wound Manage.* 2003;49(4 Suppl):2-15.

Robinson AJ, Snyder-Mackler L. *Clinical Electrophysiology.* 2nd ed. Lippincott Williams & Wilkins; 1995.

Sibbald RG, Armstrong DG, Orsted HL. Pain in diabetic foot ulcers. *Ostomy Wound Manage.* 2003;49(4 Suppl):24-29.

Wong on Web. http://www.mosbysdrugconsult.com/WOW/faces.html

History Taking

OBJECTIVES

- Based on information from a referral, take a history efficiently.
- Use the *International Classification of Functioning, Disability and Health* model to guide questions.
- Determine the priorities of the patient in terms of work, home, and community.
- Assess a patient's resources.
- Create and test hypotheses to determine a diagnosis, prognosis, and outcome measures.
- Describe the evaluation process.
- List the components of the evaluation process.
- Describe the Hypothesis-Oriented Algorithm for Clinicians model.
- Describe secondary diagnoses, medications, and risk factors.
- List critical elements in taking a history to aid in diagnosis and prognosis.
- List risk factors for developing and slow healing of wounds that may be elicited by a history.
- Describe lab studies that may aid in the development of a diagnosis and prognosis.
- Describe the impact of social and work history on wound management.
- Describe how mobility impacts wound management.
- Describe how various types of equipment may affect wound management.

Irion GL, Gardner JA, Pignataro RM.
Comprehensive Wound Management, Third Edition (pp 101-111).
© 2024 Taylor and Francis Group.

TABLE 7-1
Initial History Questions Related to Wound Quality and Wound Management

Open-ended:
- What can you tell me about your wound?

Follow-up:
- Does it hurt?
- Does it itch?
- Does it have an odor? How bad is it?
- Is the skin around your wound swollen or feel tight?
- How much is it draining? Does it get on your clothes/bedding?

Open-ended:
- Tell me about your wound dressing experiences so far.

Follow-up:
- Who has been doing your wound dressings? Why this person?
- How does it feel when your dressing is removed? Does it hurt?

Open-ended:
- Tell me about changing your dressings, or has it been changed yet?
- Why do you change the dressing/have it changed?

Follow-up:
- Were you instructed to change it at certain intervals?
- Does it fall off by itself?
- Does it come off during bathing/showering?
- Do you take it off for bathing/showering?
- Was it leaking or full?

This chapter is the beginning point of intervention with the patient. Although a patient may be referred to us with a specific diagnosis and exhibits all of the characteristics associated with the referring diagnosis, we may still not understand important aspects of their life that change the risk to integumentary integrity and may affect wound healing. Even with a complete description of the patient, we need to know what they do at work, home, and during recreational activities. Many times, the referring diagnosis is insufficient or not germane to the interventions we may use for treatment. History taking and physical examination

go hand in hand throughout our interaction with the patient. What we learn from the patient by asking questions will refine our physical examination of them, and what we learn from the physical examination may lead us to ask for more information or may uncover inconsistencies that may be due to the patient not understanding our questions; trying to give us answers they think we should hear; or concealing information because of embarrassment, moral or legal issues, or other reasons. In some cases, we will continue to learn important information about the patient throughout the episode of care, and their circumstances or resources may change.

ELEMENTS OF A HISTORY

History must be sufficiently thorough to guide the clinician to the proper tests and measures to determine the cause of the wound and to identify any characteristics of the wound, the patient, family, caregivers, living arrangements, work/school, and resources that would affect the outcomes of different intervention strategies so an optimal plan of care can be devised. Demographic data typically included are age, sex, height, weight, race/ethnicity, and primary language. Additional information could be derived from computing body mass index. The age of the patient has an impact on the rate of healing and their typical daily activities. Age and race may be related to the probability of certain etiologies of the wound (eg, sickle cell disease). Hand and foot dominance are often overlooked unless the wound is located on a hand. With wounds on a hand or foot, the patient needs to be questioned about activities involving those extremities and possible alternatives for accomplishing tasks should any limitations be placed on the extremities. Knowing hand/foot dominance may also be important in terms of any home program to ensure that the patient has sufficient dexterity to perform self-care as well as impacting their return to work and home duties. Developmental history includes any disorders that may aggravate the wound, create difficulty in carrying out a home program, or impede the patient's ability to protect the wound (Table 7-1).

USING THE FRAMEWORK OF ICF TO GUIDE HISTORY TAKING

The *International Classification of Functioning, Disability and Health* (ICF) provides a means of directing both history taking and the physical exam. Within the ICF, the clinician seeks to identify impairments, functional limitations, participation restrictions, and environmental factors and personal factors that influence issues with the patient's/client's anatomy and physiology. Typically, one thinks of taking a history before physical examination occurs. A process of obtaining a referral diagnosis, having a patient fill out a history form, following up with specific questions, and performing a standard physical exam is rigid and inefficient. Another model for evaluating a patient's condition is the Hypothesis-Oriented Algorithm for Clinicians. The Hypothesis-Oriented Algorithm for Clinicians process can be simply interpreted as a constant testing of hypotheses. Hypotheses are developed as soon as a referral diagnosis is obtained. If a patient is not referred from another clinician, the process starts with history taking. Information taken from the referral is compared with a history instrument or a history and physical note in the patient's health care record. Clinicians should be looking for triangulation of data and either asking more questions or running more tests in an effort to reach a conclusion based on hypothesis testing.

History taking and the physical exam should overlap. As the physical exam proceeds, hypotheses that were not adequately tested by the physical exam may be tested by asking more questions. In some cases, the patient is incapable of providing answers, and a reliable third party such as a family member or other caregiver must be sought. In such cases, the ability to move fluidly between the physical exam and history taking may not occur unless a reliable caregiver is available. Furthermore, history taking and physical examination often and should occur during the entire episode of care. Even as a patient is ready to be discharged, questions regarding the follow-up care to bring a wound to full healing and prevent recurrence should be asked. History needs to focus on all 5 elements of the ICF model: impairments, activity limitations, participation restrictions, personal factors, and environmental factors.

Hypotheses developed and tested throughout the process include diagnosis, prognosis, plan of care, and outcome measures chosen. The need for involvement of another party and development of a plan for emergency management should also be included in this process. Each patient/client has a role in society, and each role requires the ability to perform tasks. Moreover, task performance requires elements of the anatomy and physiology that might be impaired. Many times, available resources might be able to compensate for impairments. Resources may be part of the patient's environment or personal factors. Personal factors/internal resources include self-efficacy, knowledge, and skills that impact both prognosis and plan of care. For example, a person with knowledge of managing a wound may be able to perform more of the plan of care and require fewer visits and may have a more favorable outcome including the ability to remain working and caring for a family. Environmental/external resources such as assistance, modification of tasks or responsibilities, and

technology also impact the plan of care and prognosis. A patient may have modified work duties, technology provided for work or for treatment, and assistance at home. Part of the history should address these issues. These issues need to be evaluated along with the patient's overall degree of wellness. Wellness—physical, intellectual, emotional, and other dimensions—has a major impact on the ability to execute whatever role in society that patient may have.

During the interview and throughout the episode of care, discussions concerning the patient's need to change tasks or roles should occur and whether the employer and resources at home may allow this. Prognosis should be more than the predicted outcome related to the wound. The patient's ability to carry out roles is also part of prognosis. The plan of care needs to reconcile what we think the patient can achieve with what the patient wants to achieve. Discussion throughout the plan of care needs to focus on whether we are setting expectations that are consistent with the patient's/client's desired role in society. If a patient has a plantar ulcer and needs to be on their feet, an offloading solution needs to be discussed and agreed on to minimize the chance that the patient will walk on that foot without the clinician knowing.

Additionally, enough questions need to be asked to determine whether the patient may be underestimating or overestimating achievable goals. A patient may say that they can return to work upon discharge from the hospital and may be able to change dressings and other tasks, but a full understanding of everything that the patient needs to do and the likelihood of them being able to perform all of these tasks must be ascertained.

Medications

Patients may be taking no medications or have a long list. A list of medications being taken for the current condition, as well as other conditions, is critical information. Many individuals will forget names and dosages of drugs, whereas some will carry a list of medications with them at all times. A strategy of asking the patient to bring all prescriptions can aid in producing an accurate list. Inpatient or home therapy can be easier because all medications will be listed in the patient's health care record. Regardless of the setting, patients may be taking nonprescription drugs, including over-the-counter medicines, street drugs, herbs, or other substances, that can also affect wound healing. Particularly important for the patient with a wound are corticosteroids, nonsteroidal anti-inflammatory drugs, other anti-inflammatory or immunosuppressants drugs, antibiotics, anticoagulants, chemotherapy, insulin, and oral glycemic drugs. In addition to prescription and over-the-counter medications, is the patient using any herbal or home remedies? An issue related to medication is whether the patient is receiving other types of interventions such as radiation treatments for cancer and any allergies. Patients may be allergic to substances such as iodine, lidocaine, or specific antibiotics that may be used in their care. The effects of medications were discussed in Chapter 4.

History of Present Illness

A history of the present condition should include the date of onset (if known), course of events, pattern of symptoms, and what the patient thinks caused the wound. In the case of an acute wound, the cause is usually obvious such as a burn or laceration. In the case of a chronic wound, knowing how the wound was managed previously is imperative. For example, was the underlying venous insufficiency treated? What preventive measures have been taken to alleviate pressure? Is the present treatment causing chronic inflammation? In the case of a wound that is not easily diagnosed, learning what interventions were tried and how well they worked may assist in the diagnosis as much as knowing the past medical history and medications being used. The history of the current condition needs to include prior therapeutic interventions and careful questioning to determine why previous therapy was ineffective. Was the underlying problem addressed? Was the intervention not carried through? Was the intervention performed incorrectly? These can be delicate questions, especially when the clinician thinks the cause of the wound is obvious. The clinician needs to be prudent in implying incompetence of other health care providers, especially before a clear diagnosis can be made.

The specific concerns that led the patient to seek services and concerns or needs of the patient need to be explored. We must also determine what the patient's goals for intervention are. The plan of care may need to be modified to match the priorities of the patient rather than forcing the clinician's priorities on the patient. Many times, optimal treatment for the wound is not the optimal treatment for the individual patient because of work, home, or other concerns. The plan of care will also need to accommodate the patient's, family's, and caregiver's emotional response to the current clinical situation and possible treatments.

Social History, Living, Working, and Recreational Conditions

Social history consists of many factors related to the person's culture, resources, activities, and support system. Each patient has a unique combination of these factors that impact their risks for wounds and prognosis for healing. Over the course of an episode of care, one or more of these factors may change, so we must make an effort to keep up to date on these changes.

Social History

Cultural beliefs and behaviors may affect the patient's ability to heal from a wound profoundly and may also directly or indirectly be the cause of a wound. Some religious beliefs will limit the range of interventions available for a plan of care. Moreover, the use of home remedies that are a part of a person's heritage but are unknown to the clinician may affect wound healing. A frank discussion of family and caregiver resources, including time and not just financial resources, is important in determining what interventions are likely to be successful. Social interactions, social activities, and support systems may affect the patient's willingness to adhere to a treatment plan. Current and prior community and work (job/school) activities need to be analyzed in terms of possible causes of wounds and whether these activities are likely to help or hinder wound healing.

Social habits can be difficult to ascertain. Unfortunately, many of these social habits profoundly slow wound healing. Habits such as exercise, smoking, alcohol consumption, and drug abuse are important pieces of information to allow the clinician to develop an appropriate plan of care. Many patients will have a combination of social habits that are not conducive to wound healing. One should account for them when developing a prognosis, stating these issues explicitly in documentation. Efforts to change social habits, such as smoking, may result in frustration, and a patient may need to be referred to individuals trained specifically in this area.

Living Conditions

Living environment, community characteristics, and projected discharge destinations must be discussed. Frequently, the living environment and discharge destinations must be considered together. A patient with little support and living in an environment that is physically challenging may need to be admitted to a facility that provides the necessary support, whereas a person living in a one-floor efficiency apartment on the ground floor may be discharged to home under identical clinical conditions. Discovering who will be assisting and whether the caregiver is capable of delivering the assistance needed should be done as early as possible. Meeting with family members or volunteer or paid caregivers to discuss roles and what can be accomplished will often be critical to successful intervention. One should also try to ascertain the willingness of caregivers in addition to their abilities to avoid poor living conditions that may hamper the patient's recovery. Another issue to be explored is the patient's tidiness at home and any history of family members with skin abscesses or other infections. One can get some idea from the patient's general appearance, but the patient may have hygiene problems related to pets or housecleaning that interfere with the treatment plan.

Working Conditions

Important questions related to occupation include what tasks the job entails and whether the wound will impede the patient's ability to work or whether the tasks will prevent the wound from healing. If working is not appropriate, can the patient's work responsibilities be modified, or can they be reassigned to another job? For example, a patient with venous ulcers should be standing as little as possible, and a person with foot ulcers should minimize walking. Does the wound present a risk to coworkers (eg, a wound infected with methicillin-resistant *Staphylococcus aureus*)? As discussed with living arrangements, how tidy is the work environment? Some patients may be exposed to a work environment that is unsuitable for wound healing. For a number of reasons, a patient may not be able to return to work as quickly as desired. Many patients will have short- and long-term disability plans or sufficient sick time to stay home; however, many will lack financial resources and may feel compelled to return to work. Discussion of these issues with the patient is imperative. Rather than have them return to work without the health care provider's knowledge, adaptations to the plan of care may be possible to allow the patient to earn an income while recovering. Specific to the workplace conditions, the history should address the risk of infection from a history of skin abscesses or other infections of coworkers, cleanliness of work such as the requirement to work in dirt or sewage, and employee access to hygiene facilities (handwashing and portable toilets vs full-scale restrooms). Infection control issues determined by employer or health department regulations should also be addressed.

Family History

A number of health risks tend to occur in family members either because of genetic or lifestyle similarities. Type 2 diabetes, arterial disease, hypertension, sickle cell disease, cancer, and other diseases existing in the family may be undiagnosed in the patient. A history should include both the patient's and the patient's family's medical history.

Functional Status

The functional status and activity level prior to the problem and expectation of return to this function and activity are critical areas for an interview. Functional status and activity level may be a cause or complicating factor for a wound. For example, the person with a neuropathic ulcer on the plantar surface whose work requires walking or the person with venous insufficiency who is on their feet all day can both cause and slow healing of ulcerations.

Determining the current and prior functional status in self-care and home management activities, including activities of daily living and instrumental activities of daily living and who at home is available to assist with activities if the patient is not able or needs to desist from the activities to allow wound healing, is critical. Moreover, recreational or leisure activities and degree of physical fitness need to be considered in developing a diagnosis and tailoring a plan of care that matches the patient's needs.

Although a patient's current mobility will be explored as part of the physical examination, their mobility history is important for several reasons. The patient needs to be asked about mobility and to demonstrate mobility to the clinician. How mobile is the person in a bed or in a chair? Can the patient shift weight or get into and out of a bed or a chair independently, or is assistance needed? Is a referral to physical therapy or occupational therapy needed to aid in the prevention of more wounds or to promote healing of existing ulcers? We also need to know how long the patient has had the current level of mobility. Did the person have a gradual decline or an abrupt decline in mobility? Were certain aspects of mobility affected earlier than others? Has the patient received intervention for mobility problems previously? For example, does the patient have experience using crutches? Reduced mobility limiting a patient to a bed or a chair represents a great risk for pressure injuries. Not using an assistive device with neuropathic feet may be a risk factor as well. Any alteration in normal gait pattern also represents a risk of injury to the foot.

What equipment does the patient have? Do they know how to use it? Does the equipment suit the impairment or disability of the patient? For example, does a person with weight-bearing restrictions use a rolling walker? Does a person with diminished vision or poor balance use a rolling walker or standard walker? Why was the patient given the equipment? In many cases, the patient may have borrowed a cane, walker, or crutches from a friend or family member without being instructed in its use and is simply using the wrong type of equipment because it was convenient. Patients may have a piece of equipment but not use it for cosmetic reasons or may forget to use it. Asking a patient why they were given a walker may elicit a response that they were supposed to have weight-bearing restrictions that were not communicated to you.

Past Medical and Surgical History

Either before or during the interview, a patient should be asked about health issues that occurred earlier. Although they may not be obvious contributors to the patient's current condition, access to medical and surgical history may assist in the diagnosis of a wound or lead us to alter our plan of care for the patient. Depending on the cause of the wound, certain systems may become more important. Because of the prevalence of diabetes mellitus, all patients should be asked about endocrine/metabolic disease, especially diabetes. Patients with diabetes should also be asked about glucose control. Does the patient use insulin? What type and time of day? Does the patient manage diabetes with diet and exercise or with oral glycemic drugs?

Cardiovascular disease is also common and should be addressed. Does the patient have a history of angina, shortness of breath, or surgical interventions such as coronary artery bypass grafting? The patient should also be asked about hypertension, arrhythmia, valve disease, and any treatment for these. Gastrointestinal disorders may lead to malnutrition, anemia, or bowel incontinence; genitourinary issues include bladder incontinence leading to injury to the skin. Questions related to the integumentary system include previous wounds, dermatologic conditions, and treatments for them. A history of musculoskeletal and neuromuscular disorders can produce abnormal forces on the skin and injury. These injuries or diseases may occur in the central or peripheral nervous system. A general history of any hospitalizations and surgeries may be relevant to the patient's present condition or how the treatment plan is developed.

The risk factors listed earlier should always be explored. A simple means is to have the patient fill out a health history form. A thorough history should be available on the chart of an inpatient. Additionally, the medications taken by the patient may alert the clinician to a disease not uncovered during the history. Other health-related questions should include immune system status, which can allow wounds to develop and also impede wound healing. Some of these were discussed in greater detail previously.

Neuropathy

Similar to mobility, we need to know the history of neuropathy. We will examine the patient to determine the extent of neuropathy but will need to know the history of the neuropathy as well. A longer history of ambulation with neuropathy carries a greater risk of foot ulceration. We also need to know what interventions have been used such as off-loading devices and assistive devices. When discussing neuropathy, we should ask the patient appropriate questions about glycemic control. How often does the patient perform glucose monitoring? What are the numbers like? Does the patient know their glycated hemoglobin (HbA1c)? How often does the patient see a health care provider about their foot care?

Vascular Disease

Questions about vascular disease will follow the same approach as mobility and neuropathy in that we want a history of the severity, duration, and any interventions the patient has received related to vascular disease. We will perform vascular testing as part of the physical exam (discussed in the following chapter). Questions should be asked about any other issues related to arterial disease, such as ischemic heart disease, stroke, renal disease, amputations, and surgical interventions. A related issue is asking about any tobacco use.

Nutrition

Nutrition was discussed in Chapter 4. During a history, one may want to ask questions that will relate to the physical exam. Has the patient experienced recent weight gain or weight loss? What is the history of any weight changes? Has the patient made any changes to their diet? Depending on whether a dietitian is available for nutrition screening, we may need to ask the patient about their diet.

Continence

Incontinence of bladder or bowel is a risk factor particularly to the skin of the perineum. Any patient with erythema of the perineum and surrounding areas should be asked about incontinence and any interventions. Although this is particularly true for incontinence, we may need to discuss any of these risk factors with family or other caregivers if the patient is unable to provide the information. Many people are easily embarrassed and unwilling to discuss continence issues with others, so the health care provider must approach the topic tactfully. A simple approach is to discuss all the risk factors for skin injury, and then ask whether the patient has any of them. If patients or caregivers know why the questions about incontinence are important, they may not be as reluctant to discuss incontinence as they would if they were asked without prefacing the question by discussing incontinence as a risk factor for skin injury.

Trauma

Injuries caused by trauma are often self-explanatory; yet, some aspects of the injury could be missed if we do not ask appropriate questions. Depending on the circumstances of the injury, patients may have an emotional response, particularly if others were injured in the same incident. Traumatic injury may produce alterations in gait patterns or place unusual stress on other body parts. Questions may need to be asked as we examine different areas of the body because some more minor injuries or injuries occurring where the patient has limited sensation could be missed.

Lab Studies

Results from basic lab studies can be found on the charts of inpatients. Outpatients are unlikely to be able to provide much assistance to the clinician regarding results of lab studies. The results useful to the clinician include blood counts to determine whether anemia, thrombocytopenia (lack of platelets), or leukopenia (lack of white blood cells [WBCs]) are present. Blood chemistry including electrolytes (potassium, sodium, chloride, and bicarbonate), blood urea nitrogen (BUN) and creatinine for renal function, and blood glucose should be present on the chart of an inpatient and may be available from the referring physicians. Many sources are available for interpreting lab values such as the Academy of Acute Care Physical Therapy (https://www.aptaacutecare.org/general/custom.asp?page=ResourceGuides) and Lab Test Online (https://labtestsonline.org/).

Blood Counts

Both the total WBC count and differential white cell counts may be important in certain cases. In terms of risk for infection or diagnosis of infection, neutrophil counts are also critical. Normal WBC counts range from 4500 to 11,000/mm^3 in both men and women. Leukocytosis is a count exceeding this range. Of particular importance in the context of wound management is the diagnosis of infection. Other causes of leukocytosis that should be considered include leukemia or another form of cancer, tissue injury, and some other source of inflammation. Leukocytosis is frequently accompanied by fever, somnolence, and anorexia produced by elevated cytokines released in these conditions. As discussed in subsequent chapters, wound infection has a profound effect on decision making. Leukopenia, defined as a count less than the range listed earlier, can be produced by a number of causes including bone marrow disease (aplastic anemia), viral infection, and cancer chemotherapy. As the white cell count falls, the risk of infection increases dramatically, and additional isolation precautions must be enforced. A white cell count below 1000 or a neutrophil count below 500 usually requires reverse isolation, with gloving, gowning, donning a mask, and sterile technique even for routine wound care.

Neutrophils observed in a differential count may be termed either *segmented* (mature) or *bands* (immature). Neutrophil counts are generally elevated in the presence of bacterial infection. A large number of bands is particularly diagnostic of bacterial infection. Lymphocytes are categorized into B cells and T cells and then further classified into subcategories. B cells are responsible for antibody-mediated immunity, whereas T cells are involved in specific cell-mediated immunity against specific antigens. T-cell immunity is associated particularly with neoplasms and

viral infection but also is involved in delayed hypersensitivity reactions, including skin reactions (eg, poison ivy). Monocytes are blood cells equivalent to the tissue macrophage. These cells are responsible for later destruction of marked cells and destruction of debris following neutrophil infiltration. Eosinophils are involved in defenses against worms and are implicated in allergic responses, including asthma. Basophils are blood cells that perform some of the same functions as mast cells, releasing mediators of inflammation, particularly histamine. Normal differential counts are 50% to 60% neutrophils, 30% to 40% lymphocytes, 1% to 9% monocytes, 0% to 3% eosinophils, and 0% to 1% basophils. In addition, bands (immature neutrophils) range from 0% to 7%. Elevations in neutrophils, termed *neutrophilia*, and especially bands are usually indicative of infection by pyogenic organisms such as *Staphylococcus* or *Streptococcus* species. Lymphocytosis (excessive B or T lymphocytes) is indicative of viral infection. Monocytosis (elevated monocyte count) may occur in severe infections. Excessive numbers of eosinophils (eosinophilia) are indicative of severe allergic reactions or worm infestation, and basophilia indicates parasitic infection or hypersensitivity reactions. Neutropenia, defined as a neutrophil count less than 500, as with leukopenia, requires reverse isolation.

The normal red cell count is greater in men than women. For men, the normal ranges are 4.7 to 6.1 million/µL, a hematocrit of 42% to 52%, and a hemoglobin concentration of 14 to 18 g/dL. These ranges for women are 4.2 to 5.4 million/µL, 37% to 47%, and 12 to 16 g/dL, respectively. During pregnancy, these numbers decrease. The importance of red cell parameters, regardless of which are used, is the ability to transport oxygen to aid in wound healing. Elevations in red cell parameters (polycythemia) are rare but clinically significant. Much more common are conditions that lower these numbers, producing anemia. Causes of anemia include bleeding, diseases of red cell production (aplastic anemia, pernicious anemia, and iron and vitamin deficiencies), diseases characterized by excessive destruction of red cells (hemolytic anemias, including several autoimmune diseases, and sickle cell anemia), and genetic diseases of hemoglobin synthesis (thalassemias). Several lab tests are available for determining the cause of anemia. Another major cause is cancer chemotherapy. Regardless of the cause of anemia, decreased oxygen transport capacity of blood has a deleterious effect on wound healing, and elevating red cell parameters by correcting the cause, transfusion, or administration of erythropoietin is important to assist wound healing. Patients with renal disease or who are receiving cancer chemotherapy may be using exogenous erythropoietin to maintain red cell counts.

Platelets are fragments of cells called *megakaryocytes*. Platelets have a major role in hemostasis, which is usually the first step in acute wound healing. The normal range for platelets is 150,000 to 400,000/µL. *Thrombocytosis* is the term for an elevated count, whereas a deficiency is called *thrombocytopenia*. In terms of wound healing, the normal concern is thrombocytopenia rather than thrombocytosis. Thrombocytopenia, like anemia and leukopenia, occurs with aplastic anemia and cancer chemotherapy. Platelets can be diminished by a number of autoimmune diseases or consumed in disseminated vascular coagulation. Thrombocytopenia reduces the initial reaction to wounding and proliferation by decreasing the availability of platelet-derived growth factor. The effectiveness of platelets is also reduced in von Willebrand's disease, a genetic disorder that prevents platelets from adhering at the site of injury.

Tests related to hemostasis are the international normalized ratio (INR), prothrombin time (PT), and partial thromboplastin time (PTT). Inadequate hemostasis is a concern for several aspects of wound management, and these values and their interpretation should be understood. Thrombin is produced in the coagulation cascade as the final enzyme of the processes, converting fibrinogen to fibrin, augmenting the strength of the platelet aggregate, and trapping red cells in the thrombus.

PTT is an index of the effectiveness of the coagulation cascade only, whereas PT is affected by clotting factors, prothrombin, and fibrinogen. PT is prolonged with anticoagulation therapy, vitamin K deficiency, and genetic defects in the coagulation cascade such as hemophilias and von Willebrand's disease.

PT is tested both to screen for coagulation disorders and to determine the effectiveness of anticoagulation therapy. Because of variation in PT in different labs, the INR was developed. This index corrects for variations in testing materials and compares the results of PT to reference values; therefore, INR should be identical in different labs for the same person. Normal values for PT range from 12 to 15 seconds, PTT ranges from 25 to 40 seconds, and INR should be between 0.9 and 1.1. Note INR does not have units; it is a ratio of PT to PT reference values. Values of PT 1.5 to 2.5 times normal are desirable for patients with hypercoagulability concerns such as a history of deep venous thrombosis, coronary artery disease, or cerebrovascular disease. A PT greater than 2.5 times normal presents a risk of spontaneous bleeding, but particular care must be taken even with a therapeutic PT. Using INR numbers, concern for bleeding occurs at a value greater than 2.0. A value of 3.0 places the patient at risk of spontaneous bleeding.

Basic Metabolic Profile and Comprehensive Metabolic Profile

These 2 tests are sets of common laboratory tests. The basic metabolic profile (BMP) consists of measurements of important electrolytes, 2 indicators of renal function,

and blood glucose. Any one or more of these tests might be performed separately. The comprehensive metabolic profile (CMP) consists of the same tests but includes tests of liver and related function.

Electrolytes

The electrolytes routinely analyzed are serum sodium, potassium, chloride, bicarbonate, and sometimes calcium and magnesium. Because these are electrolytes, alterations from normal ranges can have profound effects on excitable tissues—muscle, nerve, and myocardial cells. Normal serum sodium has a range of 135 to 145 mEq/L, potassium is 3.5 to 5.0 mEq/L, chloride is 98 to 109 mEq/L, bicarbonate is 20 to 30 mEq/L, calcium is 9.0 to 10.5 mEq/L, and magnesium is 1.2 to 2.0 mEq/L. The amount of sodium in the body determines fluid volumes, and alterations can cause swelling or shrinkage of cells. Potassium is the primary determinant of membrane potentials. Excessive potassium in the extracellular fluid depolarizes cells, whereas depletion of extracellular potassium hyperpolarizes cells. In either case, serious, potentially life-threatening arrhythmias can develop with either hyper- or hypokalemia. Hypokalemia can produce fatigue, muscle weakness, or cramping. Hyperkalemia can also produce muscle weakness but additionally can lead to a sensation of numbness and palpitations, in addition to arrhythmias as discussed previously. Alterations of chloride and bicarbonate are diagnostic of fluid balance and acid-base disorders. Both calcium and magnesium are intimately involved with neuromuscular function. Ionized calcium decreases the probability of neuromuscular excitation, and, as such, both hypocalcemia and hypomagnesemia can cause muscle spasms and arrhythmias. Hypocalcemia may also produce arrhythmias due to the role of calcium in cardiac action potentials. Hypercalcemia and hypermagnesemia cause muscle weakness and arrhythmias.

Renal Function

The 2 lab values of BUN and creatinine are routinely measured. Normal kidney function eliminates these substances to produce a serum concentration within a given range. Failure of the kidneys to excrete them allows these substances to accumulate in the blood. Normal values of BUN range from 10 to 20 mg/dL in adults. Because BUN represents a balance between production of urea from breakdown of proteins and excretion by the kidney, a sharp increase in protein intake may increase BUN. Increased BUN may also result from gastrointestinal bleeding and dehydration. Decreases in BUN may be seen with liver disease because of a diminished ability of the liver to produce urea and with overhydration. Creatinine is a product of muscle tissue. The normal range for creatinine is 0.5 to 1.2 mg/dL. Creatinine excretion decreases with renal disease, causing plasma creatinine to increase above this concentration. Plasma concentration may decline with decreasing muscle mass or increase with muscle injury. Of concern with renal disease are the accompanying cardiovascular problems, including hypertension and anemia. Because erythropoietin is synthesized by renal cells, the administration of exogenous erythropoietin may be used to treat the anemia of end-stage renal failure.

Blood Glucose

Normal fasting blood glucose is considered to be 70 to 110 mg/dL, equivalent to approximately 5 g glucose circulating in the blood. Blood glucose rises with eating and decreases with insulin and exercise. A person with normal glucose metabolism will return blood glucose to the normal range within 2 hours of consumption of 75 g glucose. Blood glucose of a person with diabetes mellitus will exceed 200 mg/dL at the end of the test, and a person with impaired glucose tolerance will have a blood glucose value between 140 and 200 mg/dL. Either an oral glucose tolerance test or an elevated fasting blood sugar can be indicative of diabetes mellitus. By the older definition, hyperglycemia is present with blood glucose in excess of 150 mg/dL. Newer definitions have lowered the threshold. In 1998, the American Diabetes Association defined a new category called *impaired fasting glucose*. Impaired fasting glucose is considered to exist at a value of 110 to 125 mg/dL. This condition has been referred to as a prediabetic state. Some experts suggest that interventions at this point might be able to prevent the development of type 2 diabetes. Blood glucose exceeding 126 mg/dL on at least 2 measurements is diagnostic of diabetes mellitus.

Impaired glucose metabolism is considered a risk factor for future diabetes mellitus and macrovascular disease. A person with fasting blood glucose between 120 and 150 mg/dL is considered to have impaired glucose tolerance. As such, clinicians should be concerned about wound management for an individual with any impairment in glucose uptake. Another test commonly performed is the 2-hour postprandial blood sugar. In this test, blood glucose is measured 2 hours after eating. A normal value should be obtained within this time frame. Short-term, elevated blood glucose values up to 250 mg/dL are not considered dangerous. When blood glucose concentration exceeds this level, the ability of the renal tubules to reabsorb glucose is saturated and glucose appears in the urine. Over the long term, elevations of blood glucose above 120 mg/dL are considered a health risk. A means of monitoring long-term glucose control is to measure glycated hemoglobin. The percentage of glycated hemoglobin is an index of how well glucose has been controlled over the 120-day life span of the average red blood cell. Poor glucose control causes HbA1c to exceed 9%. This corresponds to an average value

for blood glucose greater than 210 mg/dL. Optimal control produces HbA1c values of less than 6.1%, which represents an average blood glucose value of less than 120 mg/dL.

An additional concern, and potential medical emergency, is hypoglycemia. Hypoglycemia results from an imbalance of eating, insulin, and exercise and is not uncommon in ill individuals. Symptoms of hypoglycemia may manifest at a wide range of blood glucose values. At a value of 70 or less, corrective action should be taken, usually by providing oral carbohydrates in various forms such as sugar tablets, carbohydrate snacks, or concentrated sugar drinks such as orange juice but not diet drinks. Symptoms of hypoglycemia are basically those of generalized sympathetic nervous system activation. This includes tachycardia, shaking, and excessive sweating. The patient may also complain of a headache or be apathetic and uncoordinated. Maintaining balanced eating, insulin, and activity needs to be stressed with a patient with diabetes, especially an individual who is sick or has wounds. Illness or surgery can lead to wild fluctuations in blood glucose. Frequently, stress elevates serum cortisol, which, in turn, elevates blood glucose. Insulin doses are often temporarily increased for inpatients, but often patients fail to eat regularly, and blood glucose can plummet. Clinicians must be constantly aware of this possibility and should be able to test for blood glucose and take corrective action themselves in addition to reporting the episode to the physician responsible for managing the patient's diabetes.

Comprehensive Metabolic Panel

More information can be obtained from a CMP, which consists of the tests included in the BMP with the addition of serum concentrations of markers of liver function. The tests performed as part of the CMP that are not part of the BMP may be done separately as a hepatic function panel, instead of performing them as part of the CMP.

The hepatic function panel consists of alkaline phosphatase, alanine aminotransferase (formerly called SGPT), aspartate aminotransferase (formerly called SGOT), and bilirubin. The hepatic function panel is used to detect liver damage or disease, but the results of some of this panel may indicate pathology of other systems. Alanine aminotransferase is an enzyme mainly found in the liver and as such is the primary test for detecting hepatitis. Alkaline phosphatase is related to the bile ducts and is increased when they are blocked and may indicate gall bladder, liver, and bile duct disease but may also be elevated due to increased bone turnover in chronic renal failure. Aspartate aminotransferase is found in the liver but also in the heart and skeletal muscles and historically had been used for differential diagnosis of chest pain. Bilirubin is measured as total bilirubin, which can be elevated due to liver disease or other

TABLE 7-2
Questions Related to Prognosis of Healing

How long have you had this wound?

Do you have any other infections?

Are you ambulatory? Capable of self-care? Working? Exercising regularly?

Have you had a wound like this before?

Do you have any known diseases that are not listed in your history/history form?

Follow-up:

- Diabetes (sugars), heart disease, lung disease, kidney disease?
- Do you have a list of medications that you take—prescribed, over the counter, or others?

causes such as bile duct occlusion and hemolytic anemia, or direct and indirect separately to determine the cause of elevated bilirubin. Albumin and total protein reflect the ability of the liver to synthesize proteins.

Results of Diagnostic Imaging

Patients may have diagnostic imaging for a number of reasons. Most relevant to wounds is to determine whether infection has spread to bone. Bones of the foot are particularly susceptible in those with diabetes mellitus. Osteomyelitis may show as localized destruction of bone. Free air produced by fermentation may be detected on X-ray due to deep infection with anaerobic bacteria. For example, a patient with a fracture of the humerus may develop free air around the fracture site due to *Escherichia coli* infection from being catheterized. However, early osteomyelitis without bone destruction can be missed on X-ray.

Diagnosis

Based on history, a diagnosis begins to take shape. The diagnosis may already be obvious from the history and physical examination. Typical chronic wounds such as pressure injuries, neuropathic ulcers, and venous leg ulcers; slowly healing common wounds such as surgical site infections and skin and soft tissue infections; and acute traumatic wounds such as burns, lacerations, and abrasions can be diagnosed readily. Should these common wounds not follow expected

histories (and physical examination), then unusual wounds (Chapter 18) will start to be considered. As described in Chapter 3, identifying factors slowing healing needs to be part of the diagnosis.

Prognosis

Prognosis addresses what the patient will achieve in terms of goals/outcome measures as a result of physical therapy intervention. It can be performance based, a validated clinical measure, or self-report. Prognosis will also include either or both a time frame and the number of visits. Potential prognoses related specifically to wounds include wound clean and stable and ready for patient/caregiver to manage at home; wound clean and stable and ready for grafting; wound closed; and wound managed by caregivers (home/facility). The prognosis selected from these and many other possibilities should be determined by elements from the ICF and not simply the impairment of the skin (Table 7-2).

SUMMARY

A number of factors related to the patient's health status and history can either cause a wound or impair the healing of a wound. These include the use of the *Guide to Physical Therapist Practice* to structure the history and physical examination of the patient. The terms *history, physical examination, review of systems, diagnosis, prognosis, plan of care,* and *outcomes* are defined. Deviations from normal lab values need to be interpreted for a potential influence on wound healing, especially blood cells and glucose. The clinician must also understand the social/work/play history of the patient and any medications they are taking, either prescribed by a physician or self-prescribed.

QUESTIONS

1. Why are we concerned about the use of anti-inflammatory drugs or cancer chemotherapy by patients receiving wound management?
2. What is the importance of an elevated WBC count?
3. What is the significance of neutropenia?
4. Why are thrombocytopenia and other disorders of hemostasis important in wound management?
5. Why should you ask an outpatient to show you their medications?

6. Why should you observe patients using their assistive devices?

7. What is the most difficult aspect of taking a history?

8. What should you do if you realize that you have not asked a question?

9. Are you allowed to ask more history questions after intervention starts?

10. When is the last time you should be asking the patient/client questions?

BIBLIOGRAPHY

Balon J, Thomas SA. Comparison of hospital admission medication lists with primary care physician and outpatient pharmacy lists. *J Nurs Scholarsh*. 2011;43(3):292-300.

Ross M, Zhou K, Perilli A, et al. Screening for cardiovascular disease risk factors in a physical therapist wound care practice: a retrospective, observational study. *Wound Manag Prev*. 2019;65(8):20-28.

Snyder RJ, Kirsner RS, Warriner RA 3rd, Lavery LA, Hanft JR, Sheehan P. Consensus recommendations on advancing the standard of care for treating neuropathic foot ulcers in patients with diabetes. *Ostomy Wound Manage*. 2010;56(4 Suppl):S1-S24.

Takahashi PY, Kiemele LJ, Chandra A, Cha SS, Targonski PV. A retrospective cohort study of factors that affect healing in long-term care residents with chronic wounds. *Ostomy Wound Manage*. 2009;55(1):32-37.

Physical Examination

PHYSICAL EXAMINATION

Both the referral diagnosis and history help direct the physical examination. A thorough physical examination may take several hours to complete; however, the history and careful observation should narrow the focus of the physical examination. For most patients, all aspects of the physical exam can be addressed within a few minutes if the history is done well. For other patients, a very thorough examination will be required even if the cause of the wound is very clear. An example is the patient with a history of diabetes mellitus. A very thorough examination of the

Irion GL, Gardner JA, Pignataro RM.
Comprehensive Wound Management, Third Edition (pp 113-130).
© 2024 Taylor and Francis Group.

strength, sensation, and skin quality of the lower extremities is in order regardless of the physical appearance of the wound. On the other hand, a person with an acute wound of known etiology might be examined in 10 to 15 minutes.

REVIEW OF SYSTEMS

The review of systems includes the basic elements of the examination that pertain to all patients. For physical therapy, the review of systems is generally divided into integumentary, cardiovascular and pulmonary, musculoskeletal, and neuromuscular. Each of these 4 systems will be discussed in the following sections.

Integumentary

When inspecting the skin, one examines the gross appearance of representative or at-risk areas of skin. Skin coloration, temperature, texture, turgor, and elasticity also must be examined. In addition to the skin, much may be learned by examining the hair and nails, which reflect stresses that are likely to affect the skin as well.

Skin Color

Melanin and hemoglobin are the 2 primary determinants of skin color. Melanin is the brown pigment produced by melanocytes. In individuals of sub-Saharan African descent, melanin pigmentation may be so great that variation in the hemoglobin content of the skin becomes obscured. Saturated hemoglobin with good arterial supply produces the pinkish hue typical of lightly pigmented skin. Differences in blood flow can vary skin color from a ghostly pallor to a bright red. Pallor suggests arterial insufficiency. Worse yet is a purplish hue produced by the presence of desaturated hemoglobin. This indicates severe arterial insufficiency, severe congestive heart failure, or severe pulmonary disease. A bright red color is produced by hyperemia (excessive blood flow). A reddish color (erythema) is an indication of inflammation and perhaps infection. Because blood flow also brings warm blood from the body's core to the surface, erythema is usually accompanied by skin warmth, also an indication of inflammation or infection. In heavily melanin-pigmented skin, hyperemia produces a violet or eggplant color and increased warmth that may be missed by the inexperienced clinician.

The loss of brown pigmentation may be manifested in 2 important ways. In vitiligo, patches of hypopigmented skin, usually a few centimeters across with somewhat irregular borders, are observed. Albinism produces a uniform hypopigmentation with accompanying hypopigmentation of the hair and irises of the eyes. Increased brown pigmentation occurs when melanocytes are stimulated by excessive adrenocorticotrophic hormone (ACTH). The structure of ACTH closely resembles the melanocyte stimulating hormone. High concentrations of ACTH occur with Addison's disease and pregnancy. In pregnancy, increased brown pigmentation occurs in characteristic locations such as the face, nipples, and the linea nigra, along the vertical centerline of the abdomen extending to the umbilicus.

Temperature

As discussed previously, skin temperature is altered by the magnitude of blood flow to the skin. Decreased skin temperature and pallor accompany a lack of blood flow to the skin. The clinician must determine whether the diminished temperature is localized to an area of an extremity or perhaps to the entirety of the extremity by comparing 2 extremities and along the length of each extremity. In addition, one must account for the ambient temperature, amount of clothing, and physical activity of the limb prior to examination. A single foot that feels cool compared with the other foot and the rest of the body is a clear sign of arterial insufficiency. At the other extreme, an area of skin that is warmer than expected based on a bilateral comparison or, in the judgment of the clinician, is warmer than it should be based on ambient temperature, clothing, and physical activity is a sign of inflammation or infection and is usually accompanied by hyperemia. In many cases, temperature can be assessed easily by the clinician's touch. Very poor arterial circulation and fever are readily detected by most clinicians. In some cases, quantification of local temperature is desirable. Noncontact infrared thermometers are readily available and produce quick, sufficiently accurate measurements for clinical judgment. Figure 8-1 depicts a typical device suitable for clinical practice.

Accumulations

Various materials may accumulate in the skin as a result of disease processes. When these disease processes are also the causes of wounds, identification of the accumulation in the skin is useful in determining the etiology of a wound. Hemosiderin is a particularly important accumulation. Hemosiderin (literally blood iron) is an accumulation of iron that results from the degradation of red blood cells. Hemosiderin is a storage form of iron in the tissue. Macrophages eventually pick up hemosiderin from the tissues and recycle the iron to the bone marrow. Hemosiderin produces a brownish-yellow discoloration usually referred to as hemosiderin staining. Hemosiderin staining, particularly just superior to the medial malleolus, is very predictive of venous hypertension. Many chronic wounds such as pressure injuries will have hemosiderin accumulating in

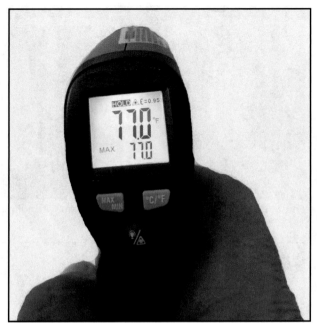

Figure 8-1. Infrared thermometer suitable for measuring skin temperature of the extremities.

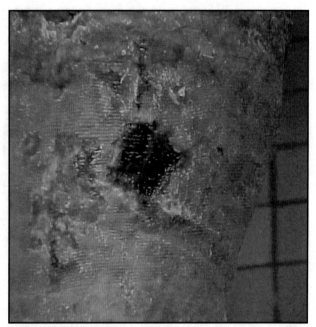

Figure 8-2. Appearance of lipodermatosclerosis in a patient with venous disease.

the skin immediately adjacent to the wound due to repetitive trauma. Bilirubin and its precursor biliverdin are also the result of the breakdown of hemoglobin. Bilirubin and biliverdin are seen in bruises. Shortly after the loss of blood directly beneath the skin (eg, a contusion), the purplish hue is due to biliverdin. As biliverdin is broken down into bilirubin, the skin takes on a yellowish tint (jaundice). Later, as bilirubin is removed by the circulation from the site of injury, the brownish-yellow hemosiderin remaining at the site of injury becomes obvious. Generalized jaundice indicates systemic overload of bilirubin. Jaundice occurs frequently in newborns due to the destruction of red cells carrying fetal hemoglobin. In adults, jaundice represents the imbalance of hemoglobin breakdown and bilirubin excretion. Jaundice may result from either hemolytic anemia (excessive breakdown of hemoglobin) or the inability to excrete bilirubin due to hepatic disease (hepatitis) or biliary obstruction.

Lipodermatosclerosis, Atrophie Blanche, Peau D'orange

Lipodermatosclerosis is considered to be a form of panniculitis, inflammation of the subcutaneous fatty tissue. Lipodermatosclerosis occurring in the lower extremity is characteristic of venous and lymphatic disease. This inflammation of the hypodermal fatty connective tissue produces what many refer to as eczema on the legs. *Eczema* is a general term for inflamed skin accompanied by a rough texture and itching. In severe cases, tissue fibrosis

accompanying lipodermatosclerosis produces an "inverted champagne bottle" appearance of the leg. The inverted champagne bottle implies a disproportionately smaller distal leg. Hemosiderin staining, erythema, and small areas devoid of any blood vessels called *atrophie blanche* often accompany this condition. An example is shown in Figure 8-2.

Atrophie blanche (translated "white atrophy") refers to characteristic skin changes observed in some patients with vascular disease termed *livedoid vasculopathy*. Healed ulcers form white, stellate scars due to the dermal sclerosis and epidermal atrophy upon wound closure. The acronym PURPLE for painful purpuric ulcers with reticular patterning on the lower extremities is used to describe livedoid vasculopathy. Atrophie blanche may be observed in patients with venous insufficiency or may be a primary disorder.

Lymphatic and venous disease results in rough, tough skin with increased pigmentation. Fibrosis from chronic skin injury shortens small areas of skin and produces puckering, which may give the appearance of the skin of an orange, thus the term *peau d'orange* (Figure 8-3). Fluid and protein leakage accumulating in the interstitial space appears to be responsible for fibrosis and puckering.

Hydration, Turgor, and Elasticity

Hydration, turgor, and elasticity are grouped together due to their association with the aging process. In senescent skin, a loss of all 3 occurs. With normal hydration,

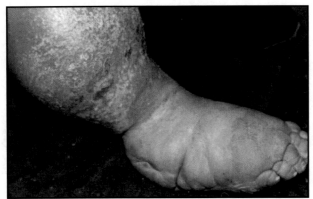

Figure 8-3. Skin changes associated with lymphedema. Note the greater puckering of skin producing the peau d'orange phenomenon. (The image is a copyrighted product of AAWC [www.aawconline.org] and has been reproduced with permission.)

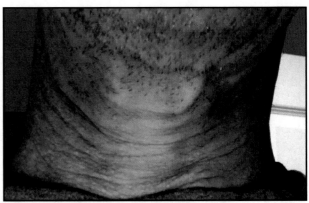

Figure 8-4. Tenting of neck skin at rest consistent with aging.

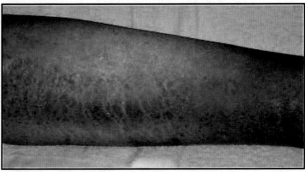

Figure 8-5. Xerosis of leg skin on patient with heavy pigmentation and diabetes mellitus.

a firm gel is evident in the dermal portion of the skin. Hydration, turgor, and elasticity can be tested by pinching the skin. With a pinch, a firm rounded skinfold can be gently lifted from the surface. This skinfold immediately retracts to its former position when released. In senescent skin, a dry, triangular skinfold can be observed, which does not immediately retract to its position upon release but remains elevated in the shape of a tent, thus the term *tenting*. Tenting can be seen at certain locations, especially the anterior neck, without pinching the skin. Turgor refers to the firmness of skin as it is pinched. This turgor is produced by resistance to compression of the gel-like property of a normally hydrated dermis in which water molecules are trapped by the glycosaminoglycans of the ground substance of the dermis. With insufficient hydration, turgor is lost as is the firm feel to the skinfold as shown in Figure 8-4. Dry skin with a flaky or cracked appearance but no loss of tissue volume or change in contour is termed *xerosis*, from the word for dry. Xerosis is more prevalent in more heavily pigmented skin and during colder weather. Xerosis is depicted in Figure 8-5.

Elasticity refers to the snapping back of healthy skin as the skinfold is released. It is partially due to skin turgor but as the name implies is also due to the presence of elastic fibers constructed of the protein elastin in the skin. The number and thickness of elastic fibers decrease with age. However, the skin of otherwise younger healthy skin can lose hydration, turgor, and elasticity in environments with low humidity, especially in the winter. Skin can rapidly lose moisture to dry, cold air and even crack in winter, requiring the use of moisturizers to maintain hydration, turgor, and elasticity.

Overhydrated skin occurs with derangements of fluid balance, resulting in edema. Edema can have many causes but basically results from excessive hydrostatic pressure in capillaries relative to the osmotic pressure across the capillary walls created by plasma proteins known as *oncotic pressure*. Edema results from congestive heart failure, venous insufficiency, and hyperemia producing excessive capillary hydrostatic pressure from excessive blood volume, failure to pump blood from veins back to the heart, or excessive dilation of arterial vessels.

With vasodilation, pressure remains high as it enters capillaries, resulting in fluid being filtered into the interstitial space. Diminished plasma protein concentration can result from a lack of production in liver disease or malnutrition or due to a loss of plasma proteins by kidney disease. Decreased plasma oncotic pressure will also allow excessive movement of water out of capillaries. Loss of plasma protein into the interstitial space whether due to injury, such as a burn, or due to very high capillary pressure creates a tremendous movement of water out of capillaries into the interstitial space, a phenomenon known as *third spacing*. Iatrogenic infiltration of fluid may occur when a line is assumed to be in a vein or a shunt used for hemodialysis and then the fluid is allowed to run into the limb. Fluid overload or edema results in damage to the epidermis and the peeling of the epidermis similar to what occurs following sunburn.

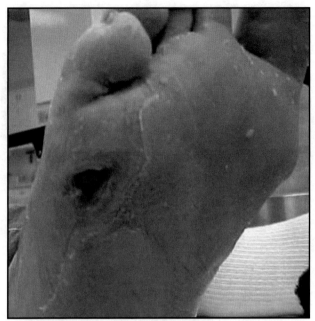

Figure 8-6. Representative plantar skin of patient with poorly controlled diabetes mellitus.

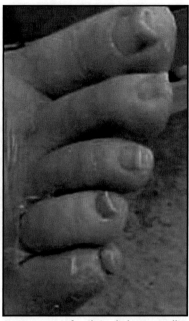

Figure 8-7. Appearance of nails in diabetes mellitus.

Hair and Nails

Loss of hair and thickening of nails are characteristic of arterial insufficiency but also occur with aging. A change in hair and nail appearance can be established by asking the patient or comparing the left and right sides. In the case of bilateral changes, the clinician may need to rely on patient recollection and personal judgment of normal hair and nail appearance. Thick, multilayered, yellowed nails are common with poorly controlled diabetes along with thick, rough skin on the soles (Figure 8-6). The characteristic appearance of nails with poorly controlled diabetes mellitus is shown in Figure 8-7.

Cardiovascular and Pulmonary

Components of the review of systems and common tests related to the cardiovascular and pulmonary systems are discussed in the following sections. Because many leg ulcers are related to arterial and venous disease, both vital signs and special tests related to them are included here.

Cardiac and Pulmonary Function

The review of systems related to cardiac function consists of vital signs and checking for clubbing, cyanosis, and edema. Heart rate and blood pressure should be measured at each opportunity. Measuring heart rate with a pulse oximeter also provides the opportunity to screen for breathing disorders; however, pulse oximetry is unreliable in the presence of vascular disease. Always check that the pulse strength is adequate before relying on the data from a pulse oximeter. Clubbing is a change in the shape of nails in which the nail shape becomes spherical as opposed to the normal cylindrical shape. Cystic fibrosis, lung cancer, and hypoxic cardiopulmonary diseases are associated with clubbing. Clubbing is not very specific because many people with no underlying disease may have detectible clubbing, but cystic fibrosis and Eisenmenger's syndrome can produce profound clubbing that is obvious to the eye. Cyanosis, a bluish tint to the skin, may be detected on the fingers, toes, around the mouth, or extend proximally if the cause is more severe. Causes may include respiratory disease or low cardiac output as may occur in severe congestive heart failure. Edema may be detected in the dependent areas, chiefly the lower extremities in congestive heart failure or other diseases that allow fluid to accumulate. Left-sided heart failure may lead to pulmonary edema, which may cause gurgling sounds with breathing, shortness of breath, frothy sputum, and orthopnea (ie, the inability to breathe when lying flat due to pulmonary edema).

Methods of assessing edema include checking for pitting (Figure 8-8) and measurements of edema. A foot volumeter may be used to compare the volume of 2 extremities and to detect changes in the volume of the same extremity (Figure 8-9). Because volumetry involves placing the extremity in water, hygiene is a concern, and an open wound should not be placed in a volumeter.

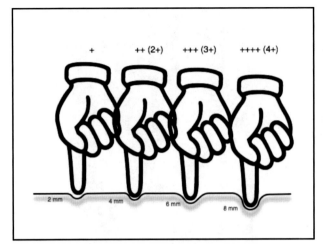

Figure 8-8. Assessment of pitting edema.

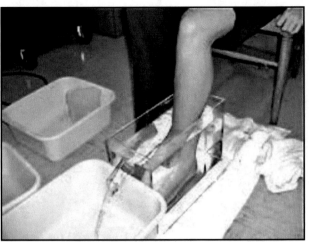

Figure 8-9. Performance of foot volumetry.

A quick and simple method that is sometimes used in place of volumetry in cases of distal edema is the figure 8 measurement shown in Figure 8-10. A tape measure is looped around the foot and ankle starting and finishing at the insertion of the tibialis anterior and passing landmarks including the head of the navicular, the styloid process of the fifth metatarsal, and medial and lateral malleoli. Reliability of the measurement is improved by using a tape measure with a spring to ensure the same tension is placed on the tape with each measurement. Another option discussed in Chapter 12 is the use of circumferential measurements along the affected extremity.

Additional tests of cardiac and pulmonary function may be performed in vascular and pulmonary function labs with referral from a physician. Cardiac catheterization can provide information about the heart's pumping ability and valvular function as well as the integrity of the coronary vessels. Arterial disease, especially in patients with diabetes mellitus, is likely to affect coronary vessels as well as cerebral and lower extremity arteries. Therefore, anyone with a history of disease in one of these areas is likely to have disease in others. For example, if a patient has a history of coronary bypass graft surgery, they are likely to be susceptible to arterial disease of the lower extremities leading to arterial ulcers or slow healing. Pulmonary function testing may be used to determine the type and severity of pulmonary dysfunction as well as assessing the effectiveness of treatment. Diminished cardiac and pulmonary function will lead to slower healing. Additionally, impairment of these functions may cause patients to lose mobility and increase the risk of ulcerations caused by decreased mobility.

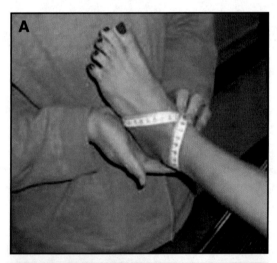

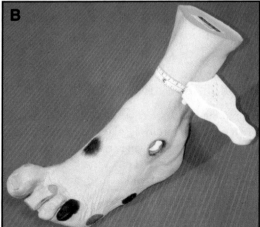

Figure 8-10. Using a tape measure to assess foot volume. (A) Using the figure 8 technique with a tape measure. (B) Spring-loaded tape measure to improve reliability of girth measurement.

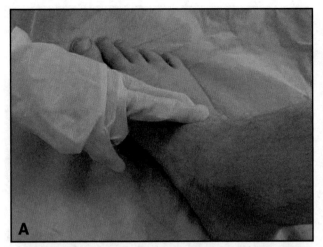

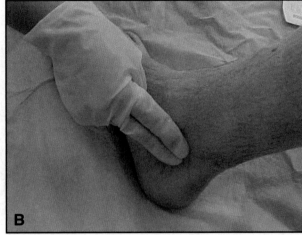

Figure 8-11. Detection of pulses. (A) Palpation of the dorsalis pedis. (B) Palpation of the posterior tibial artery. (C) Using Doppler stethoscope to detect the dorsalis pedis pulse.

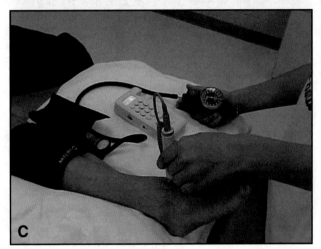

Vascular Testing

Because of the potentially serious nature of arterial insufficiency and the treatments used for venous and lymphatic diseases, the importance of arterial testing cannot be overemphasized. Compression and elevation used to treat venous and lymphatic disease are likely to exacerbate the already compromised circulation. Several tests for arterial sufficiency are available and range from highly sophisticated and expensive testing to cheap and easy but questionably valid tests.

Arterial Tests

Simple tests that do not require any equipment may be used. The simplest is palpation of the dorsalis pedis and posterior tibial pulses (Figures 8-11A and 8-11B, respectively) correlated with signs of arterial insufficiency already discussed, such as temperature and color of the limb and the appearance of hair and nails on the extremity. This examination lacks both sensitivity and specificity. Moderate arterial disease can be overlooked easily (lack of sensitivity), and many individuals with perfectly fine lower extremity blood flow may have a pulse that is difficult to palpate (low specificity). To improve sensitivity, a Doppler stethoscope (Figure 8-11C) may also be used to simply detect the presence of the lower extremity pulses. This is the same principle as palpating for a pulse but is more likely to find the pulse than simple palpation.

Ankle-Brachial Index

Measurement of the ankle-brachial index (ABI), also called *ankle pressure index* in some geographic regions, is a much better test that determines any loss of arterial pressure reaching the foot. Although this test requires several minutes to perform when making each of the 6 measurements separately, manufacturers have created machines capable of measuring all 4 extremities at once.

The ABI is based on the idea that obstruction of peripheral arteries diminishes the pressure of arterial blood as it passes distally into an extremity. Normal, healthy arteries produce little drop in arterial pressure;

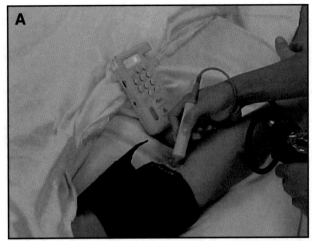 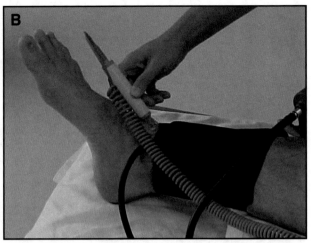

Figure 8-12. Measurement of the ABI. (A) Using a Doppler stethoscope to determine systolic pressure in the right brachial artery. This procedure is also performed on the left brachial artery. The greater of the 2 values is used in the denominator of the calculation of the ABI. (B) Measurement of systolic pressure of the right dorsalis pedis artery. The foot is positioned such that the height of the artery is the same as the brachial artery and right atrium. For measurement of the posterior tibial artery, the foot is elevated further. Both the right and left dorsalis pedis and posterior tibial arteries are measured. The 4 foot measurements are divided by the greater of the 2 brachial artery measurements to calculate the ABI.

therefore, arterial pressure measured in the brachial artery is very close to aortic pressure. Even in the arteries of the legs, very little pressure is lost. For all these measurements, pressure must be taken at the same height. Blood pressure measured in the leg needs to be done with the leg slightly elevated to raise it to the same level as the heart with the patient lying in supine. Unlike the brachial artery, which is sufficiently superficial to allow one to hear changes in flow pattern with a standard stethoscope as vessels become occluded and free to flow, the vessels of the lower extremity are generally not amenable to this technique. In the arm, we can closely approximate true systolic pressure as the pressure in the cuff at the point that blood can be heard to spurt under the cuff only at the peak systolic pressure. The lack of noise heard through the stethoscope then approximates diastolic pressure when blood is free to flow under the cuff continually through the cardiac cycle.

For the lower extremities, a Doppler stethoscope is used, typically over either the dorsalis pedis or the posterior tibial arteries. Brachial arterial pressure is also measured with the same technique, so the results can be compared. The Doppler effect is typically described as the change in pitch made as a train approaches and then moves away. As the train approaches, sound waves are compressed, increasing frequency, and as the train moves away, the sound waves are rarefied, decreasing frequency. A Doppler stethoscope emits ultrasound at 5 to 8 MHz. When the ultrasound strikes a moving medium, such as flowing blood, the shift in frequency is converted to a sound transmitted either to a speaker or earpieces. Most modern devices have built-in speakers to allow the

Doppler shift to be heard. The technique involves finding either the dorsalis pedis (Figure 8-12) or posterior tibial artery by palpation and then holding the probe at a 45-degree angle along the length of the artery as confirmed by a swishing sound.

A blood pressure cuff is placed on the calf and inflated until the swishing sound is lost. The lack of sound indicates that arterial flow is occluded. The cuff is slowly deflated as is done in sphygmomanometry. Resumption of the swishing sound indicates that pressure in the artery is just greater than pressure in the cuff. Note the lack of a unique sound to indicate diastolic pressure. The Doppler stethoscope does not work on the principle of the Korotkoff sounds. It indicates either the presence or absence of blood flow; therefore, only systolic pressure can be determined. The same technique with the Doppler device is done on both brachial arteries. If done at the same height relative to the heart, the values should be very close. Generally, the value in the leg is approximately 10% greater due to the reflection of pressure waves along the longer vessels of the leg. Therefore, we expect the ABI to be about 1.10 in a healthy person.

Any value below 0.9 is considered to be predictive of peripheral artery disease. When the ABI falls below 0.8 (ankle systolic pressure is 80% of brachial systolic pressure), some experts recommend that compression therapy not be used. Other individuals are more liberal, using a limit of 0.7. A value of 0.75 to 0.9 is indicative of moderate arterial disease; a patient with an ABI of 0.5 to 0.75 is considered to have severe arterial disease, and a value 0.4 or lower is considered to be critical limb ischemia, which is dangerous for the health of the limb and requires referral to a vascular surgeon. A value greater than 1.3 is considered to be indicative of calcification of arterial vessels. Calcification prevents the collapse of arterial vessels when cuff pressure exceeds arterial pressure. Therefore, a value greater than 1.1 in a person with risk factors for peripheral artery disease must be viewed with suspicion, and other forms of arterial testing will be needed to conclusively diagnose arterial disease.

Measurement of the ABI should be performed using 6 locations—bilateral brachial arteries, bilateral dorsalis pedis arteries, and bilateral posterior tibial arteries. The patient should be positioned in supine. The foot is elevated on a pillow or similar object such that the height of the artery is the same as the brachial artery and right atrium. For measurement of the posterior tibial artery, the foot is elevated further. Both the right and left dorsalis pedis and posterior tibial arteries are measured. The 4 foot measurements are divided by the greater of the 2 brachial artery measurements to calculate the ABI. For example, if the greater brachial artery pressure is 120 and left posterior tibial systolic pressure is 60, the ABI = 0.5.

Another use of the Doppler stethoscope is assessment of the arterial sounds without occlusion. The Doppler will produce a triphasic sound over a healthy artery. The triphasic waveform results from high forward flow during systole and brief reversal of direction from reflection of the pressure wave against resistance during early diastole, followed by forward flow again from reflection from the closed aortic valve in late diastole. Mild occlusion of the vessel being monitored produces a biphasic sound with no reversal in late systole. Greater occlusion produces a monophasic sound with systole only, and complete occlusion will produce no sound.

Transcutaneous Oxygen Measurements

This measure is performed in specialized vascular labs. The device, as the name implies, measures tissue oxygen through the skin. This measurement is performed with a special airtight sensor that heats the skin to 41°C to allow equilibration between capillary PO_2 and the sensor, taking approximately 20 minutes to perform. In particular, the device is used to determine the appropriate amputation level but can also be used to predict the likelihood of wounds healing. A value of less than 20 mm Hg carries a poor prognosis for healing, whereas a value greater than 30 predicts healing. This information can also aid the decision to debride wounds. Using the same criteria, one may decide to debride a wound with a transcutaneous oxygen reading of greater than 30 mm Hg but not if the surrounding skin produces a value of 20 mm Hg. In any case, when in doubt, a vascular surgeon must be consulted.

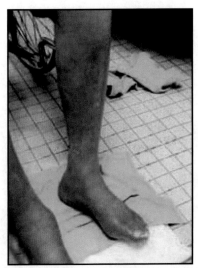

Figure 8-13. Appearance of rubor of dependency. Note the patient also demonstrates the appearances of venous disease and neuropathy.

Rubor of Dependency Test

This test is based on gravitational challenge to the arterial circulation and observation. With the patient/client placed in supine (on the back), the lower extremity is raised 60 degrees for 1 minute. Signs of arterial insufficiency may be present in this first phase as complaints of pain with elevation and an ashen appearance to the extremity. In a healthy person, a decrease in the pinkness occurs and returns as the leg is lowered to the table. In a person with arterial disease, the color of the leg goes beyond the normal pink and becomes quite red due to the phenomenon termed *reactive hyperemia*. Reactive hyperemia refers to the dilation of vessels in response to the occlusion of vessels. When the occlusion is released, blood flow is increased markedly above normal, producing the rubor of dependency. Rubor of dependency may be observed in some patients who are simply sitting. An example of rubor of dependency is shown in Figure 8-13.

Venous Filling Time Test

The venous filling time test superficially resembles the rubor of dependency test. The patient is placed in supine, and the lower extremity is elevated to 60 degrees for 1 minute. The leg is massaged to reduce leg volume as much as possible. The patient is then asked to stand, and the volume of the foot veins is observed. With normal circulation, the foot veins gradually fill through arterial inflow. Lack of filling within 10 to 15 seconds indicates arterial insufficiency. With venous insufficiency, foot veins fill rapidly through both arterial inflow and venous backflow (Figure 8-14).

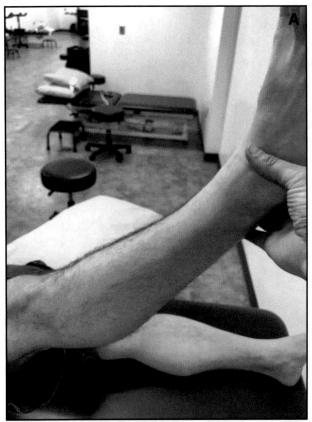
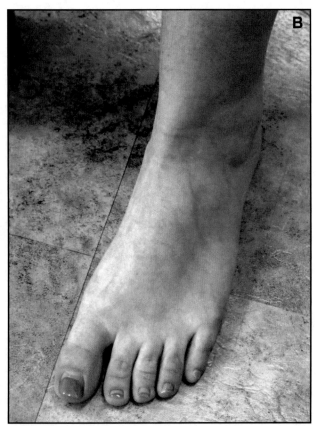

Figure 8-14. Performance of the venous filling time test. Rapid refill of the foot veins indicates venous reflux. In the presence of venous reflux, the ability to detect slow refill secondary to arterial disease cannot occur. (A) Elevation of the leg to assist in emptying foot veins; massage may be added to further empty veins. (B) Normal refilling of veins upon standing; the failure of veins to refill in 2 to 3 seconds indicates arterial disease, whereas immediate refilling indicates incompetent venous valves.

Venous Tests

Several tests for venous insufficiency are also available. Often venous disease is obvious grossly by the presence of dilated superficial veins, especially if the dilated vessels are tortuous (following a twisting path rather than a relatively straight line). Other indications include lipodermatosclerosis, hemosiderin staining, and corona (starburst) formation of smaller superficial veins. Venous tests include the percussion test, venous filling time test (nominally an arterial test), and venous plethysmography. The percussion test examines the patency of valves. A normal valve does not allow backflow from above the knee to below the knee. During this test, the examiner palpates a superficial vein below the knee and strikes the same vein above the knee. With normal valves, the pressure wave generated is baffled at the valve below, so no pressure wave is detected below the knee. With insufficient valves, the pressure wave is transmitted distally and can be palpated below the knee. The Trendelenburg test is performed in a similar manner as the venous filling time test, except for a tourniquet placed around the thigh, occluding venous but not arterial flow. The patient stands, and the examiner observes for filling of superficial veins. Immediate filling indicates incompetent valves of communicating veins. The tourniquet is then removed. Rapid filling of superficial veins demonstrates incompetence of the saphenous vein.

Venous plethysmography is a technological improvement of the venous filling time test. A plastic air chamber is placed over the lower extremity. A pressure-detecting device is attached to the chamber. The patient/client is asked to stand with the lower extremity in the chamber to provide a baseline volume. The decrease in volume that occurs in the supine position with the leg elevated is recorded. When a new baseline is reached, the patient/client is asked to stand rapidly. A progressive increase in lower extremity volume is considered normal. A rapid increase beyond the original standing baseline indicates venous insufficiency. A summary of vascular testing is provided in Box 8-1.

Imaging of Blood Vessels

Arterial blood vessels may be imaged through a number of modalities. Angiography is the use of radiopaque material injected into vessels so their presence can be

BOX 8-1
Vascular Tests

TEST	PURPOSE	TECHNIQUE
Rubor of dependency	Weak test for peripheral arterial disease	Elevate leg 60 degrees for 1 minute Ashen appearance, c/o pain may occur Lower leg and examine return of color
Capillary filling	Test for arterial or vasospastic disease	Squeeze nail bed until it blanches Release and time refill
Venous filling	Weak test for arterial disease, but can also indicate venous disease	Elevate leg Massage fluid out Rapidly lower and have patient stand Examine how rapidly veins refill Slow refill indicates arterial disease Rapid refill indicates insufficient valves
Venous percussion	Test for incompetent valve(s)	Palpate vein above and below knee Strike vein above knee Pressure wave palpated below knee indicates insufficient valve
Palpation of foot pulses	Arterial disease	Palpate between first and second ray on foot for dorsalis pedis Palpate between medial malleolus and Achilles tendon for posterior tibial Lack of pulse indicates arterial disease
Trendelenburg test	Venous disease	Elevate lower extremity to empty veins Place tourniquet around thigh in supine Patient stands Observe rate of filling of veins Rapid filling indicates venous valvular disease

viewed with routine X-ray technology. Although this is typically done for arterial vessels, it can also be used to image veins. Blood vessels may also be imaged with magnetic resonance imaging. Another technique is duplex ultrasound, which may be used for arterial or venous vessels. Any of these techniques can demonstrate occlusions of the vessels. Duplex ultrasound can also show velocity as different colors in the image. Ultrasound is a common test used when clots occluding a lower extremity wound are suspected.

Aerobic Capacity and Endurance

Simple tests of aerobic function such as upper extremity ergometry or the Balke test may be used. The Balke test consists of setting a treadmill at 3.3 mph and increasing the grade of the treadmill 1% every minute. Knowledge of aerobic capacity can be used in prescribing an exercise program when developing the plan of care. A treadmill test, whether the Balke, Bruce, or other protocol, is particularly useful for the patient with suspected arterial insufficiency. Intermittent claudication manifested as calf pain at a given intensity of exercise can be monitored through the course of treatment. Management of peripheral arterial disease is discussed in Chapter 12. Patients should undergo exercise health screening before undergoing exercise testing.

Musculoskeletal

The review of systems related to the musculoskeletal system minimally consists of strength and range of motion testing. Additional testing may be done based on the

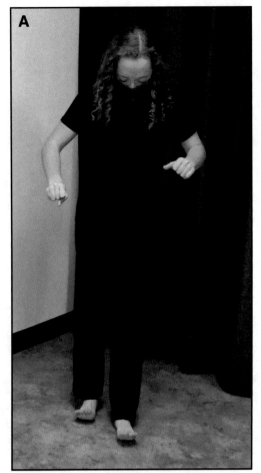
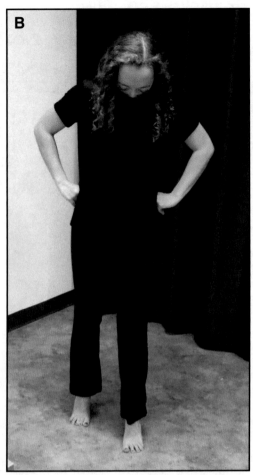

Figure 8-15. Quick lower extremity strength testing. The patient is asked to take several steps on the heels and again on the toes. The inability to maintain the position while walking indicates insufficient strength to ambulate safely and increased risk of plantar ulceration.

results of this testing. Impairments in the musculoskeletal system may lead to abnormal forces being placed on the skin or the inability to shift pressure away from certain parts of the body.

Strength and Range of Motion

These tests can be ignored when focus is totally on the wound rather than on the patient. We need to remember that we are working with a person who needs to function in a particular environment. For most patients, a rudimentary test can be conducted in less than 1 minute. Specific muscle tests can be performed as the examination or history dictates. For screening, walking on heels and toes can quickly indicate whether a person has sufficient lower extremity strength to prevent injury to the feet (Figure 8-15). More specific muscle testing is used if a patient cannot maintain more than a few steps on either the heels or toes as depicted in Figure 8-16. As

discussed in Chapter 11, limited range of motion of the toes, foot, and ankle increases the risk of injury to the skin of the foot and impairs healing of wounds on the plantar surface.

Neuromuscular

Components of the neuromuscular portion of the review of systems generally include sensory and reflex, in addition to the strength testing discussed previously. Components of a patient's balance, mobility, gait, and coordination should be tested as well. A patient may appear to be within normal limits for simple sensory, reflex, and strength testing but may not be able to perform higher-level tasks effectively. Balance, mobility, gait, and coordination problems may interfere with the healing of wounds and put other areas of the skin at risk.

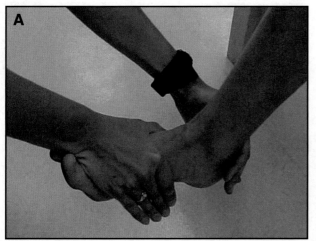
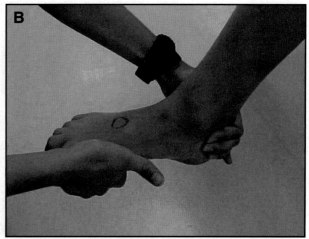

Figure 8-16. Manual muscle testing of foot muscles. The inability to walk on heels and toes requires specific manual testing of the dorsiflexors, plantar flexors, and toe muscles. (A) Testing of the dorsiflexors. (B) Testing of the plantar flexors.

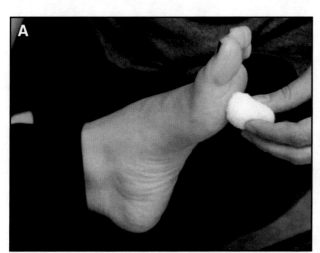
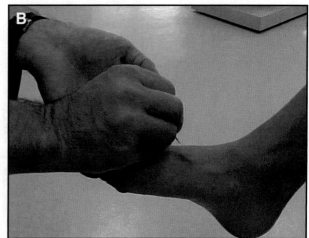

Figure 8-17. (A) Testing for light touch using a cotton ball. (B) Testing using pinprick.

Sensory Testing

Rudimentary sensory testing should also be performed routinely with every patient. Again, more detailed testing of the distal extremities is required for anyone with suspected peripheral neuropathy or other neuromuscular diseases or injuries. Several textbooks are also available to provide a detailed approach. Often a simple test of light touch with a cotton-tipped applicator or pinprick (Figure 8-17) and the patient's eyes closed is sufficient to rule out sensory deficits.

Monofilament Testing

In addition to other tools used to determine sensory integrity, diabetic foot screening commonly uses Semmes-Weinstein monofilaments to assess the risk of plantar ulceration in ambulatory, sensory-impaired individuals. These special monofilaments are designed to bend at a calibrated force. Starting with the thinnest monofilament in the set, each monofilament is touched to skin for a total of 1 1/2 seconds: bending for 1/2 second, held bent for 1/2 second, and removed for 1/2 second (Figure 8-18). Excessive callus on the foot will decrease the sensitivity of even normal feet. Once a person is able to feel a given monofilament, the clinician stops and records the value. In some cases, a clinician may wish to perform a more thorough test and actually map the entire foot.

For a screening procedure, a single 10-g monofilament may be used for a prescribed number of standardized sites. The traditional 10 sites are depicted in Figures 8-19A and 8-19B. More recent recommendations of the International Working Group on the Diabetic Foot suggest fewer sites—the first and fifth metatarsal heads and plantar first toe as shown in Figure 8-19C. The 10-g monofilament specifically tests for the loss of protective sensation. This means that a person who cannot feel this filament lacks sufficient

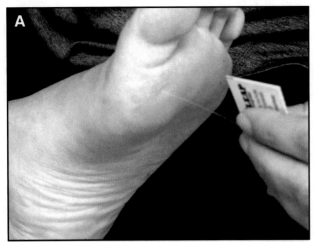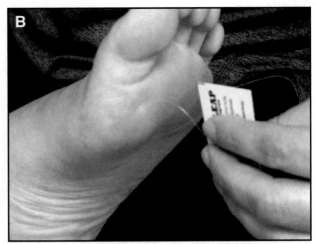

Figure 8-18. Sensory testing using a Semmes-Weinstein monofilament. Use of a 10-g monofilament tests specifically for protective sensation. Patients unable to detect this monofilament are considered to be at risk for plantar ulceration. (A) Making contact for 1/2 second. (B) Allowing the monofilament to bend for 1/2 second.

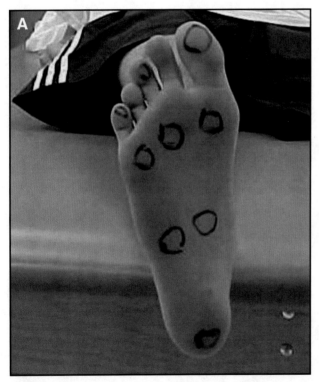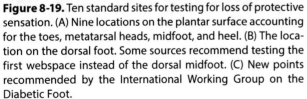

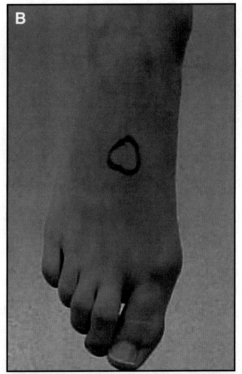

Figure 8-19. Ten standard sites for testing for loss of protective sensation. (A) Nine locations on the plantar surface accounting for the toes, metatarsal heads, midfoot, and heel. (B) The location on the dorsal foot. Some sources recommend testing the first webspace instead of the dorsal midfoot. (C) New points recommended by the International Working Group on the Diabetic Foot.

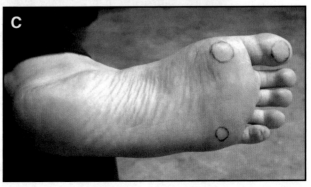

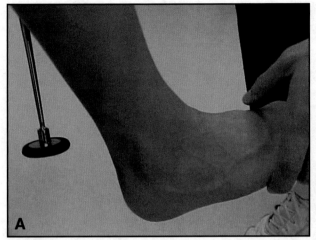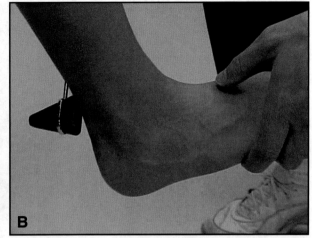

Figure 8-20. Reflex testing for lower extremities. (A) Testing ankle jerk with a Babinski hammer. (B) Testing ankle jerk with a Taylor reflex hammer.

sensation to detect impending injury to the foot. In addition, the clinician should check the foot for deformities and decreased strength, which may alter the weight-bearing pattern and gait, and should visually inspect the skin on each foot.

Further sensory testing should be done to distinguish between small and large sensory neuron loss. Reflexes and vibration are carried by large neurons, whereas monofilaments are sufficient to test for small neurons. Loss of reflexes and vibration indicates a greater degree of neuropathy because loss of neurons generally occurs first in small neurons, progressing to large neurons. Vibration can be tested with a 128-Hz tuning fork or a biothesiometer, which produces a more uniform means of testing vibration. Loss of large neurons is particularly critical. Motor neurons and position sense are carried by large neurons. Loss of the position senses, proprioception, and kinesthesia are likely to exacerbate the problems caused by sensory neuropathy. A typical gait for a person with diminished proprioception includes short, slapping steps and abnormal progression from heel strike to toe off.

Reflex Testing

Reflex testing includes the deep tendon reflexes of the biceps, triceps, brachioradialis for the upper extremities, and quadriceps (knee jerk) and gastrocnemius/soleus (ankle jerk) with a reflex hammer (Figure 8-20). The Babinski hammer is recommended for this procedure for ease of use. The long handle and weighted head allow the hammer's head to be simply dropped onto the tendon of interest as opposed to the Buck or Taylor hammers, which require more skill in striking the tendon. In addition, testing the Babinski or related reflex on the sole may be necessary given a history of upper motor neuron lesions. Testing for

resistance to quick movement and the presence of clonus with quick movement of the wrists and ankles should also be performed for individuals with upper motor neuron lesions. Increased tone manifested as either spasticity or rigidity predisposes this individual to pressure injuries.

Romberg Test

Proprioception and the dorsal columns are tested with the Romberg test. The ability to maintain balance relies on vision, proprioception, and vestibular response to acceleration. By closing the eyes, a patient relies on proprioception and vestibular response to acceleration to maintain balance. With intact proprioception and dorsal columns, a person can stand with minimal swaying. If proprioception is impaired, balance is maintained by the vestibular system responding to acceleration. A person will then have a rather noticeable sway, which is accentuated by bringing their feet closer (Figure 8-21). A patient who sways with their eyes open is likely to have ataxia, a cerebellar disorder.

Tandem Walking

The ability to walk with a narrow base of support indicates both strength and coordination required to prevent injury to feet. A person walks by placing the heel of the swinging extremity directly in front of the toes of the stance foot and repeating for multiple steps, as shown in Figure 8-22. A person with poor proprioception will walk with a wide base of support. Poor performance on tandem walking, a self-selected wide base of support, and substantial swaying on the Romberg test are all indicative of poor proprioception and increased risk of plantar ulceration.

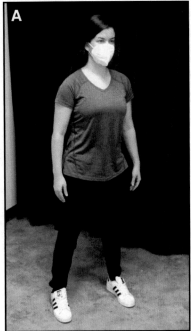
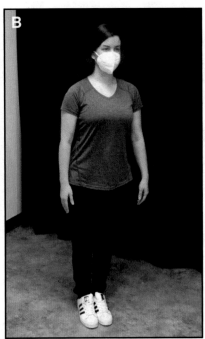
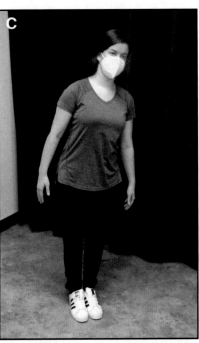

Figure 8-21. Performance of the Romberg test. Amount of sway is observed with the eyes open and feet at shoulder width. Increased sway with eyes closed indicates diminished proprioception. A more sensitive test can be performed by moving the feet closer than shoulder width. A patient with a positive Romberg test is likely to walk with a wide base of support; therefore, the clinician should be observing the patient's normal gait pattern.

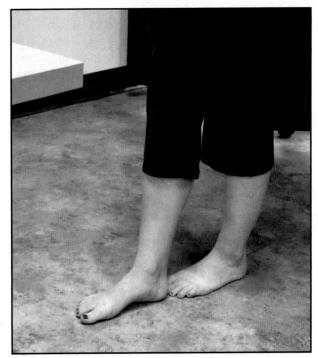

Figure 8-22. Performance of tandem walking.

MOBILITY

A brief assessment of the patient's bed mobility, transfers, and gait correlated with history including home and work environment is also commonly overlooked. Examine how the individual bears weight on different bony prominences when resting in bed, sitting, moving in bed, coming to sit, coming to stand, and ambulating. Ask about the use of assistive devices and assess the patient's ability to use the assistive device. Inquire about weight-bearing restrictions, especially those involving the wounded body part. Discussion of footwear is also covered in Chapter 11. Poor balance or coordination may require compensations that have either created or exacerbated the wound. In some cases, simply providing a walker may alleviate the problem. Other cases may require more involved interventions such as the use of total contact casts (also discussed in Chapter 11). A patient with deficits in mobility should be referred to physical therapy to improve mobility to the level consistent with their desired lifestyle.

SUMMARY

Basic tests performed during the physical examination are described in this chapter and summarized in Box 8-2. The selection of tests is driven by the history and review of systems. Four systems to be tested are the integumentary,

BOX 8-2
Components of Exam

- Color and texture of skin
  - More difficult to assess as melanin content increases
  - Blanching, cyanosis, erythema, mottling
  - Vitiligo—patches of unpigmented skin
  - ACTH—stimulates melanocytes in skin and gums; Addison's disease
  - Xerosis—dry, possibly cracking skin
  - Accumulations
    - Hemosiderin—trauma/bleeding in skin
    - Lipodermatitis with leakage of protein in skin
      - Usually lymphedema
      - Can be severe/long-standing venous hypertension
    - Peau d'orange—puckering like skin of citrus fruit
  - Callus associated with neuropathy
  - Hydration
    - Aging and tenting of skin
    - Xerosis common in darkly pigmented skin
    - Kidney disease, low humidity, low air loss mattress
- Hair and nails
- Symmetric hair and nail growth
  - Hair loss and coolness/pallor in ischemia
  - Thickened, yellow, splintering of nails with neuropathy and peripheral arterial disease
- Temperature
  - White or blue and cold
  - Red and hot
  - Use hands and infrared temperature meter
- Cardiovascular review of systems
  - Edema scale +, ++, +++, or ++++
    - Quantify with foot volumetry
    - Bilateral comparison if one extremity considered normal
    - Plateau of serial measurement if not
    - Figure 8 method is fast and reasonable for ankle

- Palpation of pulses has low sensitivity and specificity
- Ankle-brachial index (ABI) has good sensitivity and specificity
- ABI > 1.3 is inconclusive; needs further vascular testing
  - Normal is 1.1; below 0.9 considered peripheral arterial disease
  - Below 0.4 considered critical limb ischemia
    - Pain at rest
    - Nonhealing wounds
    - Gangrene
  - Toe-brachial index if ABI is inconclusive due to ABI > 1.3
- Rubor of dependency exists, but low S&S
- Musculoskeletal and neuromuscular testing
  - Strength by walking on toes and heels as quick screen
    - Measure individual muscles if patient fails
    - High risk of foot injury if patient cannot
- Sensory testing specific to foot
  - Vibration checks large sensory neurons
  - Semmes-Weinstein monofilaments
    - 10-g checks specifically for loss of protective sensation
    - Can use more monofilaments to get finer distinction
    - Total of 1.5 seconds
    - Standard sites for screening—bowling pin + dorsum
  - Ankle jerk compared with knee jerk and others
    - Quick screen for large motor and sensory
    - Can follow up with more granular testing if necessary
    - Loss of ankle jerk predicts altered gait mechanics and risk of foot injury
- Gait pattern
  - Wide base indicates loss of proprioception and risk of foot injury
- Tandem walking to challenge balance (multiple neuromuscular functions)
- Romberg to assess proprioception

cardiovascular and pulmonary, musculoskeletal, and neuromuscular. A general inspection of the skin is followed by more specific tests of the vascular system, sensation, strength, reflexes, and cardiovascular system. Tests are used to develop a diagnosis, and using the information from the history, a meaningful prognosis is developed. An excessive focus on the wound instead of the patient leads to missing out on important information gathered from examining the rest of the skin and the other 3 systems.

QUESTIONS

1. Define skin turgor. What happens to skin turgor with age? Why does this happen?

2. What are the benefits of measuring skin temperature? What does an elevated or depressed skin temperature indicate?

3. What other tests would confirm suspicions raised by a decreased skin temperature?

4. Name several tests available to test the neuromuscular aspects of the lower extremity.

5. Why do we routinely perform testing on range of motion and strength of the toes, feet, and ankle in patients with neuropathy?

6. Why do we test with tuning forks, monofilaments, and test reflexes in patients with neuropathy?

7. Why do we perform exercise screening and tests of aerobic capacity in patients with or at risk of developing wounds?

8. What are the advantages and disadvantages of volumetry vs figure 8 measurement vs circumferential measurements for quantifying edema?

9. What is the rationale for ABI testing?

BIBLIOGRAPHY

Alavi A, Hafner J, Dutz JP, et al. Atrophie blanche. *Adv Skin Wound Care*. 2014;27(11):518-524.

Bus SA, Lavery LA, Monteiro-Soares M, et al. Guidelines on the prevention of foot ulcers in persons with diabetes (IWGDF 2019 update). *Diabetes Metab Res Rev*. 2020;36(Suppl 1):e3269

Carpenter JP. Noninvasive assessment of peripheral vascular occlusive disease. *Adv Skin Wound Care*. 2000;13(2):84-85.

Kanji JN, Anglin RES, Hunt DL, Pnaju A. Does this patient with diabetes have large-fiber peripheral neuropathy? *JAMA*. 2010;303(15):1526-1532.

Lause M, Kamboj A, Faith EF. Dermatologic manifestations of endocrine disorders. *Transl Pediatr*. 2017;6(4):300-312.

Schaper NC, van Netten JJ, Apelqvist J, et al. Practical guidelines on the prevention and management of diabetic foot disease (IWGDF 2019 update). *Diabetes Metab Res Rev*. 2020;36(Suppl 1):e3266.

Scissons R. Characterizing triphasic, biphasic, and monophasic doppler waveforms. *JDMS*. 2008;24(5):269-276.

Sieggreen MY, Maklebust J. Managing leg ulcers. *Nursing*. 1996;26(12):41-46.

Sloan H, Wills EM. Ankle-brachial index: calculating your patient's vascular risk. *Nursing*. 1999;29(10):58-59.

9

Wound Assessment

OBJECTIVES

- Perform basic observations (CODES [Color of wounds, Odor, Drainage, Edges, and Size]).
- Measure dimensions of a wound.
- Document observations and measurements.
- Identify tissue types within a wound.
- Document undermining, pocketing, tunneling, and sinus tracts.
- Describe and distinguish signs of infection and inflammation both locally and systemically.
- Perform differential diagnosis of wounds of different etiology.
- Provide a prognosis for different wounds; list factors that may alter the anticipated number of visits or time for reaching goals.
- Conduct a complete wound examination/evaluation.
- Recognize the need for and utilize the results of various diagnostic imaging procedures.

Previous chapters have been directed toward assessing a patient. However, given 2 wounds with identical characteristics, patients with different cultural, work, family backgrounds, and comorbid conditions may have different goals or prognoses for that wound. A thorough examination must be performed during the initial visit with periodic re-examination appropriate for the setting. Every visit is an opportunity for re-examination, including an update on history, home, and work activities. The depth and breadth of each re-examination will be determined by a number of factors—the severity of the wound; the progress of the

Irion GL, Gardner JA, Pignataro RM.
Comprehensive Wound Management, Third Edition (pp 131-149).
© 2024 Taylor and Francis Group.

TABLE 9-1
Observations (CODES)

Color

Red, yellow, and black

Signs of infection

Extent of debridement needed

Signs of PAD

Odor

Signs of infection

Drainage

Quantitative: desiccated, min, mod, max/copious

Qualitative: color, consistency

Edges

Adherent, loose, undermined/pocketing

Surrounding skin: maceration, inflammation, hydration, nutrition, callus, induration

Size

Surface area = widest distance in any direction × widest perpendicular to first

Use clock notation for undermining and tunnels

Depth to determine volume

wound; and any signs of deterioration, such as development or worsening of odor, drainage, or pain. The purpose of this chapter is to develop a systematic method of wound examination so one can develop a differential diagnosis and a prognosis for reaching appropriate goals based on the individual needs of the patient.

WOUND CHARACTERISTICS

The 6 critical aspects are color, odor, drainage, edges, and surrounding skin and size. The acronym CODES will be used to develop a systematic examination of the wound. Methods for observing these and measurements of wounds are discussed along with the interpretation of findings. Tools for examination can be relatively simple such as cotton-tipped applicators and paper rulers; however, a thorough examination requires adequate lighting to visualize the details of the wound and surrounding skin. A dedicated exam light is useful because it can be used during debridement as well. A headlamp or pocket flashlight and magnifying glass are tremendously useful to see detail, particularly deep into a wound where an exam light might be difficult to aim. Otherwise, deeper aspects within the

wound, particularly color, could be missed. The ability to determine which tissue layers are involved in wounds and the colors deep within them can facilitate the diagnostic process greatly. A synopsis of the CODES scheme is provided in Table 9-1.

Color

This item refers to the color within the wound. The color of the surrounding skin is discussed later. The 3 basic colors that may be observed in a wound are black, yellow, and red. Within these 3 basic types, different degrees of tissue health may be reflected by the saturation. For example, a pink, or paler degree of red, indicates blood flow, and the progression from yellow to tan to brown to black indicates the desiccation of devitalized tissue.

Black

Black tissue within a wound represents desiccated necrotic tissue or eschar. The amount of eschar on a given wound can range from completely covering the wound bed (Figure 9-1A) to small quantities within the wound (Figure 9-1B) or on the edges of the wound (Figure 9-1C). With certain exceptions, black tissue should be debrided to allow migration of new cells to fill the defect and resurface it with epithelial cells. An exception to debriding blackened tissue is the presence of dry gangrene, usually on the foot, caused by severe ischemia (Figure 9-2). Such advanced arterial disease often requires amputation, and autoamputation of toes may occur. Debridement in the case of dry gangrene is unlikely to assist in healing due to the lack of delivery of nutrients necessary for healing; rather, it exposes tissue adjacent to necrotic tissue to the risk of infection. The National Pressure Injury Advisory Panel recommends leaving dry eschar on heels as long as it is stable.

Yellow

Tissue with a yellowish color may represent 1 of 3 possibilities. *Pus* (purulent exudate) within a wound has a thick texture, usually has an odor, and may have a color ranging from a greenish tint to a darker yellow, as shown in Figure 9-3. Purulence is a very specific sign of infection with pyogenic (pus-producing) organisms, which may require either the temporary use of topical antimicrobials or systemic antibiotic drugs along with more aggressive debridement of the wound. A second yellow substance is *fibrin* (Figure 9-4). Fibrinogen leaks from vessels during inflammation and is converted to fibrin. Fibrin is the end product of the blood coagulation cascade, forming an insoluble fiber that, along with platelets, creates thrombi.

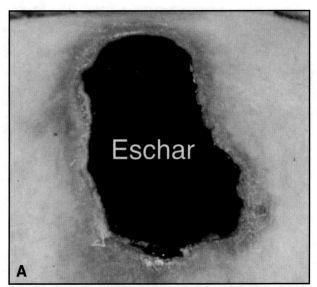

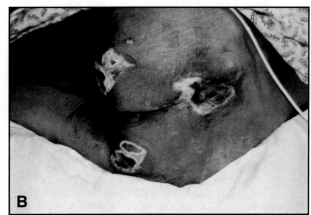

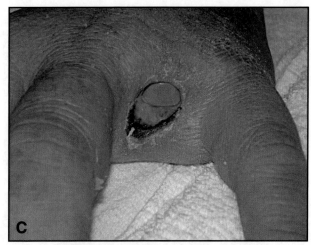

Figure 9-1. Eschar. (A) Trochanteric wound covered completely with eschar. (The image is a copyrighted product of AAWC [www.aawconline.org] and has been reproduced with permission.) (B) Individual wounds partially covered with eschar. (The image is a copyrighted product of AAWC [www.aawconline.org] and has been reproduced with permission.) (C) Eschar on the edge of the wound.

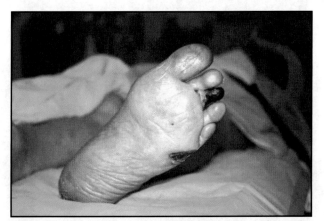

Figure 9-2. Dry gangrene of the third toe and lateral foot. (The image is a copyrighted product of AAWC [www.aawconline.org] and has been reproduced with permission.)

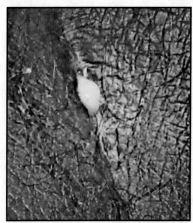

Figure 9-3. Purulent drainage from the wound.

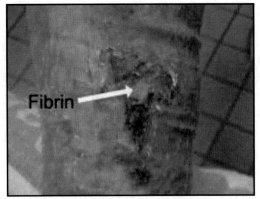

Figure 9-4. Fibrin formed over the surface of a venous ulcer.

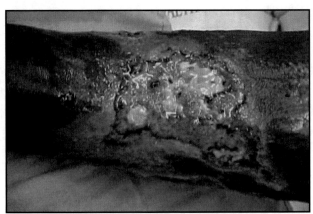

Figure 9-5. A wound undergoing autolytic debridement.

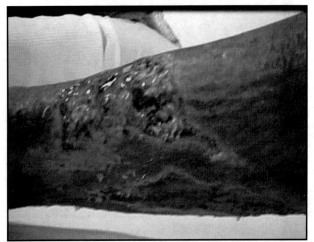

Figure 9-6. Drainage from autolytic debridement with coagulated blood on the surface.

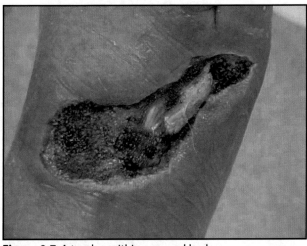

Figure 9-7. A tendon within a wound bed.

Fibrin on the surface of a wound can form a difficult-to-remove hardened sheet on wound beds, which may require debridement with specific chemicals or sharp instruments. The third material is termed *slough* (pronounced "sluff"). Slough is partially solubilized necrotic tissue. The color of slough ranges from a grayish to brownish-yellow color depending on how well autolytic debridement (breakdown of necrotic tissue by enzymes produced by cells in the wound) is proceeding (Figure 9-5). Autolytic debridement is also associated with soupy brownish drainage and stringy tissue (Figure 9-6). It should not be confused with purulence. Tendons and ligaments within a wound bed can have a yellowish color and should not be confused with necrotic tissue. Regularity of the tissue with a firm feel should cause tendon and ligamentous tissue to stand out. Moreover, the clinician can ask the patient to attempt to move the body part attached to the suspected tendon or ligament. A tendon within a wound bed is shown in Figure 9-7.

Red

A beefy red color is observed in a clean, granulating wound (most of the wound bed in Figure 9-5). A wound with this color needs to be protected from both environmental factors and harsh handling by the clinician or caregiver. Appropriate dressings for clean, granulating wounds are discussed in Chapter 16. Redness of tissue is due to the presence of hemoglobin of red blood cells circulating through tissue. As blood flow declines with arterial disease, granulation tissue becomes less red, becoming pink instead. A lighter pink color indicates poor arterial circulation (Figure 9-8). A dusky (dark) red, as seen in Figure 9-9, is an indication of impending necrosis suggesting infection of the granulation tissue, particularly in combination with weak, bleeding tissue as seen in Figure 9-8. *Friable* is the adjective used to describe tissue with a dusky, bleeding, stringy appearance. A partial-thickness wound will demonstrate a pink color characteristic of dermis (Figure 9-10). When discussing the wound color, one should simply note

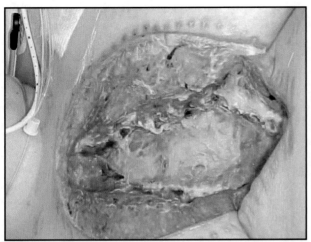

Figure 9-8. Pink granulation tissue associated with decreased blood flow.

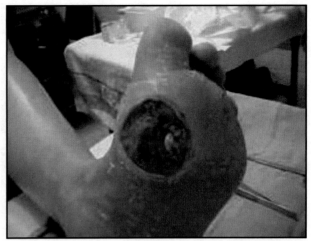

Figure 9-9. Friable tissue within the wound bed of a neuropathic ulcer indicating poor tissue health and likely infection.

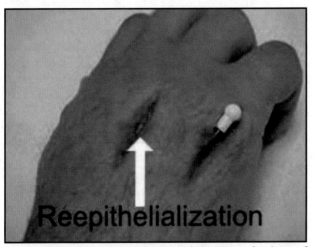

Figure 9-10. Pink-colored re-epithelialization of edges of wounds.

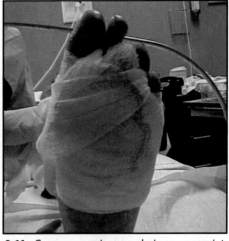

Figure 9-11. Green sanguineous drainage associated with *Pseudomonas aeruginosa* infection.

that pink dermal tissue is exposed rather than refer to the tissue as red. Red color is generally reserved for discussing the quality and quantity of granulation tissue.

Odor

Although words may fail to describe odors well, a few words are commonly used to describe them. Healthy wounds generally have no odor, but the absence of odor does not ensure the absence of infection. *Foul* is used for wounds that have an unpleasant odor that generally induces a withdrawal reaction. Putrid or fetid is reserved for a very strong, foul odor associated with decaying meat. The term *putrid* specifically applies to decaying matter, whereas *fetid* is derived from the Latin "to stink." A putrid odor may be present in a wound that has had a large amount of necrotic tissue for an extended time such as that depicted

in Figure 9-9. A venous ulcer, such as that in Figure 9-5, with relatively little necrotic tissue will have little to no observable odor.

A fruity/sweet odor is characteristic of infection with *Pseudomonas aeruginosa*. *Pseudomonas* is also characterized by a bluish-green color on the wound surface and greenish drainage (Figure 9-11). Treatment for *Pseudomonas* infection is frequently topical application of 0.25% acetic acid, the active ingredient of vinegar, which also has a characteristic odor. Proteus produces a characteristic ammonia odor. A foul-smelling wound is usually but not always infected. A wound with a strong foul odor from a distance or with the dressing still in place, however, is very likely to be infected. Large quantities of slough left in a wound over multiple hours/days may have an odor, and a clinician must be prepared to distinguish the odor of an occluded wound from infection. Slough left under an occlusive dressing (a dressing holding fluid under it)

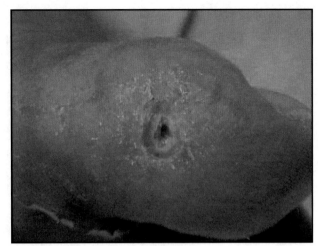

Figure 9-12. A desiccated neuropathic ulcer on the medial great toe surrounded with callus.

for a number of days may have an odor. However, this odor is typically milder than that associated with infection and will be lost when the wound is cleansed, whereas an infected wound will continue to have a foul odor after the wound is cleansed. For example, the wound in Figure 9-6 would be expected to have a mild odor when the dressings are removed after an entire week of autolytic debridement under compression bandaging, but the odor should dissipate with wound cleaning and debridement.

Drainage

Drainage should be described in terms of both the amount and quality of the drainage.

Quantitative

Terms used to describe quantity are rather subjective. A continuum of desiccated, minimum, moderate, and maximum (or copious) is used. The terms *desiccated* and *maximum* are easily identified. A wound bed that is dry needs intervention to increase its moisture to a level compatible with healing. A desiccated wound is depicted in Figure 9-12. The term *maximum* or *copious* drainage may be used when the primary dressing (dressing directly in contact with the wound) and secondary dressings are soaked with drainage. Venous ulcers frequently have copious drainage, and maceration is often present when the wounds are simply covered with dressings, as in Figure 9-6. A small area of moisture on the primary dressing may be described as minimum. Moderate drainage may be appropriate when the primary dressing is nearly full but not saturated with drainage. The wound in Figure 9-1C had moderate drainage, and some shine is seen on the surface. Making this judgment without

seeing the dressing and knowing the wear time is difficult. Moreover, the wear time for a given dressing can be inconsistent. For example, a dressing may be changed overnight or during early morning rounds with no indication of how long the dressing has been accumulating drainage. Copious drainage needs to be managed by selecting an appropriate dressing or combination of dressings to absorb drainage and protect the surrounding skin from excessive moisture. Optimizing healing is often a balancing act of maintaining wound moisture without maceration of surrounding skin and requires good clinical judgment. In general, a heavily draining wound will have more fluid than just a shine, and minimal drainage will be dry but not desiccated with dressings off. Moderate drainage will noticeably reflect light.

Qualitative

The color and consistency of drainage are also important. Clear drainage is caused by leakage of fluid from blood vessels during inflammation. By definition, a clear fluid consisting of water and small particles such as electrolytes is a transudate, whereas exudate contains larger elements such as cells and proteins. If the equivalent of serum (the fluid part of blood with the removal of proteins) is present, the adjective *serous* is used. Because serum and transudate represent the same type of fluid, the term *serous exudate* should not be used. Moreover, distinction between exudate and transudate cannot always be made visually. On the other hand, purulent exudate is acceptable terminology. This fluid obviously has cells and proteins in it. The safest term to use, rather than trying to choose between transudate and exudate, is simply *drainage*. Soupy brownish drainage is associated with autolytic debridement (breakdown of necrotic tissue using enzymes produced by macrophages and other cells). An example of copious bluish-green sanguinopurulent drainage (bloody/purulent) due to *P. aeruginosa* infection is depicted in Figure 9-11. Copious serous drainage indicates either venous insufficiency or inflammation and a need to reduce handling of the wound and to provide adequate absorption to prevent maceration. A desiccated wound indicates the need to use a dressing to retain fluid within the wound and to add moisture to a wound using dressings described in Chapter 16. Terms used to describe quantity and quality of drainage are provided in Table 9-2.

Edges and Surrounding Skin

Due to total focus on the wound itself, the edges and surrounding skin are often neglected to the detriment of wound healing. Wound edges are the primary source of new epithelial cells to resurface wounds. Unhealthy surrounding skin will slow healing tremendously, even if the wound fills with granulation tissue. Moreover, potential problems with

TABLE 9-2
Description of Drainage

QUANTITATIVE	DESCRIPTION	INTERPRETATION
Desiccated	Dry	Arterial disease, excessive absorption, lack of inflammation
Minimum	Moist wound bed, spot of drainage on dressing	Low end of normal drainage
Moderate	Wet wound bed, obvious drainage on dressing	High end of normal drainage
Maximum/copious	Strike-through, saturated dressing	Inflammation or infection, insufficient absorption, excessively long interval of dressing change
QUALITATIVE	DESCRIPTION	INTERPRETATION
Serous	Clear	Normal
Sanguineous	Bloody	Infection or trauma
Serosanguineous	Blood tinged but clear	Infection or trauma
Purulent	Thick yellow or other color	Infection
Sanguinopurulent	Thick yellow, blood tinged	Infection with subcutaneous defects
	Thin yellow	Solubilized slough

wound healing frequently show in surrounding skin first. Concerns include maceration, inflammation, hydration, nutrition, callus or hyperkeratosis, and induration. The color of skin may also provide valuable information.

Wound Edges

The edges of a wound are the only source of epidermal cells in full-thickness and deeper wounds. Partial-thickness wounds can epithelialize from hair follicles and other accessory structures lined with epithelial cells. The intact epidermis around the wound must maintain its normal hydration for epidermal cell migration onto the edge of the wound. Surrounding skin must be protected from excessive moisture coming from the wound bed. Edges must be inspected for hydration status, signs of ongoing injury, and adherence of the edge to the wound bed. Hydration status and signs of injury are described later for surrounding skin in general. The edges of the greater trochanteric wound in Figure 9-5 are adherent but demonstrate evidence of trauma on the edges with the dark edges caused by accumulation of hemosiderin in the edges.

Adherence of edges is determined both visually and by palpation. Loose, nonadherent edges are created by shearing forces on the skin and occur commonly in sacral and greater trochanteric wounds. An example of loose, nonadherent edges is shown in Figure 9-13. Epibole, as described in Chapter 3, prevents migration of epidermal cells. Lack of adherence indicates subcutaneous injury. Injury can take

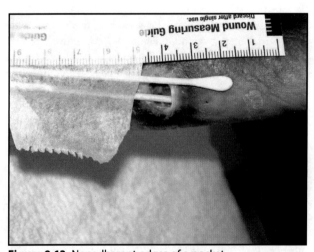

Figure 9-13. Nonadherent edges of a pocket.

the form of tunneling/tracts, undermining, and pocketing. Although patients may experience discomfort from probing, discovery of tunnels and pockets is critical. These subcutaneous defects may close prematurely, walling off bacteria and increasing the risk of abscess formation. Patients may return for a new episode of wound care due to subcutaneous cavities left along a fascial plane. Even if infection does not occur immediately, patients have developed abscesses months or years later due to introduction of bacteria into these cavities. Epibole can be seen along much of the wound edges in Figure 9-14. The reflectance on the edges indicates rounding of the tissue.

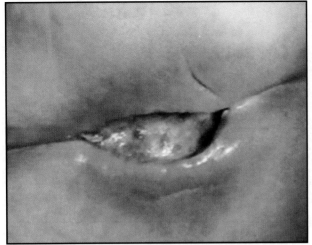

Figure 9-14. Epibole on the lower edge of the wound. Reflection of light off the curved edge and undermining below characteristic of epibole are demonstrated.

Skin Color

White indicates a lack of blood flow or arterial insufficiency. Blue coloration (cyanosis) is a sign of a severe lack of oxygen in the tissue due to arterial insufficiency, heart failure, or respiratory disease. A blackened area surrounding a wound represents necrosis, as shown on the lower surface of the trochanteric wound in Figure 9-5. A yellowish-brown, variegated coloration, especially when it is located on the lower part of a leg near the medial malleolus, is indicative of venous insufficiency (Figure 9-15). Redness indicates inflammation and possibly cellulitis (infection of the interstitial space). Inflammation is described separately later. Mottling occurs in skin with vascular disease. Areas of red, white, and blue can be seen in patches through the affected extremity. Mottling can be caused by venous thrombosis secondary to severe arterial disease accompanied by ischemia and inflammation of injured tissue in the same area. Skin atrophy results in more visible blood vessels than normal and can also cause mottling (Figure 9-16). Mottling may also be the result of necrotizing fasciitis (Figure 9-17). The administration of pressor drugs such as norepinephrine to maintain blood pressure in septic shock can lead to mottling and later gangrene, as seen in Figure 9-18.

Nutrition

A combination of dry, thin skin is indicative of a lack of nutrition to the skin, producing skin atrophy. Atrophied skin loses both dermal and hypodermal thickness as well as flattening of the rete pegs, increasing the risk of skin tears. Atrophy produces the "cigarette paper" appearance, visible blood vessels, and ecchymoses, particularly in older skin (see Figure 9-16). Long-term use of topical corticosteroids also produces skin atrophy.

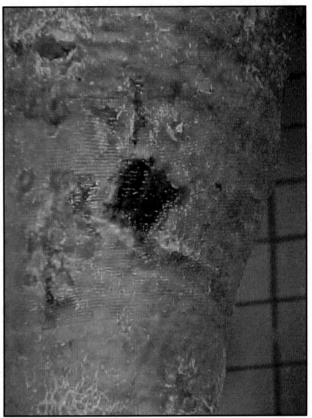

Figure 9-15. Eczema or stasis dermatitis characteristic of venous disease.

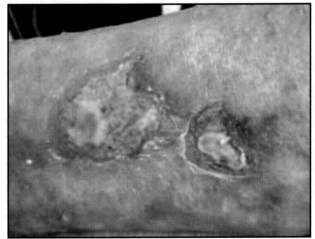

Figure 9-16. Mottling of skin with characteristic "cigarette paper" skin associated with aging, along with areas of hyperemia, blanching, and cyanosis of mottling.

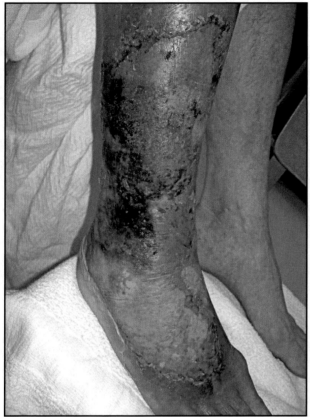

Figure 9-17. Mottling of skin in necrotizing fasciitis. Areas of hyperemia, thrombosis, and ischemia contribute to the variegated appearance of the skin. Crepitus from gas produced by anaerobes can be palpated.

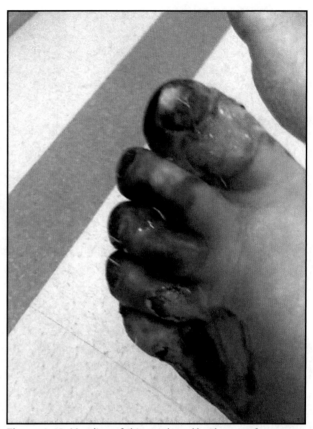

Figure 9-18. Mottling of skin produced by the use of vasopressors in septic shock. Early gangrene, thrombosis, and ischemia contribute to the variegated skin appearance.

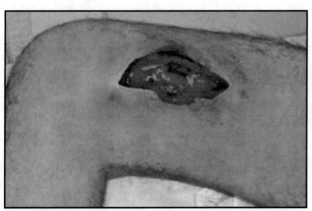

Figure 9-19. Margin of cellulitis surrounding an opened skin abscess. Also note the induration and severe edema of the surrounding skin. The brown discoloration is the remnant of skin preparation prior to surgery.

Inflammation and Infection

A small margin of a few millimeters of inflammation is expected with healing wounds. A larger margin of more than 1 cm of inflamed surrounding skin should raise suspicion of infection. An infected wound will often also be surrounded by a margin thickened by edema and fibrosis, resulting in induration, a hardening of the skin. Therefore, the surrounding skin must be examined not only visually but also by palpation. Along with induration, increased warmth may be detected (Figure 9-19). Harsh handling of a wound may also cause inflammation. A large area of inflammation beyond 1 cm may represent infection of the surrounding skin, termed *peripheral cellulitis*.

Further spread of infection may reveal increased size and firmness of lymph nodes draining the area (lymphadenitis) and red streaks in the skin (lymphangitis). Inflammation may also be caused by radiation therapy for cancer. Such an example is shown in Figure 9-14. The tight shiny skin with an extensive erythematous border was caused by radiation therapy for rectal cancer.

Skin Hydration

Skin hydration and turgor are examined together. With normal aging, both hydration and turgor may be lost. Normally hydrated skin conforms to the surface below and resists compression. Skin hydration is tested by pinching a fold of skin as described for the physical exam of the patient in general. Older skin is at high risk for damage due to trauma, in particular the use of tape and indiscriminate removal of the tape as described in Chapter 13 under skin tears.

Maceration

Maceration is a result of excessive hydration of skin (see Figure 9-6). It can be seen in normal skin following prolonged exposure to moisture, such as long baths or swimming. The macerated skin becomes swollen and lighter in color in addition to an appearance of fissuring. Surrounding skin becomes macerated from using dressings that are not absorptive enough to keep drainage off the surrounding skin, not changing dressings frequently enough, or failure to use moisture barriers or skin sealants to protect the skin from moisture. Maceration may also be caused by rough handling of the wound or placing wet cotton gauze in direct contact with the surrounding skin.

Excessive Dryness of Skin

A range of normal skin hydration may be found across individuals. The term for excessively dry skin is *xerosis*. Individuals with darkly pigmented skin have a greater propensity for xerosis, often described as being "ashy." Additionally, diabetes and arterial disease lead to skin dryness. A combination of these factors is common and can result in fissuring of the skin, a risk for infection. Xerosis can also be the result of systemic disease, especially if found in atypical areas in a person who does not have a history of "ashy skin."

Scale

Scaling may be the result of a number of disease processes that may be local or systemic. Scale represents abnormal keratinization and may be accompanied by signs of inflammation. The color of the scale may also be indicative of a specific disease. Psoriasis produces silvery scaling and may produce papules and plaques. Scaling on sun-exposed skin, especially in older individuals, may represent actinic keratosis, a precursor of squamous cell carcinoma. Eczema is generally associated with both scaling and inflammation with weeping and crusted lesions.

Chronic Injury to Surrounding Skin

Skin surrounding and near the wound should be inspected for signs of chronic injury. The presence of healed scars may suggest an ongoing or intermittent underlying problem causing wounds to occur in an area of the body. For example, multiple scarred areas may be found near the medial malleolus and other areas on the legs of a person with venous disease. Scars from old wounds near the lateral malleolus and elsewhere may be the result of sickle cell disease. Scarring is also likely to be found on problem areas in diabetic neuropathy and arterial disease. Extensive scarring decreases the extensibility of skin, making it more prone to injury in the future.

The insult responsible for creating a wound may also produce a milder, reversible injury to the skin around the wound. Bleeding into the skin may be caused by excessive shearing, pressure exerted on the skin, or venous hypertension. Red blood cells break down in the tissue, releasing hemoglobin. As hemoglobin is degraded into first biliverdin and then bilirubin, the tissue takes on a greenish and then yellow appearance from these pigments. After bilirubin is removed, iron from the hemoglobin remains in the storage form of hemosiderin, producing a yellowish-brown pigmentation. Hemosiderin is cleared slowly by macrophages leaving pigmentation in the skin for a long time. The color of the surrounding skin may, therefore, help reveal whether the injury is mild, new, continuous, or old. Measures to correct chronic injury to the skin may be taken by off-loading the area or addressing venous hypertension.

Chronic shearing, when accompanied by stiffness of the skeletal structures of the foot and dryness of the skin in diabetes, produces callus on shearing points such as the metatarsal heads and heels. However, in some cases, callus may cover the entire plantar surface of the foot and extend along the medial and lateral sides of the foot toward the dorsal side. The dorsal surfaces of toes at the interphalangeal joints may also be callused due to shearing between the skin and the tops of shoes. Callus creates increased pressure on the skin below it during ambulation and must be debrided (see Figure 9-12).

Callus is considered a form of hyperkeratosis, but hyperkeratosis may occur without external shear forces. Dry skin over extensor surfaces may become thickened by the excess accumulation of material of the stratum corneum. Normally, the stratum corneum is shed as quickly as new keratinocytes reach this layer from below. Several skin diseases are also characterized by hyperkeratosis.

Size

The extent of a wound may be assessed in many ways. The 2 basic methods are to measure representative distances and to measure volume. Within the wound, an estimated percentage of the wound bed of different tissue types or colors should be documented. One may use the following terms: (1) granulation tissue vs necrotic tissue;

(2) granulation tissue, slough, and eschar; or (3) red, yellow, and black and give percentages adding up to 100%. Examples of these ways of reporting include (1) 40% granulation tissue and 60% necrotic tissue; (2) 40% granulation tissue, 30% slough, and 30% eschar; and (3) 40% red, 30% yellow, and 30% black. The shape of the wound, if not drawn, should also be described. A round or elliptical wound is a reliable sign that the wound was caused by tissue loading such as pressure or shear. Vascular wounds tend to have irregular shapes. Arterial insufficiency produces a dry depression due to the loss of moisture from the necrotic tissue.

Measuring Wounds

Determining the size of a wound is a necessary part of the wound evaluation. Tools to measure wounds are described in the following sections. Several photographic products are available to provide surface area and depth directly from a photograph. These can be expensive and may require a photographic release. Means of measuring independent of photography are described.

Many individuals involved with wound care place great importance on wound measurements, and much research has been performed on the best practice and reliability of different techniques. However, a few important points need to be considered. In general, patients with wounds will be referred to physical therapy because of the quality of the wound rather than the quantity of the wound. Second, measurements may vary tremendously due to patient positioning. For measurements to be reliable, a patient will need to be positioned in the same manner each time a measurement is performed. Because of infection control considerations, precise measurements may not be practical. One needs to be aware that error in measurement is likely to be greater than any real day-to-day changes in wound size. Wound size will usually change little until the wound is relatively clear of necrotic tissue and infection. When wound size begins to decrease rapidly, patients may need to be discharged from the outpatient setting.

Surface Area

Wounds are measured in centimeters. If the wound is less than 1 cm across, the distance may be reported in millimeters instead of using a leading zero (0.5 cm or 5 mm). Comparisons to objects such as coins (eg, "the size of a dime") and the use of inches are not allowed. Measurement of only the surface area of a wound is suitable in the absence of subcutaneous tissue involvement. Some sources recommend measuring length and width using anatomical vertical for length and anatomical horizontal for width. Medicare requires using the greatest distance across the wound regardless of the orientation and the greatest distance

perpendicular to the first measurement. See Figure 9-20 for examples of different methods. Using any of these methods, the 2 measurements may be multiplied to determine a crude number to describe the cross-sectional area of the wound. Multiplying length × width will overestimate the true surface area depending on how much the shape deviates from a rectangle. Error in this computation is 21.6% when a wound is round and may be overestimated even more with a highly irregular wound circumference. In cases of a highly irregularly shaped wound, measurements may need to be taken at multiple locations. A map of irregularly shaped wounds should be drawn in the medical record with representative distances marked clearly on the map.

Clock Notation

A means of establishing consistent directions for wound measurement is clock notation. Using clock notation, we indicate the cephalic direction on the trunk and proximal direction on a limb as 12:00 and the caudal direction on the trunk or distal direction on a limb as 6:00. Using this notation, the term *length* refers to the distance from 12:00 to 6:00, and *width* is measured from 9:00 to 3:00. Clock notation is also used to document undermining and tunneling.

Tools

Measuring the distance across the wound may include disposable paper rulers, sterile cotton-tipped applicators, transparent grids, and plastic materials such as sandwich bags. Disposable paper rules and sterile cotton-tipped applicators offer the advantage of low cost. A quick, simple method is to hold a paper ruler over the wound and read directly from it. Moreover, one can place a paper ruler next to a wound and take a photograph with the ruler visible to document both the size and condition of the wound. However, the paper ruler is not useful for documenting depth, whereas sterile cotton-tipped applicators can be used for all 3 dimensions. To use this technique, the wooden end is held to one edge of the wound as the thumb of a gloved hand is slid to the opposite side of the wound. The cotton-tipped applicator is then held close to a ruler to measure the distance in centimeters (see Figure 9-20C).

A simple method to provide a more accurate cross-sectional measurement involves placing a plastic sheet material such as plastic wrap or a sandwich bag with the 2 sides cut to trace a wound for a permanent record. The wound tracing can be digitized to compute surface area. The problem with using a single sheet of plastic is the potential for contamination. A sandwich bag or a doubled-over piece of plastic wrap allows the top layer to be kept and the surface in contact with the wound to be discarded. Wound tracings may be photocopied or scanned to be placed in a paper or electronic record permanently (see Figures 9-20D to 9-20F). Software to allow computation of the surface area may also be used.

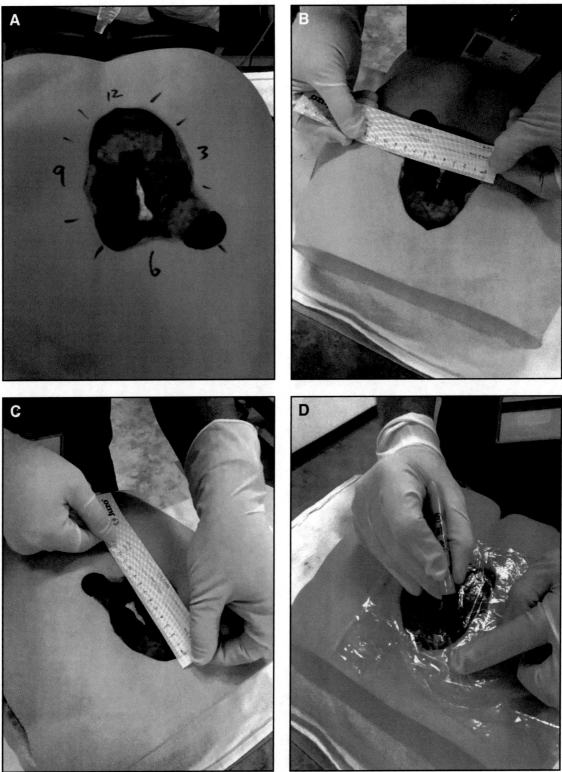

Figure 9-20. Wound measurement. (A) Clock orientation on a wound model. 12:00 is toward head on trunk and toward the proximal joint on an extremity. (B) Measuring wound width from 3:00 to 9:00 using a paper ruler on a wound model. (C) Using a paper ruler to measure length from 12:00 to 6:00. (D) Using a plastic sandwich bag to trace the wound on a model. Double layer placed over the wound and using a marker to trace the wound. *(continued)*

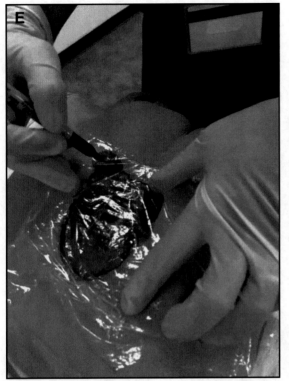
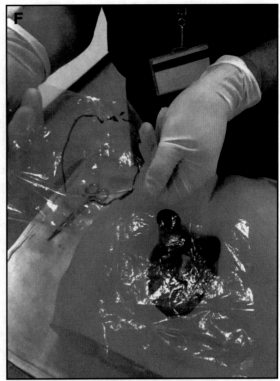

Figure 9-20 (continued). (E) Completing tracing of the wound edges. (F) Top layer being removed. The layer contacting the wound is left.

Depth

Depth of a wound should be determined for wounds with significant subcutaneous involvement, such as stage 4 pressure injuries. Determining the volume of shallow wounds such as burns without subcutaneous involvement, stage 2 pressure injuries, arterial ulcers, or venous ulcers is generally not practical because the depth is not much greater than the error in measurement.

The simplest means of providing an index of volume is to measure wound depth with a cotton-tipped applicator in a way that is similar to measurement of the cross-sectional area (Figure 9-21). To reduce error in means of localizing the skin surface, one cotton-tipped applicator is placed across the wound, and another is placed in the wound with the wooden stick end into the wound next to the cotton-tipped applicator lying across the wound. The point at which depth is measured depends on the configuration of the wound. Generally, one should use the deepest spot. If a wound has multiple depths such that one number could not accurately describe the wound, a map of the wound may need to be drawn with depths indicated on the map.

Obtaining measurements of length, width, and depth allows a crude approximation of wound volume to be made. More precise means of volume determination can be performed by filling the wound with a suitable material. Sterile saline from a premeasured syringe may be used. Volume

of the syringe is recorded before and after the wound is filled from the syringe. Volume is simply calculated by subtracting the final volume of the syringe from its initial volume. This method is only effective if the patient can be positioned in such a way that the surface of the wound is parallel to the floor. If this position is not practical, hydrogel, a more viscous material, may be infused instead. A more involved procedure is to use dental impression gel, such as Jeltrate (Dentsply International). An equal volume of warm water is added to the powder from the canister and mixed. Before the material hardens, it can be placed into the wound and allowed to become firm. Jeltrate is biocompatible and is easily removed from a wound after it hardens. The impression of the wound can be placed in a graduated cylinder to determine wound volume. The volume of the impression gel must be measured before it dries completely and loses volume from evaporation.

Tunnels/Tracts

The locations of tunnels and sinus tracts are documented using clock notation for direction and the distance a cotton-tipped applicator can be inserted beneath intact skin. An example of appropriate notation is a 2.5-cm tunnel at 11:00 (Figure 9-22). However, in many cases, one cannot be certain that the end of the tunnel can be reached. Failure to find the end of the tunnel may also occur in cases in

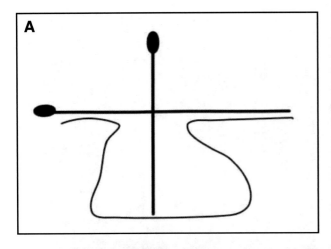

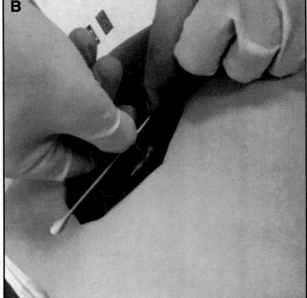

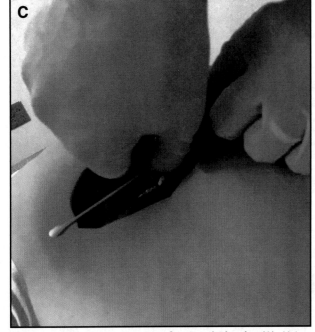

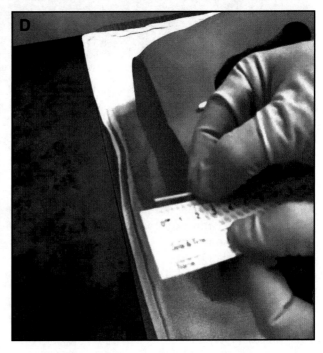

Figure 9-21. Measurement of wound depth. (A) Using 2 cotton-tipped applicators. One is used to measure depth, and the second is used to aid in determining the upper edge of the wound. (B and C) Demonstration on a wound model. (D) Measuring length of a cotton-tipped applicator from the surface of the wound to the wound bed.

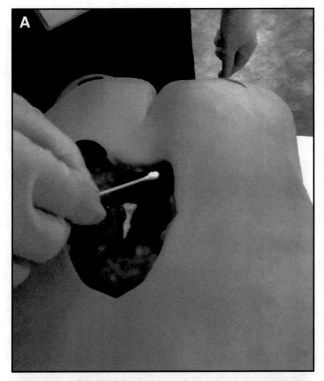

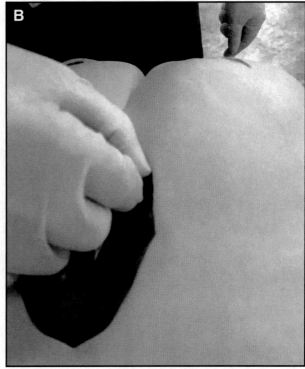

Figure 9-22. Demonstration of tunnel measurement on a wound model. (A) Holding a cotton-tipped applicator just outside the tunnel. (B) Reaching the bottom of the tunnel and using the thumbnail along the cotton-tipped applicator to determine tunnel's length. (C) Depth of tunnel is documented as 2.5 cm at 7:00.

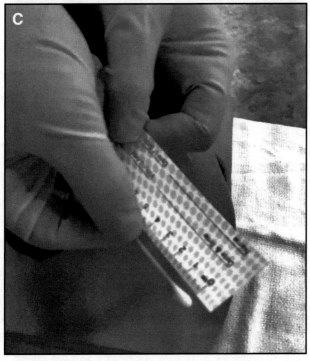

Undermining/Pocketing

Undermining resembles an overhanging cliff caused by necrosis of tissue beneath intact skin. It is commonly associated with pressure injuries produced by shearing. This phenomenon is depicted in Figure 9-23. Undermined areas tend to have a maximal distance at a certain point and symmetrically decrease in an arc of the wound's perimeter. To document undermining, a broken line is drawn to indicate the distance of undermining and to denote the arc involved. If not drawn, one may use clock notation to indicate the location and extent of undermining. For example, in Figure 9-23A, undermining is present from 11:00 to 2:00 with a maximum undermining being measured in Figure 9-23B. In some cases, the term *pocket* may be used to describe a type of subcutaneous defect that extends under intact skin where the edge of the wound is nonadherent but does not have a clifflike appearance. These are generally the remnants of abscesses that may be found incidentally when drainage is found emanating from the pocket. Pockets should be found during the initial and subsequent wound assessment by checking for whether the edges of the wound are adherent. Should undermining exist in such a way that clock notation might be ambiguous, such as from 12:00

which 2 wounds communicate subcutaneously. One may not be able to move a cotton-tipped applicator from one wound to the other, but fluid may be observed coming out of one wound while pulsed lavage is being applied to the other. In such cases, one may note that probing completely between the 2 wounds could not be accomplished, but the 2 wounds appear to be connected beneath intact skin.

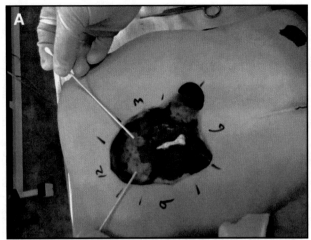

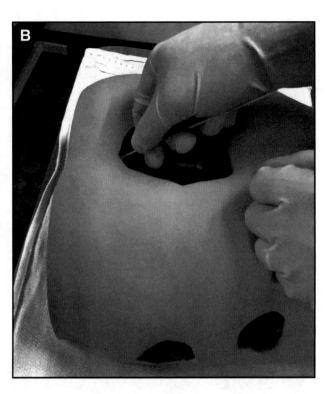

Figure 9-23. Demonstration of undermining measurement on a wound model. (A) Cotton-tipped applicators demonstrating arc of undermining from 11:00 to 2:00. (B) Finding the deepest area of undermining with a cotton-tipped applicator.

to 6:00 or 3:00 to 9:00, one can simply document which side of the wound has the undermining (eg, the right or left side using the anatomical position).

QUALITY OF WOUND BED

Issues with the wound bed include the relative health and turgor of the wound. A healthy wound bed is red, firm, and does not bleed with trivial trauma. Unhealthy wound beds may result from infection or critical colonization, ischemia, and lack of moisture. Pink tissue is indicative of diminished blood flow to the wound bed. Dusky, bleeding, stringy, weak tissue without turgor (friable tissue) indicates injury most likely caused by infection or critical colonization. Brown, darkened areas within the wound bed are caused by tissue necrosis, frequently due to infection. Boggy tissue either under intact skin or within the wound indicates deep necrosis and edema. Such wounds require further exploration. Hardness of the wound surface results from either desiccation or the presence of hardened fibrin on the wound surface.

The percentages of red, yellow, and black and the quality and quantity of drainage are factors in determining the plan of care regardless of the etiology. The type of debridement, dressings used, and frequency of visits are among issues that will depend on the quality of the wound bed.

INFECTION AND CRITICAL COLONIZATION/LOCAL INFECTION

Determining the level of bioburden is critical in developing a plan of care. Signs of infection have been described by the acronym IFEE, which stands for Induration, Fever, Erythema, and Edema, as described in Chapter 3. Copious drainage exceeding the expected amount for the size and location of the wound is also suggestive, whereas the presence of purulence is considered sufficient to diagnose infection. In wounds with large subcutaneous components, purulence may be missed. During palpation of the wound and surrounding skin, one should gently attempt to express drainage to determine whether purulence is present. Purulence may also be initially detected within tracts and pockets during probing with a cotton-tipped applicator. Many patients may indicate exquisite pain during the first few treatments due to inflammation, but this pain should resolve with the removal of bacteria and necrotic tissue during these initial visits. A return or increase in odor that persists after wound irrigation and increased pain in the wound should make the clinician suspicious of infection or reinfection.

TABLE 9-3

Systemic Inflammatory Response Syndrome Criteria for Sepsis

- Heart rate greater than 90 beats/min (tachycardia)
- Either hypothermia or fever
  - Core temperature less than 36°C (96.8°F)
  - Core temperature greater than 38°C (100.4°F)
- Increased respiration as either tachypnea or hypocapnia/hyperventilation
  - Respiratory rate (RR) greater than 20 breaths/min (tachypnea)
  - PaCO$_2$ less than 32 mm Hg (hypocapnia/hyperventilation)
- White blood cell (WBC) count shows elevation, depression, or increased bands (immature neutrophils)
  - WBC count greater than 12,000/mm^3 (leukocytosis)
  - WBC count less than 4000/mm^3 (leukopenia)
  - Bands greater than 10% (bandemia)

Sepsis is present if infection is either present or highly suspected and 2 or more of the criteria exist.

Fever and leukocytosis are part of the acute phase reaction along with anorexia and somnolence.

Tachycardia and tachypnea indicate cardiovascular and metabolic disturbances.

For children, HR, RR, and WBC count must be compared with norms for age.

Criteria for HR and RR are greater than 2 standard deviations above mean. Criterion for hypothermia is the same as adult, but criterion for fever is 38.5°C. Bandemia is also 10%.

Data source: Bone et al, 1992.

Infection may take one or more of several forms beyond purulence within a wound bed and subcutaneous defects. Infection may spread to bone (osteomyelitis), particularly in wounds that can be probed to a bone's surface. Cellulitis is the spread of infection through the interstitial space, producing erythema, warmth, and pain. Lymphadenitis and lymphangitis may also be present. Erysipelas is a specific type of cellulitis that is most commonly caused by group A *Streptococcus*. This type of infection is more common when venous or lymphatic drainage of the area is compromised. Facial (cheek and bridge of nose) and leg erysipelas account for almost all cases. In addition to localized heat, pain, and erythema, systemic effects (fever, chills, decreased appetite, and somnolence) are commonly present at diagnosis. Spread of infection through the blood is given the general terms *sepsis* or *septicemia*, although the more specific terms of *bacteremia, viremia*, and *fungemia* may be used. Although the terms sepsis and septicemia may also be used interchangeably, sepsis may also be used to indicate local infection. Septicemia may be considered a more specific type of sepsis to indicate infection spread to the blood.

Indicators of systemic infection include increased blood glucose, including wide fluctuations of blood glucose from hypoglycemia to values of 400 mg/dL or greater, elevated white blood cell count, increased sedimentation rate, and elevated C-reactive protein. Recently, procalcitonin has been identified as a way of distinguishing whether a patient requires systemic antibiotics. Clinical signs of sepsis are produced by the patient's immune response to the infection. The collection of signs accompanying sepsis is called the *systemic inflammatory response syndrome*. Criteria for sepsis based on systemic inflammatory response syndrome are listed in Table 9-3.

DETERMINING PROGRESS/ REGRESSION

Throughout the episode of care, the clinician must determine the current phase of healing and whether a wound is progressing normally or becomes chronic in a given stage of wound healing. A nonhealing wound may be chronically in the inflammatory, proliferative, epithelializing, or remodeling stage. The wound may fail in one of the following steps: inflammation, proliferation, epithelialization, or remodeling.

Critical decision-making points are whether the wound is infected; whether the wound requires debridement; requires filling of depth, undermining, tunnels, or sinus tracts; and the degree of drainage. Many of these points are addressed together; however, in some cases, the clinician may need to work with competing goals to optimize wound

TABLE 9-4
Scoring Scheme for PUSH Tool

CROSS-SECTIONAL AREA	DRAINAGE	TISSUE TYPE
0 points for 0 cm^2	0 points for no exudate	0 points for closed
1 point for < 0.3 cm^2	1 point for light exudate	1 point for epithelial tissue
2 points for 0.3 to 0.6 cm^2	2 points for moderate exudate	2 points for granulation tissue
3 points for 0.7 to 1.0 cm^2	3 points for heavy exudate	3 points for slough
4 points for 1.1 to 2.0 cm^2		4 points for necrotic tissue
5 points for 2.1 to 3.0 cm^2		
6 points for 3.1 to 4.0 cm^2		
7 points for 4.1 to 8.0 cm^2		
8 points for 8.1 to 12.0 cm^2		
9 points for 12.1 to 24.0 cm^2		
10 points for > 24.0 cm^2		
Data source: Stotts et al, 2001.		

healing. For example, sharp debridement accomplishes the goals of treating infection and the presence of large quantities of necrotic tissue. On the other hand, the use of autolytic debridement and preventing maceration of surrounding skin at the same time may be difficult. The assessment for wound infection has been described frequently by the acronym IFEE. An infected wound often has the characteristics of induration, fever, erythema, and edema. The odor and color of drainage from the wound can aid in this determination. The presence of dusky or brownish patches within the wound is also very suggestive of wound infection.

PRESSURE ULCER STATUS FOR HEALING TOOL

The pressure ulcer status for healing (PUSH) tool is a validated tool for assessment of the severity of pressure injuries. It has been used for other types of wounds in an effort to demonstrate an improvement in the quality of wounds. Scores range from 0 for a closed, epithelialized wound without drainage to 17 points for a wound greater than 24 cm^2 in an area with heavy exudate and necrotic tissue. The scoring scheme is depicted in Table 9-4. Scores for each element are added to produce a total score. Higher scores are worse than lower scores. Note that exudate is used in the place of drainage, although "light" could apply to transudate, and a distinction is made between necrotic tissue being worse than slough. In this case, necrotic tissue implies that specific tissues within the wound bed can be identified as opposed to solubilized necrotic tissue.

SUMMARY

Assessment of the wound requires clinical judgment based on objective tests, history provided by the patient or caregiver, and direct observation by the clinician. Although acute wounds usually present no problem with determining the cause, many chronic wounds may not present an obvious cause. In addition, the clinician needs to determine why the wound failed to heal and why any previous treatment failed. Observation of the wound can be based on the CODES system described previously. Measurement of the surface area is sufficient for superficial or full-thickness wounds. For wounds with substantial subcutaneous involvement, either wound volume or depth characteristic of the wound needs to be documented. A discussion of the systems for characterizing wounds of different types is provided.

QUESTIONS

1. What significance do different colors of the wound bed carry?
2. What is the progression of the wound bed color in the deterioration of a wound?
3. What is the progression of subcutaneous fat color change in the deterioration of a wound?
4. What are the different possibilities of yellow/brown color in a wound?
5. What is the significance of the odor of a wound?
6. What is the significance of a wound retaining a foul odor after cleaning/debridement?
7. What is the significance of a dry wound?
8. What is the significance of a very wet wound?
9. What is the significance of a wound wet with odor and deterioration?
10. What is the significance of a wound wet with granulation tissue and no odor?
11. What is purulent drainage and what does it typically mean?
12. What is sanguineous drainage and what does it typically mean?
13. What is serosanguineous drainage and what does it typically mean?
14. What is sanguinopurulent drainage and what does it typically mean?
15. Why does anybody care about the size of a wound?
16. What are Medicare requirements for measuring wounds?
17. What does maceration indicate?
18. What constitutes normal inflammation with respect to skin surrounding a wound?
19. What does callus indicate? Is it good or bad? Why? What interventions are used to control callus formation?
20. What does induration indicate?
21. What do tunnels, tracts, and undermining indicate?
22. What is the purpose of clock notation?
23. Should you rely completely on the physical appearance of the wound to diagnose the cause of the wound?

BIBLIOGRAPHY

Bilgin, M, Güneş UY. A comparison of 3 wound measurement techniques: effects of pressure ulcer size and shape. *J Wound Ostomy Continence Nurs.* 2013;40(6):590-593.

Bone RC, Balk RA, Cerra FB, et al. Definitions for sepsis and organ failure and guidelines for the use of innovative therapies in sepsis. The ACCP/SCCM Consensus Conference Committee. American College of Chest Physicians/Society of Critical Care Medicine. *Chest.* 1992;101(6):1644-1655.

Ding S, Lin F, Gillespie BM. Surgical wound assessment and documentation of nurses: an integrative review. *J Wound Care.* 2016;25(5):232-240.

Ebright JR. Microbiology of chronic leg and pressure ulcers: clinical significance and implications for treatment. *Nurs Clin North Am.* 2005;40(2):207-216.

Fierheller M, Sibbald RG. A clinical investigation into the relationship between increased periwound skin temperature and local wound infection in patients with chronic leg ulcers. *Adv Skin Wound Care.* 2010;23(8):369-381.

Hsu JT, Chen YW, Ho TW, et al. Chronic wound assessment and infection detection method. *BMC Med Inform Decis Mak.* 2019;19(1):99.

Keast DH, Bowering CK, Evans AW, Mackean GL, Burrows C, D'Souza L. MEASURE: a proposed assessment framework for developing best practice recommendations for wound assessment. *Wound Repair Regen.* 2004;12(3 Suppl):S1-S17.

Kirsner RS, Vivas AC. Lower-extremity ulcers: diagnosis and management. *Br J Dermatol.* 2015;173(2):379-390.

Langemo DK, Melland H, Hanson D, Olson B, Hunter S, Henly SJ. Two-dimensional wound measurement: comparison of 4 techniques. *Adv Wound Care.* 1998;11(7):337-343.

Lorentzen HF, Gottrup F. Clinical assessment of infection in nonhealing ulcers analyzed by latent class analysis. *Wound Repair Regen.* 2006;14(3):350-353.

Serena TE, Hanft JR, Snyder R. The lack of reliability of clinical examination in the diagnosis of wound infection: preliminary communication. *Int J Low Extrem Wounds.* 2008;7(1):32-35.

Shah A, Wollak C, Shah JB. Wound measurement techniques: comparing the use of ruler method, 2D imaging and 3D scanner. *J Am Coll Clin Wound Spec.* 2015;5(3):52-57. doi:10.1016/j.jccw.2015.02.001

Smollock W, Montenegro P, Czenis A, He Y. Hypoperfusion and wound healing: another dimension of wound assessment. *Adv Skin Wound Care.* 2018;31(2):72-77.

Stotts NA, Rodeheaver GT, Thomas DR, et al. An instrument to measure healing in pressure ulcers development and validation of the pressure ulcer scale for healing (PUSH). *The Journals of Gerontology Series A: Biological Sciences and Medical Sciences.* 2001;56(12):M795-M799.

van Rijswijk L. The fundamentals of wound assessment. *Ostomy Wound Manage.* 1996;42(7):40-46.

Woo KY, Sibbald RG. A cross-sectional validation study of using NERDS and STONEES to assess bacterial burden. *Ostomy Wound Manage.* 2009;55(8):40-48.

Pressure Injuries

DEFINING THE PRESSURE INJURY

This chapter discusses issues related to wounds created by static tissue loading. The vast majority of this type of wound occurs in bedbound individuals and historically were termed *bedsores*. A more technical term, *decubitus ulcer*, was developed with the same meaning—an erosive type of wound that would develop in a person lying down for extended periods. The journal *Advances in Wound and Skin Care* was previously called *Decubitus*. However, the old terms of decubitus ulcer and bedsore should have been

discouraged for more than 30 years. Unfortunately, young clinicians tend to pick up language used by mentors, and these terms still have not disappeared. The body formerly known as the National Pressure Ulcer Advisory Panel (now the National Pressure Injury Advisory Panel [NPIAP]) recently encouraged the use of the term *pressure injury*. The NPIAP and the European Pressure Ulcer Advisory Panel (epuap.org) are authorities that disseminate information, including definitions, and provide recommendations regarding the prevention and treatment of pressure injuries.

Irion GL, Gardner JA, Pignataro RM.
Comprehensive Wound Management, Third Edition (pp 151-179).
© 2024 Taylor and Francis Group.

Unfortunately, terminology changes alone have not helped in terms of understanding the mechanisms of pressure injury. One issue with the terminology related to lack of movement is that persons with neurologic and cognitive deficits can also develop the same type of ulcerations. Additionally, some wounds associated with being bedbound are not ulcers. As typically defined, ulcer refers to an erosion/sloughing out of necrotic tissue, whether produced by mechanical forces as in pressure ulcers and neuropathic ulcers, or by chemicals as in esophageal, gastric, and duodenal ulcers caused by stomach acid, vascular disease, or infectious disease.

Pressure injuries are caused by excessive static loading of tissue. They can produce injuries similar to compartment syndrome with a positive feedback cycle of tissue injury, pressure, and further injury until skin necrosis occurs, leaving an ulcer in the skin that may sometimes appear rather suddenly. Pressure injuries and neuropathic ulcers are both produced by excessive tissue loading, and both require suitable off-loading for both prevention and healing. As discussed in the next chapter, neuropathic ulcers are caused by dynamic tissue loading, as opposed to the static loading of pressure injuries.

According to the NPIAP, a pressure injury is

localized damage to the skin and underlying soft tissue, usually over a bony prominence or related to a medical or other device. The injury can present as intact skin or an open ulcer and may be painful. The injury occurs as a result of intense and/or prolonged pressure or pressure in combination with shear. The tolerance of soft tissue for pressure and shear may also be affected by microclimate, nutrition, perfusion, co-morbidities and conditions of the soft tissue.[1]

The NPIAP periodically refines definitions. The change in terms from *pressure ulcer* to *pressure injury* was not universally welcomed because the term *injury* could be construed to imply negligence.

Pressure injuries have an incidence of approximately 2.5 million per year, with a greater incidence in intensive care units and long-term care where patients may be unable to reposition themselves. The greater incidence in these settings also appears to be due to poorer health and more use of medical devices with patients in these settings. Further discussion of these populations can be found in Chapter 18.

Types of Tissue Loads

One particular problem with the emphasis on terminology is the misconception that these injuries are produced by only one cause—excessive pressure over a bony prominence for extended periods. While this may be the cause of many wounds of dependent people, especially the very deep wounds, other causes must be addressed to prevent these wounds and promote their healing. According to the NPIAP, pressure and shearing are the 2 types of tissue loading that can produce pressure injuries. Friction contributes to skin injuries in people who also have risk factors for pressure injuries. Although excessive pressure may compress blood vessels and compromise blood flow, this concept misses the idea that compression produces tensile stress on the tissue. Cyclic tensile forces can strengthen connective tissue, whereas prolonged tensile stress leads to connective tissue breakdown and ulceration. In addition to body weight alone, medical devices, adhesives, and excess moisture can also place stresses on tissue, leading to similar injuries.

Pressure

Anyone incapable of repositioning is at risk of exerting excessive pressure over bony prominences. This includes patients with mobility, sensory, or cognitive issues. *Interface pressure* is the term used to express the effects of the body's weight and surface area resting on a support surface. Pressure refers to force per unit surface area. In a static situation in which one object rests on another, force is due to its weight (mass × acceleration produced by gravity). An object of a given weight will produce less pressure if the area in contact with the support surface is greater and more pressure if the weight is supported on a smaller area. However, the human body is much more complex than a single object of uniform density. As noted in Chapter 1, tissues can deform and diminish pressure. Dissipation of force primarily occurs due to the deformability and septation of subcutaneous adipose tissue. Therefore, lack of adipose tissue increases the risk of pressure causing tissue injury. However, excessive adipose tissue increases the skin's tautness, negating the ability of adipose tissue to deform.

Bone has negligible deformability, and as such, skin overlying bony prominences is trapped between an unyielding surface and the support surface. Although not noted in the NPIAP pressure injury definition, the skin overlying other tissues with minimal deformability such as tendons, cartilage, and teeth is also at risk. The skin overlying the Achilles tendon, dorsiflexor tendons, the external ear, nose, and lips is also particularly subject to injury. Extended use of an endotracheal tube can cause substantial injury to the lips and teeth as well as tracheal injury.

The tissue between the hard tissue and support surface is believed to have reduced perfusion. Should the pressure be relieved in time, the buildup of metabolites produces reactive hyperemia, allowing restoration of the tissue's metabolism. Extended pressure may lead to tissue necrosis.

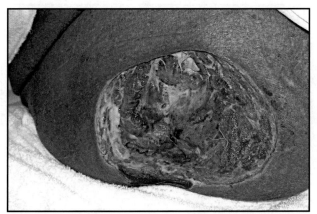

Figure 10-1. Photograph of stage 4 pressure injury of right greater trochanter.

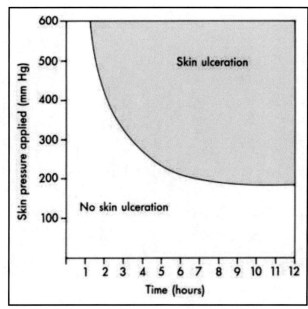

Figure 10-2. Pressure distribution curve. The combination of time and pressure above the curve represents the risk of injury. In some versions of this curve, a line is drawn from 250 mm Hg and the y-axis, joining the curve at 200 mm Hg to represent tissue failure at high pressures.

Injury can occur in deep tissue before skin ulcerates and can even damage bone, as seen in Figure 10-1. Delayed removal of pressure may create a worse situation by superimposing reperfusion injury. Reperfusion injury is caused by restoring blood flow to damaged tissue, which generates free radicals when oxygen is brought to inflamed tissue.

Commonly, pressure injuries result from both overt injury and disruptions in blood flow to the skin from the underlying tissue. Prolonged pressure and abnormal forces, such as friction and shear, can occlude and possibly damage microvascular structures within the dermis. When cells are deprived of oxygen, anaerobic cellular respiration occurs, leading to tissue acidosis and cell death. Edema also occurs, leading to further impairments in blood flow, and the combination of tissue necrosis and edema can rapidly propagate injury, likely accounting for very deep ulcerations. These factors may be exacerbated by repeated reperfusion injury and the accumulation of free radicals.

Most tissues can withstand relatively high pressures for short periods, but low pressures can lead to extensive damage over extended periods. For example, many tissues that experience pressure injuries can have blood flow restricted by a tourniquet during surgery without tissue necrosis. However, a tracheostomy tie secured around the neck for weeks can produce a full-thickness ulcer. This relationship is known as the pressure distribution curve (Figure 10-2).

Muscle tissue and adipose are less tolerant to ischemia than the skin, which can survive long periods of transient circulatory impairment if blood flow is restored in a timely manner. These properties may lead to significant damage to deeper tissues, even when the skin's surface shows relatively minor signs of injury. The presence of minor visible skin damage despite significant underlying tissue destruction is sometimes referred to as the "iceberg phenomenon." For this reason, pressure injuries often evolve, developing over many hours or even days before the full extent of destruction becomes visible at the surface of the wound. Therefore, dead space and necrotic tissue within the wound bed are common in pressure injuries.

However, the individual dosing of pressure required to produce an injury is still not clear. Some patients develop pressure injuries following surgery, particularly if they are kept in the same position in preoperative holding, during surgery, and during recovery from anesthesia. In contrast, some people may be bedbound for years without ever developing a skin injury. Historically, the combination of pressure and time is commonly expressed as pressure > 30 mm Hg for 2 hours. However, the reality is that nobody knows what combination of pressure and time will produce an injury in a given person. Additional factors and mechanisms described in the following sections increase the risk of injury.

Friction

Friction produces superficial skin injuries that are round and red because abrasion has removed the epidermis from the skin and exposed the dermis. In many cases, people susceptible to pressure injury receive injuries from friction due to passive repositioning that drags the person across the support surface. In previous pressure ulcer definitions, friction was included, but the current definition excludes friction. However, frictional injuries should be considered a major risk factor because the factors leading to frictional injuries from repositioning also lead to pressure and the next risk factor—shearing.

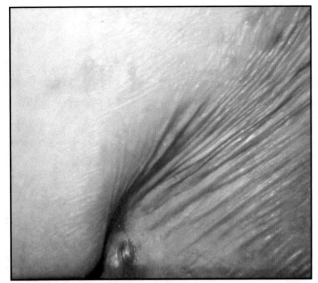

Figure 10-3. Effect of shearing on the skin. Note the bunching effect of shearing forces on the skin. In this example, the skin has been injured by the distortion of the skin superior to the gluteal cleft on the right side. Erythema of the injured skin is present, along with small ulcers.

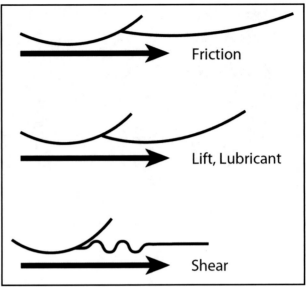

Figure 10-4. Tissue loads other than pressure placing skin at risk.

Shearing

Shearing refers to a force tangential to the skin surface. Although this superficially resembles friction, friction is caused by a dynamic force of the skin moving across a surface. In contrast, shearing is a tangential, static force on the skin that typically occurs during the process of positioning. The term *pressure injury* does not capture that shearing forces placed on the skin can be equally devastating as pressure. In particular, heads-up positioning > 30 degrees is associated with shearing. Most commonly, shearing occurs over the sacrum with a person either reclined in a chair or in the Fowler's position in bed (head up with feet elevated). When skin adheres to the reclined surface, the patient's body weight places a force on the skin that deforms the skin into wrinkles that, in turn, kink blood vessels. Blood flow to the involved tissue is compromised in the same way as a garden hose's flow is compromised when bent back on itself. Shearing injury is a major problem in dependent, obese patients who cannot be easily repositioned. If such a person is rotated among positions, the skin under the patient may not slide but become wrinkled underneath. An example of shearing injury is shown in Figure 10-3. Erythema and ulceration are shown on the right buttocks where the wrinkling can be seen. A comparison of friction and shear is shown in Figure 10-4.

At-Risk Regions

Common sites for the development of pressure injuries are depicted in Figure 10-5. Heels are among the most likely area for pressure injuries to develop. A disproportionate amount of weight is supported on a small, rounded area with *the skin under tension* as it is pulled around the calcaneus. Heels are mostly at risk when positioned in bed as opposed to sitting. Heels are protected when the patient is in the prone position, but dependent patients are rarely positioned this way. In the prone position, the dorsum of the foot and toes are at risk instead. Heel injuries are easily avoidable by a technique known as *floating the heels*. Pillows are placed under the legs as depicted in Figure 10-6 such that the heels are not in contact with the bed's surface. Several devices are available that float the heels and maintain the foot in dorsiflexion. These will be discussed later in the chapter.

The greater trochanter is placed at risk with a dependent person in sidelying. Regardless of a person's body composition, the greater trochanter acts as a bony prominence with little subcutaneous fat to protect the overlying skin. A dependent person should never be placed in sidelying. Instead, foam wedges (Figure 10-7), pillows, or other devices can be used to position a person in three-quarters supine (midway between sidelying and supine) with body weight placed directly over the soft tissue posterior to the greater trochanter instead of directly over the bony prominence.

The ischial tuberosities are a high-risk area for those in prolonged sitting. This typically involves a person with a

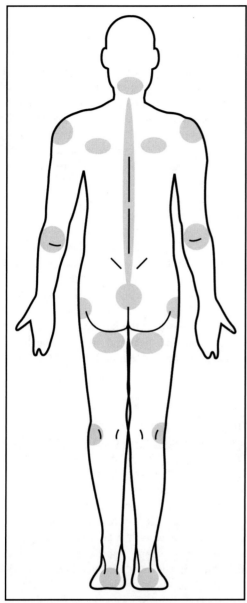

Figure 10-5. At-risk areas for skin breakdown.

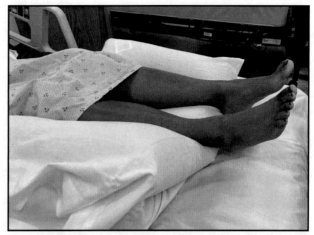

Figure 10-6. Floating heels on a pillow. Raising the heels off the support surface greatly reduces the risk of injury to the skin on the heels.

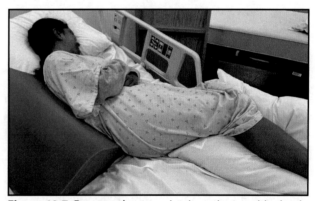

Figure 10-7. Foam wedge to maintain patient positioning in three-quarters supine.

spinal cord injury (SCI) seated in a wheelchair. Individuals with full sensation will not stay in the same seated position for more than a few minutes due to the nociceptive messages received by an intact nervous system. A person with normal sensation but either decreased cognition or lack of strength to reposition may also be at risk. Even more so than on the heels, skin over the ischial tuberosities will be stretched simply by hip flexion required to be in the sitting position. Leaning forward increases the tension placed on the skin, and leaning backward decreases it.

Additionally, the degree of support on the feet and the thigh's length resting on the support surface will alter the pressure placed on the ischial tuberosities. Optimized seating allows pressure redistribution. Greater pressure will exist over the skin of the ischial tuberosities when knees are higher than hips. A deeper seat will distribute more pressure on the thighs.

An often overlooked area is the occiput in patients with immobilization of the cervical spine. The occiput is round, and the skin has more tension at rest than many other places on the body; therefore, the occiput does not distribute the weight of the head well. Gel devices are manufactured specifically to distribute weight along more surface area of the head.

Medial epicondyles in supine; the lateral malleolus and medial malleolus in sidelying; and the knee's medial condyles, scapular spines, and inferior angles in either supine or supported sitting are common sites of pressure injury. Although round bony prominences with disproportionate weight distribution are at great risk, any skin area over a bony prominence, tendon, cartilage, or medical device is at risk for injury.

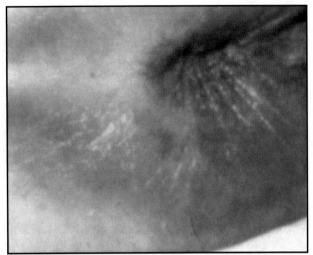

Figure 10-8. Skin injury caused by incontinence.

Contributing Factors Increasing Susceptibility

The risk of injury can be depicted as a hyperbolic curve, as shown in Figure 10-2. A hyperbolic curve implies that the product of 2 variables is a constant. In the case of pressure injuries, the constant represents the risk of tissue injury. This means that a high pressure applied for a short time carries the same risk as a low pressure applied for a long time. Note, however, that the curve touches the pressure axis but not the time axis. This means that a threshold amount of pressure is required to produce an injury, even if that pressure is infinite. Newer diagrams have been developed that vary from the theoretical hyperbolic curve, taking into account that an injury will occur at large pressures regardless of how short a time the tissue is exposed to the pressure.

In Figure 10-2, the curve will be shifted downward with contributing factors. The minimal pressure to produce an injury is reduced. The amount of pressure for a given time to cause an injury or the amount of time for a given amount of pressure necessary to cause an injury are reduced by these factors. Unfortunately, these are strictly conceptual, and actual numbers needed to produce injuries in any given individual are unknown. Factors that depress the curve in Figure 10-2 may be categorized as the skin's microenvironment, malnutrition, and excessive skin tension.

Microenvironmental factors include moisture, temperature, and the presence of harmful chemicals on the skin. Skin that is either too warm or too cold or too dry or too wet is at greater risk. A support surface that allows moisture to move off the skin or conducts heat from the skin can either aid or contribute to damage. A surface that traps heat and moisture against the skin, such as a foam or gel cushion or the presence of skinfolds, increases the risk

of injury. Surfaces that conduct too much heat and moisture away from the skin, such as low-air-loss beds, also increase risk. Both urinary and fecal incontinence produce chemical injury to the skin in addition to holding heat and moisture.

Many people who are already susceptible to pressure injury have the additional burden of incontinence. The caustic nature of urine and feces combined with excessive moisture, temperature, dependency, and potentially the weight of the genitalia increases the risk of injury. Incontinence is also frequently comorbid with malnutrition. Tube or parenteral feedings often lead to a liquid stool that may contact the skin for multiple hours per day or enter a sacral or ischial wound. In such cases, a rectal tube or similar device may capture liquid stool to prevent injury. Some patients may also be candidates for Foley catheters to reduce the risk of perineal injury and pressure. Incontinence injuries such as shown in Figure 10-8 may be inappropriately labeled as a pressure injury. This is discussed later in this chapter. Additionally, incontinence disrupts normal integumentary flora and alters the skin's pH, which may increase the susceptibility to injury from pressure, friction, and shear and increases the likelihood of tissue breakdown and infection.

Moisture-Associated Skin Damage

This category was also recently added due to the prevalence of misdiagnosis of skin injury produced by moisture as stage 2 pressure injury. The definition of stage 2 (see the following) explicitly states that it should not be confused with moisture damage, whether due to moisture in general or more specifically by incontinence or intertrigo, which are discussed next. Moisture injury can be produced by wound drainage, sweating, leakage of fluid from the skin, support surfaces that prevent evaporation of fluid, or any combination resulting in the skin's maceration. Maceration, as defined in Chapter 3, refers to softening and whitening of skin constantly exposed to water. Urine and feces also result in excess moisture on the skin, but the chemical composition leads to greater skin injury. Skinfolds that remain in contact with each other also lead to skin injury called *intertrigo*. Note that patients may have stage 2 pressure injury, moisture-associated skin damage (MASD), or both. Recognizing the difference aids in providing the correct treatment.

Incontinence-Associated Dermatitis

Just as MASD has been confused with pressure injuries so has incontinence-associated dermatitis (IAD). The chemical composition and pH of urine and feces and prolonged contact lead to skin injury equivalent to diaper rash. Both MASD and IAD increase the risk of pressure injury. An example of IAD is shown in Figure 10-8.

Intertriginous Dermatitis

The term *intertrigo* is used as well as intertriginous dermatitis. It is produced within skinfolds due to constant contact creating a moist, warm environment that promotes the growth of fungal species. The reddening produced by intertriginous dermatitis could be confused with other injuries but occurs in locations unlikely to develop pressure injuries. Antifungal medications and absorbent material with antifungal properties can be used to mitigate the effect of overlapping skinfolds.

Malnutrition

Malnutrition has 2 effects on risk. The inability to maintain the nutritional needs of tissue diminishes the tissue's ability to overcome stresses and repair themselves. Moreover, unintentional weight loss diminishes the cushioning effect of soft tissue over bony prominences. Emaciated individuals have more prominent bony prominences, and more bones such as ribs act as bony prominences. The skin over inferior angles of the scapulae, ribs, iliac spines, and vertebral spines can become ulcerated in such individuals.

Excessive Tension

Tension may create injury either through a direct effect of tensile force on the connective tissue or by distortion of blood vessels. Excessive tension on the skin results from obesity; devices and wrinkled/bunched bedding under the patient; and methods of securing devices, such as hook and loop bands, elasticized garments, and tape on the edges of bandages. Obesity is particularly problematic because repositioning may not clear an area of skin from the support surface. Instead, it may result in stretching the skin on one side of the body and wrinkling it on the other side. In particular, obesity creates taut skin on the low back and upper gluteal areas. Edema from dependency, especially the sacrum from prolonged Fowler's positioning, contributes to the high incidence of sacral pressure injuries within individuals with obesity. In addition to the tension placed on the skin adjacent to the tape, excessive tension placed on tape used to secure dressing can also injure the skin beneath the tape by shearing.

Medical Device–Related Pressure Injury

This term was also added recently due to increased emphasis on medical devices' role in skin injury. Previously, medical devices were only considered to be contributory. Devices such as Foley catheters that are left under patients produce focal pressure at the device's apex where the skin is also stretched over the device, producing a tensile force on the skin. Interface pressure can become very high over a device. Some care providers may assume that the support surface will give sufficiently to prevent pressure and leave the device under the patient. Ordinarily, a person would complain of discomfort and either move the device or have it moved. However, a patient with diminished sensation, communication, cognition, or level of consciousness will not be in a position to rectify the situation. Patients have received very deep injuries over tissue remote from a bony prominence. Pressure injuries can also be caused by devices that rest on the skin, such as nasal cannulas over the ears, tracheostomy ties around the neck, and endotracheal tubes on the lower lip. Drawing attention to this problem by creating a new category has led to changes in equipment and foam dressings under devices that rest on the skin. The NPIAP defines medical device–related pressure injury (MDRPI) as follows:

> Medical device-related pressure injuries result from the use of devices designed and applied for diagnostic or therapeutic purposes. The resultant pressure injury generally conforms to the pattern or shape of the device. The injury should be staged using the staging system.[1]

A related term specific to mucus membranes is *mucosal membrane pressure injury*. The NPIAP defines this as follows:

> A mucosal membrane pressure injury is found on mucous membranes with a history of a medical device in use at the injury location. Due to the anatomy of the tissue, these ulcers cannot be staged.[1]

The NPIAP has provided materials for dissemination to health care providers in an effort to reduce these types of injuries (https://npiap.com/store/ViewProduct.aspx?id=14128515). Best Practices for Prevention of Medical Device-Related Pressure Injuries with photographs of different injuries and stages for them is available on the NPIAP website. The practices consist of the following:

- Choose the correct size of medical device(s) to fit the individual.
- Cushion and protect the skin with dressings in high-risk areas (eg, nasal bridge).
- Remove or move removable devices to assess skin at least daily.
- Avoid placement of device(s) over sites of prior or existing pressure injury.
- Educate staff on the correct use of devices and prevention of skin breakdown.
- Be aware of edema under device(s) and potential for skin breakdown.
- Confirm that devices are not placed directly under a patient who is bedridden or immobile.

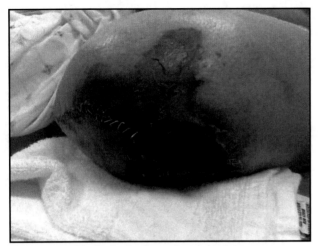

Figure 10-9. Medical adhesive–related skin injury.

MDRPIs often resemble the shape of the responsible instrument. Examples of devices that may cause MDRPIs include oxygen masks and tubes, continuous positive airway pressure and bilevel positive airway pressure devices, endotracheal tubes, nasogastric tubes, electrocardiogram leads, urinary catheters, compression stockings/thromboembolism deterrent stockings, bedpans, cervical collars, and other types of casts and splints. The incidence of pressure injuries is 2.4 times higher in people who require medical devices compared with those who do not. Pediatric patients may be even more vulnerable due to delicate skin, particularly in premature infants. Common areas for these injuries include the ear, sacrum, coccyx, and heel.

In addition to these practices, anyone who has sensory or cognitive deficits or is unable to communicate should not have devices placed under them. This includes neonates and children too young to draw attention to tissue injury.

Medical Adhesive–Related Skin Injury

Adhesives are used for convenience in cases where no good alternatives exist or due to a lack of creativity in securing devices or dressings. As much as possible, adhesives should be avoided, especially on older adults' and newborns' skin and in places where the skin cannot be monitored easily. Alternatives to adhesives for securing dressings are discussed explicitly in Chapter 16. Adhesive-related injury can manifest on a continuum from redness caused by a hypersensitivity reaction to skin breakdown. With repeated application, even hypersensitivity can produce severe injury leading to skin breakdown. An example of skin injury from adhesives is shown in Figure 10-9. In this example, a person with a dehiscent amputation site wound had dressings secured with tape despite her repeated requests not to use tape. Repeated application

of adhesive, even with great care, can remove epidermal cells, and with sufficient force, a flap of epidermis can be torn, resulting in a skin tear. Skin tears are addressed in Chapter 13. Skin can also be damaged by the shearing force placed on the skin either because tape is stretched before application to the skin or because edema occurs after the tape is applied. Additionally, adhesives may hold moisture and heat against the skin.

Definitions of Stages of Pressure Injuries

Pressure injury staging has a long history, and the purpose beyond documentation itself remains dubious. As discussed in Chapters 2 and 9, a system for wounds, in general, is already in place using the epidermis, dermis, and fascia to describe them. The NPIAP has developed and refined definitions of stages. Briefly, stage 1 is unblanchable erythema with no ulceration. Stage 2 is a partial-thickness injury. A full-thickness, suprafascial ulceration is stage 3, and stage 4 has greater depth than fascia.

Stage 1

The definition of the NPIAP at the time of writing is subject to change but appears as follows below. The NPIAP has consistently identified non-blanchable erythema of intact skin as stage 1 but has added details and disclaimers to the definition over the years. Figure 10-10A demonstrates the difference between blanchable and non-blanchable redness, while Figures 10-10B and 10-10C demonstrate stage 1 in lightly pigmented and darkly pigmented tissue.

> Stage 1 Pressure Injury: Non-blanchable erythema of intact skin. Intact skin with a localized area of non-blanchable erythema, which may appear differently in darkly pigmented skin. The presence of blanchable erythema or changes in sensation, temperature, or firmness may precede visual changes. Color changes do not include purple or maroon discoloration; these may indicate deep tissue pressure injury.[1]

The major issue with this description is the implication that pressure injuries begin on the skin surface, and inspection for non-blanchable erythema will somehow prevent pressure injuries. Although the purpose of the description may be to bring attention to the patient before skin injury occurs, superficial knowledge of stage 1 may lead to complacence in the absence of any non-blanchable erythema rather than focusing on the risk of the individual. Depictions of blanchable vs non-blanchable erythema characteristic of a stage 1 injury are shown in Figure 10-10A.

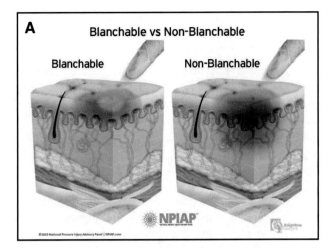

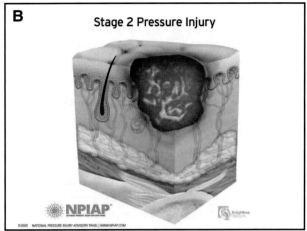

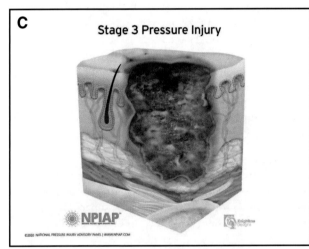

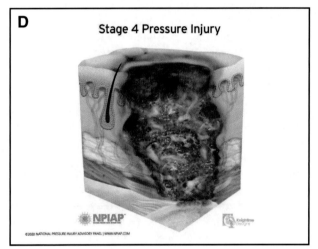

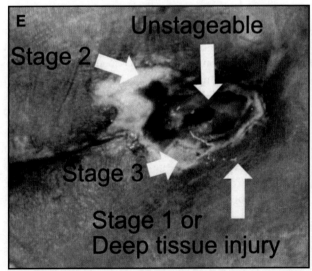

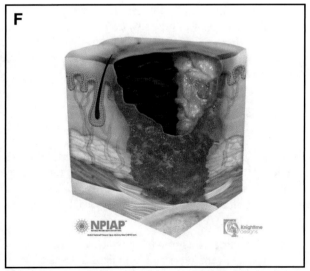

Figure 10-10. Appearance of different stages of pressure injuries. Stage 1 is characterized by non-blanchable erythema. (A) Blanchable vs non-blanchable erythema. (B) Stage 2 demonstrates ulceration through the epidermis and partly into the dermis. (C) Stage 3 extends through the entire dermis down to the fascia level. (D) Stage 4 pressure injuries include subfascial structures such as muscle, tendon, ligament, and bone. (E) Multiple depths of injury are depicted in a wound over the sacrum. (The image is a copyrighted product of AAWC [www.aawconline.org] and has been reproduced with permission.) (F) Unstageable with slough and eschar covering the wound bed.

Stage 2

This definition has changed substantially over the years but remains a characterization of a partial-thickness injury in which the dermis is exposed but tissues below are intact. The NPIAP definition is as follows:

Stage 2 Pressure Injury: Partial-thickness skin loss with exposed dermis. The wound bed is viable, pink or red, moist, and may also present as an intact or ruptured serum-filled blister. Adipose (fat) is not visible, and deeper tissues are not visible. Granulation tissue, slough, and eschar are not present. These injuries commonly result from adverse microclimate and shear in the skin over the pelvis and shear in the heel. This stage should not be used to describe moisture-associated skin damage (MASD), including incontinence-associated dermatitis (IAD), intertriginous dermatitis (ITD), medical adhesive–related skin injury (MARSI), or traumatic wounds (skin tears, burns, abrasions).[1]

The basic message is that damage from causes other than pressure has been conflated with stage 2 injuries. The newest definition is an effort to bring attention to the differences from injuries caused by tape, urine, and other causes now addressed in the recently introduced terms discussed under contributing factors. The definition also indicates that granulation tissue is not present in the wound. By definition, slough and eschar are not present in these partial-thickness injuries. Therefore, the presence of granulation tissue, slough, and eschar would immediately direct the clinician to a stage consistent with full-thickness wounds. However, the definition can still be confused with a friction injury rather than tissue necrosis due to pressure, shear, or tension on the skin. A depiction of a type 2 injury is shown in Figure 10-10B.

Stage 3

The definition of stage 3 is similar to the general definition of a full-thickness dermal wound, except that it explicitly states that fascia is not visible. Therefore, a stage 3 injury is a suprafascial wound. This definition also begins to describe an unstageable injury. The official NPIAP definition is as follows:

Full-thickness loss of skin, in which adipose (fat) is visible in the ulcer and granulation tissue and epibole (rolled wound edges) are often present. Slough and/or eschar may be visible. The depth of tissue damage varies by anatomical location; areas of significant adiposity can develop deep wounds. Undermining and tunneling may occur. Fascia, muscle, tendon, ligament, cartilage and/

or bone are not exposed. If slough or eschar obscures the extent of tissue loss, this is an Unstageable Pressure Injury.[1]

Therefore, full thickness of the dermis has been removed from the injury site, exposing fat but not fascia. Fascia or any subfascial structures present in the wound indicate a stage 4 injury. A depiction of a stage 3 injury is shown in Figure 10-10C.

Stage 4

The NPIAP definition indicates a subfascial injury. The only recent change has been the emphasis on the unstageable ulcer. The definition is as follows:

Stage 4 Pressure Injury: Full-thickness skin and tissue loss with exposed or directly palpable fascia, muscle, tendon, ligament, cartilage, or bone in the ulcer. Slough and/or eschar may be visible. Epibole (rolled edges), undermining, and/or tunneling often occur. Depth varies by anatomical location. If slough or eschar obscures the extent of tissue loss, this is an Unstageable Pressure Injury.[1]

Stage 4 injuries are common in high-pressure areas such as the sacrum, ischial tuberosities, greater trochanter, and heels where pressure is likely to severely limit blood flow to the tissue, producing edema, thrombosis, and necrosis that propagate from deep to superficial. A depiction of a stage 4 injury is shown in Figure 10-10D.

Unstageable

This definition has existed for several years now. It was created to handle the situation in which the tissue at the base of the wound cannot be visualized to distinguish between stages 3 and 4. Based on the definition of stage 2, an unstageable wound could not be a stage 2 because the presence of eschar or slough eliminates the possibility. The definition is as follows:

Obscured full-thickness skin and tissue loss. Full-thickness skin and tissue loss in which the extent of tissue damage within the ulcer cannot be confirmed because it is obscured by slough or eschar. If slough or eschar is removed, a stage 3 or stage 4 pressure injury will be revealed. Stable eschar (i.e., dry, adherent, intact without erythema or fluctuance) on the heel or ischemic limb should not be softened or removed.[1]

Debridement of the wound will eventually remove tissue obscuring the base of the wound, allowing staging to be performed. A photo of a wound with an unstageable area is shown in Figure 10-10E and a depiction in Figure 10-10F.

Deep Tissue Pressure Injury

This stage was previously termed *suspected* deep tissue pressure injury. The latest set of definitions dropped the word "suspected." This definition was added simultaneously as unstageable to manage the situation of subcutaneous necrosis in the absence of a skin ulcer. We had no language to describe this condition before this definition as the original terms were only created for ulcerated skin.

Persistent non-blanchable deep red, maroon or purple discoloration. Intact or non-intact skin with localized area of persistent non-blanchable deep red, maroon, purple discoloration, or epidermal separation revealing a dark wound bed or blood-filled blister. Pain and temperature change often precede skin color changes. Discoloration may appear differently in darkly pigmented skin. This injury results from intense and/or prolonged pressure and shear forces at the bone-muscle interface. The wound may evolve rapidly to reveal the extent of tissue injury or resolve without tissue loss. If necrotic tissue, subcutaneous tissue, granulation tissue, fascia, muscle, or other underlying structures are visible, this indicates a full-thickness pressure injury (unstageable, stage 3, or stage 4). Do not use DTPI to describe vascular, traumatic, neuropathic, or dermatologic conditions.[1]

Deep tissue pressure injury commonly precedes stage 4 injuries in areas such as the sacrum, ischial tuberosities, greater trochanter, and heels. The photo in Figure 10-10E shows multiple depths of pressure injury, including deep tissue injury, stages 2 and 3, and an unstageable area.

Pathophysiology of Pressure Injuries

Although pressure injuries are commonly described as the result of too much pressure for too long, this view is overly simplistic and may lead to poor management. The underlying assumption is that pressure injury results from compression of blood vessels, and tissue becomes ischemic due to the product of time and pressure. While high pressures due to weight being distributed over a limited area such as a medical device under a dependent patient or thighs dangling over the edge of a wheelchair may be responsible for tissue injury, these situations also have a great deal of tensile stress that damages connective tissue and may narrow blood vessels. Neighboring areas of shearing can kink vessels and produce necrosis. Even conditions in which pressure is not present, such as adhesives creating a shearing force, can produce devastating injuries. In general, pressure caused by tissue compression between a bony prominence and support surface creates deep injuries to the tissue stretched over the prominence.

In some cases, tissue necrosis can be present while the skin remains healthy. Ultrasound and other imaging techniques are being developed to detect these injuries before skin breakdown occurs. These injuries are known as *deep tissue injuries*. Shearing can produce varying depths of injury depending on the depth to which blood vessels become kinked. In contrast, tension will be greatest at the surface where the radius from the bony prominence stretching the skin is greatest.

The development of pressure injuries has been described as occurring in 4 stages: hyperemia, edema and thrombosis, necrosis, and ulceration. In cases of deep tissue injury, only the first 3 stages have occurred.

Hyperemia

After approximately 1 hour of unrelieved pressure, mild tissue injury is believed to occur. This manifests as the release of inflammatory mediators. Blood vessels in the area of injury dilate. However, one should realize that tissue compression has likely already resulted in vasodilation in the compressed area due to the accumulation of vasodilatory mediators. Vasodilation of arterioles in the compressed area may mitigate compression depending on the degree of compression and shearing of blood vessels. Tissue injury increases the volume of tissue experiencing vasodilation, extending beyond the site of injury. Unfortunately, this contributes to the fallacy that pressure injuries are always preceded by non-blanchable surface erythema because generally the site of injury is too deep to visualize any erythema. Tools under development may become widely deployed to detect injury of at-risk individuals earlier.

Edema and Thrombosis

Within a few hours of unrelieved pressure, sluggish blood flow combined with tissue injury promotes thrombosis. When pressure is relieved in the face of vasodilation and increased venous resistance due to thrombosis, precapillary pressure is elevated, resulting in leakage of fluid into the interstitial space. Furthermore, reperfusion injury can occur when oxygen flow is restored to the inflammation site, exacerbating the injury. A critical combination of thrombosis, edema, and reperfusion injury can lead to a positive feedback cycle of injury and the propagation of the injury laterally and superficially. Blood vessel injury promotes further thrombosis, injury caused by edema promotes further edema, and a cascade of injury to surrounding tissue is created.

Necrosis

After about 6 hours of unrelieved pressure, the tissue color changes from red to blue-gray similar to the appearance of surface gangrene, resulting in a condition comparable to compartment syndrome.

Ulceration

As tissue injury and necrosis continue due to the positive feedback cycle of injury and thrombosis/edema, the skin may remain intact. In some cases, skin can be severely discolored and be unmistakably necrotic, but no open wound is visible. Eventually, the necrotic skin degrades into an ulcer. The true extent of necrosis is often underestimated due to the size of the opening in the skin. One particular case may illuminate this situation. A patient was referred to one of the authors to address a wound over the sacrum that was referred to as "just a small opening, the size of a dime." However, the entirety of the skin over the sacrum was dark, and as necrotic tissue was removed, necrotic tissue was found completely to the sacrum, about 10 cm deep, 10 cm wide, and 12 cm long. No healthy tissue whatsoever could be found in the vicinity of the sacrum, and the patient was referred to a surgeon for further debridement.

"Sudden" Development of Pressure Injuries

Because necrosis occurs deep in tissues immediately stretched and compressed under a bony prominence, skin on the surface may appear intact, especially if the skin is darkly pigmented. However, the tissue below feels boggy and warm. As discussed in Chapter 8, normal tissue is firm. A boggy, giving, squishy feel indicates the loss of connective tissue and normal turgor of cells replaced by degraded cells. Eventually, inflammation and necrosis spread to the skin over the course of perhaps several weeks. When necrosis finally produces ulceration of the skin, liquefied malodorous slough leaks, and eventually skin over the necrotic tissue necroses itself, resulting in the sudden appearance of a large wound. In some cases, an acute care hospital may admit a patient from either home or a long-term care facility where the pressure injury had been under way for a long time. If the pressure injury suddenly ulcerates the skin after 48 hours and deep tissue was not previously identified and documented, the hospital is responsible for the cost of the care for that ulcer.

Issues and Limitations of Using Stages

The notion of stages of pressure injuries creates the impression that stages are progressive, which they are not. Stage 1 injuries do not progress through a process of stage 1 to stage 2, then 3, and 4. Unrelieved pressure over a bony prominence is likely to produce stage 4 and may never show non-blanchable erythema until ulceration is about to occur. However, a person who does experience non-blanchable erythema should be viewed as being at high risk of developing ulceration. The most recent iteration of the definitions uses stages 1 to 4. However, throughout the literature and among clinics, the terms *stage*, *grade*, or *category* may be used, and Roman numerals are still frequently used in some sources.

The erythema of stage 1 may be easy to observe in lightly pigmented skin but becomes progressively more difficult to ascertain as skin pigmentation increases. In darker pigmented skin, a more purplish/eggplant color and warmer temperature than the surrounding skin indicate a stage 1 injury. Another limitation is the use of staging by agencies to report the status of wounds. In some cases, clinicians are encouraged to perform reverse staging, which is an illogical attempt to show healing of a wound by calling a partially granulated stage 4 injury a stage 3 injury and later, when it is nearly fully granulated, calling it a stage 2. One should logically refer to a partially granulated stage 4 and a fully granulated stage 4 pressure injury. Finally, we already have terminology for wounds in general that would clearly identify the wound's status. Additionally, some clinicians inappropriately use pressure injury stages for wounds with etiologies other than pressure.

The biggest problem with using pressure injury stages is the pervasive belief that surface hyperemia indicates a reversible injury, and at that point, one can then prevent injuries. Relying solely on the detection of non-blanchable erythema to guide prevention efforts is problematic because 80% of those with deep tissue injuries do not first demonstrate surface erythema.

Four Basic Causes of Pressure Injuries

Prevention of pressure injuries is dependent on understanding what leads to pressure injuries. People who can detect excessive tissue loading will process the information and do something to relieve the problem if they have the physical and cognitive capacity. Responding to injurious tissue loading requires information going in, being processed, and going out to effectors that change the situation. The inability to respond can be attributed to 4 factors:

1. Lack of sensation—neuropathy, SCI, peripheral nerve injury, other injuries/disease
2. Lack of cognitive awareness/communication deficits—critical illness, coma, delirium, sedation, neonates, stroke, head injury, non-native speaker
3. Unwillingness to reposition—dementia, psychosis
4. Inability to reposition—restraints, paralysis, paresis, devices, motor neuron diseases

Skin Failure

At the end of life, patients will sometimes develop a characteristic type of pressure injury called a *Kennedy terminal lesion*, decubitus ominosus, Trombley-Brennan terminal tissue injury, and Skin Changes at Life's End (SCALE). Although most pressure injuries can be preventable, Kennedy terminal lesions may be considered unavoidable. This type of injury tends to occur primarily at the sacrum or coccyx and appears as yellow, red, or black tissue discoloration. Patients who develop this type of injury tend to expire within 6 weeks of onset, and, as such, it represents "skin failure." Skin failure may reflect hypoperfusion due to microvascular dysfunction as a part of multiorgan dysfunction and/or sepsis marked by renal failure, respiratory insufficiency, cardiac failure, and critical hepatic impairments. Low blood volume/hypovolemia is another contributing factor in the development of Kennedy terminal lesions.

Prevention of Pressure Injuries

In addition to the burden placed on the patient by the wounds themselves, pressure injuries are associated with poor outcomes, decreased quality of life, and elevated health expenditures. Pressure injuries contribute to longer episodes of care; higher pain levels; and greater risk of infection, morbidity, and mortality. These wounds are among the costliest preventable injuries, with conservative annual estimates of at least $9.1 billion to $11.6 billion in the United States or $20,900 to $151,700 per patient depending on pressure injury stage or severity. The incidence of pressure injuries varies based on patient population and setting. The incidence in public hospitals worldwide is 6.3%, with a point prevalence of 14.8%. Within the United States, the estimated prevalence of pressure injuries in health care facilities is 4.5%. For patients treated in community settings, including home care and outpatient facilities, the prevalence of pressure injuries is approximately

7.4%. Each year, pressure injuries affect more than 2.5 million Americans and are responsible for 60,000 deaths. However, the incidence and prevalence of pressure injuries appear to be on the downward trend. The overall prevalence of pressure injuries declined from 13.5% in 2006 to 9.3% in 2015, decreasing 31% across all care settings.

The most important part of prevention is admitting that a problem exists; complacency is responsible for avoidable pressure injuries. Most clinicians should realize that anyone who is not capable or motivated to reposition is at risk. However, knowing the risk factors and doing something about them are not the same. Many people with risk factors never develop a pressure injury, and prevention is labor intensive. As a result, staff tasked with inspection and repositioning dependent patients may become complacent. Patients also may want to stay in a given position regardless of the consequences. They may either refuse or undo positioning, which leads to the question of whether all pressure injuries are avoidable. This question had been debated for years, but in recent years, the federal government has used the terminology of avoidable and unavoidable pressure injuries in its regulations. An unavoidable pressure injury is one that occurs when the patient receives a score on a standardized tool indicative of high risk and receives the standard of care for a high-risk individual.

Risk Factors for Pressure Injuries

One or a large number of factors may be responsible for developing pressure injuries in any given individual. Potential risks for the development of pressure injuries are listed in Table 10-1. Typically, a combination of lack of mobility, lack of cognition or motivation to move, and exacerbating factors of malnutrition and incontinence is responsible. In particular, individuals with SCIs, diabetes mellitus, hip replacement surgery, femoral fractures, intensive care unit patients with hypotension, and older patients with multiple diseases are at risk. In severe cases, the prevention of pressure injuries may become extremely difficult and perhaps impossible. The lack of volitional repositioning, whatever the cause, is associated with a great risk of pressure injuries. This was demonstrated in a paper published in 1961 showing 90% of those with 20 spontaneous movements or fewer during sleeping hours developed pressure injuries. In contrast, no subjects observed with greater than 50 spontaneous movements developed injuries. A related problem is the failure to protect skin during prolonged surgical procedures and the extended time spent in emergency departments on inadequate pressure-redistributing stretcher mattresses.

TABLE 10-1
Risk Factors for Pressure Injuries

- Physical causes of immobility
  - Altered neuromuscular integrity
  - Diminished strength
  - Altered muscle tone (spasticity, rigidity, dystonia, athetosis, flaccidity, etc)
- Altered musculoskeletal integrity
  - Decreased range of motion
  - Traumatic injury
  - Muscle disease
  - Other
- Devices
  - Splints
  - Casts
  - Orthoses
  - Restraints
- Cognitive causes of immobility
  - Altered state of consciousness, stupor, coma
  - Prolonged anesthesia
  - Diminished motivation to self-reposition
- Diminished sensation
  - Spinal cord injury
  - Spina bifida
  - Head injuries
  - Peripheral neuropathy
- Excessive moisture
  - Use of moisture-resistant support surface
  - Urinary incontinence
  - Fecal incontinence
- Emaciation
  - Malnutrition
  - Dehydration
- Management
  - Inappropriate turning/repositioning schedule
  - Inappropriate support surface
  - Neglect of immobility issues
  - Failure to off-load at-risk areas
  - Failure to clean following episodes of incontinence
  - Harsh cleaning procedures
  - Failure to moisturize/protect dry skin

At-Risk Populations

Certain patient populations are known to be at greater risk of developing pressure injuries. People with multiple comorbidities housed in nursing homes, long-term acute care, and intensive care units have a much greater risk than patients in typical med-surg hospital units. Immobile, tube-fed, incontinent individuals with cognitive problems have tremendous risk. Patients on prolonged ventilation with sedation or paralysis and those with delirium or profound weakness are also at great risk. Within palliative care settings, the estimated prevalence of pressure injuries is almost 20%. People with SCIs that result in loss of sensation to the skin over the ischial tuberosities are at very high risk even if they can reposition and know the risk of developing injuries due to sensory loss.

Factors that increase the risk of pressure injury include advanced age, dehydration, diabetes, malnutrition, and respiratory and cardiovascular disease. Movement impairments that contribute to increased risk of pressure injuries may come from various causes, including neurologic damage, dementia, decreased levels of consciousness, pharmacologic sedation, and the use of anesthesia. These mobility issues may be temporary or permanent. Body mass index (BMI) also affects the risk of pressure injuries for individuals who are underweight, overweight, and obese. Rates of pressure injuries among individuals who are normal-weight were 7.8%; 12.7% in individuals who are underweight; and 5.7%, 4.8%, and 12% in individuals who are overweight, obese, and morbidly obese, respectively. Nutritional factors can exacerbate the risk of pressure injury. Despite excess body weight, people with higher BMIs may exhibit just as many signs of malnutrition as underweight people because additional caloric intake may not meet the dietary requirements for integumentary health and adequate wound repair. Among bariatric patients, the risk of MDRPIs is often exacerbated by poorly fitting devices not made for the patient's size.

Patients with SCIs have one of the highest prevalence rates for pressure injuries, estimated at 10% to 48% within inpatient rehabilitation settings. Risk factors associated with pressure injuries in patients with SCI include the loss of sensory and motor function and changes in circulatory perfusion and soft tissue composition. Patients with SCI tend to exhibit muscle atrophy and increased intramuscular adipose tissue due to movement dysfunction. These changes render subcutaneous tissue less resilient to pressure and other types of applied stress. Skin injuries among patients with SCI may also be linked to mechanical forces exerted on the skin during transfers. Within patients with SCI, pressure injury risk could also be predicted using the following aspects of the Functional Independence Measure: bathing, bladder and bowel management, lower body dressing, toileting, bed and chair transfers, tub/shower transfers, and toilet transfers, with bed/chair transfers having the greatest predictive value.

TABLE 10-2
Scoring Based on the Norton Scale

	4	3	2	1
Physical condition	Good	Fair	Poor	Very bad
Mental condition	Alert	Apathetic	Confused	Stupor
Activity	Ambulant	Walk/help	Chairbound	Stupor
Mobility	Full	Slightly limited	Very limited	Immobile
Incontinent	Not	Occasional	Usually/urine	Doubly

Data source: Agency for Healthcare Research and Quality.

In neonates, the occipital area is often at risk for pressure injuries because of the infant's larger head size relative to the rest of the body. Infants who are born at less than 32 weeks of gestation have scarce amounts of subdermal adipose tissue. The skin of premature infants also has a less developed dermis, with shorter, thinner collagen and elastin fibers than older children and adults. Also, neonates have much thinner stratum corneum, rendering infants more susceptible to temperature changes, evaporative fluid loss through the skin and integumentary damage from antiseptic skin cleansers, and a greater risk of skin infection.

Older adults represent another vulnerable population with increased susceptibility to pressure injuries. Integumentary changes associated with aging include thinning of the epidermis and dermis and atrophy of subcutaneous adipose tissue.

Other factors addressed are the type of support surface and patient positioning that may not be well matched to the individual's characteristics.

Risk of Pressure Injury During Surgery

Pressure injuries during surgery have been a recent emphasis of the NPIAP. Known risk factors include the surgical procedure's length, hypotensive episodes during the procedure, low core temperature, and reduced mobility postoperatively. In particular, obese individuals are more likely to experience resedation due to general anesthetic stored in adipose tissue during surgery. The obese person is, therefore, likely to remain immobile significantly longer.

Strategies to reduce risk include using a pressure redistribution mattress during surgery; elevating heels; and positioning differently before, during, and after the surgical procedure. Use of a pressure-reducing mattress before and after surgery may also reduce risk.

Risk Assessment

Knowledge of risk factors allows the clinician and caregivers to reduce the risk of developing pressure injuries. In the clinical situation, rather than simply assessing the risk factors informally, several standardized tools have been developed in an attempt to quantify risk. Quantification allows clinicians and caregivers to speak a common language in terms of risk factors and provides the clinician with an objective means of decision making. The goals for the tools described later are to identify individuals in need of prevention measures and address specific factors that put them at risk.

Three standardized instruments for assessing risk have been developed. These are the Norton scale, the Braden scale, and the Gosnell scale. The Norton scale is a sum of ordinal scale values for overall physical condition, mental condition, activity level, bed mobility, and continence. Each item is scored between 1 and 4, and the 5-item scores are added. The sum then determines risk. The scoring system for the Norton scale is shown in Table 10-2. The lowest possible score is 5, and the highest is 20. A score of 14 or less indicates a risk for developing pressure injuries, and a score of 12 or less indicates high risk. Based on the risk, prevention and intervention strategies may be undertaken. Although some of the items require the clinician's judgment, the reliability of the scale is sufficient for most needs. As with any instrument using ordinal scales, the numerical differences cannot be treated mathematically. For example, a score of 7 does not necessarily represent 30% more risk than a score of 10.

The Braden scale is the most commonly used scale and has proven reliability and validity. It has 6 items, which are rated on an ordinal scale of 1 to 4. Categories include sensory perception, skin moisture level, activity level, mobility level, nutritional status, and exposure to friction and shear. With this scale, risk also increases with a lower score. This scale uses sensory perception rather than mental condition and moisture rather than incontinence.

TABLE 10-3
Scoring Based on the Braden Scale

	1	2	3	4
Sensory perception	Completely limited	Very limited	Slightly	No impairment
Moisture	Constantly moist	Moist	Occasionally	Rarely
Activity	Bedbound	Chairbound	Walks occasionally	Walks frequently
Mobility	Completely immobile	Very limited	Slightly	No limitations
Nutrition	Very poor	Probably inadequate	Adequate	Excellent
Friction and shear	Problem	Potential problem	No apparent problem	
Data source: Agency for Healthcare Research and Quality.				

Similar to the Norton scale, it also uses mobility and activity level. The Braden scale scores 2 additional items that are not on the Norton scale. The risk of friction and shear, which are somewhat related to bed mobility, and nutrition are addressed in this scale but not in the Norton scale. The Braden scale does not give a score to the clinician's overall impression of physical condition. The scale gives a maximum score of 23; one item (friction and shear) only scores between 1 and 3. Scoring is shown in Table 10-3. For this scale, a person with a score of 16 or below is generally considered to be at risk. However, for certain populations, a score of 17 to 18 is considered at risk for the development of pressure injuries.

The Gosnell scale is an adaptation of the Norton scale. One major difference is the reversal of the scores, such that a high number represents a greater risk. With this adaptation, 5 is the lowest possible score, indicating the least risk, and a score of 20 represents the greatest risk. Another difference between the Gosnell scale and the Norton scale is replacing "physical condition" with nutrition. Other items appear on the tool but are not used in the scoring directly. Also, very detailed instructions are included in the tool.

Nutritional Assessment

A clear association between malnutrition and new injury development has been observed. Particular risk factors cited include low dietary protein and hypoalbuminemia. Nutrition is addressed specifically in Chapter 4. The Agency for Healthcare Research and Quality (AHRQ) guidelines recommend an evaluation of nutritional status using a nutrition-screening manual. Preferably, a clinical dietitian would be available to perform a thorough nutritional assessment. The AHRQ also recommends that a reassessment be made every 3 months. Nutritional risk factors addressed in the guidelines include the inability to take food by mouth, a history of involuntary weight loss, immobility, altered mental status, and educational deficit.

The guidelines recommend encouraging dietary intake and supplementing the diet if the person is malnourished, including nutritional support by tube feed or other means. An intake of 30 to 35 kcal/kg of body mass each day with 1.25 to 1.50 g of protein/kg per day is recommended.

Pain Assessment

Pain management was discussed in Chapter 6. For an individual with limited mobility, complaints of pain from a body surface should be treated as a sign of imminent skin injury. A thorough investigation of the pain's cause, rather than simply treating the pain, needs to be performed. Routine assessment of pain is recommended by the AHRQ, although they also recommend further research into this topic. Specifically addressed is the potential for intensified pain during dressing changes and debridement. They suggest that pain should be managed by eliminating or controlling its source and providing analgesia during painful procedures such as debridement. All patients should be assessed for pain related to the pressure injury or its treatment. Controlling the source of pain may include covering wounds, adjusting support surfaces, and repositioning.

Psychosocial Assessment

In many situations, health care professionals cannot provide all of the care; the patient or other caregiver must take a major role. Even in the acute care hospital, psychosocial issues may promote or impair the efficacy of provided services. Issues that need to be addressed include whether the patient comprehends the care plan and if the patient is motivated to adhere to the plan. The clinician needs to understand the values, lifestyle, psychosocial needs, and goals of the patient and the family or caregiver. The AHRQ guidelines specifically mention mental status, learning ability, depression, social support, polypharmacy or overmedication, alcohol and drug abuse, goals, values, lifestyle, sexuality, culture and ethnicity, and stressors. With these issues in mind, the clinician, patient, family, and other caregivers should collaboratively set treatment goals. When developing a home plan of care, the clinician needs to determine whether the patient and family have the resources available to be treated at home. This includes not only financial resources but also the ability to understand and follow through on the treatment plan. Periodic reassessment is also recommended by the AHRQ, and follow-up should be planned in cooperation with the individual and caregiver.

INTERVENTIONS FOR PREVENTION AND HEALING

While assessing and understanding a patient's risk factors for developing pressure injuries is important, none of that matters if the clinician does not address the patient's risk. Interventions may then follow directly from addressing the factors. Physical therapy may be prescribed to improve mobility and instruct the patient to use assistive and adaptive devices. Specialized support surfaces and orthoses may be ordered. Also, incontinence issues may be addressed. The AHRQ recommends that bed- and chair-bound individuals and anyone with an impaired ability to reposition be systematically evaluated for risk factors.

Furthermore, the AHRQ recommends that individuals be assessed on admission to acute care and rehabilitation hospitals, nursing homes, home care programs, and other health care facilities and should be reassessed at periodic intervals. As recommended by the AHRQ, all assessments of risk should be documented. This provides legal protection for the clinician and the facility and allows changes in the patient's status to be evaluated easily. In addition to the ethical issues with the prevention of pressure injuries, an additional financial incentive has been put in place by the Centers for Medicare & Medicaid Services. The Centers for Medicare & Medicaid Services will no longer provide additional payment to treat pressure injuries not present on admission to a hospital. The admitting facility will be responsible for all additional treatment costs.

Skin Care

Those identified as having risk factors need interventions, including education of patient, family, and caregivers, to maintain and improve tissue tolerance to pressure to prevent injury. The AHRQ recommends that all individuals at risk have a systematic skin inspection at least once per day, paying particular attention to the bony prominences. The results of skin inspection should be documented. Historically, trying to toughen the skin has been proposed as a means of increasing tissue tolerance to tissue load. On the contrary, this practice has been shown to cause damage rather than prevent injury. The AHRQ guidelines state clearly that the practice of massaging over bony prominences should not be used.

Incontinence presents 2 problems. First is the presence of excessive moisture on the skin; second is the physical composition of urine and feces. Both are generally acidic. Urine pH can range from 6 to 3, and feces can contain a large quantity of bile acids. Because incontinence is such an important risk factor, skin cleansing should occur at the time of soiling and at routine intervals. Hot water and harsh detergents should not be used. Instead, many mild cleansing agents are available that can both minimize irritation and maintain appropriate moisture of the skin. Although removing acidic urine and feces is important, minimizing force during cleansing and friction applied to the skin is equally important to prevent skin injury. On the other hand, excessive skin dryness can also lead to injury.

Prevention of injury must also include minimizing low humidity (< 40%) and exposure to cold. Moreover, dry skin should be treated with appropriate moisturizers. Various moisturizers are available. These moisturizers vary in their concentration of solids. Watery lotions with a low concentration of solids are not as effective as emollients with a higher concentration of oil and solids. An effective moisturizer will retain fluid within the skin while protecting the skin from excessive external sources of moisture such as incontinence, perspiration, or wound drainage. Skin care products are discussed in Chapter 16. On occasion, sources of moisture may not be controllable. Various absorptive pads or garments may be necessary under these conditions. However, all underpads and briefs are not suitable for this purpose. Only those made of materials that absorb moisture and wick it away from the skin should be used. General purpose underpads may be suitable for those at low risk for a few days, such as individuals at low risk for pressure injuries after surgery with copious drainage from surgical wounds. Moisture barriers should be used for the individual who frequently has moisture on the skin. For the person at risk, extra care, including referral to physical therapy, becomes necessary to prevent skin injury due to friction and shear forces.

The patient, family, and caregivers should be instructed in proper positioning and transferring techniques. As lack of mobility is the most important cause of pressure injuries, referral to physical therapy to improve mobility should be made if the potential for improvement exists and improved mobility is consistent with patient and family goals. In some cases, simply maintaining current activity level, mobility, and range of motion is an appropriate goal, which may also require a course of physical therapy.

Turning Schedules

Any bedbound individual with compromised mobility or other risk factors should be repositioned according to an individualized schedule that should be written, posted, and carried out by the patient's caregivers. Historically, a recommendation of turning on a schedule rotating among sidelying to one side, supine, and sidelying to the other side every 2 hours has been made. Rather than using a directly sidelying position, pillows or wedges should be used to turn the patient 30 degrees to avoid positioning directly on the greater trochanter. For individuals at high risk, especially those who are emaciated and malnourished, 2 hours in one position may be too long and more frequent repositioning might be necessary.

Blindly repositioning without regard to neurologic deficits, musculoskeletal injuries, or particular skin areas at high risk is a disservice to the patient. Moreover, a patient should never be positioned directly over an injury if possible, and if not possible, the patient should be on a pressure-redistributing surface. To prevent injury caused by bony prominences contacting each other, pillows, foam wedges, or other devices should be used to keep the knees or ankles apart. Anyone with impaired mobility or who is bedbound should have a device that totally relieves pressure on the heels, usually by raising the heels off the bed (floating the heels). This may consist of simply placing pillows under the legs or may include more complex devices such as Multi Podus (Restorative Care of America, Incorporated) or heel lift boots (Figures 10-11A to 10-11D). Donut devices should never be used on anyone at risk for pressure injuries. These devices are designed only for temporary comfort use in individuals not at risk for pressure injuries.

While pillows and wedges are effective in turning, Sage has developed the TAP (turn and position) system to assist staff with turning patients (Figures 10-12A to 10-12C). The system is used to help achieve a 30-degree turn for a patient with 2 wedges. The system also has a glide sheet that helps decrease friction and shear. The benefit of this system is 2-fold. Not only does it help prevent sacral pressure injuries, but it also helps with proper caregiver mechanics, thus decreasing staff injuries, which add to the overall cost of treating pressure injuries.

In addition to pressure, shear must be minimized. Shear stress increases directly in proportion to the incline of a bed or chair. In the case of reclining, shear is placed on the skin over the sacrum when the skin adheres to the support surface as body weight pulls downward. These forces also occur during transfers, turning, and bed mobility. To minimize injury due to shear, the clinician should maintain the head of the bed at the lowest degree of elevation consistent with medical conditions and other restrictions, such as increased intracranial pressure, pulmonary edema, congestive heart failure, and gastroesophageal reflux. To

further decrease shearing, the patient can be placed in the Fowler's position. Raising the foot of the bed puts a patient in hip and knee flexion such that weight is placed on the posterior thigh to stop the patient from sliding downward in bed when supine. However, prolonged Fowler's position needs to be avoided due to the risk of hip and knee flexion contractures. Using a trapeze or draw sheets to lift and avoid dragging individuals in bed who cannot assist during transfers and position changes is recommended. Recently, the NPIAP has advocated using foam dressings for the prevention of pressure injuries: "Consider placing foam dressings on body areas and pressure injuries at risk for shear injury." Many intensive care units have a protocol for applying sacral foam dressings to all patients at admission to the unit. Typically, foam dressings with silicone borders provide adhesion but are very gentle to the skin. Another benefit of these dressings is that the edges can be lifted to inspect the skin underneath and then laid back down.

Some recent technology has been developed to assist health care professionals in either understanding if a patient has been turned sufficiently to prevent skin breakdown or determining patient position. The first product is VU by Wellsense (Figures 10-13A and 10-13B). The VU is a mat that goes inside the hospital mattress covering and shows health care providers where pressure is under a patient to assist with effective repositioning. This is done via an Advanced Pressure Visualization System. Live images are shown of tissue interface pressures on a tablet at the foot of the bed. Staff are educated that they want to stay away from ROY (red, orange, and yellow), indicating elevated pressure areas. Another system is Leaf Patient Monitoring System by Smith & Nephew, which is used to determine the patient position (Figures 10-14A and 10-14B). The Leaf system is the first Food and Drug Administration–cleared medical technology that continuously monitors patients' activity and position to help identify patients who could benefit from repositioning. This system can track patients in both the bed and the chair and when they are ambulating.

Support Surfaces

Support surfaces are used to redistribute pressure or reduce the amount of pressure on any given body part, particularly for areas where bony structures are compressed. A large number of support surfaces have been created to reduce the risk of pressure injuries. Several terms associated with them are discussed here. The terms *pressure relief* and *pressure reducing* have been used to suggest appropriate use. A pressure-relieving surface provides an interface pressure measurement below 25 mm Hg. Pressure-reducing devices provide an interface pressure of 26 to 32 mm Hg. Interface pressure refers to the pressure measured between a support surface and bony prominences

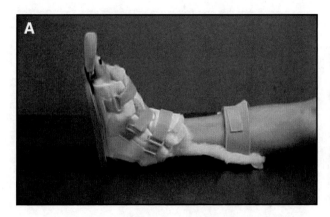

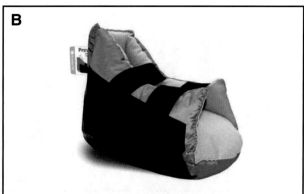

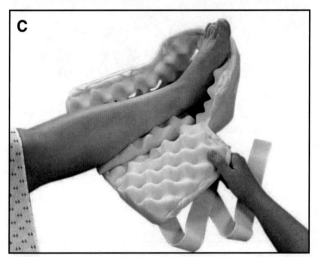

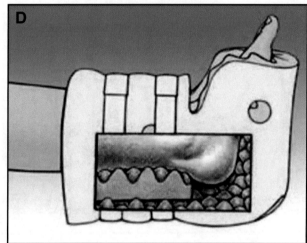

Figure 10-11. (A) Multi Podus boot: The heel is protected from the weight of the patient's leg. (B) Prevalon (Sage) heel lift boot. (Reproduced with permission from Stryker.) (C) Foam heel lift boot. (Reproduced with permission from Stryker.) (D) Application of foam heel lift boot.

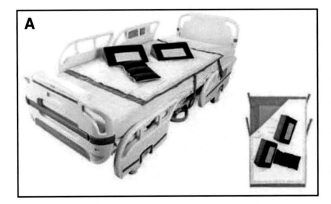

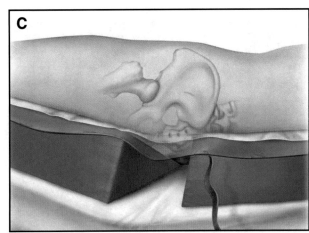

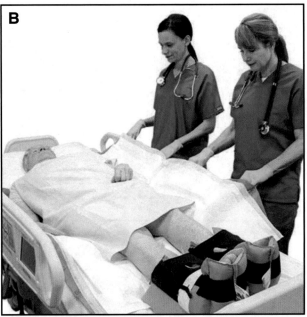

Figure 10-12. Tap and turn device. (Reproduced with permission from Stryker.)

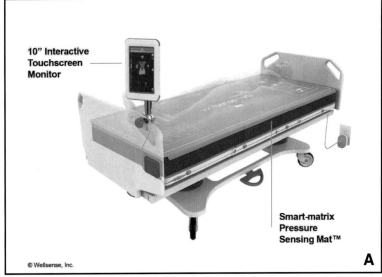

Figure 10-13. VU device. (Reproduced with permission from Wellsense.)

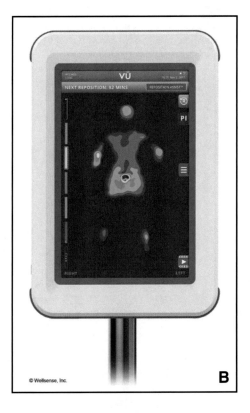

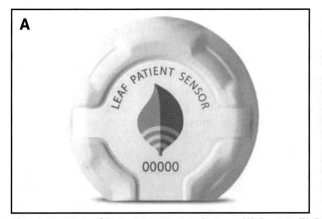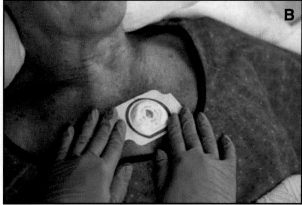

Figure 10-14. Leaf Patient Monitoring System. (A) Device. (B) Device applied to a patient. (Reproduced with permission from Smith & Nephew.)

such as greater trochanters. The purpose of definitions based on 32 mm Hg is to avoid pressures greater than the accepted standard for capillary closing pressure. This number is based on assuming that an interface pressure greater than 32 mm Hg deforms capillaries sufficiently to cut off blood supply to the tissue between the support surface and the bony prominence. This number is based on a 1930 study of healthy, younger men and may vary tremendously between men and women and with age and cardiovascular status. More recently, the term *pressure redistributing* has been used to describe more adequately what the device can offer the patient.

Several terms are used to evaluate support surfaces. *Indentation load deflection* is tested with specific equipment and testing procedures. A standard test of 25% indentation load deflection examines the load necessary to compress a surface to 75% of its original height. This load is expected to be within the range of 25 and 35 pounds (lb). The 65% deflection is determined similarly. The ratio of the load necessary to compress the surface to 35% of its original height to the load necessary to compress the surface to 75% of its original height is termed the *support factor*. A high ratio indicates a surface that initially gives to provide comfort but maintains firm support. The density of foam refers to the weight in pounds of a cubic foot of foam. Density should be greater than 1.8 lb/ft^3 to prevent bottoming out and premature fatigue of the foam. In addition, several terms are used to describe the performance of support surfaces. *Immersion* allows bony prominences to sink into the support surface so that pressure can be borne by tissues surrounding the bony prominences (Figure 10-15). A support surface with low immersion places more pressure against a bony prominence as the surrounding tissues make little contact with the support surface.

The term *envelopment* refers to the ability of the support surface to deform around any irregularities. Superficially, these 2 terms seem similar. Both are related to

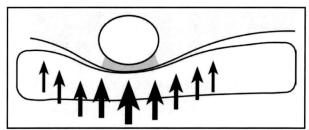

Figure 10-15. Pressure redistribution provided by a seat cushion.

the property of deformation. Immersion refers more specifically to the "give" of the surface, whereas envelopment refers to the contouring of the surface to what is placed on it. A surface may have both good immersion and envelopment or may be good in just one property. *Postural stability* refers to the ability of the patient to be held in place by the surface. A high immersion may provide good postural stability. However, a support surface with good envelopment provided by allowing material in the support surface to flow beneath the cover may produce poor postural stability. Many support surfaces may be constructed of combinations of materials to optimize these 3 characteristics.

To provide different properties, seat cushions may be created in several shapes other than flat. Precontouring a cushion to the general shape of a person's supporting tissues can provide more postural stability for a given amount of envelopment or immersion. A segmented cushion has the equivalent of cuts in both horizontal directions to allow movement among the different segments and provide better envelopment for a given immersion. A third strategy is cutting out a pressure-relief area. The Isch-Dish (Span America Medical Systems, Inc) has a cutout area in the back of the cushion. The sacrococcygeal region and ischial tuberosities areas are floated. More weight is borne on the posterior thighs, which can tolerate the pressure better than the tissue over the bony prominences of the sacrococcygeal spine and ischial tuberosities. Covers used on the support surface influence the overall performance of the support surface. A tight cover reduces both immersion and envelopment. A cover designed to lower friction and shear may reduce postural stability.

Moisture and temperature control may also be important considerations. Certain materials have a low heat transfer rate, allowing retention of heat by the skin surface, whereas others may have a high heat transfer rate, which reduces the skin/body temperature. Moisture vapor transmission rate refers to the movement of moisture through the surface. The ability of specific materials to allow accumulation of moisture should also be considered when determining the most appropriate support surface for a given individual. Choice of support surface may become an exercise in compromise as a support surface with one good characteristic may become less useful because of a poor characteristic. For example, some materials used in fluid-filled cushions can provide excellent envelopment but provide poor postural stability and cause heat and moisture retention.

Pressure-Redistributing Devices

Any individual assessed to be at risk for developing pressure injuries should be placed on a pressure-redistributing device appropriate for the individual's amount of time sitting on a chair or lying in bed. These devices may be discussed as pressure-reducing devices or pressure-relief devices. The devices do not reduce or relieve pressure across the support surface as a whole. Instead, redistributing it to areas that can withstand a greater pressure reduces pressure in areas that might be injured. For example, a cushion might be created that decreases pressure on the ischial tuberosities by redistributing some of the pressure to the posterior thigh and some of the medial and lateral surfaces of the thigh. Pressure relief may be produced by cutting an area from a cushion (or another device) such that the body part does not contact a support surface. This procedure of removing material from a specific location is also known as "cutting a relief" in the device. Unless otherwise specified by a device's characteristics as a pressure-relief or pressure-reducing device, a pressure-distributing device (PRD) will imply pressure redistribution by exploiting some of the properties of the available materials.

Anyone determined to be at risk for developing pressure injuries should avoid uninterrupted sitting in a chair or wheelchair. Appropriate cushions or chair bottoms should be supplied commensurate with risk. For the individual with lower extremity musculoskeletal injuries but otherwise can reposition, a simple wheelchair with a sling seat may be sufficient. At the other extreme, a person with quadriplegia who cannot reposition and lacks sensation should have a specialized pressure-redistributing cushion. In addition to redistributing pressure, seating arrangements must also consider postural alignment, weight distribution, balance, and stability. The AHRQ guidelines recommend that an individual be repositioned, shifting the points under pressure at least every hour while sitting or being put back to bed if consistent with overall patient management goals. However, allowing a person to remain in bed also carries the risk of pressure injuries. Some areas at risk in sitting will have pressure reduced when lying in bed, but some locations may continue to have pressure or shear as while sitting, particularly the sacrum.

Moreover, lying in bed presents a tremendous risk to general health, including the risk of thromboembolism, pneumonia, gastrointestinal and renal disease, and bone demineralization. Individuals should be taught to shift weight while seated every 15 minutes if they have the physical and cognitive abilities. A written plan for the use of positioning devices should be supplied and reviewed with each individual. A patient who has a pressure injury on a sitting surface should avoid sitting. If pressure on the injury can be relieved, limited sitting may be allowed.

Several classifications of PRDs have been described. Surfaces can be categorized by their mechanisms as alternating pressure pads, beds, mattress overlays, mattress replacements, and enhanced overlays and mattresses. Alternating pressure pads consist of a pump that periodically directs air to one set of cells while simultaneously allowing air to be released from another set, resulting in alternating pressure points over a given time. To be effective, these devices must be at least 2 inches in depth.

Mattress overlays fit over a standard mattress. These include air, foam, gel, or water. Air overlays should be at least 3 inches in depth and can be either powered or nonpowered. Foam features include a density of 1.35 to 1.8 lb/ft^3 and a 25% indentation load deflection of 25 to 35 lb. A waterproof and friction-reducing cover should be part of the overlay. A minimum depth of 2 inches is recommended for gel overlays and 3 inches for water.

Mattress replacements are designed to fit into standard bed frames, replacing a standard mattress, as opposed to an overlay or dedicated bed. These, like overlays, may be air, foam, gel, or water. Because they replace a mattress, the recommended thickness is greater than that of an overlay. For air, it is 3 inches, foam is 5 inches, and it includes the features also mentioned for the overlay. Recommended gel depth is 5 inches, as is that of water mattress replacements.

Enhanced overlays and mattresses include alternating pressure mattresses, low-air-loss overlays, nonpowered adjustable zone overlays, low-air-loss mattresses, and low-air-loss mattresses with adjuvant features. Classes of support surfaces are listed in Table 10-4.

By definition, beds are integrated systems, including a frame and any control devices for the support surface. These may be further categorized as air-fluidized beds, low-air-loss beds, and low-air-loss beds with adjuvant

TABLE 10-4
Classes of Support Surfaces

GROUP	DESCRIPTION	PRODUCTS	CHARACTERISTICS	USES
1	Designed to replace standard hospital or home mattress or an overlay. All in this group are unpowered devices.	Mattresses Pressure pads Mattress overlays Foam, air, water, gel	Least expensive devices Only distribute pressure over a larger area	Dependent in mobility or limited mobility with any stage PI on trunk/pelvis and at least one of the following: Impaired nutrition Incontinence Altered sensory perception Compromised circulation
2	Also designed to replace standard hospital or home mattress but all are powered with the exception of nonpowered advanced pressure-reducing mattresses	Powered air flotation beds Powered pressure-reducing air mattresses Nonpowered advanced pressure-reducing mattresses	More expensive than group 1 devices Redistribute pressure Require power, except one nonpowered device Require prior authorization from Medicare	Higher-risk person with limited ability to reposition Large or multiple ulcers on trunk/pelvis that have not improved on a group 1 device or has a flap or graft
3	Complete bed system	Air-fluidized beds	Very expensive Heavy Require power May not be appropriate for some homes	Full-thickness wounds on trunk/pelvis Completely dependent in mobility Requires 24-hour caregiver Has received at least 1 month of conservative therapy

features. Air-fluidized beds consist of a tank filled with silicone microspheres circulated with an air pump and a sheet to contain the microspheres. The features of this support surface are described in greater detail later in this chapter as a pressure-relieving device.

Low-air-loss beds consist of interconnected air cells monitored for pressure that allow air to be lost as pressure increases within a cell. An air pump replaces air as needed when weight is shifted from a cell. These have a minimum depth of 5 inches and may require a stool to allow the patient to move in and out of bed. Low-air-loss beds with adjuvant features are basically the same type of support surface but include features such as percussion, vibration, or periodic movement of a patient across the surface to reposition the patient to improve respiratory status.

Another way to categorize support surfaces is what material makes up the surface. Elastic foam is designed to deform to accommodate a load placed on the support surface and may consist of a series of layers, may be contoured, or may be combined with another material such as gel- or air-filled chambers. A combination of foam and either gel or air chambers allows postural stability because of the properties of immersion and the gel or air chambers' envelopment. Foam alone loses its resilience and bottoms out as the foam degrades with time, a property called *impression set*, and foam has a limited ability to envelope and allows immersion. Foam is absorbent, so it can retain heat and moisture against the skin and can become contaminated. A porous cover and construction with open-cell foam allow some moisture to move through the surface away from the skin. Foam cushions and mattress overlays are useful only for patients' comfort when they are at low risk of developing injuries; they should never be used for a patient with any injuries present. The stiffness of foam must strike a compromise between envelopment of soft foams and bottoming out. Pre-contouring a foam support surface provides immersion and envelopment with improved postural stability. Viscoelastic foam is constructed of open-cell foam and is temperature sensitive. The foam nearest the skin becomes softer due to the increased temperature of the

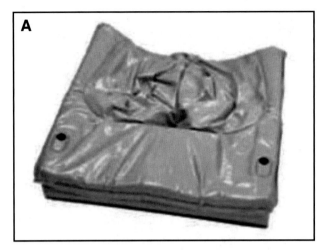

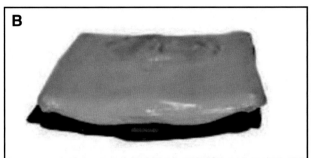

Figure 10-16. Support surfaces for chairs. (A) Jay J2 Deep Contour gel cushion. (B) Jay J2 gel cushion (Sunrise Medical).

foam. The viscoelastic nature helps the foam conform to the body surface and reduce interface pressure. Solid-gel support surfaces function in the same way as viscoelastic foam, but gel has the disadvantage of retaining heat and moisture if the surface is used for more than 2 hours.

Fluid-filled support surfaces have the advantage of being deformable without the large restoring force of surfaces such as foams. This property allows very low interface pressures to occur if the surface is maintained properly. Fluid-filled support surfaces may be filled with air, water, or viscous fluid materials and may have interconnected chambers. Pressure is redistributed by the flow of the fluid between chambers, permitting envelopment and immersion. Proper redistribution only occurs with proper inflating; over- or underinflating negates their effectiveness.

Moreover, their effectiveness for sufficient pressure reduction at the greater trochanters and heels is questionable. They tend to bottom out easily and may become cold or leak. Like foam, water flotation is useful for patients with lower risk and only if the injury is not on the heel or greater trochanter. They should be reserved for patients who are independent in mobility and weight shifting. Air-filled cushions must also be inflated optimally to prevent bottoming out with underinflation and excessive pressures with overinflation.

Gel overlays and seat cushions are more useful than foam and water flotation. In particular, these overlays are capable of dispersing both pressure and shearing forces. However, these overlays and cushions are costly, heavy, and allow moisture to accumulate. Gel overlays are useful for minimal- to moderate-risk patients and patients with manageable injuries and independent mobility. They are frequently used on operating tables for prevention during long procedures that carry the risk of pressure injuries. Although gel seat cushions (Figures 10-16A and 10-16B) can be very expensive, they can be very effective for a person with an SCI or other loss of sensation below the waist. Gel-filled surfaces may periodically require redistribution of the gel through the surface to prevent bottoming out.

The most effective type of PRD for seat cushions is static air. These devices allow the movement of air among channels to redistribute pressure and, to some extent, shear. Drawbacks include the potential for over- or underinflating, seams' potential to fatigue and leak, and accidental puncture. Static air cushions and bed overlays can be useful for minimal- to moderate-risk patients and patients with manageable injuries and independent mobility. They are easy to clean and transport, as opposed to water flotation and gel PRDs.

Dynamic air systems consist of adjacent compartments that alternately inflate and deflate, reducing the time that any area is exposed to high pressure. These can be very useful for moderate-risk, mobility-dependent patients and those with manageable injuries. Dynamic air systems may take the form of a specialty bed or an overlay system placed on a standard bed. Specialty beds consist of either low-air-loss or air-fluidized or combination units. These beds or overlays are recommended for stage 3 or 4 injuries on multiple turning surfaces. Because of the expense of providing support surfaces, most facilities have developed specific criteria for determining medical necessity, such as a specific score on one of the risk assessment tools or the guidelines elaborated in the AHRQ publication. Low-air-loss devices are now available in overlays as well as the traditional bed. In either case, the unit consists of compartments inflated separately with sensors and a pump to maintain proper pressure in each segment as air is lost slowly through the compartments to dissipate pressure. The cover is water vapor permeable; therefore, clinical decisions for managing wound drainage must consider the greater evaporation of moisture from the wound. Pressure and airflow may be adjustable for individual compartments.

Some higher-end units provide airway clearance by either vibrating or rotating through an arc of movement to reduce the time any given lung segment is left in a dependent position. Low-air-loss beds are very expensive; large hospitals may own a small number, or the beds may be rented for hospital or home use. These devices are particularly useful for mobility-dependent, moderate- to maximum-risk patients and patients with difficult-to-manage injuries. The air segments' compressibility would make mobility and cardiopulmonary resuscitation difficult without the safety mechanisms built into the units. Air can be let out rapidly in emergencies by use of a cardiopulmonary resuscitation switch. Deflating the bed can be useful for transfers into and out of bed depending on the patient's height. Mobility can be improved by temporarily increasing the segments' pressure by using a "maximum inflation" or equivalent function. Deflation of the bed is generally more useful for shorter patients and maximum inflation for taller patients.

Air-fluidized beds are the only true pressure-reducing devices. These beds consist of a tank containing ceramic silicon-coated soda-lime beads, a pump to drive air through the beads, and controlling mechanisms including temperature control. A vapor-transmitting sheet is placed over the beads in the tank. Because the tank's beads are 1.5 times as dense as water, the suspended beads cause the patient to be floated, reducing the pressure between the body and support surface. The bed is also designed to minimize friction, shear, and maceration. Body fluids drain into the tank, clumping the beads, which then settle out and are removed.

Moreover, drainage causes sodium ion release from the beads, rendering the medium bacteriostatic. Also, the temperature of the microspheres is controllable. Appropriate dressings need to be placed on the wound to avoid desiccation, in contrast to beds with vapor-impermeable sheets. Because these beds support the patient with the least pressure, they are indicated for patients with the greatest risk of developing pressure injuries or for patients whose pressure injuries may not heal due to problems with positioning. These problems may include the inability to be repositioned or the presence of pressure injuries on multiple turning surfaces (eg, pressure injuries on both greater trochanters and the sacrum). As with low-air-loss beds, airflow can be turned off for emergencies, such as cardiopulmonary resuscitation administration. A combination of air-fluidized and low-air-loss bed is available from Hill-Rom. The upper section uses low air loss, and the lower section uses an air-fluidized tank. The upper section protects the upper body from pressure, while the lower section provides optimum pressure relief where pressure injuries are most likely to develop. Air-fluidized beds may also be used for patients with extensive burns to promote healing of burned posterior regions and graft donor sites, Stevens-Johnson syndrome, necrotizing fasciitis, and other skin conditions that are discussed in the following section and may be used for end-stage cancer. A summary of devices, their selection criteria, and groupings is given in Table 10-4.

Selection of Pressure-Redistributing/-Reducing/-Relief Devices

The selection criteria that the AHRQ suggests for making decisions on support surfaces include providing an increased support area, low moisture retention, reduced heat accumulation, shear reduction, and pressure reduction properties. Other properties to be considered are the dynamic vs static properties and cost per day. The panel recommended that clinicians assess all patients with existing pressure injuries to determine their risk for developing additional pressure injuries. If the patient remains at risk, a pressure-reducing surface should be used. Static support surfaces are recommended for patients who can assume various positions, stay off the injury, and do not cause the device to bottom out. Bottoming out is defined as a distance of less than 1 inch between the surface below the specialized support surface and bony prominences.

Dynamic support surfaces are recommended for patients who cannot assume various positions, who cannot stay off the injury, or who cause a static support surface to bottom out. Having a wound that does not show evidence of healing is another indication for a dynamic support surface. Air-fluidized beds are indicated for patients at high risk for developing pressure injuries and patients with difficult-to-manage injuries. Low-air-loss beds are indicated for moderate-risk patients and those with manageable injuries. Overlay-type PRDs are indicated for patients at minimum to moderate risk and injuries that do not require pressure relief to heal. When the AHRQ guidelines were written, panel members could not find any compelling evidence that one support surface for beds performed better under all circumstances.

In the original guidelines, kinetic therapy beds were not addressed. These beds were designed primarily to assist with respiratory issues by improving clearance of pulmonary secretions with a gentle rotation from side to side, also known as *continuous lateral rotation therapy*. Newer specialty beds from KCI, Hill-Rom, and Huntleigh accomplish the equivalent of rocking motion by rhythmically inflating and deflating air chambers across the bed from side to side. Also, these newer beds can provide airway clearance by vibrating the support surface. The RotoProne bed (Arjo) turns the patient into a prone position safely, without having staff turn the patient. However, this therapy is very expensive given the bed's rental cost and the need to have a dedicated health care professional with the patient at all times. Therefore, the RotoProne bed should only be used on the sickest of patients with no other viable alternatives. The use of kinetic therapy beds, however, does not eliminate the need for a turning schedule.

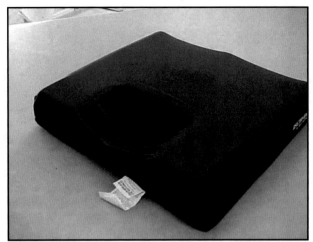

Figure 10-17. Support surface for a chair: Isch-Dish (Span-America Medical Systems).

The AHRQ recommended several considerations specific to sitting. These include an assessment of postural alignment and interventions such as instruction, orthoses, or cushions to provide postural alignment. Positioning should be used to ensure optimal distribution of weight, balance, stability, and continuous pressure relief. Although more favorable from a cardiopulmonary standpoint, sitting even in a well-cushioned chair causes very high interface pressures. Recommendations from the AHRQ guidelines include avoiding sitting if an injury develops on a sitting surface, such as the sacrum or the ischial tuberosities. Bear in mind, however, that these guidelines were developed before the development of newer seating cushions. One type in particular, the Isch-Dish, takes weight completely off the ischial tuberosities and sacrum and redistributes it to the posterior thighs (Figure 10-17). If pressure can be relieved totally, the guidelines recommend that the patient sits for a limited time. As with the bedbound individual, the person should have an individualized written plan. Each person should have an individually prescribed cushion, be repositioned every hour, and shift weight every 15 minutes while sitting if possible.

Medicare Part B Support Surface Guidelines

Medicare Part B Support Surface Guidelines Policies for reimbursement for support surfaces are divided into groups I, II, and III. Criteria for group I devices are either complete immobility or limited mobility or any stage injury on the trunk or pelvis and at least one of the following contributing factors: impaired nutritional status, fecal or urinary incontinence, altered sensory perception, or compromised circulatory status. The need for a PRD should be included in a plan of care established by the patient's physician or home care nurse and documented in the medical records, including education of the patient or caregiver on prevention or management of pressure injuries, regular assessment by a health care practitioner, appropriate turning and positioning, appropriate wound care, appropriate management of moisture (incontinence), and nutritional assessment and intervention consistent with the overall plan of care; a written order must be provided by the physician. In group I, devices include alternating air pressure mattresses and overlays, gel mattresses or overlays, and water pressure mattresses and overlays.

Group II products include low-air-loss beds noted as "powered air flotation bed." This group includes powered pressure-reducing air mattresses, nonpowered advanced pressure-reducing overlays for mattresses, powered air overlay for mattresses, and nonpowered advanced pressure-reducing mattresses. Requirements for a group II product include multiple stage 2 pressure injuries located on the trunk or pelvis, when the patient has been using a group I support surface as part of a comprehensive treatment program with worsening or no improvement over the past month, large or multiple stage 3 or 4 pressure injuries on the trunk, or recent myocutaneous flap or skin graft for a pressure injury on the trunk or pelvis with surgery within the past 60 days, and when the patient has been on a group II or III support surface immediately before discharge. Coverage is limited to 60 days for operative repair of injuries. Again, a written order and a comprehensive plan as described earlier for group I surfaces are required. Use of the group II surface is allowed until the injury is healed or documentation in the medical record shows that other aspects of the plan of care are being modified to promote healing or that the group II surface is medically necessary for wound management.

Group III only includes air-fluidized beds. Requirements include the presence of stage 3 or 4 pressure injury, the patient is bed- or chairbound due to severely limited mobility, the patient would require institutionalization without the air-fluidized bed, and failure of more conservative treatment. A comprehensive plan of care, including the air-fluidized bed, is required as described under group I devices. In general, a more conservative plan of care should have been in effect for at least 1 month with failure to heal before using an air-fluidized bed. Other limitations also need to be addressed. These include the presence of coexisting pulmonary disease, lack of a caregiver willing and able to provide the care required by a patient on an air-fluidized bed, and an inadequate electrical system or structural support for these extremely heavy beds.

Possible Surgical Interventions

Patients with pressure injuries may experience difficulty in healing using conservative treatment methods. The goal is for wound resolution as early as possible to prevent complications. Multiple types of surgical options are available for nonhealing pressure injuries. Patients may require surgical debridement to treat necrotic soft tissue, osteomyelitis, and advancing necrotizing infections, or they may require surgical closure such as split skin graft and flaps. Elective surgical closure procedures may be selected to increase the quality of life, improve daily living activities, and promote a faster resolution. Screening patients before these surgical interventions will decrease the risk of wound complications. Healing rates may vary depending on the patient's health condition. Successful surgical outcomes depend on an individualized assessment investigating factors such as nutrition, glucose control, and infection presence. Lifestyle factors should also be considered, such as altering tobacco and alcohol consumption and promoting patients' adherence to pressure injury prevention strategies and incontinence management.

Once a pressure injury has been completely debrided, wound closure options include pedicle muscle, myocutaneous or fasciocutaneous flaps, and, less commonly, free flap. Skin grafts are available, but they may have higher failure rates and lower short-term durability. A surgical flap's goal is to fill the wound cavity by obliterating dead space using vascularized tissue from the donor site. Donor site and type of flap selection are based on multiple factors, including the wound's location, the need for ambulation, prior history of pressure injuries, previous surgical interventions, and patient comorbidities.

Typical pressure injury locations that may require surgical closure include the ischium, sacrum, greater trochanter, and the distal leg. Postoperative management also includes removing shear, avoiding excessive moisture, optimizing nutrition, and promoting tobacco cessation. Support surface evaluation is required because postoperative instructions will include 6 to 8 weeks of complete bed rest until the healing wound site's maximum tensile strength has been reached. Failure to manage pressure effectively increases the risk of wound recurrence. Support surfaces are recommended for at least 2 to 4 weeks following surgery. A sitting tolerance program may be instituted in cases involving areas of skin impacted by sitting. Patients may sit up in bed for 15 minutes at a time, up to 3 times per day. If the surgical flap does not have redness, induration, or drainage, patients may begin sitting in a chair with a pressure-relief cushion, with sitting time increasing in 15-minute increments every 2 to 3 days. After 2 weeks of following this program, the goal is for patients to tolerate 2 hours of sitting each session. If the skin or wound is deteriorating or drainage is observed, the sitting protocol must be suspended, and the physician must be notified. Follow-up visits with the surgeon should occur monthly for at least 3 months and then every 3 to 6 months.

Common complications from pressure injury surgical closure procedures include hematoma, seroma, infection, and wound dehiscence. The incision line's dehiscence has been reported in rates up to 48.5%; the risk of dehiscence increases with poorly controlled diabetes, age, and previously failed flaps in the same location. Flap failure may also occur due to circulatory impairment. Monitoring the flap by observing the skin color and capillary refill is considered the gold standard.

Strategies for preventing pressure injury recurrence are similar to prevention strategies, recognizing that the risk for future pressure injuries is increased in people with a previous history of chronic wounds. Patients and caregivers must be aware of the importance of pressure redistribution, the proper support surface, and frequent repositioning. Caution is required to prevent or reduce friction and shear during bed mobility and transfers. Also, diligent skin care can help reduce vulnerability to injury by keeping pressure areas dry and healthy. Daily skin inspection helps with the early identification of impending injury with timely medical attention when needed. Potentially harmful lifestyle behaviors, such as diet, tobacco, and alcohol use, should be addressed using appropriate patient education methods.

SUMMARY

Pressure injuries are caused by several factors, including pressure, shear, friction, excess moisture, heat or skin dryness, and lack of nutrition. Both time and pressure on a body surface must be considered in assessing the risk of skin injury. Staging of pressure injuries is based on the tissue involved, and, therefore, reverse staging cannot be done logically. Positioning must account for pressure, the patient's body composition, mental status, and the support surface. Guidelines for appropriate support surfaces are discussed, as is the need for adequate nutritional and psychosocial assessment. Methods to enhance the healing of pressure injuries are discussed in subsequent chapters. The NPIAP has offered revised guidelines on their website with the latest being the 2019 version. The Quick Reference Guide is free from their e-store, whereas the full guidelines require payment at https://guidelinesales.com/page/NPIAP.

QUESTIONS

1. Contrast the terms *pressure* and *shear*.
2. Contrast the terms *shear* and *friction*.
3. What else can cause tissue injury besides a patient's weight?
4. List common contributing factors for pressure injuries.
5. What is the commonly held belief of the pressure and time required to damage skin?
6. What is the most common cause of shearing over the sacral skin?
7. Which parts of the body are most susceptible to passive loading in the following?
   a. Supine/recumbent
   b. Sidelying
   c. Prone
8. Why should dependent patients never be put in sidelying?
9. What is the alternative position for sidelying? How is it achieved?
10. Is friction a part of the definition of a pressure injury? What is the value in detecting injury created by friction?
11. Define medical device–related pressure injury, medical adhesive–related skin injury, and moisture-associated skin damage?
12. Why is body composition important in the risk of developing pressure injuries?
13. Why are the occiput and lateral condyles of the elbows at such high risk for skin breakdown?
14. Why is reclining such an important risk factor in sacral injuries?
15. List reasons that a person might require a specialty bed.
16. What options are available for reducing the risk of pressure injuries in a person during sitting?
17. Why are psychosocial factors important in preventing pressure injuries?
18. What is the pathophysiology of pressure injuries?
19. Why do they start deeply?
20. Why do they seem to appear suddenly?
21. Define the classic 4 stages of pressure injuries 1 to 4 (currently accepted) or I to IV.
22. Define unstageable and suspected deep tissue injuries.
23. What are the 4 basic causes of pressure injuries?
24. What is the practical value for staging pressure injuries?
25. Why is pressure injury prevention so difficult? What needs to be done to keep incidence as low as possible?
26. Why do pressure injuries occur during surgery? What can be done to minimize risk?
27. Which health care provider plays the most important role in preventing pressure injuries? Why?
28. Contrast the following pressure-reducing support surfaces: foam, gel, air, water, air-fluidized, and low-air-loss.
29. Define and list the advantages/disadvantages of the following.
   a. Support factor
   b. Envelopment
   c. Immersion
   d. Reticulated
   e. Precontoured
30. What are the most commonly used tools for predicting pressure injury risk?
31. What are the major components of these tools?
32. What are the redundancies in these tools?
33. What is the value of these tools that obligate their use in health care environments?
34. What are the cutoff scores for these instruments?
35. What are common issues that typically place patients at high risk for these 2 tools?

REFERENCE

1. Edsberg LE, Black JM, Goldberg M, McNichol L, Moore L, Sieggreen M. Revised National Pressure Ulcer Advisory Panel Pressure Injury Staging System: Revised Pressure Injury Staging System. J Wound Ostomy Continence Nurs. 2016;43(6):585-597. doi:10.1097/WON.0000000000000281

BIBLIOGRAPHY

Agency for Healthcare Research and Quality (US). Air-fluidized beds used for treatment of pressure ulcers in the home environment [Internet]. Nov 7, 2001. Technology Assessment. https://www.ncbi.nlm.nih.gov/books/NBK285388/

Agency for Healthcare Research and Quality. https://www.ahrq.gov/patient-safety/settings/hospital/resource/pressureulcer/tool/index.html

Barry M, Nugent L. Pressure ulcer prevention in frail older people. *Nurs Stand*. 2015;30(16):50-60. doi:10.7748/ns.30.16.50.s46

Black JM. Prophylactic dressings for pressure injury prevention: how do they work? *Adv Skin Wound Care*. 2019;32(7S Suppl 1):S2-S3. doi:10.1097/01.ASW.0000558696.45433.30

Black JM, Cuddigan JE, Walko MA, Didier LA, Lander MJ, Kelpe MR. Medical device related pressure ulcers in hospitalized patients. *Int Wound J*. 2010;7(5):358-365. doi:10.1111/j.1742-481X.2010.00699.x

Black JM, Edsberg LE, Baharestani MM, et al. Pressure ulcers: avoidable or unavoidable? Results of the National Pressure Ulcer Advisory Panel Consensus Conference. *Ostomy Wound Manage*. 2011;57(2):24-37.

Cox J. Risk factors for pressure injury development among critical care patients. *Crit Care Nurs Clin North Am.* 2020;32(4):473-488. doi:10.1016/j.cnc.2020.07.001

Demarré L, Van Lancker A, Van Hecke A, et al. The cost of prevention and treatment of pressure ulcers: a systematic review. *Int J Nurs Stud.* 2015;52(11):1754-1774. doi:10.1016/j.ijnurstu.2015.06.006

Edsberg LE, Black JM, Goldberg M, McNichol L, Moore L, Sieggreen M. Revised National Pressure Ulcer Advisory Panel pressure injury staging system: revised pressure injury staging system. *J Wound Ostomy Continence Nurs.* 2016;43(6):585-597. doi:10.1097/won.0000000000000281

Fowler E, Scott-Williams S, McGuire JB. Practice recommendations for preventing heel pressure ulcers. *Ostomy Wound Manage.* 2008;54(10):42-57.

Hajhosseini B, Longaker MT, Gurtner GC. Pressure injury. *Ann Surg.* 2020;271(4):671-679. doi:10.1097/SLA.0000000000003567

Harmon LC, Grobbel C, Palleschi M. Reducing pressure injury incidence using a turn team assignment: analysis of a quality improvement project. *J Wound Ostomy Continence Nurs.* 2016;43(5):477-482. doi:10.1097/WON.0000000000000258

Kottner J, Balzer K, Dassen T, Heinze S. Pressure ulcers: a critical review of definitions and classifications. *Ostomy Wound Manage.* 2009;55(9):22-29.

Kottner J, Cuddigan J, Carville K, et al. Prevention and treatment of pressure ulcers/injuries: the protocol for the second update of the international Clinical Practice Guideline 2019. *J Tissue Viability.* 2019;28(2):51-58. doi:10.1016/j.jtv.2019.01.001

Langemo D, Haesler E, Naylor W, Tippett A, Young T. Evidence-based guidelines for pressure ulcer management at the end of life. *Int J Palliat Nurs.* 2015;21(5):225-232. doi:10.12968/ijpn.2015.21.5.225

Mervis JS, Phillips TJ. Pressure ulcers: pathophysiology, epidemiology, risk factors, and presentation. *J Am Acad Dermatol.* 2019;81(4):881-890. doi:10.1016/j.jaad.2018.12.069

Mervis JS, Phillips TJ. Pressure ulcers: prevention and management. *J Am Acad Dermatol.* 2019;81(4):893-902. doi:10.1016/j.jaad.2018.12.068

Munoz N, Posthauer ME, Cereda E, Schols JMGA, Haesler E. The role of nutrition for pressure injury prevention and healing: the 2019 International Clinical Practice Guideline Recommendations. *Adv Skin Wound Care.* 2020;33(3):123-136. doi:10.1097/01.ASW.0000653144.90739.ad

National Clinical Guideline Centre (UK). The prevention and management of pressure ulcers in primary and secondary care. National Institute for Health and Care Excellence (UK); 2014. (NICE Clinical Guidelines, No. 179.) https://www.ncbi.nlm.nih.gov/books/NBK248068/

Pittman J, Gillespie C. Medical device-related pressure injuries. *Crit Care Nurs Clin North Am.* 2020;32(4):533-542. doi:10.1016/j.cnc.2020.08.004

Preventing pressure ulcers in hospitals. Content last reviewed October 2014. Agency for Healthcare Research and Quality. https://www.ahrq.gov/patient-safety/settings/hospital/resource/pressureulcer/tool/index.html

Reger SI, Ranganathan VK, Sahgal V. Support surface interface pressure, microenvironment, and the prevalence of pressure ulcers: an analysis of the literature. *Ostomy Wound Manage.* 2007;53(10):50-58.

Young M. Medical device-related pressure ulcers: a clear case of iatrogenic harm. *Br J Nurs.* 2018;27(15):S6-S13. doi:10.12968/bjon.2018.27.15.S6

Neuropathic Ulcers

DIABETIC FOOT ULCERS

The term *diabetic foot ulcers* (DFUs) is widely used, and these wounds account for a large majority of wounds addressed in this chapter. However, other neuropathies can produce the same ulcer type. Additionally, many DFUs are arterial, and interventions specific for neuropathy would be inappropriate for arterial ulcers. One of the major reasons for using the term is that the Centers for Medicare & Medicaid Services provides payment for some Current Procedural Terminology codes if a diagnosis of DFU is provided, rather than covering them for neuropathic ulcers.

Irion GL, Gardner JA, Pignataro RM.
Comprehensive Wound Management, Third Edition (pp 181-209).
© 2024 Taylor and Francis Group.

DIABETES AND THE RISK OF FOOT INJURY

In the United States, care costs for diabetic foot complications have been estimated at $15 billion annually. Based on data collected between 2005 and 2010, approximately one-third of the cost of care for people with diabetes in the United States comes from the treatment of foot ulcers, with hospitalization for foot ulcers accounting for half of the overall financial burden. In addition, approximately 85% of all nontraumatic lower-limb amputations are secondary to DFUs. Loss of limb has devastating consequences on function and quality of life. The estimated 5-year mortality rate accompanying amputation is 39% to 68%. Diabetes is a risk factor for many health conditions in addition to neuropathy leading to foot injuries, which is the focus of this chapter. The 2 main forms of diabetes leading to neuropathy are type 1 (DM1) and type 2 diabetes mellitus (DM2). DM1 usually emerges in childhood and adolescence and constitutes approximately 5% of all diabetes cases. DM1 results from immune injury, destroying beta cells of the pancreas that normally produce insulin and the requirement for insulin replacement. DM2 has a greater genetic component and is linked to a constellation of symptoms, including obesity, hypertension, insulin resistance, and other endocrine changes that produce anabolic resistance. Lifestyle behaviors, such as poor diet and lack of physical activity, are largely responsible for its development. The prevalence of these factors in society is increasing, along with the number of people who are overweight and obese. This has contributed to the increasing prevalence of DM2, including in children. In the United States, the estimated prevalence of DM2 was 37 million in 2022, slightly less than 10% of the population.

Neuropathy and peripheral artery disease are common conditions associated with diabetes, and both can lead to the wounding and delayed healing of the foot. Most people with DFUs (80%) have both neuropathy and arterial insufficiency. For this chapter, peripheral neuropathy is a major emphasis, whereas arterial disease is addressed in the next chapter. Peripheral neuropathy is the most common complication of diabetes. Approximately 50% of people with diabetes will eventually develop distal neuropathy. Among people with DFUs, about half are primarily caused by neuropathy, whereas approximately 20% are caused by inadequate blood flow. People with diabetes also experience increased vulnerability to infection and delayed wound healing as a consequence of metabolic dysfunction.

Although 60% to 80% of DFUs eventually heal, these types of wounds carry many serious consequences. The lifetime rate of foot ulceration in people with diabetes is estimated at 10% to 25%.[1] Unfortunately, in people with diabetes, other complications such as vision problems, end-stage kidney disease, and other issues tend to take precedence over foot care. Unless the damage to the sensory nerves results in pain, most of the problems associated with neuropathy can be easily ignored. However, the effects of neuropathy and glycosylation/stiffening of joints of the foot can progress into a major health problem that can lead to loss of the limb.

Recurrence of ulcers is also a major issue, with approximately 40% of patients developing a subsequent wound within 1 year. The chance of wound recurrence increases with the duration of diabetes and inadequate glycemic control, as reflected by higher hemoglobin A1c (HbA1c) levels.

NEUROPATHY, PERIPHERAL ARTERIAL DISEASE, AND DIABETIC FOOT ULCERS

In people with diabetes, one of the greatest risk factors for developing peripheral neuropathy is poor glycemic management. HbA1c levels are an important prognostic indicator, with recommended goals of 7% or less in nonpregnant individuals with diabetes. However, providers may set tailored glycemic management goals depending on other health-related concerns. Unfortunately, for many individuals, diabetes is a silent disease; 50% of people may not even be aware that they have diabetes until complications cause them to seek medical attention. Risks for developing neuropathy and foot ulceration include hypertension, dyslipidemia, and tobacco use. The prevalence of neuropathy also increases with patient age, duration of diabetes, history of peripheral vascular disease, kidney disease, foot deformity, prior foot ulcerations, and previous lower extremity amputation.

Adopting the term *diabetic foot ulcer* has worsened the issue of conflating neuropathy and arterial disease. Although neuropathy and arterial disease are frequently comorbid with diabetes, a given individual with diabetes mellitus can have one, both, or neither. Neuropathy creates a condition of abnormal dynamic loading of the foot. Arterial disease starves the tissues of resources, increasing the foot's susceptibility to injury from any stressor, especially abnormal dynamic loading and infection. Moreover, arterial disease can produce foot ulcerations in the absence of neuropathy. As discussed in the following sections, neuropathy and arterial disease produce characteristic wound appearances and locations. Because those with neuropathy also often have diminished immunity, the combination of neuropathy, arterial disease, and infection frequently leads to amputation.

NEUROPATHIC ULCER PROPERTIES

Diabetes is the predominant but not the sole cause of neuropathy. Although many neuropathic ulcers are attributable to diabetes, possible causes of peripheral neuropathy include trauma, infection, vascular impairments, vitamin or nutrient deficiencies, spinal stenosis, peripheral nerve injury, infectious and genetic diseases, Hansen's disease (leprosy), Guillain-Barré syndrome, Charcot-Marie-Tooth disease, chronic inflammatory demyelinating polyneuropathy, chronic alcohol use, and chemotherapy-induced peripheral neuropathy, which is most common in cancer survivors who have received platinum-based medications such as oxaliplatin and cisplatin, vinca alkaloids (vincristine), or taxanes (paclitaxel). Much of the research on the management of neuropathy comes from the Hansen's Disease Research Center in Baton Rouge, Louisiana.

Peripheral neuropathy carries several major consequences. Both large- and small-diameter nerve fibers can be affected, leading to sensory, motor, and autonomic dysfunction. Some patients with peripheral neuropathy may experience discomfort related to small-fiber sensory changes, including decreased ability to distinguish normally painful stimuli, temperature, and crude touch. Symptoms of small-neuron disease may include burning and tingling. Symptoms associated with large-fiber sensory changes may include diminished or lost sensation in fine touch and vibration. However, loss of protective sensation is particularly devastating because it leads to reduced ability to detect and respond to stimuli that can potentially damage the integument.

Motor neuropathy affects muscles of the toes, foot, and ankles, often resulting in an imbalance between flexor and extensor muscle groups and wasting of the foot's intrinsic muscles. Over time, muscle imbalances contribute to bony deformities and abnormal pressure points during weight-bearing activities and ambulation. In turn, these abnormal pressure points can contribute to callus formation. The presence of calluses further increases the risk of damage to the skin and underlying tissue, especially under repetitive stress. Bony deformities and calluses correspond to the most common locations for foot ulcerations to occur, the plantar and medial aspect of the great toe and the metatarsal heads.

Consequences of autonomic neuropathy include abnormalities in blood flow due to inefficient vasodilation and vasoconstriction in response to changes in temperature and activity. Autonomic neuropathy can lead to drying and cracking of the skin, contributing to callus formation, cracks, and fissures that can allow bacteria and other pathogens to enter the skin.

Because people with peripheral neuropathy are vulnerable to inadvertent skin injury of the feet, repetitive mechanical forces can sometimes lead to skin injury from innocuous events such as breaking in new shoes. Although a person with normal protective sensation would limit wearing new shoes, repetitive minor trauma can result in blisters that can develop into a wound. The combination of motor neuropathy leading to bony foot deformities and autonomic changes with dry skin and callus exacerbates the effect of repetitive minor trauma.

Because neuropathy creates a biomechanical issue, wounds tend to be elliptical to round, created by the compression and shearing of tissue over bony prominences during the gait cycle. The plantar surface's pressure/shear points under metatarsal heads and on the toes are the most susceptible to neuropathic injury. Additionally, the loss of protective sensation may allow frictional injuries on the foot surfaces—such as the fifth metatarsal styloid process, lateral and dorsal surfaces of the toes, tips of the toes, and heel—to occur.

Moisture within neuropathic ulcers varies. Often, neuropathic ulcers are dry due to comorbid arterial disease; however, they can have normal moisture and even become quite wet due to infection. With the eradication of infection, the wound bed may shift rapidly from wet to dry, and the clinician must be prepared to switch to a different dressing to accommodate the change in the wound's moisture.

The ulcers are often painless due to neuropathy. However, some patients may have intermittent dysesthesia (painful, short duration, electrical or burning sensations), or they may experience more constant paresthesia, a pins and needles type of sensation. Loss of protective sensation as determined by the inability to sense the bending/unbending of a 10-g monofilament is extremely likely to be present in a person with neuropathic ulcers. Other sensory changes characteristic of neuropathic feet include loss of vibration sense (large sensory neurons), loss of position sense (Romberg test), and diminished or absent ankle jerk (large motor and sensory neurons). Distinctions between arterial and neuropathic ulcers are highlighted in Table 11-1.

ARTERIAL ULCER PROPERTIES

Blood flow restrictions due to peripheral arterial disease tend to have a greater effect on smaller-diameter arterial vessels. These smaller vessels generally supply the distal extremities. For this reason, arterial ulcers tend to start on the toes, although they can form wherever capillary blood flow becomes slow enough for tissue necrosis to occur. Because ischemia reduces tissue's tolerance to stress,

TABLE 11-1

Differential Diagnosis of Ulcers Caused by Neuropathy and Arterial Disease

CHARACTERISTICS	NEUROPATHIC	ISCHEMIC (ARTERIAL INSUFFICIENCY)
Appearance	Round or elliptical	Dry surrounding skin Irregular, wet or dry gangrene Atrophy of skin, thickened nails, loss of hair Rubor of dependency
Location	Sites of pressure or shear during weight-bearing and ambulation	Distal, especially toes and heels, but may occur anywhere arterial vessels occlude
Pain	None, but may have dysesthesia	Painful
Tests	Sensory testing shows loss of protective sensation, loss of vibration, position sense, reflexes	Low ankle-brachial index Low transcutaneous oxygen Claudication during treadmill

mechanical forces placed on tissues with compromised circulation can lead to roundish ulcers similar to those produced by neuropathy. However, while many arterial ulcers have a characteristic, round "punched out" appearance, the shape of the ulceration can vary based on the shape of the tissue area supplied by the affected arterial field. Therefore, clinicians should not rely on the shape alone to distinguish arterial disease from neuropathy as a cause of the wound.

Arterial ulcers are dry, except for wet gangrene. Wet gangrene occurs when blood flow is insufficient for tissue survival but is enough that osmosis produced by dead tissue can drive some water movement from whatever tissue and circulation remain. In general, a patient with arterial insufficiency will complain of pain in the affected extremity (claudication). The clinician usually will be able to observe atrophy of the skin and muscle in the area. Skin will take on a glossy appearance with loss of fat, and the blood vessels within the skin can be visualized. Hair loss on the extremity, thickening of nails, and yellow discoloration from fungal infection are commonly seen with arterial disease. The ankle-brachial index is a common test used outside the vascular lab to determine foot perfusion status. Arterial ulcers will be accompanied by a low ankle-brachial index value, as discussed in Chapter 8.

PATIENT MANAGEMENT

Prevention of foot ulcers in a person with diabetes starts with the management of blood glucose. Two types of information concerning blood glucose are the moment-by-moment (snapshot) value and the long-term, "average" value. Measuring blood glucose with a glucometer should yield a value near 90 mg/dL (70 to 99 mg/dL is considered normal fasting glucose according to Lab Tests Online). However, many people, especially those with wildly fluctuating blood glucose, become uncomfortable with such low levels due to fear of hypoglycemia/insulin shock. HbA1c (or more simply A1c) is the result of glucose in the blood attaching to hemoglobin within red blood cells. The process of attaching glucose molecules to proteins is called *glycosylation*. Too much glycosylation can result in altered protein function and is responsible, to a large degree, for the changes in the foot that predispose individuals to ulceration. HbA1c obtained during a single measurement reflects an "average" value of blood glucose control over approximately 3 months, whereas a glucometer only provides a "snapshot" of current glucose control.

Glycosylation is an important piece of the pathophysiology of diabetes mellitus. Glycosylation of joints and endothelial cells, in particular, are responsible for much of the injury to the feet. Stiff joints, atherosclerosis, and arteriolosclerosis (stiffening of arterioles) are largely due to chronic hyperglycemia.

HYPERGLYCEMIA AND DIABETIC NEUROPATHY

Hyperglycemia damages all 3 types of neurons. Many people focus solely on the sensory issue, which, although important, only allows people to let the injury go relatively un-noticed. Motor and autonomic neuropathy are at least equally important as sensory in causing foot

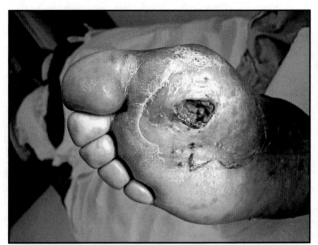

Figure 11-1. Crowding and molding of toes to the shape of the shoe's inside due to sensory neuropathy.

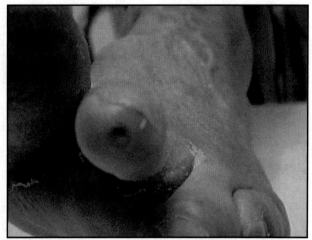

Figure 11-2. Tip-top-toe syndrome. Ulceration of the tip of the second toe has occurred secondary to the crowding of toes.

injury. Glycosylation of joints results in hallux rigidus and limitus, a stiffer foot that cannot dissipate forces during the transition from the midfoot to the forefoot, and creates an abnormal toe off, which leads to the classic ulceration beneath the first metatarsal head and, less commonly, one of the other metatarsal heads. Loss of proprioception leads to a wide base of support, placing further abnormal forces on the foot.

TRIPLE NEUROPATHY

The term *triple neuropathy* is used to bring greater attention to the effects of motor and autonomic damage. Sensory neuropathy has multiple effects in addition to the person being unaware of potential injury to the foot. Unusual forces on the foot such as objects left in shoes, seams, objects penetrating the shoe, and breakdown of the shoe components that then rub against the foot will not be detected. Patients have been known to spend an entire day walking in a shoe with broken glass and creating substantial acute injury to the foot. The other major aspect of sensory loss is wearing shoes that are too small or laced too tightly. As sensory loss progresses, the shoe's normal feel on the foot can be compensated by initially lacing them more tightly and, later on, by purchasing smaller shoes. This feels appropriate to the patient as the deep pressure produced by the smaller shoes provides the perception of normal fit. One of the results of wearing shoes that are too small is the crowding of toes and molding of toe shape to the inside of the shoe and into adjacent toes, as shown in Figure 11-1. Both crowding of the toes and motor neuropathy can lead to the deformities of claw toes and hammertoes.

Motor neuropathy weakens the intrinsic muscles of the foot prior to affecting the longer dorsiflexors. The imbalance

of muscle forces contributes to the altered shape of the foot already created by forcing toes into too-small shoes. Claw toes and hammertoes increase the susceptibility to injury to the skin over the toes' interphalangeal joints and tips, known as *tip-top-toe syndrome*, as shown in Figure 11-2.

Autonomic neuropathy decreases sweating of the feet, leading to dry skin with potential cracking and fissuring and, when combined with arterial disease, increases susceptibility to injury. Moist skin remains supple and able to dissipate forces, whereas dry, stiff skin can both become injured itself and create a harder surface that damages the tissue between bone and the hard skin. The situation becomes progressively worse each time a plantar ulcer is healed by scarring, and more elasticity of the foot's plantar skin is lost.

AT-RISK AREAS OF THE FOOT

More than half of plantar foot injuries occur along the first ray, which should be expected as about half of the plantar forces during gait are placed on the first ray. These injuries are nearly always preceded by callus formation. As with scarring, callus formation decreases the ability of the skin to dissipate forces. Thirty percent of DFUs occur on the plantar surface of the first toe; 22% on the first metatarsal head; 13% on the dorsum of the toes; 10% on the plantar surfaces of other toes; 1% on the heel; and 9% and decreasing percentages on the second, third, fourth, and fifth metatarsal heads.

Although pressure is often blamed for creating the injuries, most of the problem can be traced to the tangential, shearing forces that occur during walking and lead to callus formation. Callus is a normal response to the skin of the palms and soles being exposed to excessive shearing forces. Pressure alone is unlikely to cause plantar ulceration

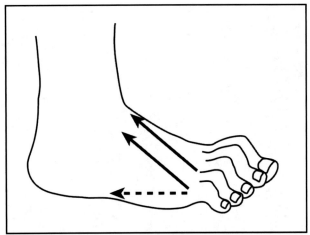

Figure 11-3. Forces producing hammertoes. Normal strength of long extensors of the toes, weakness of the intrinsic toe flexors, and sensory neuropathy leading to wearing shoes that are too small for the foot contribute to the formation of hammertoes.

because those without diabetes can stand all day or march with heavy backpacks without developing plantar ulcers. However, cycles of deforming the skin with little dissipation of forces have been shown to lead to ulceration. In particular, a stiff first toe greatly increases the susceptibility of the first ray to ulceration.

FOOT DEFORMITIES ASSOCIATED WITH DIABETIC NEUROPATHY

Several deformities can contribute to foot injury. Hammertoes, claw toes, hallux rigidus, and hallux limitus are more common with diabetes mellitus.

Hammertoes and Claw Toes

Diabetic neuropathy is described as glove and stocking distribution, implying that the longest neurons are affected first. Neurons that reach the toes are injured first, and those innervating muscles in the leg will be affected later than neurons supplying intrinsic muscles of the foot. The very strong dorsiflexor muscles combined with the smaller toe muscles of the foot produce the toe's shape with respect to the metatarsophalangeal and interphalangeal joints' positioning. When the smaller muscles within the foot become weak from neuropathy, the large dorsiflexors pull the metatarsophalangeal joints into extension, and the interphalangeal joints are passively pulled. In hammertoes, the pull is less than in claw toes, resulting in passive positioning of the second through the fifth proximal interphalangeal joint in flexion and the distal interphalangeal joints

into extension such that the pulp of the second through fifth toes remain on the support surface. The forces leading to hammertoes or claw toes are depicted in Figure 11-3.

Claw toes result from greater metatarsophalangeal joint extension than that of hammertoes. The proximal interphalangeal joints become so elevated that the second through fifth toes must rest on their tips. In both hammertoes and claw toes, the great toe with only a single interphalangeal joint will typically rest on its tip. As noted earlier, sensory loss commonly results in wearing shoes that are too small. Muscle force imbalance combined with small shoes increases the likelihood of developing hammertoes or claw toes. Ulceration of the dorsum of the toes created by hammertoes or claw toes rubbing against the top of the shoe can be managed by wearing extra-depth shoes that create more room for the toes.

Tip-Top-Toe Syndrome

Damage to the skin on hammertoes or claw toes produces the tip-top-toe syndrome. The interphalangeal joint skin develops calluses, commonly called *corns*, that may subsequently ulcerate. Tips that are pushed against the end of the shoe in hammertoes or rest on the shoe's bottom in claw toes ulcerate. Crowding and molding of toes are commonly seen along with tip-top-toe syndrome. Damage to a second toe tip is shown in Figure 11-2.

Hallux Rigidus

Loss of articular cartilage at the first metatarsophalangeal joint produces a stiff first toe that prevents the normal rolling action at toeoff. The stiff toe places excessive wear on the skin under the first toe and metatarsal head. Hallux rigidus may also occur in the absence of diabetes mellitus. Glycosylation of the joints producing stiffness increases the likelihood of the condition. Additionally, glycosylation of joints proximal to the hallux further loads the first toe and increases skin injury risk.

Hallux Limitus

Although somewhat similar to hallux rigidus, people with hallux limitus may have a full passive range of motion of the first toe when not weight-bearing. In stance, the person cannot move the toe through its range of motion, and like hallux rigidus, excessive forces are placed on the first ray. Hallux rigidus and limitus may be present before neuropathy occurs, but abnormal stresses placed on the foot that occur with neuropathy may either exacerbate or initiate these conditions.

TABLE 11-2
Causal Pathway to Amputation With Diabetic Neuropathy
Neuropathy
Minor trauma
Ulceration
Faulty healing
Gangrene
Amputation

TABLE 11-3
Risk Factors for Foot Ulceration and Amputation According to ADA
Diabetes mellitus for more than 10 years
Poor glucose control
Presence of cardiovascular, retinal, or renal complications
Peripheral vascular disease
History of ulcers or amputation
Peripheral neuropathy
Altered biomechanics
Evidence of increased pressure manifested as callus, erythema, hemorrhage under a callus
Limited joint mobility
Bony deformity
Severe nail pathology

NEUROPATHY AND RISK OF INFECTION

Infections are a common complication in neuropathic foot ulcers. People with diabetes experience immunologic changes that increase this risk. In skin areas with sensory loss, the rate of leukocyte infiltration is compromised. In addition, macrophage function is diminished, resulting in less phagocytosis. Wound healing and immunologic dysfunction are further complicated by the limited blood supply to the area caused by macro- and microvascular disease. Due to these complex impairments, the risks of deep tissue and bone infection increase, thereby increasing the risk of bone infections, or osteomyelitis, and the risk of amputation. As a result of diminished or absent sensation and altered circulation, people with diabetes sometimes fail to manifest typical signs and symptoms of infection, such as pain, tenderness, redness, and elevated skin temperatures. Careful monitoring of healing time with delays in wound closure is sometimes the only indication that infection exists.

FOOT WOUNDS AND CAUSAL PATHWAY TO AMPUTATION

The National Hansen's Disease Program developed the LEAP (Lower Extremity Amputation Prevention) program in 1992. The program was originally developed to prevent amputation for those with Hansen's disease but has been extended to any condition that results in loss of protective sensation of the feet, including diabetes. Their website is https://www.hrsa.gov/hansens-disease/leap/index.html. The object is to prevent escalation along the causal pathway to amputation. The pathway begins with neuropathy and minor trauma leading to ulceration. People with minor trauma of the feet usually do not have any problem healing, but those with neuropathy are already at a disadvantage

for healing. Continued trauma, decreased immune function associated with diabetes, the presence of vascular disease, and lack of attention to the injury increase the risk of faulty healing. Gangrene is generally a consequence of severe arterial disease. However, the increased metabolic demands of infection superimposed on those of healing can produce gangrene in a person who would not have developed it without the foot injury. However, vascular disease that might otherwise lead to gangrene and amputation might be prevented by revascularization or even more conservative earlier interventions. The lack of sensation to motivate the person to seek attention combined with rapid onset of infection and tissue damage results in the need for amputation. The pathway is highlighted in Table 11-2.

Amputation Prevention

Amputation is more than the loss of the limb. A second amputation risk is very high, as is the risk of mortality with a second amputation. The amputation alone does not lead to mortality, but the underlying disease processes that led to amputation also increase the risk of stroke, myocardial infarction, and kidney failure. Nonetheless, making lifestyle changes, including better glycemic control and disease surveillance, may lead to a healthier future. Risk factors for amputation are highlighted in Table 11-3. The prevention components include annual foot screening, patient education, daily self-inspection, footwear inspection, and management of simple foot problems.

FOOT SCREENING

A specific tool for screening for neuropathy is the Michigan Neuropathy Screening Instrument (Table 11-4). This consists of a historical document completed by the patient and a physical examination consisting of foot inspection, detection of vibration, ankle jerk, and monofilament testing. Each of these is described within the instrument and within this section. Several of these were presented in Chapter 8. Foot screening addresses all 3 components of neuropathy and their consequences. Heel and toe walking are used to assess whether the person has sufficient strength to walk without undue stresses on the feet. The ability to transition from heel strike, relax the foot, and then transition from midstance to toe off reduces shearing on the plantar surface's soft tissue. Ankle and foot range of motion can be checked simultaneously by observation during walking and comparing to active and passive range of motion.

Shoe inspection includes determining whether the shoe fits properly. Due to lack of sensation, many of those with neuropathy will wear shoes that are too small. Smaller shoes provide the degree of sensation on the foot to which the person has been accustomed. However, wearing such small shoes leads to several problems. First, the shape of the person's foot will take on the shape of the shoe's inside, the so-called molding of the foot, as depicted in Figure 11-1. The toes may be pushed into metatarsophalangeal extension resulting in hammertoes or claw toes depending on the shoe's fit, especially when combined with the intrinsic foot muscles' weakness. Claw toes and hammertoes then predispose the person to injury to the toes' tips and tops (tip-top-toe syndrome). Shoes may not have the same shape as the shoe last (the mechanical form on which the shoe is built). A tight shoe on the forefoot may be loose on the hindfoot, resulting in pistoning of the heel in the shoe and frictional injury to the skin. Frictional injuries can occur on additional locations, such as the fifth toe's styloid process, depending on mismatches in foot and shoe shapes.

A weight-bearing tracing or template of the foot can be drawn, as shown in Figure 11-4, and placed gently inside the patient's shoe. The clinician then looks for gaps where the shoe is too large and the paper's crinkling where the shoe is too small. The patient can take the pair of templates for shoe shopping to purchase appropriately fitting shoes. Once traced, the words right and left should be written on the appropriate template, so the wrong one is not used upside down. Shoes should be held at both ends and pushed to force the shoe into bending. The shoe should bend at the metatarsal heads to allow normal transition from midstance into toe off without undue resistance. The shoe's top is pinched to determine whether the shoes have sufficient give to allow the foot to move within the shoe. Heel height should be minimal to flat to avoid excessive loading of the forefoot. Patients should be advised to avoid wearing high-heeled shoes, particularly those with narrowed toes.

Several methods can be used to map pressure points. A simple method is the Harris mat or foot imprinter, as shown in Figure 11-5. This device utilizes a rubber mat with ink on the back, which is then placed over a sheet of paper in the tray below. The inked side of the mat has grids that correspond to the pressure placed on the mat. The widest grid requires the least pressure, and the narrowest grid requires the most pressure. High-pressure areas will look dark, and areas with very low pressure will not register on the paper. The results can indicate a high arch, a flat foot, and, to some degree, the pathway of pressure along the foot. Frequently, "hot spots" will correspond to calluses on the foot. More information can be obtained from computer-based devices. These range from shoe inserts to a walking mat.

In addition to lack of strength altering gait and, therefore, stresses on the feet, sensory input and sensory processing should be considered. Tandem walking by placing the heel of one foot directly in front of the other toes, as depicted in Figure 11-6, produces a very narrow base of support and requires good motor control to perform. Inability to perform tandem walking does not implicate one system but does indicate the likelihood of the patient placing abnormal stresses on the foot during ambulation.

The Romberg test specifically tests proprioception. The patient is asked to stand with feet at shoulder width and then close their eyes. With vision removed, balance can be maintained by proprioception or the vestibular system. Proprioception incorporates stretch and compression of many structures and becomes integrated in the cerebellum. Small errors are corrected quickly but not as quickly as visual input; therefore, closing the eyes leads to a small amount of sway even with intact proprioception. The vestibular system, however, requires acceleration to initiate an error correction. Therefore, the vestibular system in isolation produces more sway than proprioception, which may be overcorrected, leading to substantially greater sway and risk of falling; therefore, spotting the patient is required. If eyes are closed, and a person exhibits little sway, the patient is considered to have intact proprioception. Substantial sway indicates that the person's proprioception is impaired, as shown in Figure 11-7. Generally, impaired proprioception can also be inferred by a wide base of support during ambulation. One should expect a patient who has substantial wear on the soles' inner sides and walks with a wide base of support to perform poorly on the Romberg test.

TABLE 11-4
Michigan Neuropathy Screening Instrument—Patient Version

A. History (To be completed by the person with diabetes)

Please take a few minutes to answer the following questions about the feeling in your legs and feet. Check yes or no based on how you usually feel. Thank you.

1.	Are your legs and/or feet numb?	Yes	No
2.	Do you ever have any burning pain in your legs and/or feet?	Yes	No
3.	Are your feet too sensitive to touch?	Yes	No
4.	Do you get muscle cramps in your legs and/or feet?	Yes	No
5.	Do you ever have any prickling feelings in your legs or feet?	Yes	No
6.	Does it hurt when the bed covers touch your skin?	Yes	No
7.	When you get into the tub or shower, are you able to tell the hot water from the cold water?	Yes	No
8.	Have you ever had an open sore on your foot?	Yes	No
9.	Has your doctor ever told you that you have diabetic neuropathy?	Yes	No
10.	Do you feel weak all over most of the time?	Yes	No
11.	Are your symptoms worse at night?	Yes	No
12.	Do your legs hurt when you walk?	Yes	No
13.	Are you able to sense your feet when you walk?	Yes	No
14.	Is the skin on your feet so dry that it cracks open?	Yes	No
15.	Have you ever had an amputation?	Yes	No

Total:

HOW TO USE THE MICHIGAN NEUROPATHY SCREENING INSTRUMENT

History

The history questionnaire is self-administered by the patient. Responses are added to obtain the total score. Responses of "yes" to items 1 to 3, 5 to 6, 8 to 9, 11 to 12, 14 to 15 are each counted as 1 point. A "no" response on items 7 and 13 counts as 1 point. Item 4 is a measure of impaired circulation, and item 10 is a measure of general asthenia—they are not included in scoring. To decrease the potential for bias, all scoring information has been eliminated from the patient version.

Physical Assessment

For all assessments, the foot should be warm (> 30°C).

Foot Inspection

The feet are inspected for evidence of excessively dry skin, callus formation, fissures, frank ulceration, or deformities. Deformities include flat feet, hammer toes, overlapping toes, hallux valgus, joint subluxation, prominent metatarsal heads, medial convexity (Charcot foot), and amputation.

Vibration Sensation

Vibration sensation should be performed with the great toe unsupported. Vibration sensation will be tested bilaterally using a 128 Hz tuning fork placed over the dorsum of the great toe on the bony prominence of the DIP joint. Patients, whose eyes are closed, will be asked to indicate when they can no longer sense the vibration from the vibrating tuning fork.

In general, the examiner should be able to feel vibration from the hand-held tuning fork for 5 seconds longer on his distal forefinger than a normal subject can at the great toe (eg, examiner's DIP joint of the first finger versus patient's toe). If the examiner feels vibration for 10 or more seconds on his or her finger, then vibration is considered decreased. A trial should be given when the tuning fork is not vibrating to be certain that the patient is responding to vibration and not pressure or some other clue. Vibration is scored as (1) present if the examiner senses the vibration on his or her finger for <10 seconds, (2) reduced if sensed for >10, or (3) absent (no vibration detection).

(continued)

TABLE 11-4 (CONTINUED)
Michigan Neuropathy Screening Instrument—Patient Version

Muscle Stretch Reflexes

The ankle reflexes will be examined using an appropriate reflex hammer (eg, Tromner or Queen square). The ankle reflexes should be elicited in the sitting position with the foot dependent and the patient relaxed. For the reflex, the foot should be passively positioned and the foot dorsiflexed slightly to obtain optimal stretch of the muscle. The Achilles tendon should be percussed directly. If the reflex is obtained, it is graded as present. If the reflex is absent, the patient is asked to perform the Jendrassic maneuver (ie, hooking the fingers together and pulling). Reflexes elicited with the Jendrassic maneuver alone are designated "present with reinforcement." If the reflex is absent, even in the face of the Jendrassic maneuver, the reflex is considered absent.

Monofilament Testing

For this examination, it is important that the patient's foot be supported (ie, allow the sole of the foot to rest on a flat, warm surface). The filament should initially be prestressed (4 to 6 perpendicular applications to the dorsum of the examiner's first finger). The filament is then applied to the dorsum of the great toe midway between the nail fold and the DIP joint. Do not hold the toe directly. The filament is applied perpendicularly and briefly (<1 second), with an even pressure. When the filament bends, the force of 10 grams has been applied. The patient, whose eyes are closed, is asked to respond yes if he or she feels the filament. Eight correct responses out of 10 applications is considered normal, 1 to 7 correct responses indicates reduced sensation, and no correct answers translates into absent sensation.

B. Physical Assessment (To be completed by health professional)		
1. Appearance of feet	Right a. Normal 0 Yes 1 No b. If no, check all that apply: __Deformities __Dry skin, callus __Infection __Fissure __Other (specify):	Left a. Normal 0 Yes 1 No b. If no, check all that apply: __Deformities __Dry skin, callus __Infection __Fissure __Other specify:
2. Ulceration	Right Absent Present 0 1	Left Absent Present 0 1

3. Ankle reflexes	Present Present/ Absent
	             Reinforcement
	0 0.5 1
		Present Present/ Absent
		             Reinforcement
		0 0.5 1

4. Vibration perception at great toe	Present Decreased Absent 0 0.5 1	Present Decreased Absent 0 0.5 1
5. Monofilament	Normal Reduced Absent 0 0.5 1	Normal Reduced Absent 0 0.5 1
Signature:		Total Score: /10 Points

Courtesy of the Michigan Diabetes Research and Training Center, Ann Arbor, Michigan.

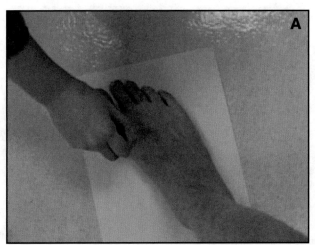
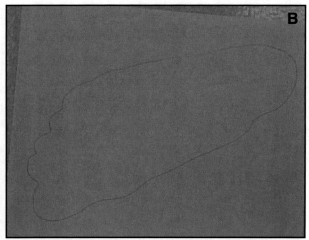

Figure 11-4. Drawing a foot template to choose appropriately fitting shoes. (A) Drawing the template. (B) Finished product. The template is cut with scissors and placed inside prospective shoe purchases to ensure proper fit.

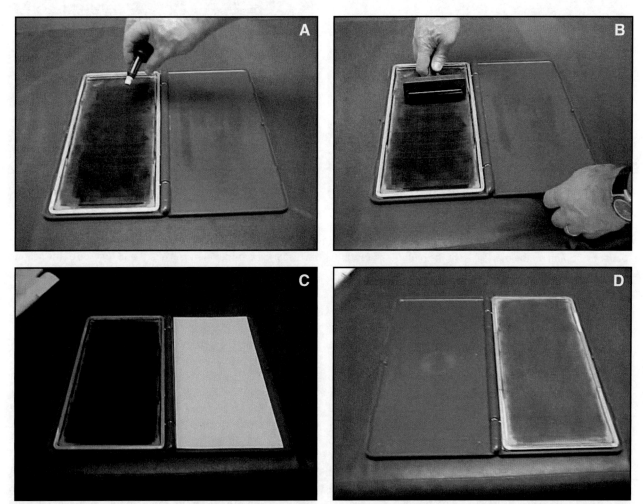

Figure 11-5. Harris foot mat. (A) Application of ink to the grid on the underside of the mat. (B) Ink being spread evenly across the grid. (C) Paper is placed on the tray beneath the mat. (D) The mat is rotated into its tray with the smooth side up and the inked, grid side down. *(continued)*

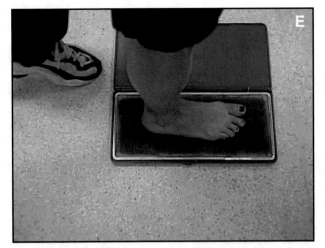
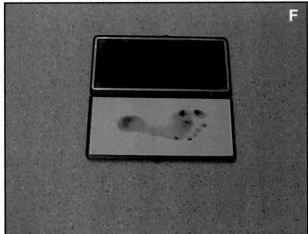
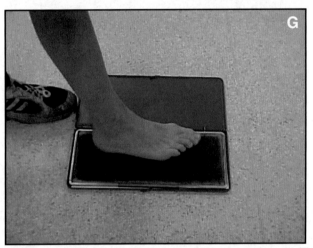
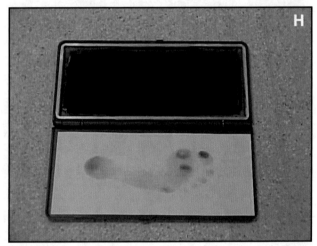

Figure 11-5 (continued). (E) Patient stepping onto the mat. (F) High-pressure areas are indicated by more densely marked portions of the paper. Higher pressures are necessary for the grid's progressively closer portions to come in contact with the paper below it. Note the high pressures on the head of the first metatarsal and proximal lateral portion of the first toe. (G) Second patient stepping on the mat. (H) Note the high pressures under the first and second metatarsal heads and first toe of the second patient.

GAIT ASSESSMENT

Normal ambulation relies on an intricate balance between sensory input and motor control; sensory and motor damage due to peripheral neuropathy leads to changes in gait and abnormal plantar pressures. These pathomechanics contribute to foot ulceration and delayed healing. In addition to foot ulcers, changes in the walking patterns of people with peripheral neuropathy are a leading cause of falls and loss of function. During gait, the peripheral nerves provide input about joint position and weight acceptance by transmitting signals regarding proprioception, pressure, touch, and vibration. For this reason, sensory deficits can affect foot placement, balance, shock attenuation, and the ability to adapt to uneven surfaces.

Volitional control of muscles of the lower limb also plays an important role in gait. In people with diabetic peripheral neuropathy, distal leg muscles are most often affected. These changes result in weakness at the foot and ankle. During the gait cycle, weakness of the tibialis anterior and toe extensors can result in decreased dorsiflexion. Ineffective eccentric control of the dorsiflexors causes the foot to rapidly decelerate, causing it to slap the ground. This contrasts with the smooth, well-controlled motion that should occur from initial contact to weight acceptance as the gait cycle transitions from the swing to the stance phase in people with normal motor strength and control. Decreased concentric contraction of the ankle dorsiflexors can manifest as foot drop or steppage gait during the swing phase. This occurs when the tibialis anterior cannot effectively raise the toes to clear the ground when advancing the affected leg. Some patients with dorsiflexor weakness compensate by increasing the amount of hip and knee flexion during swing, whereas others may drag their toes or trip when moving

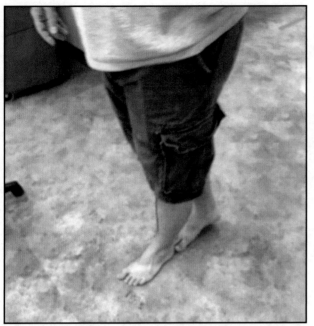

Figure 11-6. Tandem walking is used to determine the patient's proprioception, coordination, and ability to protect the foot.

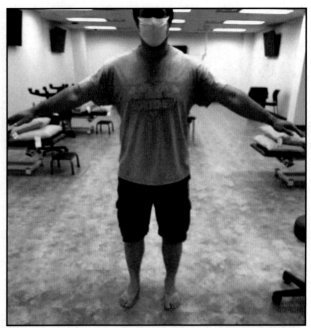

Figure 11-7. Performing the Romberg test to determine the patient's proprioception. Swaying indicates the loss of proprioception and excessive reliance on the vestibular system to remain upright in the absence of visual input.

the leg forward. Because most people with diabetes have symmetrical symptoms, these gait impairments commonly occur bilaterally. Other common gait issues in people with peripheral neuropathy include greater step-to-step variation, presumably due to unsteady balance. Increased stance time, decreased step length, and reduced gait speed and cadence can also be observed.

Reduced ankle dorsiflexion can cause an increase in friction and shear at the forefoot and metatarsal heads during ambulation, making these common locations for neuropathic ulceration. Gait deficits and abnormal plantar pressures can also be exacerbated by obesity and advancing age.

Sensory testing for a foot screening includes Semmes-Weinstein monofilaments (Figure 11-8) using the 5.07 or 10 g (either label might be used) on the 10 sites depicted in Figure 11-9. The ability to feel the 10-g monofilament indicates that the patient has adequate sensation to determine that the feet are experiencing potentially damaging forces. Failure to feel the 10-g monofilament is classified as "loss of protective sensation." This is an important term in assessing the risk of a foot injury. Using an array of monofilaments can give a better picture of the sensory status of the foot. However, we are interested in whether the patient has a loss of protective sensation for a foot screen. Note that some sources use fewer than 10 sites and may use alternative sites.

For sensory testing, the patient's eyes must be closed, and they should say when the sensation is being perceived rather than being asked, "Can you feel this?" Additionally,

the rhythm and sequence of placements should be randomized (spatial and temporal variation) so that the patient does not answer that the monofilament or other sensory test can be felt despite the sensory loss. Other sensory tests applicable to foot screening are vibration with a 128-Hz tuning fork and ankle jerk.

VIBRATION TESTS FOR LARGE SENSORY NEURONS

A patient is asked to distinguish whether the tuning fork is vibrating. The patient's feet should be randomly touched with either a vibrating or nonvibrating tuning fork in several locations with a random rhythm and sequence of locations of vibrating and nonvibrating tuning forks. A pause should always occur to give the patient adequate time to state that touch or vibration was felt. A tuning fork will slow after 2 to 3 touches, so one of the tuning forks will need to be struck several times. Do not always strike a tuning fork and then touch with the vibrating tuning fork; randomize their presentations. An alternative to the tuning fork is the biothesiometer. This device determines vibration thresholds and therefore is easier to use and more reliable than using a tuning fork. However, the biothesiometer is not a standard device in most clinics.

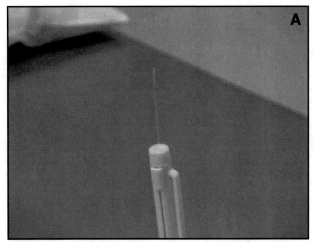
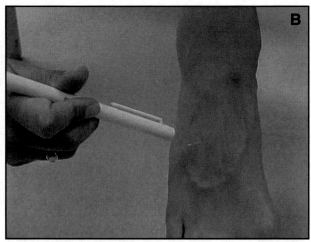

Figure 11-8. Sensory testing with a 10-g monofilament. (A) Appearance of a typical 10-g monofilament for testing protective sensation. (B) Testing procedure showing the bending of the 10-g monofilament on the dorsal foot location.

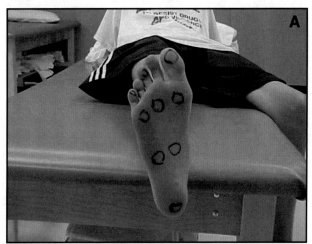
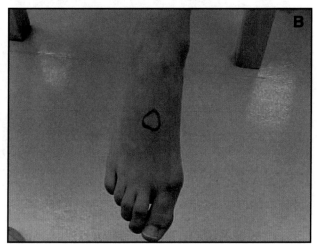

Figure 11-9. (A) Standard locations for monofilament screening on the plantar surface of the foot. (B) Standard location for monofilament screening on the dorsum of the foot. Some testers will use a location proximal to the webspace between the first and second toe.

Ankle jerk tests both large sensory and motor neurons. It should be compared minimally with a knee jerk and preferably with multiple convenient reflex testing sites rather than just bilateral ankle jerk because the magnitude of the response tends to be more consistent within than among different people.

Foot deformities as described previously and Charcot foot (described in the following section) are additional risk factors. The skin condition is also part of foot screening. Autonomic neuropathy impairs sweating and leads to dry skin on the foot. Dry skin to the point of cracking and callus formation places the foot at high risk of breakdown. Arterial disease may contribute to dry skin as well as living in cold and dry environments. Nail condition is also assessed as part of the foot screening. Thickened, yellow nails are common with diabetes and arterial disease. Thick nails can place tremendous pressure on the toes and lead to subungual hematoma and risk of infection. A summary of tests related to neuropathic feet is shown in Table 11-5.

CHARCOT FOOT

A particularly devastating complication of neuropathy is the complex of sensory, motor, and autonomic changes that lead to structural and vascular changes known as *Charcot foot*. Charcot arthropathy was named for a prominent French neurologist and was first described as a consequence of syphilis. An acutely swollen foot with no significant radiographic changes may represent the early stage of Charcot foot, requiring careful observation, rest, elevation, immobilization, and referral to a specialist experienced in treating Charcot foot. Charcot foot occurs most commonly with diabetes mellitus but may occur with other neuropathic diseases. Up to 13% of patients seen in high-risk diabetes mellitus clinics have this condition. In the diabetic foot, the term Charcot foot is used to describe a progressive condition of multiple osteo-arthropathies characterized by joint dislocation, pathologic fractures, and deformities. The most common deformity is a rocker-bottom or boat-shaped foot in which the concavity of

TABLE 11-5

Components of Foot Screen and Physical Exam for Suspected Neuropathy

TEST	PURPOSE
Strength testing—initially heel and toe walking If unsuccessful, manual muscle testing of foot and ankle	Determine whether patient has sufficient strength to smoothly transition through gait cycle to avoid damage to foot.
Ankle and toe range of motion—initially during gait If abnormalities suspected, specific range of motion of foot and ankle, particularly the hallux	Determine whether patient has sufficient range of motion to smooth transition through gait cycle to avoid damage to foot, especially the hallux.
Romberg	Determine whether patient has sufficient proprioception for proper gait. Should correlate with observed gait pattern.
Tandem walking	Determine whether patient has sufficient motor control for ambulating safely. May be inadequate due to either sensory deficits or central planning.
5.07/10-g monofilament	Determine whether patient has loss of protective sensation.
Vibration	Determine whether large sensory neurons are intact.
Ankle jerk bilaterally and compared with at least knee jerk, preferably with upper extremity reflexes	Determine whether large sensory or motor neurons are damaged.
Footwear assessment: Heel height, condition of sole, uneven wear medially or laterally, give of material, whether foot pistons in shoe during gait	Determine whether shoes are correct material to avoid injury to shoes; whether abnormal gait pattern is evident in wear pattern on sole.
Foot template inserted into shoe; examine for areas with gaps and crinkling of the paper	Determine whether the shoe is the correct size and shape for the patient's feet.
Harris mat/foot imprinter	Determine whether the patient has any "hot spots" indicative of excessive pressure during weight-bearing.
Foot assessment: Hammertoes, claw toes, bunions, hallux limitus, hallux rigidus, prominent metatarsal heads, prior amputation, Charcot foot	Determine whether the patient has any foot deformities indicative of damage or risk of injury.
Skin and nail assessment: Dry, cracked skin vs turgor and appropriate moisture; skin atrophy, callus, ecchymoses, ulcers, erythema, maceration, fissures; thick, yellow nails, ingrown, other nail deformities; need for nail care	Determine whether the patient has any risk factors or damage to the skin.
Ankle-brachial index	Determine whether the patient has arterial insufficiency to the feet.
Venous filling test	Determine whether the patient has arterial or venous insufficiency of the feet.
Capillary refill	Gross screening test for arterial or vasospastic disease; whether any compression device is excessively tight.
Venous percussion test	Determine whether the patient has incompetent venous valves.

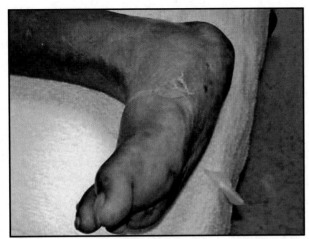

Figure 11-10. Example of a Charcot foot. Note the boat-shaped deformity and healed forefoot wound. The foot now has an open wound on the heel.

the arch of the foot is not only lost, but also the bottom of the foot becomes convex (Figure 11-10). The toes frequently lose contact with the foot's support surface, and tremendous shear forces are exerted at the metatarsal heads.

Charcot foot was originally believed to be due to lack of sensation and accumulated trauma but was later shown to have a neurovascular component. This includes an increased blood flow due to denervation accompanied by demineralization of the foot's bones. Osteopenia, combined with the loss of sensation, leads to pathological fractures of the foot. Moreover, motor denervation and resultant muscle imbalance lead to a very high risk of ulceration of the plantar surface and dorsal surfaces of hammertoes.

Diagnosis of Charcot Arthropathy

Unilateral swelling, elevated temperature, and erythema are early signs of Charcot foot development. These events are associated with the increased blood flow caused by denervation of blood vessels of the lower extremities. Further examination may reveal joint effusion, bone resorption by imaging techniques, an insensate foot, and usually some degree of pain. Approximately 40% of patients with Charcot foot have already experienced ulceration. Because of the swelling, heat, erythema, and pain of Charcot arthropathy, this condition may be confused with osteomyelitis. Differential diagnosis can be performed with a bone scan, blood work, white count, and bone biopsy. Charcot arthropathy is described as having 4 stages. The first stage of Charcot arthropathy is characterized by a hot, red, swollen foot with bounding pulses. During stage 1, the resorption of bone produces severe osteopenia.

For diagnosis, an increase of 2°C is considered necessary, but the temperature elevation may greatly exceed that

number. During the second stage, dissolution, fragmentation, and fracture of bone occur as osteopenia weakens bones too much to support the foot's biomechanics. A patient is considered to be in stage 3 with the development of a rocker-bottom foot deformity. Stage 4 consists of plantar ulceration with possible progression to infection, gangrene, and amputation. Interventions to prevent progression of Charcot foot during stage 1 are non–weight- bearing of the affected extremity, and, if appropriate, the use of total-contact casting until skin temperature is normal. If the disease progresses to stage 3, the patient will need molded shoes or special Charcot shoes with molded inserts and possible surgery to repair deformities to prevent the progression to stage 4. Unfortunately, the process may progress to stage 4, and damage to the foot may become so severe as to require amputation. Another classification of Charcot arthropathy is based on radiographic, thermometric, and clinical signs into either the acute phase or postacute phase.

Acute Episodes

Patients and clinicians working with a patient with a history of Charcot should be vigilant for signs of early episodes characterized by edema, elevated temperature, and risk of fracture. The patient should be placed in a total-contact cast until the temperature returns to within 1°C of normal. Acute Charcot arthropathy may be treated with immobilization and stress reduction, including decreased weight-bearing with crutches. Unfortunately, unloading one foot overloads the contralateral foot. With the likelihood of bilateral disease, the other foot is placed at greater risk of fracture. Other options that do not overload the contralateral extremity include using a total-contact cast for 5 to 6 months, arthrodesis, open reduction, and internal fixation of the fractures. Long-term solutions can be instituted during the postacute phase. The postacute phase classification may be given after the affected foot's temperature is within 1°C of the contralateral foot. At this time, the patient may be fitted for orthotic shoes and use a removable cast walker until a custom shoe is ready. Some patients may be fitted for a Charcot restraint orthotic walker to prevent injury after the acute episode subsides. In about 25% of cases, reconstructive foot surgery is performed.

Chronic Charcot Foot

The accumulation of deformities results in the chronic Charcot foot. Initially, a Charcot shoe may be adequate protection for the foot. In some cases, fractures and dislocations may become too extreme for the foot to fit in a standard Charcot shoe. At this point, the patient is at very high risk of future amputation.

CLASSIFICATION OF NEUROPATHIC FOOT INJURY

Neuropathy, like pressure injury, has its own method for describing the severity of the injury. The Wagner grades are well established and well known to clinicians, but the grades actually represent 3 different types of injury, and the grades do not directly state the type of injury. The University of Texas classification system does not appear to be widely adopted, but it is an alternative means of classification that provides more information than the Wagner grades in that it accounts for both the severity of the injury and the etiology. Because Wagner grades appear to be better known universally, interventions are described based on Wagner grades. The classification of neuropathic ulcers helps document wound severity and predicted response to treatment and create a plan of care that matches the wound's characteristics and addresses barriers to healing. It also helps predict the response to treatment and facilitates interprofessional communication and coordination of care across settings. However, the plan of care should not be based solely on a single assigned grade. The complete record of observation and testing should be used for treatment planning. The SINBAD system provides a score between 0 and 6 based on characteristics of the wound. Site, Ischemia, Neuropathy, Bacterial infection, ulcer Area, and Depth create the name of the system. A score of either 0 or 1 is assigned for each of the 6 items; a score of 3 or greater is associated with delayed healing. For site, 0 is assigned for forefoot and 1 for midfoot or hindfoot. Evidence of reduced pedal blood flow is given 1 point for ischemia. Lost protective sensation is given 1 for neuropathy. One point is given for bacterial infection; for ulcer area > 1 cm^2; and for an ulcer reaching muscle, tendon, or deeper.

Wagner Classification

The Wagner grades are frequently used for prognosis and intervention decisions for neuropathic ulcers. The scale does not represent a given wound's progression; rather, it represents an increase in the severity and invasiveness required to treat the wound. As the descriptions detail, neuropathy, infection, and ischemia are progressively involved. The scale ranges from grade 0 to grade 5. A grade 0 ulcer represents either damage to the foot, but the skin remains intact or the high risk of ulceration. Severely injured subcutaneous tissue may be present, and as such, minor trauma to the foot may lead to a serious infection of the necrotic tissue within the foot. Grade 1 is used to describe a partial-thickness or superficial ulcer (Figure 11-11A). A full-thickness wound with subcutaneous involvement is classified as a grade 2 neuropathic ulcer (Figure 11-11B). Note that only 2 grades are used to denote the depth of the ulcer. A wound is classified as grade 3 when an infection is present, manifested as either an abscess or osteomyelitis (Figure 11-11C). Progression to forefoot gangrene is documented as a grade 4 ulcer, and grade 5 represents gangrene of most of the foot.

University of Texas Classification

This system uses both a number from 0 to 3 to indicate the wound's depth and a letter to indicate the presence or absence of infection and/or ischemia. The lowest grade of 0 indicates that the patient either appears to be in the process of developing an ulcer (preulcerative lesion) or has re-epithelialized an ulcer. Grade 1 is a superficial wound that does not involve any subfascial structures. Grade 2 is used for ulcers that penetrate to the tendon, capsule, or bone. Wounds that penetrate bone or a deep abscess between bones are given grade 3. One of the letters A through D will also be assigned, with the implication that the presence of ischemia is worse than infection. A is assigned to a wound that has neither infection nor ischemia. B designates an infected wound, C is given to a wound with ischemia, and D is assigned to a wound with both infection and ischemia. The Wagner grades and University of Texas classifications are shown in Table 11-6.

INTERVENTIONS

Interventions for neuropathic ulcers include patient education, local wound care, periodic screening of the feet and footwear as described previously, and off-loading of the affected foot. In cases of bilateral involvement, off-loading options may be limited. Of all possible interventions, metabolic control is the most important factor for long-term health. Patients must be reinforced and rewarded by all health care team members to maintain blood glucose as close to normal (< 100 mg/dL) as possible. Fear of the consequences of hypoglycemia may undermine efforts to achieve normal blood glucose. In many cases, patients seem content with random blood glucose substantially higher than 90 mg/dL (140 to 200 mg/dL). With multiple demands on the patient's life, blood glucose control can be difficult before ulceration, but glucose control only becomes more challenging with infection. Rising blood glucose itself is suggestive of infection.

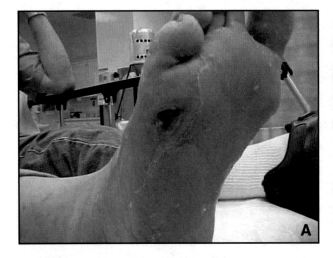
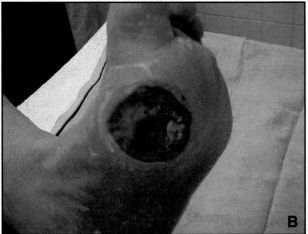
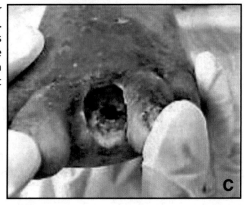

Figure 11-11. Wagner classification. (A) Shallow ulcer characteristic of Wagner grade 1. Note the dryness and callus formation over the entire plantar surface. (B) Deep ulcer characteristic of Wagner grade 2. Note the thick rim of callus around the wound. Also, note the presence of hammertoes, which increase the shearing forces under the metatarsal heads during gait. (C) Infection with subsequent third ray amputation (toe and metatarsal). Infection is characteristic of Wagner grade 3.

Off-Loading

A multitude of off-loading options is now available. Technological advances have increased options available. In addition, total-contact cast kits have simplified the process of casting. Although some of these alternatives approach its effectiveness, total-contact casting remains the gold standard of neuropathic foot off-loading.

Total-Contact Casting

The device is called *total contact* to distinguish from a common orthopedic cast used to set a fracture. Although it does not truly produce total contact, the padding is minimal. A thin stockinette material is applied to the extremity that will be casted, and padding is placed over the toes with insertion of the Achilles tendon, malleoli, and tibial crest as demonstrated in Figure 11-12. The felt padding over the tibial crest is much thinner than the foam typically used over the other areas. Ideally, the cast is created with the patient prone and the knee at 90 degrees in order to produce a neutral ankle. Achieving a neutral ankle with the patient in sitting requires constant vigilance. Multiple

plaster-casting bandages with or without fiberglass-reinforcing tape are required to create a quality cast. Training with an experienced clinician is recommended. Ideally, quick-setting plaster bandages are used. An experienced clinician can form a good cast in the time the plaster sets, but a less experienced clinician may be too slow. Using slower-setting plaster may allow the ankle to move out of neutral or gaps to form in the cast.

Total-contact casts provide a combination of benefits that is not available in any alternative. The cast controls ankle motion, a common mechanism of action among off-loading devices. Locking the ankle in neutral and creating a rocker bottom eliminate most of the shearing forces on the plantar surface. A snug fit of the total-contact cast distributes a substantial amount of body weight along the cast walls, thereby diminishing pressure on the plantar surface; shoes cannot provide this benefit. The fit also counteracts swelling. The initial cast is generally in place for 1 week, and the extremity is carefully examined for any injury possibly caused by the cast. Subsequent casts may be worn for longer periods as the clinician develops confidence that the cast will not cause injury. Many patients with neuropathic ulcers are not good candidates for total-contact casting.

TABLE 11-6

Wagner Grades and University of Texas Classification of Diabetic Foot

WAGNER GRADE	MEANING	UT CLASSIFICATION	MEANING
0	No open ulcer but high risk	0	Pre- or postulcerative or completely re-epithelialized
1	Superficial ulcer of skin or sub-cutaneous tissue	1	Superficial wound not involving tendon, capsule, or bone
2	Ulcers extend into tendon, bone, or capsule	2	Wound penetrating to tendon or capsule
3	Deep ulcer with osteomyelitis or abscess	3	Wound penetrating to bone or joint
4	Partial foot gangrene	A (added to #)	No infection or ischemia
5	Whole foot gangrene	B (added to #)	With infection
		C (added to #)	With ischemia
		D (added to #)	With infection and ischemia
Data source: Armstrong et al, 1998.			

Along with the advantages, total-contact casts carry significant risks that must be weighed against the rewards of using this approach. The cast adds substantial mass to the end of the leg and produces an awkward gait in a person who may already have a gait deviation. Sleeping in the cast risks injury to the contralateral limb and the lower extremities of another person in the same bed. Although an experienced clinician can create a cast in only a few minutes, the cost in terms of supplies and clinic time is substantial. However, the major problem is the difficulty in monitoring the limb's condition with the cast in place. Patients must be educated about the dangers of ignoring the limb for the period between visits. They must be warned not to put sharp objects into the cast to scratch an itch. Patients must also be educated on how to maintain the integrity of the cast until the next visit. For example, bathing/showering without protecting the cast will degrade the cast quickly, resulting in an inadequate cast with the potential for damaging the skin. The total-contact cast is not a panacea. Significant injuries have occurred to patients wearing total-contact casts that have resulted in amputation; therefore, patient selection is critical. If a patient is not a good candidate for maintaining the cast's integrity and monitoring their limb's health, other options are available. The greatest problem with the alternatives is that they are all removable and can be left off the limb for extended periods.

Bivalved Total-Contact Cast

The bivalved total-contact cast is constructed slightly differently to increase its wear time. It is reinforced with fiberglass tape and cut along the sides and then along the medial and lateral sides of the foot so the anterior piece, including the dorsum of the foot, can be separated from the rest of the cast. The cut edges are covered with moleskin or some other soft, adhesive material, and hook and loop straps are attached to allow the 2 pieces to be approximated. This device is somewhat less effective than a total-contact cast, but we do not know whether the decreased effectiveness is due to the device itself or a lack of compliance in wearing in real clinical practice. With a total-contact cast, wearing is enforced as the cast cannot be removed and donned for office visits. Bivalved casts and the other devices can be simply removed once the patient leaves the clinic and put back on for the next visit. A major advantage of removable devices is the ability to bathe, sleep, dress, and so on without the cast as long as the bivalved cast is donned after that. An example of a bivalved cast is shown in Figure 11-13.

Controlled Ankle Movement Walker

Orthopedic boots for stable fractures known as controlled ankle movement (CAM) walkers give a good combination of effectiveness, cost, and safety. They are easily donned and doffed, control ankle motion, provide a rocker bottom, and are designed to take substantial weight from

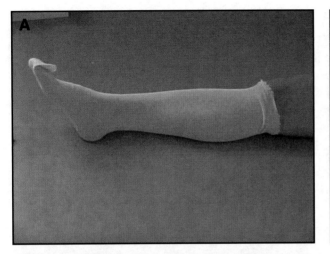

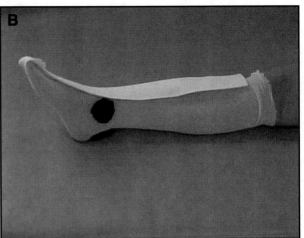

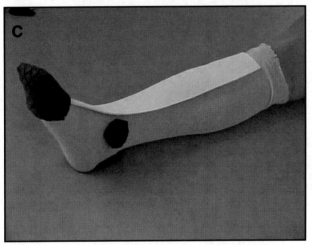

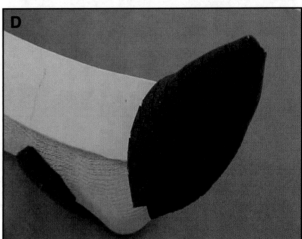

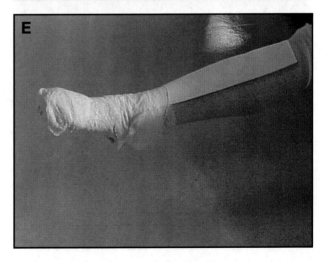

Figure 11-12. Total-contact casting. (A) Stockinette applied from the knee, beyond the toes, and folded onto the dorsal surface. (B) Padding required for total-contact casting. A thin layer of felt is placed over the tibial crest, and foam is placed over both malleoli and the heel cord's insertion. (C) Foam is placed over the toes, including the metatarsals, with beveling of the edge under the metatarsal heads to improve foot biomechanics. (D) Close-up view of foam over the forefoot. (E) The first plaster bandage is applied. Several turns around the ankle are necessary to maintain rigidity. The ankle must be maintained in neutral as plaster or fiberglass bandages are applied. Positioning the patient in prone is preferred but not always possible.

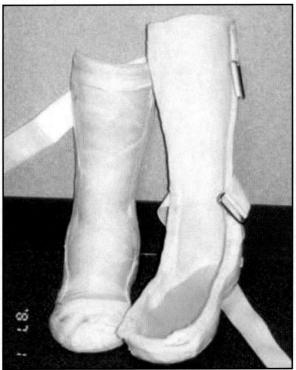

Figure 11-13. Bivalved total-contact cast. The cast is made sturdier than a typical total-contact cast and cut as shown to allow the cast to be donned and doffed by the patient. (The image is a copyrighted product of AAWC [www.aawconline. org] and has been reproduced with permission.)

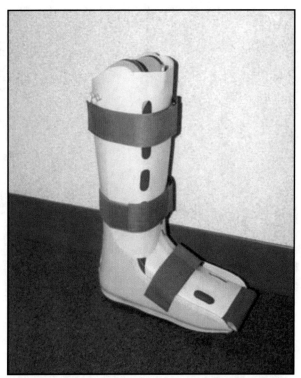

Figure 11-14. CAM walker used as a substitute for a total-contact cast. (The image is a copyrighted product of AAWC [www. aawconline.org] and has been reproduced with permission.)

the foot and ankle. They are off-the-shelf items, which makes them very accessible but also limits their fit. Newer versions of CAM walkers are better than previous generations in terms of fit, but the fit is dependent on the ability and care of the wearer. In many cases, the same person we might not want to put in a total-contact cast may also not demonstrate the ability to fit the boot well. Careful patient education is still needed along with demonstration to mitigate issues with fit. A typical CAM walker is shown in Figure 11-14.

Charcot Restraint Walker

This device is considered a semipermanent orthosis that is custom fit, mimicking a total-contact cast. These are very expensive due to the custom fitting and more rugged materials used. They have the appearance of a bivalved cast but with much higher-end and durable components, as depicted in Figure 11-15.

DH Offloading Walker

Another option that provides a novel feature is the DH Offloading Walker (Össur). Its construction is similar to a CAM walker, but the insole has detachable hexagonal

pieces, as shown in Figure 11-16. A clinician can choose to remove a number of these to provide a pressure relief beneath an ulcer. It is designed to fit either the right or left. The open construction does not control edema, and it uses uprights attached to straps to control weight-bearing rather than an exoskeleton.

Enforcing Wear of Off-Loading Devices

The advantage of removable off-loading devices is the ability to take them off, including during sleep. Many individuals with DFUs may awake multiple times during the night to urinate and are unlikely to take the time to don an off-loading boot. This can progress to walking throughout the home, then to the mailbox, then just a short trip to the store, or just to go to church, and so on. The more this happens, the more complacent the patient becomes to the point of wearing the off-loading device to the clinic only. Options to enforce wearing include zip ties and fiberglass casting tape. These are extreme measures to enforce wearing in the situation in which a patient swears they are wearing the device when, in fact, they are not. Using such strategies stretches the limits of autonomy unless the patient agrees to resort to this measure. Although zip ties are easily obtained and could be replaced by the patient

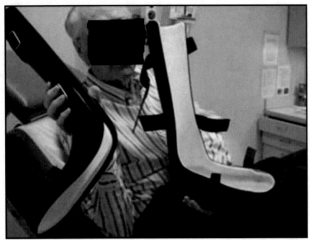

Figure 11-15. Charcot restraint walker custom fit to the patient. (The image is a copyrighted product of AAWC [www.aawconline.org] and has been reproduced with permission.)

before the next clinic visit, removing fiberglass casting tape is more difficult.

Half Shoes

Shoes with either the rearfoot or forefoot elevated are available, as are rocker-bottom shoes. The OrthoWedge shoe (Darco) depicted in Figure 11-17A is designed for forefoot ulcers. Half shoes with a built-up forefoot can be used for removing weight-bearing from the heel. Half shoes for forefoot ulcers provide 10 degrees of dorsiflexion but not a rocker bottom because this would defeat the purpose of limiting weight-bearing to the rearfoot. Although this device eliminates weight-bearing and shearing forces on the forefoot, gait can be difficult. The patient is limited to a step-to gait; attempting to step through will cause the half shoe to roll onto the forefoot, thus defeating its purpose, as shown in Figure 11-17B. The built-up rearfoot is difficult to match with the other shoe, adding to the difficulty of gait. Given that many potential users of these devices already have gait impairments, these devices must be matched to the correct patient.

Shoes

Once an ulcer is healed, a patient must consider the use of "diabetic" shoes. In some cases, a prescription for diabetic shoes might be written for a high-risk individual who has not yet developed a plantar ulcer. A pedorthist is a specialist in dispensing diabetic footwear. For individuals who have not yet ulcerated but have diminished protective sensation, a good-quality pair of shoes that match the foot template described previously may be sufficient.

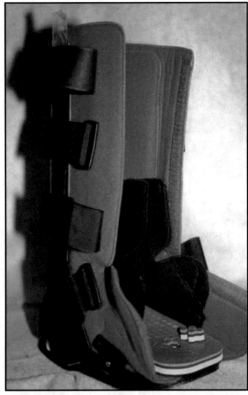

Figure 11-16. DH Offloading Walker used as an alternative to a total-contact cast. (The image is a copyrighted product of AAWC [www.aawconline.org] and has been reproduced with permission.)

Those with moderate deformities such as hammertoes may require extra-depth shoes to accommodate the foot's increased height. Off-the-shelf Charcot shoes can be used for moderate Charcot deformity, but custom shoes need to be molded to the shape of the patient's foot/feet with severe Charcot deformity. Medicare provides one pair of shoes annually. In general, patients are advised to rotate shoes and gradually increase the wear time of new shoes. Often an initial limit of 1-hour wearing time is suggested, with daily increments until the shoes can be worn daily but rotated with older shoes. Shoes should be discarded if they show excessive wear that could injure the feet.

Molded Inserts

Medicare also provides 2 pairs of molded inserts for diabetes annually but not other neuropathies. These can also be obtained from a pedorthist. Molded inserts are shaped to the plantar surface to distribute plantar forces more evenly. They are made of a dense foam that will eventually compress and lose its effectiveness, requiring replacement.

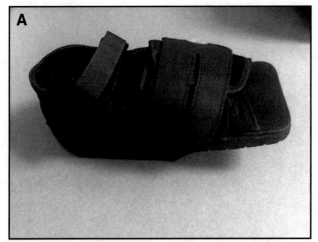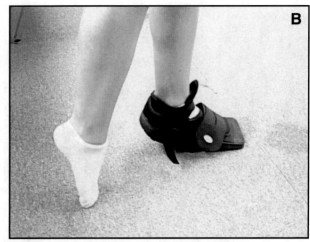

Figure 11-17. OrthoWedge shoe. (A) Note the dorsiflexion imposed by the shoe and the lack of weight-bearing on the forefoot. (B) Walking in an OrthoWedge shoe. A patient can place weight on the forefoot without an appropriate gait pattern.

Walking Patterns

Another strategy for managing the load on the injured foot is altering the gait pattern. Complete off-loading can only be achieved by not allowing weight-bearing on the involved foot. Non–weight-bearing gait with a 3-point pattern can be achieved with either a standard walker or crutches. Knee scooters are a possibility for some patients with sufficient skill. The patient's ability to use these assistive devices must be assessed, and the ability to use it when waking at night must be considered. A given patient might manage crutches or a knee scooter when fully awake but struggle and possibly fall when sleepy and in the dark. Such an individual might use crutches during the day and a walker at night. The patient will more likely walk to the bathroom by holding onto walls, but appropriate assistive devices should be offered nonetheless. If a patient needs to be non–weight-bearing bilaterally, a scooter or wheelchair could be used. Depending on the individual, partial weight-bearing may be sufficient using heel touch instead of toe touch with crutches or a walker. A cane could be offered in select cases, but the patient will need to be trained to use it on the unaffected side.

Instead of reducing weight-bearing with an assistive device, the gait pattern can be altered to reduced shear on the foot by avoiding the transition from midfoot to toe off. As shown in Figure 11-18, a step-to gait pattern is created by the patient, bringing the affected extremity even with the unaffected extremity, advancing the unaffected extremity, and again bringing the affected extremity even. This way, no rolling from midstance to toe off can occur. Another option is to allow the affected foot to be advanced in a step-through pattern but lift the foot from midstance and advance it using hip flexion instead of rolling from midstance to toe off (Figure 11-19).

NEUROPATHIC ULCER MANAGEMENT

Wagner grades are useful for developing a plan of care for the management of neuropathic ulcers. As noted in the earlier discussion of classifications of neuropathic ulcers, one should utilize all possible information to determine a care plan. A grade 0 ulcer has intact skin and must be protected by off-loading the foot by total-contact casting or other methods described previously, including orthotic or special shoes. The foot needs to be inspected for the presence of subcutaneous necrosis and potential breach of the skin. Subcutaneous necrosis below intact skin frequently produces a greenish hue to a circumscribed region beneath at-risk skin.

Management of grade 1 and 2 ulcers includes local wound care, edema management, protection from maceration, and foot protection by total-contact casting or another method. Total-contact casting both off-loads and controls edema. The control of edema, however, presents 2 serious challenges to the clinician. Resolution of edema may compromise the total-contact cast's fit, causing damage to the skin under the cast. On the other hand, increased swelling within the cast may cause ischemic injury. Patients must be taught to monitor the cast carefully and to seek immediate care if swelling causes vascular compromise within the cast and to return for recasting if the cast becomes too loose.

Grade 3 ulcers require referral to an orthopedic surgeon or podiatrist who may perform resection of bone or bony prominence with osteomyelitis and incision and drainage of the abscess. The surgeon may decide that selective removal of foot bones may be required to rid the foot of infection. Oral or parenteral antibiotics, but not topical, are recommended by the American Diabetes Association.

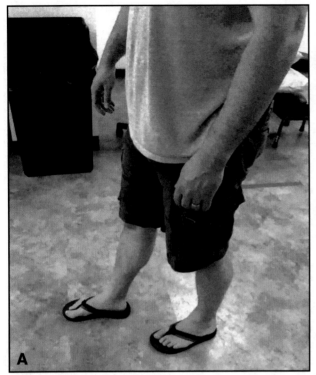 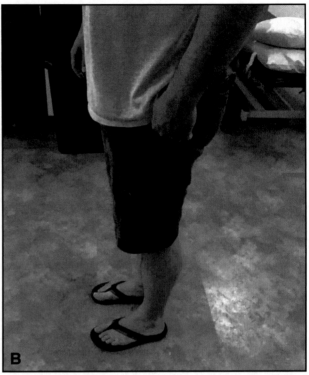

Figure 11-18. Step-to gait pattern used to minimize shearing forces on the affected foot. The patient only brings the affected foot even with the unaffected foot but steps through with the unaffected foot. Note inappropriate footwear. Patients with neuropathy should avoid such footwear to prevent foot injury.

Total-contact casting is contraindicated for Wagner grades 3 to 5. Local wound care includes removing as much necrotic tissue by sharp debridement as quickly as feasible. Sharp debridement may be supplemented with pulsatile lavage with concurrent suction. Whirlpools and wet-to-dry dressings are discouraged by the American Diabetes Association, whose guidelines indicate immediate sharp debridement due to infection risk.

Grades 4 and 5 neuropathic feet with dry gangrene require referral to a vascular surgeon with possible revascularization or amputation of the limb. The choice of dressing is determined by several factors, which is discussed in Chapter 16. Often, neuropathic ulcers are dry and need to be moisturized with hydrogel. If the wound is wet initially, one should consider that it may be infected and use an absorbent dressing. More discussion occurs in Chapters 16 and 20 when the plan of care is discussed.

Overload vs Underload Model

An overlooked part of treating a neuropathic foot is rehabilitation and prevention. Once the wound is healed, the patient is at risk of developing another ulcer, and measures to prevent recurrence and improve the patient's quality of life must be part of the care plan. Rehabilitation is based on shifting from the overload model of neuropathic ulceration to the underload model. Simply put, the overload model considers neuropathic ulcers to be the result of excessive loading of an insensate foot. Based on this model, one strives to decrease loads through footwear and decreasing mobility. However, recent thought of continually protecting injured structures has led to the consideration of the need to rehabilitate gait and tissue biomechanics. Neuropathic ulcers appear to be a consequence of a lack of protective sensation and altered biomechanics that must be restored. For example, one would not have a patient continually wear a cervical collar after a neck sprain, so why should we continually protect the foot instead of attempting to rehabilitate it?

The underload model is based on the idea that neuropathic ulcers result from the lack of stimuli to maintain tissue integrity. In addition to wound management, the underload model aims to provide a well-prescribed loading relative to individual biomechanics. In particular, the midfoot-forefoot transition with active arch support and metatarsal-toe transition is targeted. Reliance on passive arch support and lack of toe off place excessive forces on metatarsal heads that could be improved.

Preventive Therapy

Prevention begins with an understanding of the individual's foot biomechanics. Patients should always be asked to walk as part of the initial physical examination, if possible. Not all patients are good candidates for foot rehabilitation. If the patient has been ambulatory, the biomechanics should be assessed. Footwear should also be assessed and potentially replaced or adapted. Standard foot-strengthening exercises can be initiated before the wound is closed and should be performed at home as well as in the clinic. Biomechanical retraining should normalize the dissipation of forces, particularly the transition from midfoot to forefoot. The range of motion both passively and actively and in weight-bearing needs to be assessed. A rigid foot, especially the hallux, places substantial shear on the skin over the metatarsal heads and toes.

REHABILITATION FROM FOOT ULCERATION

Once the wound is closed, the rehabilitation process continues with standard foot-strengthening exercises, including towel curls, marble pickup, ankle alphabet, golf ball rolls, curling and spreading toes, and others (Figure 11-20). Some patients can be advanced to more difficult exercises such as toe raises on a slant board, standing on an unstable surface such as a BOSU (BOSU Fitness, LLC), and resistance bands for dorsiflexion and plantar flexion. This foot exercise program is done concurrently with a graduated walking program and a lower extremity balance and strengthening program. A foot-strengthening program usually involves barefoot walking for a person without neuropathy, including walking on sand or smooth rocks. This is a difficult decision for a person with neuropathy. One needs to weigh the risks and benefits of such a program. For the person with diabetic neuropathy, barefoot walking is likely to be too advanced. It should be considered only for the exceptional person.

SUMMARY

Although arterial disease and neuropathy are frequently comorbid, the astute clinician needs to separate the effects of each and recognize the effects of combined arterial disease and neuropathy. Triple neuropathy increases the risk of plantar ulceration due to biomechanical changes. Sensory neuropathy prevents pain from stopping the problem, and autonomic neuropathy weakens the skin. Total-contact casting is the gold standard for off-loading but also creates the risk of injury, particularly for the patient who

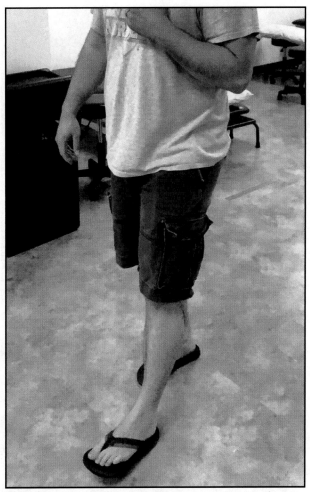

Figure 11-19. Hip flexion gait strategy to minimize shearing forces on the affected foot. Note inappropriate footwear. Patients with neuropathy should avoid such footwear to prevent foot injury.

cannot be trusted to monitor and maintain the cast between visits. Removable off-loading devices allow inspection, but patients can take them off and only put them back on for outpatient visits. The Wagner and University of Texas classification systems are useful for contemplating a care plan, but the inter-rater reliability is only moderate. Off-loading is one of the treatment plan components for intact skin, small or large ulcers but not for infected wounds or gangrene. Immediate sharp debridement is recommended for all neuropathic ulcers due to the risk of infection. Footwear suitable for the patient's feet and lifestyle is commonly the domain of a pedorthist. Prevention of ulceration and rehabilitation from ulceration require a program of foot exercises with an emphasis on improving the biomechanics of shifting from midfoot to forefoot.

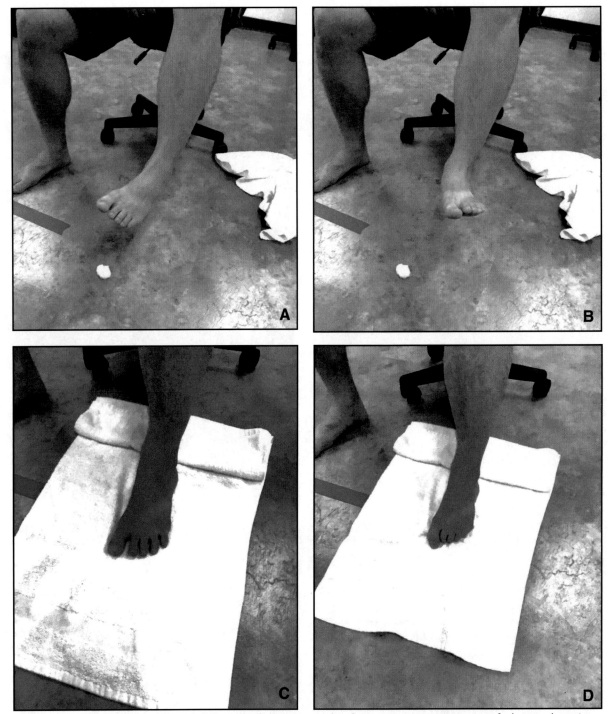

Figure 11-20. Exercises used for rehabilitation of the neuropathic foot to prevent recurrence of plantar ulcerations. (A) Inversion. (B) Eversion. (C) Towel crunches beginning. (D) Towel crunches end. *(continued)*

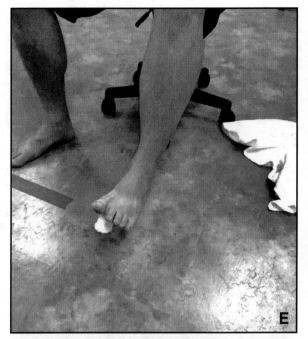

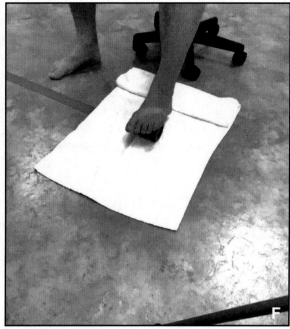

Figure 11-20 (continued). (E) Picking up a cotton ball with toes. (F) Rolling foot over cylinder. (G) Toe ups.

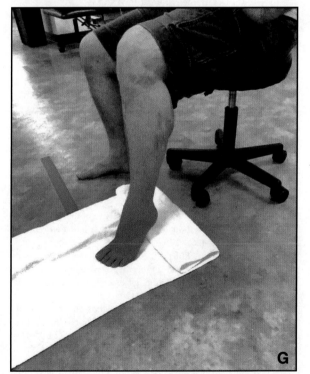

QUESTIONS

1. Distinguish among the terms *neuropathic*, *arterial*, and *diabetic foot ulcer*.

2. What is considered to be the normal range for fasting blood glucose?

3. What is considered to be a better test that indicates long-term glycemic control?

4. What are the manifestations of musculoskeletal glycosylation?
   a. Nerves
   b. Musculoskeletal structures of the foot
   c. Gait

5. What are the manifestations of the following?
   a. Sensory neuropathy
   b. Motor neuropathy
   c. Autonomic neuropathy

6. List the most common locations for neuropathic ulcers.

7. What are the differences between claw toes and hammertoes?

8. What are the elements of tip-top-toe syndrome?

9. What are the consequences of hallux rigidus and limitus?

10. What are the elements of the causal pathway to amputation as related to neuropathy?

11. What are the 3 elements of physical therapy intervention for neuropathic ulcers?

12. Describe the Charcot foot. What happens during the acute stage?

13. What are the 5 Wagner grades? What is the significance of the progression of grades?

14. Why does the American Diabetes Association recommend immediate sharp debridement for neuropathic ulcers?

15. What is the purpose of off-loading?

16. What is the gold standard for off-loading?

17. How long is the first cast typically left in place? How long for subsequent casts?

18. What are the advantages and disadvantages of removable off-loading devices?

19. What other options are available? How effective are they?

20. What is the appropriate long-term footwear for the following?
    a. Low risk
    b. Moderate deformity/hammertoes/claw toes
    c. Moderate Charcot deformity
    d. Severe Charcot deformity

21. What does Medicare allow for footwear for people with diabetic neuropathy?

22. What gait patterns/assistive devices are available for off-loading an affected foot?

23. Why is a total-contact cast contraindicated for Wagner grade 3?

24. Why is a vascular consult needed for Wagner grades 4 and 5?

REFERENCE

1. Hicks CW, Selvin E. Epidemiology of peripheral neuropathy and lower extremity disease in diabetes. *Curr Diab Rep*. 2019;19(10):86. doi:10.1007/s11892-019-1212-8

BIBLIOGRAPHY

Amemiya A, Noguchi H, Oe M, et al. Shear stress-normal stress (pressure) ratio decides forming callus in patients with diabetic neuropathy. *J Diabetes Res*. 2016;2016:3157123.

American Diabetes Association. Standards of Medical Care (living document). Accessed June 15, 2021. https://care.diabetesjournals.org/content/43/Supplement_1

Armstrong D, Lavery LA, Harkless LB. Validation of a diabetic wound classification system: the contribution of depth, infection and ischemia to risk of amputation. *Diabetes Care*. 1998;21(5):855-859.

Boyko EJ. How to use clinical signs and symptoms to estimate the probability of limb ischaemia in patients with a diabetic foot ulcer. *Diabetes Metab Res Rev*. 2020;36(Suppl 1):e3241.

Braun LR, Fisk WA, Lev-Tov H, Kirsner RS, Isseroff RR. Diabetic foot ulcer: an evidence-based treatment update. *Am J Clin Dermatol*. 2014;15(3):267-281.

Bus SA. The role of pressure offloading on diabetic foot ulcer healing and prevention of recurrence. *Plast Reconstr Surg*. 2016;138(3 Suppl):179S-187S.

Chin YF, Yeh JT, Yu HY, Weng LC. Knowledge of the warning signs of foot ulcer deterioration among patients with diabetes. *J Nurs Res*. 2018;26(6):420-426.

Cowley MS, Boyko EJ, Shofer JB, Ahroni JH, Ledoux WR. Foot ulcer risk and location in relation to prospective clinical assessment of foot shape and mobility among persons with diabetes. *Diabetes Res Clin Pract*. 2008;82(2):226-232.

Eraydin Ş, Avşar G. The effect of foot exercises on wound healing in type 2 diabetic patients with a foot ulcer: a randomized control study. *J Wound Ostomy Continence Nurs*. 2018;45(2):123-130.

Fard AS, Esmaelzadeh M, Larijani B. Assessment and treatment of diabetic foot ulcer. *Int J Clin Pract*. 2007;61(11):1931-1938.

Hamatani M, Mori T, Oe M, et al. Factors associated with callus in patients with diabetes, focused on plantar shear stress during gait. *J Diabetes Sci Technol*. 2016;10(6):1353-1359.

International Working Group on the Diabetic Foot. Accessed June 6, 2021. https://iwgdfguidelines.org/guidelines/guidelines/

Kee KK, Nair HKR, Yuen NP. Risk factor analysis on the healing time and infection rate of diabetic foot ulcers in a referral wound care clinic. *J Wound Care*. 2019;28(Suppl 1):S4-S13.

Lavery LA, Higgins KR, LaFontaine J, Zamorano RG, Constantinides GP, Kim PJ. Randomised clinical trial to compare total contact casts, healing sandals and a shear-reducing removable boot to heal diabetic foot ulcers. *Int Wound J*. 2015;12(6):710-715.

Lavery LA, LaFontaine J, Higgins KR, Lanctot DR, Constantinides G. Shear-reducing insoles to prevent foot ulceration in high-risk diabetic patients. *Adv Skin Wound Care.* 2012;25(11):519-524.

Ledoux WR, Shofer JB, Cowley MS, Ahroni JH, Cohen V, Boyko EJ. Diabetic foot ulcer incidence in relation to plantar pressure magnitude and measurement location. *J Diabetes Complications.* 2013;27(6):621-626.

Lott DJ, Zou D, Mueller MJ. Pressure gradient and subsurface shear stress on the neuropathic forefoot. *Clin Biomech (Bristol, Avon).* 2008;23(3):342-348.

Miranda-Palma B, Sosenko JM, Bowker JH, Mizel MS, Boulton AJM. A comparison of the monofilament with other testing modalities for foot ulcer susceptibility. *Diabetes Res Clin Pract.* 2005;70(1):8-12.

Monteiro-Soares M, Boyko EJ, Jeffcoate W, et al. Diabetic foot ulcer classifications: a critical review. *Diabetes Metab Res Rev.* 2020;36(Suppl 1):e3272.

Park JH, Suh DH, Kim HJ, Lee YI, Kwak IH, Choi GW. Role of pro-calcitonin in infected diabetic foot ulcer. *Diabetes Res Clin Pract.* 2017;128:51-57.

Reiber GE. The epidemiology of diabetic foot problems. *Diabet Med.* 1996;13(Suppl 1):S6-S11.

Shin JY, Roh SG, Sharaf B, Lee NH. Risk of major limb amputation in diabetic foot ulcer and accompanying disease: a meta-analysis. *J Plast Reconstr Aesthet Surg.* 2017;70(12):1681-1688.

Stang D, Young M. Selection and application of a diabetic foot ulcer classification system in Scotland: part 2. *Diabet Foot J.* 2018;21(2):100-106.

Tay WL, Lo ZJ, Hong Q, Yong E, Chandrasekar S, Tan GWL. Toe pressure in predicting diabetic foot ulcer healing: a systematic review and meta-analysis. *Ann Vasc Surg.* 2019;60:371-378.

Waaijman R, de Haart M, Arts ML, et al. Risk factors for plantar foot ulcer recurrence in neuropathic diabetic patients. *Diabetes Care.* 2014;37(6):1697-1705. doi:10.2337/dc13-2470

12

Vascular Ulcers

OBJECTIVES

- Discuss diagnostic criteria for venous ulcers.
- Describe the pathophysiology of venous ulcers.
- Discuss the interventions available for venous disease and criteria for their use.
- Discuss diagnostic criteria for lymphatic ulcers.
- Discuss the interventions available for lymphatic disease and criteria for their use.
- Discuss diagnostic criteria for arterial ulcers.
- Discuss the interventions available for arterial disease and criteria for their use.

Venous disease accounts for a large number of wounds. Venous leg ulcers can be a major component of a wound practice. Arterial disease can also lead to ulcerations, but the interventions for them are somewhat limited beyond surgical intervention. Lymphatic disease is often treated by specialists in this practice and is not discussed in detail in this chapter. An awareness of the characteristics of lymphatic disease and treatment of ulcers secondary to lymphedema are the emphasis.

VENOUS AND ARTERIAL ANATOMY AND PHYSIOLOGY

Venous leg ulcers are the result of the anatomical and physiologic differences between arterial and venous vessels. An arterial ulcer is a straightforward consequence of ischemia, whereas leakage of fluid from the microvasculature secondary to venous hypertension sets the stage for venous leg ulcers.

Irion GL, Gardner JA, Pignataro RM.
Comprehensive Wound Management, Third Edition (pp 211-236).
© 2024 Taylor and Francis Group.

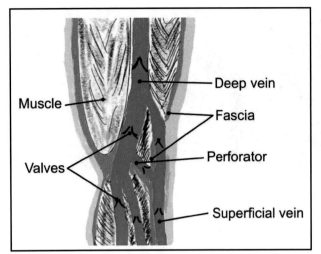

Figure 12-1. Types of veins based on anatomical depth. Deep veins are located deep to the fascia, superficial veins are located superficial to the fascia, and perforators (communicating) allow superficial veins to drain into the deep veins.

Large veins and arteries are paired and usually given the same name. These named paired vessels are deep to the fascia. Veins are considerably redundant due to the need to return the blood under low pressure. The cross-sectional area of veins is much larger than the accompanying arteries, with a resulting low velocity and greater opportunity for coagulation to occur. Arterial blood flow is driven by pumping of the heart, creating arterial pressure with a relatively small effect of gravity. Venous blood flow has little pressure to drive it back to the central circulation, and, therefore, gravity has much more of an effect on venous flow. Moving blood against gravity is aided by the combination of valves and muscle pumping. Unfortunately, issues with coagulation, venous valve dysfunction, and muscle pumping can produce venous disease, leading to venous leg ulcers.

Venous Anatomy

In addition to the increased number of venous vessels compared with the accompanying arterial vessel, a large number of venous vessels must drain the skin to the large subfascial veins. For the sake of discussing function, venous vessels are divided into deep, superficial, and communicating. Another term for communicating is *perforator*. This term expresses the idea that these veins perforate the fascia and allow the superficial veins to drain into the deep veins. Superficial veins have greater pressure than deep veins, which allows the superficial veins to drain through the perforators into the deep veins. The relationships among superficial, communicating/perforator, and deep veins are depicted in Figure 12-1.

Vein Function

Put simply, the function of systemic veins is to collect nutrient-depleted, waste-containing blood from capillaries and return it to the right atrium to unload wastes and replenish the blood. Competent one-way valves prevent reflux, the backward flow of blood. With normally functioning valves, pressure applied to the outside of a vein will only drive blood flow forward. Any difficulty in emptying a vein will increase both venous and capillary pressure as blood enters faster than it exits. Pressure will build as high as necessary to drive blood flow out of the vein at the same rate that it flows in from the arterial side. Therefore, anything that slows the exit of blood from a vein relative to the entry of blood will cause venous pressure to increase.

Capillary Leakage

Forces described by Starling are used to explain capillary leakage. Hydrostatic pressure is the result of pumping blood into a vessel, producing the potential energy that is then converted to kinetic energy in the form of flow. The rate at which blood is forced into a vessel segment, the rate at which it is allowed to move out of the segment, and the compliance of the vessel determine hydrostatic pressure in a vessel. Hydrostatic pressure in the interstitial space is normally slightly negative. As fluid accumulates in the interstitial space, hydrostatic pressure increases. The difference between capillary and interstitial hydrostatic pressure drives substantial fluid outward until capillary and interstitial fluid pressures become equal.

A second force is created by the presence of plasma proteins, primarily albumin. Plasma proteins decrease the propensity of fluid to leave the capillary, producing what is known as *oncotic pressure*, the pressure necessary to stop swelling. Plasma oncotic pressure is normally slightly less than hydrostatic pressure entering the capillary, but slightly higher than hydrostatic pressure at the end of the capillary due to loss of hydrostatic pressure in driving flow through the capillary. Therefore, Starling forces predict net leakage at the arteriolar end of a capillary and absorption of fluid at the venular end of the capillary. This model, however, is oversimplified. A given capillary may leak or gain fluid along a portion of its entire length, and the rate of leakage of any given capillary may vary over time. Any net leakage is generally managed by the lymphatic system, which returns any net leakage of fluid to the subclavian veins.

Three major factors are responsible for capillary fluid leakage—the difference in hydrostatic pressure (capillary pressure vs interstitial pressure), the difference in oncotic pressure (concentration of plasma proteins vs interstitial protein), and the tightness of endothelial cells. Edema can be divided into the categories of inflammatory and non-inflammatory. Inflammation creates edema due to both arteriolar dilation and opening of spaces between venular endothelial cells. Noninflammatory edema is caused by unbalanced Starling forces, which can be normal or pathologic. An example of normal, temporary edema is intense exercise. During exercise, arteriolar dilation increases capillary pressure, resulting in more leakage than lymphatics can handle. However, edema resolves gradually at the end of exercise, as arteriolar dilation ends, leakage slows, and the lymphatics have the opportunity to restore interstitial volume. With inflammation, edema continues until interstitial pressure becomes opposite and equal to the pressure driving fluid out, which can produce long-lasting, profound edema.

Another factor that becomes important in the context of this chapter is the effect of venous pressure. Capillary pressure is increased by both low arteriolar resistance, allowing blood to enter capillaries, and high venous resistance, preventing blood from exiting capillaries. Both reflux (backward flow due to an incompetent valve) and obstruction of venous vessels decrease the outflow of capillaries and can drive venous pressure to an unmanageable degree. Thus, venous disease can create substantial leakage that exceeds the ability of the lymphatic system to maintain interstitial volume. With venous disease, the degree of edema will be proportionate to the degree of venous outflow resistance (Figure 12-2).

Venous Hypertension

Most people are familiar with the term *hypertension* as it applies to the systemic circulation. In arterial hypertension, excessive pressure occurs in the systemic arteries, which leads to damage to both the arteries themselves and tissues served by them. Similarly, excessive pressure in veins leads to injury to both the veins and the tissue surrounding them. Stereotypical changes occur in both the skin and vein as a consequence of venous hypertension.

Roles of Types of Veins

Deep veins of the extremities are subfascial, carrying blood back from skeletal muscle, bone, and other subfascial structures. Walking and other muscle activities increase the flow within deep veins, but deep vein pressure actually becomes lower than it is in standing due to the venous muscle pump. Superficial veins are suprafascial and primarily carry blood back from the skin. Superficial veins drain readily into deep veins through perforators even during exercise when the valves are functioning properly and veins are unobstructed. Incompetent

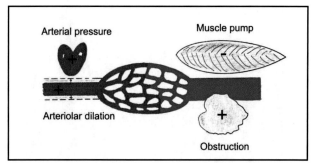

Figure 12-2. Determinants of venous pressure. Venous pressure is increased by factors that allow more blood in from arterioles due to arterial pressure and arteriolar dilation. Venous pressure is decreased by factors that empty veins, such as muscle pumping, and increased by factors that prevent emptying of veins, such as occlusion and valve dysfunction.

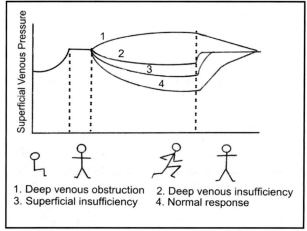

1. Deep venous obstruction   2. Deep venous insufficiency
3. Superficial insufficiency   4. Normal response

Figure 12-3. Effect of muscle pumping on superficial venous pressure. The normal response to muscle pumping produces a decrease in venous pressure below that found during sitting. Reflux from diseased superficial veins reduces the response. Reflux from deep veins produces a greater attenuation of the muscle pump effect. With occlusion of deep veins (upper curve), reflux back through perforators from working muscles causes superficial venous pressure to rise above that occurring with standing alone.

perforators/communicators allow the deep veins to flood superficial veins, resulting in elevated superficial venous pressure. This increased superficial venous pressure results in severely dilated and tortuous varicose veins.

Muscle Pump

The muscle pump mechanisms augment the emptying of veins against gravity, thereby preventing excessive pressure from developing in the veins. Each contraction of muscle compresses deep veins, either within muscles or between muscle and fascia. A brief elevation of pressure

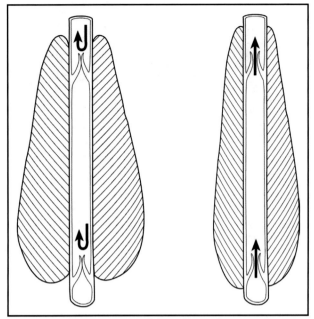

Figure 12-4. Components of the calf muscle pump. Pumping requires the presence of unobstructed vessels, valves to ensure unidirectional flow, and a source of energy (muscle contraction).

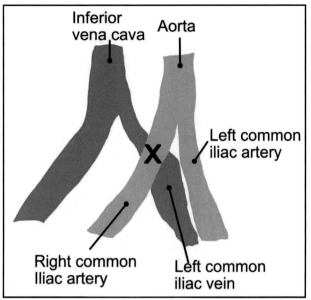

Figure 12-5. May-Thurner syndrome. Occlusion of the left common iliac vein by the right common iliac artery produces this syndrome.

against the vein could potentially drive blood flow in both directions, but competent venous valves will only allow blood to move out of the extremity. Without competent valves, venous pressure must rise to drive blood forward and out of the dependent limb. As a result of muscle pumping, venous pressure during walking is less than it is in sitting.

In the case of superficial veins, muscle contraction creates pressure between the skin and fascia. Where skin and fascia are tight, more pressure is generated than where the skin is loosely attached to fascia, and the venous pump is less effective. Additionally, the lowering of deep vein pressure by muscle pumping aids the emptying of superficial veins. Effective muscle pumping requires 3 components—unobstructed veins, competent valves (no reflux), and muscle activity. Failure of one or more of these components compromises the venous pump. The components of the venous pump are shown in Figure 12-4.

Obstruction

Veins are at greater risk for obstruction than arterial vessels due to their lower pressure, slower velocity, greater likelihood of coagulation, and more compliant walls. Veins can be obstructed from either the inside or outside. Internal causes of obstruction include clots due to slow flow velocity or hypercoagulability and thrombi from damage to vessel walls.

External obstruction may occur due to masses compressing a vein. Tumors may occur anywhere along venous

drainage, but inguinal lymph nodes filling with cancer cells may cause severe compression of the iliac arteries. Obesity and pregnancy may also compress iliac veins. Another cause is May-Thurner syndrome, also known as *iliac vein compression syndrome*. The anatomy of the common iliac arteries and veins are offset with the aortic branches to the left of the common iliac veins, as shown in Figure 12-5. As the right common iliac artery traverses the midline to enter the right lower extremity, it crosses the underlying left common iliac vein. In some individuals, the right common iliac artery can significantly compress the left common iliac vein, requiring stenting of the left common iliac vein to restore blood flow to the left lower extremity.

Reflux

Reflux is the backward flow created by incompetent valves. A competent valve will allow only enough backflow to close the valve distal to its segment. With muscle contraction, venous pressure increases sufficiently to open the valves above each segment between adjacent valves to create forward flow. As pressure diminishes between muscle contractions, valves close, preventing backflow (regurgitation). With dysfunctional valves, the pressure created by muscle contraction drives blood flow in both directions, and gravity allows blood to move from proximal to distal. Venous pressure builds and may damage additional venous valves, resulting in progressive failure of venous valves. The increase in pressure causes leakage of both fluid and small molecules from the microcirculation and the lengthening and widening of veins. Because the distance between

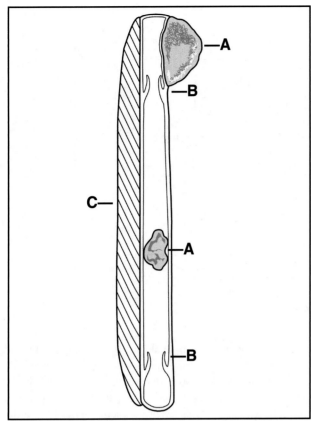

Figure 12-6. Potential causes of pump failure. (A) Obstruction of the vein from outside by a mass, such as a tumor, or from inside by a blood clot. (B) Incompetent venous valves. (C) Loss of muscle function due to atrophy in this example.

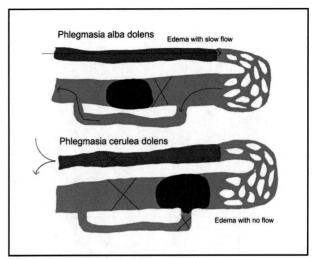

Figure 12-7. Phlegmasia. In the case of deep venous occlusion only, venous and capillary pressure rise, but drainage may still occur by reflux through superficial veins, resulting in severe edema but sufficient blood flow to preserve the limb. In the more severe form, both superficial and deep venous occlusion become great enough to impair or stop arterial inflow to an extremity.

capillaries and the next confluence of veins is fixed, the lengthening of a vein can only be accomplished by the vein repeatedly changing directions. When superficial veins become longer and wider, the classic appearance of dilated, tortuous varicose veins can be seen. Reflux through perforators is especially damaging to superficial veins. The large volume of blood moving through the deep veins into superficial veins can produce severe varicose veins when allowed to reflux into the superficial veins. Mechanisms that cause the muscle pump to fail are summarized in Figure 12-6.

Phlegmasia

Phlegmasia represents the ultimate degree of venous insufficiency, resulting in failure to allow arterial flow into an extremity. An example of phlegmasia is shown in Figure 12-7. Phlegmasia usually occurs in the lower extremities but can also occur in upper extremities secondary to a complication of subclavian central catheters. Two types of phlegmasia are described in the literature. Phlegmasia alba dolens (white, painful) produces a

swollen, white extremity due to a lack of venous outflow in deep veins only. Phlegmasia cerulea dolens (blue, painful) is characterized by severe swelling and cyanosis. This type involves both deep and superficial veins and can lead to gangrene. It has a high risk of amputation and mortality due to pulmonary embolism.

Effectiveness of Venous Pump

All potential venous pump mechanisms are not equally effective. Some properties of the pump mechanism vary due to anatomy. Most discussions of the venous pump are limited to the calf muscle pump. The foot, leg, and thigh have muscle-pumping mechanisms that differ due to their anatomy and involvement of subfascial and suprafascial pumps. Compression against an unyielding surface such as bone or fascia produces more pressure than compression against skin, which is more yielding than fascia. Therefore, the pumping of deep veins is more effective than superficial veins. When comparing different areas of the extremities, some places, such as the wrist and ankle, have much tighter skin that performs better as a part of the pumping mechanism. Additionally, longer veins will need to pump against greater pressure. As a general rule, long superficial veins running through loose skin are the most likely to fail. In particular, the greater saphenous vein just above the ankle is the most prevalent site of venous insufficiency and its problems.

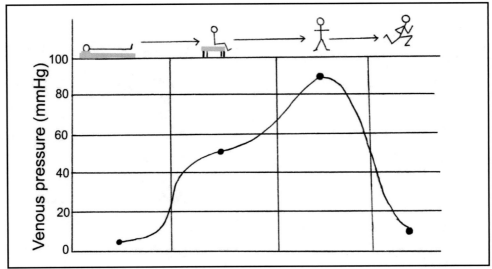

Figure 12-8. Effects of posture and walking on venous pressure. Note that venous pressure during walking with competent muscle pumping produces less pressure than that occurring with sitting. In those with venous disease, ambulatory venous hypertension can be produced.

Effects of Posture and Movement

Pressure within the circulatory system is produced in 2 ways. The pressure head generated by cardiac pumping is depleted as blood passes through arterioles and reaches low values by the time blood enters the veins. A column of fluid also produces pressure. A column above the heart, such as raising the arm overhead, decreases pressure in the extremity, whereas a column of fluid below the heart is additive. For this reason, arterial pressure is measured at the level of the heart regardless of the person's position so that the pressure generated by cardiac pumping is measured without any contribution from a column of fluid above or below the heart level. Pressure measured in leg and foot arteries is measured in supine with the leg slightly elevated to position the artery being measured at the height of the aorta (or right atrium), the so-called phlebostatic axis. This column of fluid will impact any position above or below the phlebostatic axis.

Increased pressure in the veins causes distention (ie, widening), and, therefore, for a given flow rate, velocity will slow. Chronic widening of veins produces damage to venous valves. Some individuals have a large number of superficial veins that fail to support this column of fluid, producing varicose veins. In normal lower extremity vein function, muscle pumping overcomes the effects of this column of fluid, but long periods of standing still predispose one to venous disease. A history of prolonged standing is a standard part of taking history for a person with leg ulcers.

As shown in Figure 12-8, leg venous pressure is lowest in a recumbent position, less than 20 mm Hg, and lowered further by elevating the legs. As a person raises the rest of the body higher than the legs, venous pressure increases

and reaches its maximum of about 100 mm Hg upon static standing. Venous pressure increases more in taller individuals. Walking activates the muscle pump to the point of bringing leg venous pressure close to its supine value of about 20 mm Hg. In people with inadequate muscle pumping, leg venous pressure decreases only slightly depending on the cause. If the person has superficial venous insufficiency, we expect leg pressure to decrease moderately. However, the person with deep venous insufficiency will see little drop due to the reflux of deep venous blood coming from the exercising muscle into the superficial veins, as shown in Figure 12-3.

The situation becomes worse with deep venous obstruction leading to shunting of muscle venous blood through superficial veins. In this case, superficial venous pressure can increase during exercise. Additionally, depending on the cause, the return of leg venous pressure postexercise to static standing is very short with insufficient leg veins, as shown in Figure 12-3. With normal muscle pumping, the person's superficial veins are spared the elevated pressure for several minutes postexercise. The person with deep vein obstruction will have elevated pressure for several minutes, and those with incompetent valves will experience static standing pressure within seconds of the end of exercise. This effect has practical significance for those who are required to stand for long periods. Short periods of muscle activity in standing can diminish venous pressure for those with healthy veins. However, those with venous insufficiency will need to rhythmically contract their leg muscles almost constantly to combat elevated venous pressure.

Causes of Venous Hypertension

When venous disease causes venous pressure to remain high despite walking, the term *chronic ambulatory venous hypertension* is used. The muscle pump has 3 components that must function to allow optimal pumping. Thus, causes of ambulatory venous hypertension include insufficient valves that allow reflux, obstruction of veins, and insufficient muscle pump activity. Because obstruction can occur from either within or outside a vein, patients should be evaluated by the referring physician to determine the cause of the obstruction and initiate treatment if possible. Insufficient muscle pumping can be caused by disease or injury to the nervous system or temporary immobilization. The cause of this lack of muscle activity should be determined before the referral is made. Causes of venous hypertension are highlighted in Table 12-1.

HISTORY AND PHYSICAL EXAM

The diagnosis of a venous leg ulcer is generally straightforward. The person's history often reveals long periods of uninterrupted standing either for work or recreation. The patient will complain of "heaviness" in the legs, but some patients may describe a moderate bursting type of pain. Patients frequently state an acute onset, mentioning trauma to the leg that caused the skin to open. Although trauma may be responsible for tearing necrotic tissue from the leg, trauma is unlikely to be the primary cause. When everything else points to venous insufficiency, the report of trauma should not influence the diagnosis.

A previous history of a venous leg ulcer and a family history of varicose veins or small "spider veins" are expected. Because of its length, lack of surrounding muscle, and suprafascial depth, the greater saphenous vein is the most likely to fail and lead to venous leg ulcers. The skin distal to the malleoli is sufficiently tight to provide compression. However, the lack of tightness above this point allows dilation and failure of the veins just proximal to the medial malleolus. Venous leg ulcers can occur near the lesser saphenous and other places on the leg. However, approximately two-thirds of venous leg ulcers are observed proximal to the medial malleolus in the so-called "gaiter region" between the calf muscles and ankle.

Skin Changes

During observation of the involved extremity, one should expect to see one or more of the following: edema, telangiectasia (spider veins), lipodermatosclerosis, and hemosiderin staining surrounding the ulcer. Edema is produced by the elevated capillary pressure created by venous insufficiency. Spider veins are small dilations produced by

TABLE 12-1
Causes of Venous Hypertension

Insufficient valves

Insufficient valves of deep veins

Insufficient valves of communicating veins

Insufficient valves of superficial veins (varicose veins)

Obstruction of lower extremity veins

Pregnancy

Obesity

Clotting/thrombosis of veins

Insufficient calf muscle activity

Prolonged standing

Neuromuscular disease affecting the leg muscles

Musculoskeletal injury or disease affecting the leg muscles

Immobilization of the lower extremity

superficial vein insufficiency. Large, tortuous distended superficial veins can be produced by perforator reflux from deep veins into the superficial veins. With elevated pressure, veins will grow longer and can only do so by periodic turns. Although their cosmetic appearance would give the impression that varicose veins are the worst case of venous disease, people with severe disease approaching phlegmasia may not exhibit this tortuosity and distention as long as the perforators remain competent. Lipodermatosclerosis is the thickening and tightening of the skin shown in Figure 12-9. Erythema, flaking skin, and proteinaceous crusts on the skin cause some clinicians to refer to the skin appearance as "eczema," but *lipodermatosclerosis* is the preferred term. This appearance has a high specificity for venous disease. The skin appearance will worsen with comorbid lymphedema.

Appearance of Venous Ulcers

In general, the venous leg ulcer will appear wet and shiny. The wound bed generally appears well granulated with a variable amount of slough depending on how soon after the onset of skin necrosis the patient is seen. In Figure 12-10, a typical venous leg ulcer is seen. Characteristics include a red, wet appearance; irregular margins; and adherent, macerated edges. A small amount of yellow slough and clotted blood are also present in this particular wound at the time of photography.

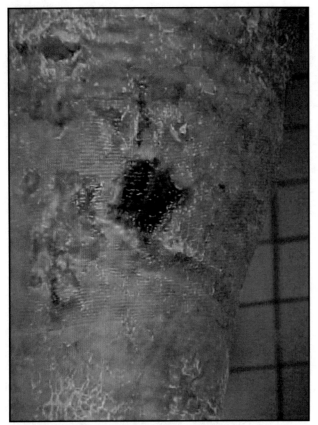

Figure 12-9. Appearance of skin in venous disease.

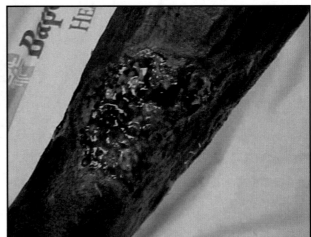

Figure 12-10. Appearance of a typically wet venous ulcer.

PATHOPHYSIOLOGY OF VENOUS ULCERS

For blood to move from capillaries into the engorged veins, the outflow pressure of capillaries increases until pressure within capillaries exceeds pressure within the draining veins. This high pressure causes the leakage of water, electrolytes, and small molecules. As pressure increases even further, larger constituents of blood including proteins and cells may leak from capillaries. Edema of venous disease results from both high hydrostatic pressure and the high concentration of protein in the interstitial space. As protein leaks from capillaries into interstitial space, the osmotic gradient that normally opposes movement of fluid out of capillaries is decreased, allowing fluid to escape at an even greater rate.

Normal loss of fluid and plasma proteins can be handled by lymphatic drainage; however, with venous hypertension, proteins leak out faster into the interstitial space than they can be taken up, resulting in accumulation of plasma proteins in the interstitial space. Although edema alone increases the diffusion distance for nutrients, the presence of proteins, particularly fibrinogen, has been blamed for tissue injury. Interstitial fibrinogen may be converted to the insoluble protein fibrin, which is the major component of thrombi. Excessive water and protein combined with decreased numbers of capillaries diminish diffusion of oxygen and nutrients required for the health of tissue surrounding the vein. Within the capillaries, hypertension produces dilation, elongation, tortuosity, and frequently thrombosis, similar to the effect hypertension has on superficial veins as they become varicose veins. These changes in capillaries are most pronounced in areas with hyperpigmentation and lipodermatosclerosis. Capillary changes are also most often observed in patients with insufficient perforator and deep veins.

Chronic leakage of large molecules and red blood cells into the interstitial space results in tissue injury and ulceration. Proinflammatory cytokines and iron overload create changes in fibroblasts and macrophages that predispose tissue to injury. Fibroblasts are converted to myofibroblasts, which increase tension in the dermis, and iron overload maintains the macrophage in a mode that promotes tissue breakdown instead of repair. Microangiopathy resulting from elevated pressure leads to rarefaction of capillaries (Figure 12-11).

Microangiopathy

Elevated venous pressure due to muscle pump failure causes elevated pressure and dilation of capillaries. Capillary distention can be observed before the tissue injury characteristic of venous hypertension can be observed, and the severity of skin damage and capillary injury are highly correlated. A severe reduction in the number of capillaries can be observed within the ulcer itself and at the edge of the ulcer. A large number of damaged capillaries characterized by dilation, elongation, tortuosity, stasis, and thrombosis can be observed. Thus, avascular areas develop resulting in tissue injury, progressing to tissue death and ulceration of the skin. Wound healing would also be expected to be slow or absent given the lack of nutritive circulation. A correlation between loss of capillaries and decreased transcutaneous oxygen ($TcPO_2$) has been demonstrated in a series of patients with chronic venous insufficiency. During healing, capillary density improved in all cases in both the ulcer and surrounding skin on the ulcer's edge. A greater increase in capillary density was observed in patients with relatively rapid healing compared with patients with relatively slow healing. In addition, $TcPO_2$ increased rapidly in the fast healers and was initially lower in slow healers. Healing was accompanied by an increased $TcPO_2$ in both groups but was higher in the fast healers. Although healing occurred in these patients, the deranged capillary morphology remained. This, in part, may explain the high recurrence of ulceration in patients simply receiving treatment for ulcerations but not for venous hypertension.

Surgical Treatment

Several options are available for the treatment of venous insufficiency. The old treatment of stripping through a large incision has been modified such that only smaller incisions are sufficient for performing the procedure. Other options include ultrasound-guided sclerotherapy and endovascular thermal ablation with either a laser or radiofrequency device. Sclerotherapy involves the injection of an agent that causes the vessel walls to collapse. Ablation of incompetent perforators is particularly useful for alleviating varicose veins.

CEAP Classification of Venous Disease

A classification scheme for venous disease uses a grading and categorical system to describe the severity, etiology, and the type of vein involved. The CEAP categories are Clinical appearance (7 gradations for severity), Etiology (congenital, primary, secondary), Anatomy (superficial, deep, or perforating), and Pathophysiology (obstruction or reflux). For the anatomy and pathophysiology components of this classification scheme, any or all of the terms may be used. Etiology may be congenital (rare) or may be either or both primary and secondary. Primary refers to the cause being attributable to a defect in the vein itself, not secondary to another phenomenon. For example, *primary* and *reflux* would be used together to describe a vein with failing valves occurring without any injury to the vein (assumed to be hereditary). The terms *secondary* and *obstruction* are frequently used together because conditions such as compression of veins due to obesity, pregnancy, tumor, improperly applied elastic bandage or cast, or clotting within a vein are

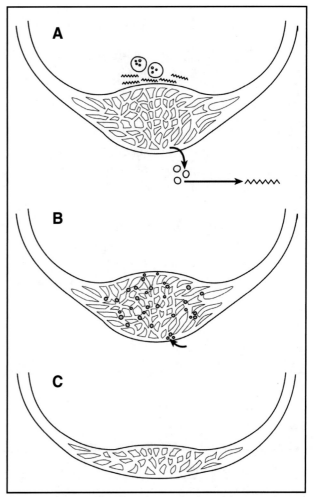

Figure 12-11. Pathophysiology of ulcers due to chronic venous insufficiency. (A) Leakage of proteins from capillaries. (B) Inflammation caused by trapped leukocytes. (C) Rarefaction of capillaries secondary to venous hypertension.

responsible for the obstruction (the obstruction is secondary to another problem). The definitions for clinical picture are provided in Table 12-2.

INTERVENTIONS

Interventions for venous leg ulcers include local wound management for debridement of any slough on the wound surface and protecting the surrounding skin from drainage. Compression therapy is used to treat the underlying venous disease. Gentle cleansing of wounds should be done with each dressing change along with any debridement that might be required. Using whirlpool therapy creates more problems with venous insufficiency. Typical whirlpool temperatures increasing arterial inflow and the dependent position with the thigh compressed over the edge of the whirlpool tank exacerbate venous insufficiency.

TABLE 12-2
Descriptions Used for the CEAP System

CLINICAL PICTURE

C0: No visible or palpable signs of venous disease

C1: Telangiectasias or reticular veins

C2: Varicose veins; distinguished from reticular veins by a diameter of 3 mm or more

C3: Edema

C4: Changes in skin and subcutaneous tissue secondary to CVD

      C4a: Pigmentation or eczema

      C4b: Lipodermatosclerosis or atrophie blanche

C5: Healed venous ulcer

C6: Active venous ulcer

S: Symptomatic

A: Asymptomatic

ETIOLOGY

Ec: Congenital

Ep: Primary

Es: Secondary

En: No venous cause identified

ANATOMY

As: Superficial veins

Ap: Perforating veins

Ad: Deep veins

An: No venous location identified

PATHOPHYSIOLOGY

Pr: Reflux

Po: Obstruction

Pr,o: Reflux and obstruction

Pn: No venous pathophysiology identifiable

Reproduced with permission from Lurie F, Passman M, Meisner M, et al. The 2020 update of the CEAP classification system and reporting standards [published correction appears in *J Vasc Surg Venous Lymphat Disord.* 2021 Jan;9(1):288]. *J Vasc Surg Venous Lymphat Disord.* 2020;8(3):342-352. doi:10.1016/j.jvsv.2019.12.075

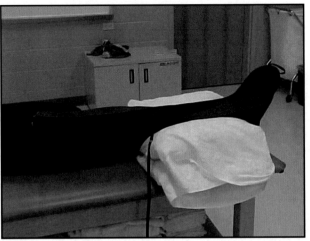

Figure 12-12. Single-cell compression pump. A single air chamber is alternately inflated and deflated. An on time and off time must be set as well as the pressure.

External compression counteracts the capillary hydrostatic pressure that produces the edema. Therefore, patients must have compression in place for as much of the day as possible. For venous leg ulcers, any dressing strategy employed must also provide compression. Several companies have developed kits that include dressings and compression bandages. In addition to compression bandaging, compression may be performed with a clinical or home compression pump. Some older compression pumps are single-cell units in which a single sleeve inflates and deflates rhythmically (Figure 12-12). Most newer devices are sequential, multicell pumps in which 3 or more cells inflate sequentially from distal (over the foot) toward the knee and then over the thigh. The cells deflate in reverse order and begin inflation distally toward proximally again (Figure 12-13). Any wounds should be covered with an appropriate dressing and a plastic bag to prevent soiling the compression sleeve. The bagged extremity is then placed into the compression sleeve, and the affected extremity is elevated. Pumping is done for 1 hour with pressure at 50 mm Hg, or less than diastolic pressure. Pressure higher than 50 mm Hg is believed to compress lymphatic vessels, and pressure less than diastolic ensures some circulation into the extremity throughout the entire cardiac cycle. If using a single-cell sleeve, 90 seconds on and 30 seconds off is commonly used, although no definitive evidence exists for a particular compression protocol. A sequential pump is simply allowed to run continuously as described earlier. If the patient needs to be seen in a clinic, treatment may be done 2 to 3 times per week. A more cost-effective strategy is for a rental of a home unit for more frequent treatments up to twice per day. In many cases, compression is achieved solely with bandaging rather than the use of compression pumps.

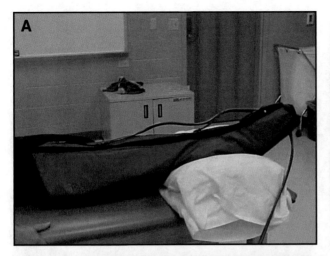

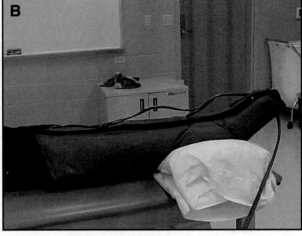

Figure 12-13. Sequential compression pump. (A) Four air chambers are sequentially inflated in the distal-to-proximal direction. For this model, only the pressure exerted by the pump is adjustable. All 4 chambers are deflated. (B) The chamber around the foot is inflated. (C) All 4 chambers are inflated.

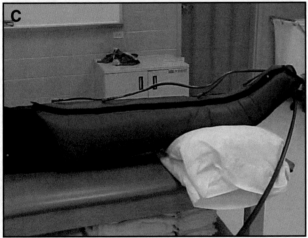

Options for compression bandaging are an Unna's boot and multilayer compression. An Unna's boot is still available, but multilayer compression bandaging is now considered to be a standard of care. An Unna's boot can be applied quickly, but it is messy to apply (Figure 12-14), and regulating the pressure within it is difficult. It is considered to be only useful in ambulatory patients in whom the semirigid dressing aids the calf pump mechanism. Moreover, the Unna's boot loses effectiveness as volume of the leg decreases, the bandage material cannot absorb much drainage, and maceration of the periwound skin may occur unless other steps are used to manage drainage from the wound.

Multilayer bandaging systems consist of either 2 (Figure 12-15), 3, or 4 layers (Figure 12-16). Some systems, such as that depicted in Figure 12-15, have indicators on the bandages to assist the clinician in stretching the bandage to the correct tension. All of the commercially available kits provide a layer for absorption of drainage and utilize short-stretch bandages. Short-stretch bandages provide compression effectively both at rest and during muscle contraction. Long-stretch bandages, such as ACE

wraps (3M), must be pulled with great tension and may provide excessive pressure at rest. During exercise, these bandages give too easily and do not provide as much compression as a short-stretch bandage. Regardless of the type of compression system used, the clinician must ensure that the bandaging does not create excessive pressure and must provide the patient with emergency information of how and under what conditions to remove the compression bandaging. A simple test is to check capillary refill (Figure 12-17). Compression pumps and bandages should be used until the clinician is certain that edema has been removed as much as possible. This is determined most objectively by serial measurements with a foot volumeter, although multiple girth measurements along the leg or the figure 8 measurement may be used. When volume of the leg is no longer decreasing with compression, the patient should be fitted for custom compression stockings (Figure 12-18). The clinician must check the other leg to determine if venous insufficiency is also present in that extremity.

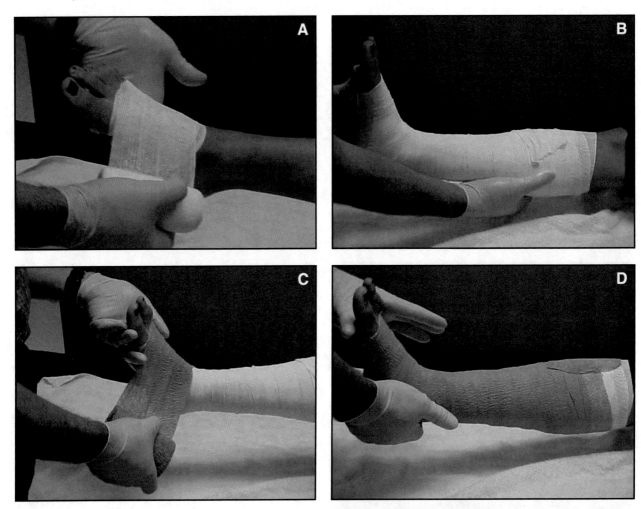

Figure 12-14. (A) Application of an Unna's boot. Application begins around the metatarsal heads with the bandage applied in a figure 8 fashion proximally. (B) Completed application of the Unna's boot paste bandage. (C) Second layer consists of cohesive bandaging. (D) Complete Unna's boot application with paste bandage and cohesive bandage. (E) Residue left on patient's leg and foot from the Unna's boot.

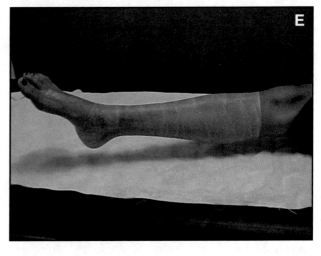

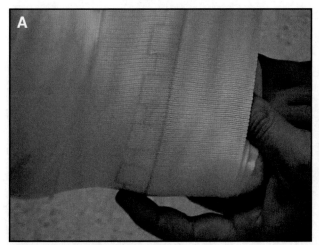
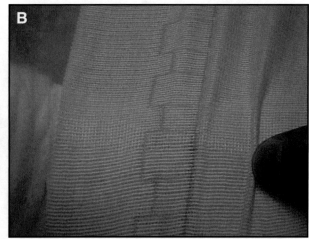

Figure 12-15. (A) Two-layer bandage application. Markings on the elasticized bandage indicate appropriate tension to produce the desired pressure when applied in the half-overlapping spiral technique. Short quadrangles are stretched into squares to produce approximately 30 mm Hg pressure on the leg. (B) Further stretching causes larger quadrangles to form squares and produce approximately 50 mm Hg pressure.

Applying Multilayer Bandaging

In multilayer bandaging systems, the first layer is a layer of absorbent batting that absorbs drainage and fills irregular areas such as those around the malleolus where pressure may be low without appropriate padding. Another layer is a short-stretch bandage; therefore, the minimal multilayer bandage has 2 layers. Some short-stretch bandages have calibrated markings to indicate the amount of pressure that will be exerted by the bandage at a given length as shown in Figure 12-15. Typically, rectangles are elongated into squares when the appropriate tension is achieved. An outside layer of cohesive bandage is frequently the last component of the multilayer bandage system. This layer prevents the short-stretch bandage from becoming dislodged and sliding down the leg. In a 4-layer system, the second layer, which goes over the absorbent batting, is a moderate-stretch bandage; the third layer is a short-stretch bandage; and the fourth layer is a cohesive bandage. This type of bandage should be left in place as long as feasible, which, typically, is about 7 days. Both half-overlapping spirals and figure 8s have been suggested for various layers of the bandaging systems. Half-overlapping spirals are simpler to apply but unravel more readily and may not control venous hypertension as well. A figure 8 is difficult for the novice but can be performed almost as quickly as a spiral wrap by an experienced clinician. The figure 8 method appears to control venous hypertension more effectively. Kits are generally designed such that the short-stretch bandages are wrapped in a figure 8 and other layers are applied in half-overlapping spirals. When using a kit, follow the manufacturer's directions for wrapping each layer. The length of each bandage supplied is based on whether a half-overlapping spiral or figure 8 technique is to

be used. The figure 8 technique uses much more bandage length. Using a figure 8 for a layer that the manufacturer instructs using a half-overlapping spiral is likely to result in having insufficient bandage length.

Unna's Boot

Several techniques have been used to apply an Unna's boot. A figure 8 allows some movement between layers and dissipation of excessive pressure. Other options include creating a figure 8 with strips instead of rolling the bandage around the limb. This technique is suggested to allow more give than a figure 8 being rolled. Others simply use half-overlapping spirals and go up, back down, and up again as the length of the bandage allows. Periodic smoothing of the paste on the Unna's boot should be done as the bandage is applied to provide more even distribution of the paste.

General Wrapping Considerations

Bandaging should produce a greater pressure at the ankle and be progressively decreased as the bandage is wrapped more proximally. This pressure gradient can be automatically developed during the bandaging process by applying equal tension to the bandage as wrapping proceeds. Based on the law of LaPlace, tension equals pressure times radius ($\tau = P \times r$, where τ = tension in the bandage, P = pressure generated by the bandage on the limb, and r = radius of the limb). Therefore, wrapping the bandage with a constant tension on the bandage as it is advanced from the foot toward the knee results in a greater pressure at the foot where the radius of the turns of the bandage is

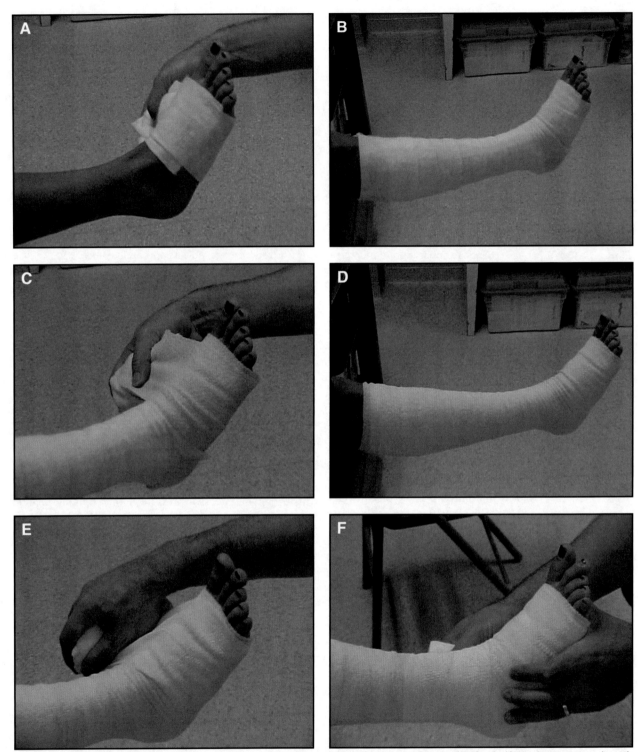

Figure 12-16. Four-layer compression bandaging. (A) First layer of absorbent material is applied in half-overlapping spirals with particular attention to filling areas around the malleolus. (B) Completion of the first layer. (C) Beginning of half-overlapping spiral technique with the light-stretch bandage. (D) Completion of the second layer. (E) Beginning of third layer, the short-stretch bandage, in a figure 8 technique. (F) Foot completed; starting up the leg with the short-stretch bandage. *(continued)*

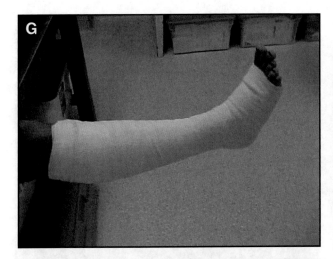

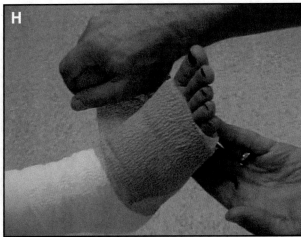

Figure 12-16 (continued). (G) Completion of third layer. Note the diamond pattern generated by the figure 8 technique. (H) Beginning of fourth layer, the cohesive bandage. (I) Completion of the fourth layer.

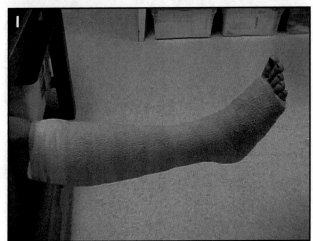

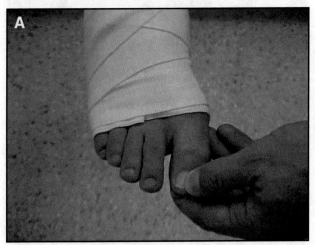

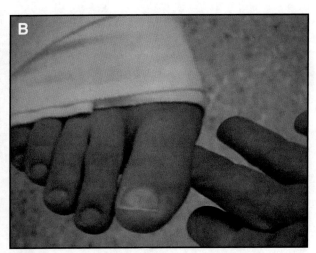

Figure 12-17. Compressing the great toenail for testing capillary refill.

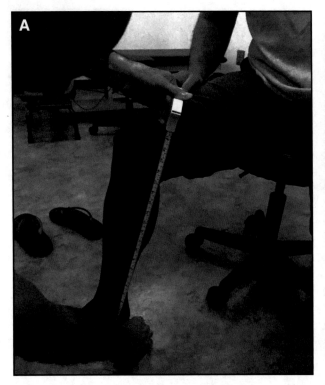

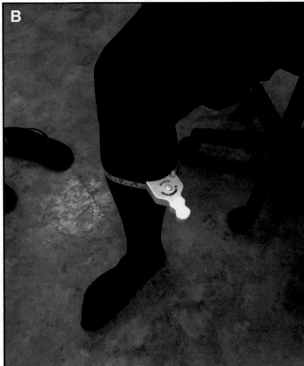

Figure 12-18. Measurement for knee-high compression stockings. (A) Measuring from the floor to the crease of the knee. (B) Measuring the widest circumference around the leg. (C) Measuring the smallest circumference around the ankle. A spring-loaded tape is used to ensure consistent measurements.

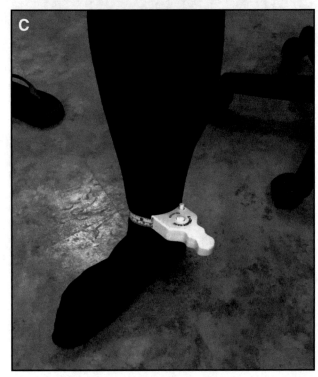

small, and pressure is lower approaching the knee where the radius of the leg becomes largest.

Using multiple bandages or layers of bandages creates a somewhat more complex situation. An equation used to account for multiple layers and different widths of bandages is given as $P = NTk/CW$, where N = number of layers, T = tension, k is a constant, C = circumference, and W = width of the bandage. The practical implications of this equation are (1) more layers create a greater pressure on the limb; (2) with increasing circumference, pressure is reduced; (3) narrower bandages create more pressure; and (4) if one desires to create less pressure proximally, greater-width bandages may be used as one proceeds from distally to proximally. The last implication is the constant in the equation. The actual pressure generated on the limb during simple compression bandaging is not known but can only be estimated. Experience is needed to ensure that bandaging produces an effective pressure on the limb.

Contraindications for Compression Therapy

The most important aspect of treating venous insufficiency is to first rule out arterial insufficiency. Although a clear diagnosis of venous insufficiency may be made, arterial insufficiency must be ruled out thoroughly because some people may have both. Compression therapy will exacerbate arterial insufficiency and may threaten the limb. Various experts suggest that an ankle-brachial index (ABI) of < 0.8 to 0.7 is a contraindication for compression. Some sources suggest using a lighter compression between 0.7 and 0.8. Others express confidence in using light compression down to an ABI of 0.6. As a practical rule, do not apply compression when a patient has an ABI value between 0.7 and 0.8 unless you are certain that the patient will be attentive to any problems that might occur with the compression. If the ability of the patient or caregiver to recognize and act on an emergency situation is questionable, compression should be reserved for a limb with an ABI of 0.8 or greater. Other absolute contraindications for compression include phlebitis and suspected deep venous thrombosis. Relative contraindications include conditions in which mobilization of fluid would occur from the lower extremities to a central circulation that cannot handle the extra fluid (congestive heart failure and pulmonary edema). Diminished sensation is considered a relative contraindication because of the lack of ability to detect conditions that could injure the patient.

Although an episode of care with a patient may end, compression therapy does not. In a patient with unilateral disease, the patient should be switched from multilayer compression bandaging to compression stockings when either both limbs are the same size, or limb volume or

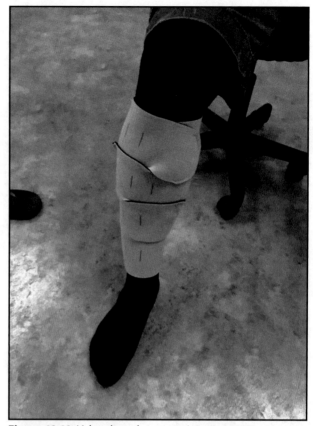

Figure 12-19. Velcro-based compression garment.

circumference reaches a steady value and does not decrease further. In patients with bilateral disease, multilayer bandages are discontinued when there is no further change in limb volume. Patients have many more palatable choices for compression stockings now. Many are not obvious to laypeople and can be quite fashionable.

For patients needing continued higher compression, a number of strap and Velcro-based options are available, including the Circaid Juxtalite (Medi) depicted in Figure 12-19.

Exercise

Exercise programs have been used to improve skin blood flow and reduce edema in patients with chronic venous insufficiency. Another study also demonstrated a greater rate of wound closure. A period of 3 months of exercise, regardless of compression, improved skin perfusion relative to compression alone or a control group. Exercise can involve simple dorsiflexion exercise (10 contractions per hour while awake); however, a more comprehensive program of combined treadmill walking, stationary cycling, and lower extremity resistance exercise may produce improvements in both muscle-pumping activity and venous function.

LYMPHEDEMA

Although wounds are usually not considered to be the primary problem with lymphedema, many individuals, especially those with severe lower extremity lymphedema, will develop ulcers. A brief description of the lymphatic system and lymphedema and its treatment as it relates to ulcers follows.

Lymphatic Anatomy

The lymphatic system consists of small blind-end lymphatic capillaries that tend to follow small arterioles, venules, and blood capillaries. The ends of the lymphatic capillaries consist of flaplike structures that close off the vessel when the interstitial fluid volume is low and open as fluid accumulates. The presence of valves within lymphatic vessels allows forward movement of lymph to occur. Propulsion of lymph toward the subclavian veins is due to intrinsic contractility of lymphatic vessels, external compression of lymphatic vessels by muscle contraction or other forces, the negative pressure in the thorax during inspiration, and pulsation of the descending aorta and other arteries.

From lymphatic capillaries, lymph moves proximally through progressively larger lymphatic vessels. These larger vessels enter lymph nodes in several characteristic locations where lymph is exposed to elements of the immune system. Under normal conditions, pathogens are destroyed, but in some cases, the persistence of bacteria or other pathogens stimulates the proliferation of immune cells in the nodes and the swelling termed *lymphadenitis*. Should lymphatic defenses be overwhelmed, erosion of the lymph node and overlying skin may occur. Infection spreading along lymphatic vessels produces the red streaks in the skin known as *lymphangitis*. Failure of the lymphatics to clear pathogens allows them to enter the bloodstream and produce septicemia.

Lymphatic drainage from the right upper quadrant of the body drains into the right lymphatic duct and then into the right subclavian vein. The remainder of the drainage enters the thoracic duct and then into the left subclavian vein. Lymphatic drainage is increased with increased interstitial volume and may increase by a factor of approximately 10-fold. Other factors that stimulate drainage are muscle contraction and deep breathing. Creating a robust negative pressure within the thorax creates a pressure gradient driving lymph flow proximally.

Lymphatic Terminology

An area of the body between sites of lymphatic drainage is called a *watershed*, analogous to an area of land that might drain into one or another body of water. Watersheds have been mapped out through the body, and one can obtain various charts demonstrating them. Obstruction of lymphatic vessels within a watershed produces lymphedema in characteristic locations. One of the theories of lymphedema treatment is that lymphatic drainage can be redistributed to different watersheds that are not obstructed. A segment of lymphatic vessel between valves is termed a *lymphangion*. Like veins, valves allow external forces to move lymph into the next proximal lymphangion by only allowing the external force to move the lymph forward.

Lymphatic Pathophysiology

In many places in the world, lymphedema is usually caused by a worm passed through mosquitoes. *Wuchereria bancrofti* infests the lymphatic system, causing obstruction. In Western civilization, most lymphedema is due to injury to the lymphatic system from surgery and radiation therapy for cancer. Breast cancer and uterine cancer treatment are common causes of upper and lower extremity lymphedema, respectively. Because another disorder causes these types of lymphedema, they are termed *secondary lymphedema*.

A small number of cases of lymphedema are primary. In primary lymphedema, the lymphatic system does not develop normally, compromising the ability to return fluid and protein from the interstitial space. Primary lymphedema may be present at birth (congenital lymphedema, 10% of primary lymphedema). A specific type of congenital lymphedema called *Milroy's disease* accounts for 2% of primary lymphedema. In Milroy's disease, lymphatic vessels fail to develop normally due to a genetic defect (autosomal dominant) in a specific type of vascular endothelial growth factor. Lymphedema may be delayed until later in childhood or young adulthood in the disorder called *lymphedema praecox*. By definition, lymphedema praecox, the most common primary lymphedema, is not apparent at birth but develops before the age of 35. Lymphedema developing after the age of 35 represents 10% of primary lymphedema. It is termed *lymphedema tarda* or *Meige disease*. In all forms of primary lymphedema, lymphatic vessels fail to develop normally.

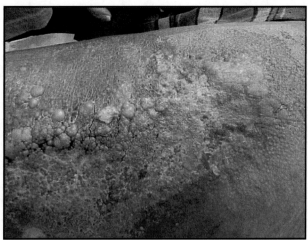

Figure 12-20. Appearance of skin in lymphedema. (The image is a copyrighted product of AAWC [www.aawconline.org] and has been reproduced with permission.)

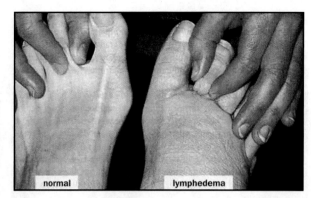

Figure 12-21. Stemmer sign. (The image is a copyrighted product of AAWC [www.aawconline.org] and has been reproduced with permission.)

Characteristics of Skin Injury Secondary to Lymphatic Disease

Skin impairment with lymphedema is generally more severe than with the edema of venous disease, although wounds may not develop until severe skin injury is evident. In the most severe cases, the skin eventually becomes thick, redundant, and wrinkled, similar to the skin of elephants, leading to the term *elephantiasis*. The greater loss of protein into the interstitial space produces much of the appearance of the skin, as shown in Figure 12-20. Along with retention of fluid, excessive protein in the interstitial space causes fibrosis and puckering of the skin in a pattern known as *peau d'orange* (orange peel–like). Hemosiderin staining and bacterial and fungal infections of the skin are also common. Maintaining dry, clean skin may become impossible with severe lymphedema, leading to fungal infection and bacterial superinfection.

A common diagnostic test for lymphedema is the Stemmer sign. The edema secondary to lymphatic disease frequently prevents the lifting of the skin distal to the metacarpophalangeal joints. A positive Stemmer sign, as shown in Figure 12-21, results when one cannot grasp the skin on the dorsum of the second toe or finger distal to its metacarpophalangeal/metatarsophalangeal joint or grasping the skin is difficult compared with grasping the same area on an uninvolved side. By definition, only the second digit is used for the Stemmer sign. A positive Stemmer sign is virtually predictive of lymphedema. However, a negative Stemmer sign (one is able to grasp the skin) does not rule out early or mild lymphedema.

Stages of Lymphatic Disease

For diagnosis and treatment, lymphedema is categorized into 4 stages. Stage 0 represents a preclinical presentation, and stage 3 is the most advanced form. A person in stage 0 has a diminished lymphatic transport capacity, but the diminished functional reserve has not yet been challenged to allow manifestations of lymphatic disease to become evident. For example, consider a patient who received surgical and radiologic intervention for uterine cancer many years ago. For all of this time, she has had a diminished capacity to transport lymph from the right lower extremity. However, the need to transport lymph (lymphatic load) had not exceeded its reserve. At this point, she would be said to be in the latency substage of stage 0. Patients in this stage must be counseled about risk factors that could allow them to exceed their lymphatic drainage capacity. However, after many years, people in this stage may begin to ignore this counseling.

As a consequence, a stressful event may tip the balance of lymphatic load to a point exceeding reserve. For example, the woman described needs to mow her lawn after many consecutive rainy days. The grass becomes progressively longer and does not dry sufficiently. The weather is also hot and humid. The heat combined with the physical effort of pushing a lawn mower through long, wet grass results in a much greater lymphatic load than she has experienced since her uterine cancer treatment. After more than 10 years of no consequences of subclinical lymphatic disease, demand finally exceeds lymphatic transport, and lymphedema becomes clinically evident.

Stage 1 is also termed the *reversible stage*. Simple elevation allows the edema to resolve. Pitting edema occurs, but tissue properties are unaltered. No changes in skin color or texture have occurred. Appropriate therapy at this stage is expected to result in a return to normal limb volume. Lack of appropriate therapy may allow the disease to progress to stage 2. Another term for stage 2 is *spontaneously*

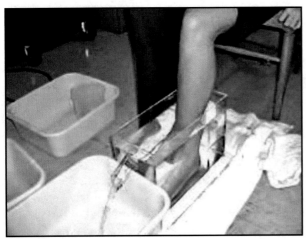

Figure 12-22. Use of a foot volumeter.

irreversible lymphedema. The name implies that simple elevation is no longer sufficient to return the limb to its premorbid volume. At this stage, a positive Stemmer sign is expected. Tissue fibrosis and cellulitis are also expected at this stage. Often, lymphedema stabilizes at stage 2. Therapy may be effective in reducing limb volume, but lack of appropriate therapy and development of chronic cellulitis may allow progression to stage 3 lymphedema. Stage 3 is known as *lymphostatic elephantiasis.* Skin becomes hardened to the extent that pitting becomes difficult or no longer occurs, and the Stemmer sign becomes more evident. Skin creases become very deep and pronounced to the point of disfigurement. Hyperkeratosis, fungal infections, and darkening of the skin are common. Papillomas and cysts frequently appear as well as open wounds in the forms of ulcers and fistulas. Treatment at this stage is possible, but restoring limb volume will require more extensive treatment than if it had been initiated during stages 1 or 2.

History

In addition to routine questions for anybody with an open wound, the patients should be asked about the onset of the lymphedema. Lymphedema can be a primary disease or, much more commonly, secondary to surgical and radiation treatment for cancer. Primary lymphedema can occur early in life or much later. In addition, secondary lymphedema can be somewhat remote from the event responsible for it. Recent overexertion, particularly in the heat; infection; or wearing clothing or jewelry that is too tight might convert latent lymphedema to overt lymphedema. History should include events such as surgery that might have been responsible as well as recent events that may have caused the lymphatics to be overwhelmed. Issues that the patient is having with work or home, such as dressing, ambulation, and others, should be ascertained.

Physical Examination

Specific to lymphedema, a patient should be examined for any impairments that might affect the performance of activities. For lower extremity lymphedema, gait should be examined. Range of motion, strength and sensation, posture, and performance of activities of daily living should be assessed. The Stemmer sign is a test specifically for lymphedema. The clinician attempts to pinch the skin on either the second toe or finger of the involved extremity. The inability to pinch a fold of skin is a positive test for lymphedema.

Either volume or girth is performed as an outcome measure. Volumeters are available for both upper and lower extremities and just a hand or foot. A foot volumeter and its use are depicted in Figure 12-22. Various formulas for estimating volume based on measurements at specific sites along an extremity have been developed. Another option is to measure at specific sites before treatment and repeat at intervals during an episode of care. Volumetry is more accurate in determining volume, but it is time consuming and creates extra work due to infection control. As an alternative, girth measurements need to be performed at standardized locations that are repeatable, and a tape measure with a calibrated spring improves the reliability of the measurements.

Treatment of Lymphatic Disease

Many therapies have been developed for lymphatic disease. Like venous disease, successful treatment involves an intensive period of compression therapy followed by lifetime maintenance of compression.

Complete Decongestive Therapy

Complete decongestive therapy (CDT) is an involved program requiring extensive and expensive training. Training programs require several weeks and may be divided into specific course levels. The CDT treatment regimen consists of manual lymph drainage (MLD), compression bandaging, "remedial exercises," and patient education on skin care.

Compression Pumping

Practitioners of CDT discourage the use of compression pumps due to the risk of rare cases of genital edema. Home units of sequential compression pumps are routinely used to treat lymphedema. Pressure is kept at 50 mm Hg or below to prevent compressing lymphatics for 2 to 4 hours/day. Compression garments or bandaging are used between compression pumping.

Patient Education

Skin care is a significant element of patient education. Keeping the skin moist and healthy is emphasized as well as avoiding any injuries or swelling. Patients are instructed to avoid the excessive activity of the affected limb, avoid excessive heat, and elevate the limb whenever feasible. Patients are also instructed to wear gloves when gardening, avoid any activity that might injure the extremity, and promptly address any injury to the skin of that extremity.

Compression Bandaging

Compression bandaging commonly used for lymphedema is somewhat different in terms of the materials used for venous disease. Foam sheets are frequently used in the place of absorbent batting material with the hope of breaking up fibrosis. Short-stretch bandages of different widths are used depending on the girth of the limb. Unlike compression bandaging for venous disease, the digits are also wrapped as demonstrated in Figure 12-23.

Exercise

Exercise of the affected extremity(ies) is encouraged with compression bandaging in place. Compression bandages produce the counterpressure necessary to offset capillary hydrostatic pressure and encourage fluid uptake from the extremity. Exercise without compression may lead to exacerbation of edema. Practitioners of CDT have specific exercises, but any exercise that generates a muscle-pumping action without unduly increasing arterial inflow and capillary leakage of fluid may be used. Like MLD, which is described in the following section, a strategy of clearing the lymphatic pathway at its most proximal point and moving distally is applied for exercise as well. As a consequence, neck and then shoulder exercises precede elbow exercises; the wrist and hand should be last. Moderate weights that can be lifted for at least 30 repetitions should be used, and the patient should be wearing compression bandaging during exercise. Deep breathing is also incorporated into the exercise program to move lymph from the cisterna chyli into the thorax.

Manual Lymphatic Drainage

MLD is touted as the primary component of CDT. It uses specific massagelike skin strokes with light pressure to encourage the movement of lymph and the development of alternate pathways around obstructed vessels. MLD is begun at the neck to clear the appropriate duct (right or thoracic) or both to encourage the movement of lymph through both sides based on the analogy of traffic on a road that needs to be cleared ahead before the traffic behind can

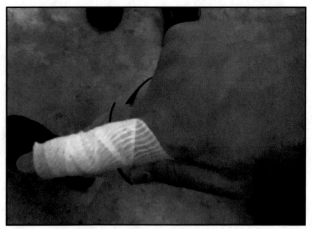

Figure 12-23. Wrapping of fingers for lymphedema.

move. MLD is progressed distally as vessels ahead of the obstruction are "cleared." MLD must be immediately followed by compression bandaging that needs to be left in place between MLD treatments to be effective.

LIPEDEMA

Lipedema is a condition that can be confused with lymphedema but is believed to be more prevalent than lymphedema. Lipedema is an accumulation of adipose tissue that affects the person below the waist, but in some individuals, it can affect the upper extremities. The feet are spared, and the Stemmer sign is negative. Lipedema affects women, whereas lymphedema can affect men and women, but women in developed countries are more likely to develop lymphedema than men because of the treatment of breast cancer. Liposuction can be used, but removing large quantities of tissue may damage the lymphatics, leading to lymphedema. However, without treatment, lipedema can lead to lymphedema, venous insufficiency, or both. When both lipedema and lymphedema are present, the term *lipolymphedema* is used. An individual could also have venolymphedema, venolipedema, or venolipolymphedema. Therefore, the evaluation needs to distinguish among lipedema, lymphedema, venous insufficiency, a combination of 2 of them, or all 3 of them.

ARTERIAL DISEASE

Although we commonly discuss arterial disease in terms of either intermittent claudication or gangrene of the toes, it is frequently asymptomatic, particularly in early, mild disease with an ABI just below 0.9. In addition, denial of symptoms by curtailing activity to avoid leg pain may contribute to "asymptomatic" arterial disease. Lack

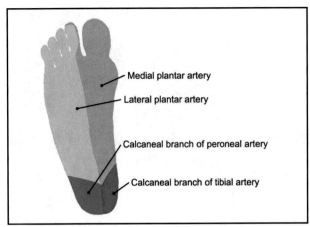

Figure 12-24. Angiosomes of the foot.

of perfusion to tissue can lead to a number of early symptoms discussed in Chapter 8 that can be confused with normal aging because peripheral arterial disease itself is associated with aging. Thus, arterial disease can often be ignored up to and even in the presence of tissue necrosis.

Atherosclerosis is, by far, the most common cause of peripheral arterial disease. Common risk factors include smoking, hypertension, diabetes mellitus, hypercholesterolemia, and lack of physical activity. As arterial disease progresses, tissue served by the involved vessels may progress through loss of reserve function, atrophy, and finally necrosis. In addition to atherosclerosis, blood vessels may be diseased by infection or autoimmune disease, including infectious arteritis, polyarteritis nodosa, hypersensitivity vasculitis, and Buerger's disease (thromboangiitis obliterans). The smaller arterial vessels, arterioles, may also be injured, particularly with hypertension and diabetes mellitus.

The degree of vascular impairment can be described using Fontaine's clinical classification. Grade I is used for a person who is asymptomatic, but disease can be detected with testing, such as the ABI being less than 0.9. Grade II is used to describe a person who experiences intermittent claudication. Grade II is further divided into IIa, in which leg pain does not limit the person's lifestyle, and IIb, in which leg pain does limit what the person can do. Grade III is used to describe a person with pain or paresthesia at rest, whereas established gangrene or trophic lesions are evident in grade IV.

Wounds Associated With Arterial Disease

Ischemic ulcers are the result of tissue necrosis secondary to arterial insufficiency of a limb, usually due to atherosclerosis. In addition to tissue necrosis, arterial disease also slows the healing of wounds of other etiologies. In particular, the combination of neuropathy and foot ischemia increases the risk of developing foot ulcers that heal very slowly or not at all, requiring amputation. Other causes of ischemic ulcers include sickle cell disease, Buerger's disease (thromboangiitis obliterans), Raynaud's disease, Raynaud's phenomenon secondary to scleroderma and other autoimmune diseases, and primary forms of vasculitis. Types of primary vasculitis include Wegener's granulomatosis, microscopic polyangiitis, Henoch-Schönlein purpura, polyarteritis nodosa, cryoglobulinemia, Kawasaki disease, giant cell arteritis, Takayasu's arteritis, and Behçet's disease.

Because the most common form of arterial disease encountered is atherosclerotic, measurement of the ABI should be performed to assess the severity of arterial disease. A value below 0.8 to 0.7 is indicative of arterial disease. In a patient with an ABI below 0.45, healing is unlikely. Claudication is likely to occur before the ABI becomes this low in physically active individuals. However, many with arterial disease do not exert themselves enough physically to experience claudication until the ABI falls below 0.5. Segmental blood pressure measurements along the extremity may isolate the area of occlusion noninvasively. A time-consuming but functional test is TcPO$_2$. This test should be available in a vascular lab to determine the point along the extremity at which oxygen delivery to tissues is compromised. Imaging studies including duplex ultrasound, magnetic resonance angiography, and angiography using contrast may be required for surgical planning.

Large-vessel atherosclerosis of the iliac, femoral, popliteal, and tibial arteries may be detected and repaired by bypass surgery or removal of specific blockages. However, smaller-vessel disease can produce ischemia within specific areas of tissue supplied by these smaller arterial branches. These tissue areas are known as *angiosomes*. Angiosomes are analogous to dermatomes in that a map of blood vessels serving regions of the skin is analyzed for the source of the blockage. Just as one would test dermatomes to determine which nerve root may be responsible for a problem, angiosomes indicate which artery might be occluded. This way, a vascular surgeon could attempt to reopen a specific small artery rather than performing a bypass of one of the large arteries such as the popliteal or anterior tibial. Proponents of this approach state a decrease in the number of amputations. An angiosome map of the plantar foot is shown in Figure 12-24.

In the most common case of atherosclerosis of the lower extremity, tissues at the highest risk of necrosis are the most distal structures. Normally, blood pressure does not dissipate much as flows travels along blood vessels of the lower extremity. However, with the obstruction of arterial vessels characteristic of atherosclerotic plaque and thrombosis, necrosis occurs in tissues distal to the obstruction, usually on the foot, especially the toes. However, small arteries anywhere in the extremities can be involved. Ischemia of the posterior heel due to obstruction of the small branches serving this tissue has been misdiagnosed as pressure injuries due to the location despite abundant history pointing to arterial disease. These wounds tend to be deep wounds with irregular borders outlining the arterial distribution involved.

Manifestations of Arterial Disease

The 3 major types of ischemic necrosis of the extremities are wet gangrene, dry gangrene, and mummification. In wet gangrene, liquefactive necrosis is possible due to the presence of enzymes capable of degrading necrotic tissue. In dry gangrene, necrosis occurs too quickly for any breakdown. The tissue loses fluid volume and becomes progressively discolored. Early gangrene may produce a subtle purple color indicative of deoxygenation caused by thrombosis of vessels with the sluggish flow. The gradual loss of tissue volume is accompanied by the progressive darkening/black color of dry gangrene. In mummification, the tissue outline is relatively preserved, with a wrinkled appearance of the skin. Examples of the effects of arterial disease are shown in Figure 12-25.

Many authorities recommend that dry gangrene not be debrided because it acts as dressing to protect the tissue beneath it. Debridement of dry gangrene is discouraged because debridement exposes necrotic tissue that can quickly support pathogenic organisms and allow disseminated infection. Severe ischemia requires revascularization or surgical amputation. In some cases, autoamputation occurs in which the necrotic tissue, often a toe, withers and falls off the limb.

Conservative treatment for arterial disease consists of local wound care, but dry gangrene should not be debrided. Reduction of risk factors such as smoking, elevated blood glucose, hypertension, hyperlipidemia, and limb protection can be offered to the patient. Seemingly trivial mechanical trauma may produce ulcers. Padding, lotions, absorption of excess moisture, and the use of assistive and adaptive devices may help protect limbs at risk for developing infection or injury.

Pharmacologic treatment for arterial insufficiency includes thrombolytic drugs, anticoagulants, vasodilators, and pentoxifylline (Trental). Surgical treatment provided

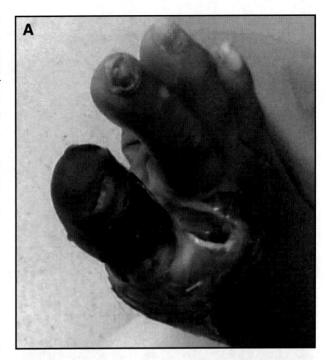

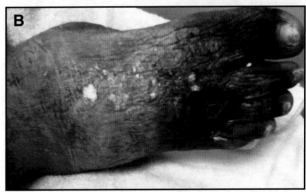

Figure 12-25. Arterial disease of feet. (A) Dry gangrene on great toe with wet gangrene in webspace. (B) Mummification.

by vascular surgeons or interventional radiologists includes bypass surgery, endarterectomy, and percutaneous transluminal angioplasty.

Exercise for Peripheral Arterial Disease

Exercise recommendations for improving claudication and function are described in the 2016 American Heart Association/American College of Cardiology guideline for management of lower extremity peripheral arterial disease. Basic components are walking 3 or more times/week at an intensity that elicits pain of 3 of 4 on the claudication pain scale (moderate pain) for 30 to 45 minutes per session, excluding rest breaks. Rest breaks are necessary to allow the

TABLE 12-3
Characteristics of Arterial, Venous, and Lymphatic Wounds

CHARACTERISTIC	ARTERIAL	VENOUS	LYMPHATIC
Location	Distal, especially toes	Mostly superior to medial malleolus	Affected extremity
Appearance	Depression, loss of skin volume with dry gangrene; poor quality tissue with wet gangrene	Wet, often with good granulation; may have some quantity of slough	Hyperpigmented, thickened skin; may have fissuring
Pain	Painful	May range from uncomfortable to bursting type of pain	Variable
History and physical exam	Hypertension, diabetes, smoking, skin atrophy, loss of hair on extremity, complaints of claudication	Standing, varicose veins, aching legs	Cancer, radiation, lymph node removal, swelling that initially resolved with position

individual to tolerate the exercise training. Improvements in circulation are likely from the response to ischemia; therefore, exercise while experiencing claudication appears to be necessary for optimum outcomes. Seated rest breaks should last until pain is resolved. In addition, resistance and flexibility exercises are recommended for improving general health.

Martorell Ulcer

The Martorell hypertensive ischemic leg ulcer occurs near the ankle (posterolateral leg) in older men and women (mean age of 74) who have a long history of hypertension. Subcutaneous arteriolosclerosis causes small arterial vessels to become calcified and narrowed, leading to a shallow, necrotic, rapidly enlarging wound. All patients with this type of ulcer have hypertension, and 58% have diabetes. However, this type of ulcer is much less prevalent than hypertension. These data indicate that hypertension is necessary but not sufficient for the development of this ulcer. The ABI is normal. A biopsy is needed to confirm the diagnosis.

SUMMARY

Arterial, venous, and lymphatic disease can create ulcers requiring skilled assessment and therapy. A thorough differential diagnosis is critical. Arterial disease can create an emergent surgical problem, and treatment for chronic venous insufficiency may need to be modified or may be contraindicated in the presence of arterial insufficiency. Arterial insufficiency may occur anywhere but is most common where vessels are the most distal (ie, on the toes and heels). Venous ulcers are located most commonly just proximal to the medial malleolus, sometimes proximal to the lateral malleolus, and rarely elsewhere. Arterial insufficiency can be painful at rest, increasing with elevation, and the wounds tend to be pink rather than red. Venous insufficiency may cause uncomfortable pressure in the leg, which is relieved by elevation, and the wounds tend to be red and very wet with hemosiderin staining of the skin surrounding the ulcer. Failure to treat the underlying venous hypertension is a frequent cause of failure to heal or recurrence of the venous leg ulcers. Compression therapy includes compression bandaging, pumping, and fitting for custom stockings when edema is removed. A comparison of the 3 major types of vascular disorders is given in Table 12-3.

QUESTIONS

1. Contrast venous and arterial anatomy.
2. What is the role of the venous valve, particularly in the lower extremities?
3. What are the roles of the deep, superficial, and perforator veins?
4. How does fascia interact with the 3 types of veins?
5. What should happen to venous pressure when one
   a. Stands from sitting or lying
   b. Sits
   c. Walks
6. What mechanisms prevent venous reflux?

7. What is venous hypertension?

8. What is meant by chronic ambulatory venous hypertension?

9. What are the 3 underlying causes of venous hypertension?

10. What is typically in the history of a patient with a venous ulcer?

11. Why are the greater saphenous veins particularly susceptible to venous hypertension?

12. What is the most common location of a venous ulcer?

13. What is the usual appearance of a venous ulcer?

14. What is lipodermatosclerosis?

15. Why does skin injury result from venous hypertension?

16. What surgical options are available for venous disease?

17. What is the CEAP system?

18. Why do primary venous disease and reflux usually go together?

19. Why do secondary venous disease and obstruction usually go together?

20. Why is compression the major component of the plan of care for venous ulcers?

21. Why is the ABI measured in patients with venous disease?

22. What values of ABI are considered safe for compression therapy?

23. What is the risk when patients have neuropathy as well as venous hypertension?

24. What is the implication of the law of Laplace with respect to applying a compression bandage?

25. What is considered the gold standard for venous leg ulcer compression?

26. What are the advantages and disadvantages of using an Unna's boot for compression?

27. Where should bandaging for venous insufficiency start? Why?

28. What should be done to ensure that compression bandaging is not too tight?

29. How do we know when compression bandaging or pumping should end?

30. When the leg's volume is stabilized, what must be done next? For how long?

31. Why is whirlpool therapy contraindicated for venous ulcers?

32. What is the typical appearance of lymphedema?

33. Contrast pitting edema of venous disease with brawny edema of lymphedema.

34. What are the typical problems with lymphedema?

35. Define the 3 stages of lymphedema.

36. What is the Stemmer sign?

37. What options are available for measuring limb volume?

38. What are the advantages and disadvantages of limb circumference measurements and volumetry?

39. What is the relationship between lymphedema and edema associated with venous disease?

40. How is lipedema distinguished from lymphedema?

41. What is the gold standard for peripheral arterial testing by physical therapists?

42. What is the normal value for ABI?

43. What does a value of ABI greater than 1.3 mean?

44. Peripheral arterial disease is diagnosed at what value of ABI?

45. What value of ABI is considered to be critical limb ischemia?

46. What are the typical symptoms of peripheral arterial disease?

47. What are the typical signs of peripheral arterial disease?

48. What can physical therapists do for arterial disease?

BIBLIOGRAPHY

Aggarwal S, Moore RD, Arena R, et al. Rehabilitation therapy in peripheral arterial disease. *Can J Cardiol*. 2016;32(10 Suppl 2):S374-S381.

Andriessen A, Apelqvist J, Mosti G, Partsch H, Gonska C, Abel M. Compression therapy for venous leg ulcers: risk factors for adverse events and complications, contraindications—a review of present guidelines. *J Eur Acad Dermatol Venereol*. 2017;31(9):1562-1568.

Bauer AT, von Lukowicz D, Lossagk K, et al. New insights on Lipedema: the enigmatic disease of the peripheral fat. *Plast Reconstr Surg*. 2019;144(6):1475-1484.

Bonkemeyer Millan S, Gan R, Townsend PE. Venous ulcers: diagnosis and treatment. *Am Fam Physician*. 2019;100(5):298-305.

Couch KS, Corbett L, Gould L, Girolami S, Bolton L. The international consolidated venous ulcer guideline update 2015: process improvement, evidence analysis, and future goals. *Ostomy Wound Manage*. 2017;63(5):42-46.

Cowan T. Strategies for improving outcomes in venous leg ulcer care. *J Wound Care*. 2018;27(7):456-457. doi:10.12968/jowc.2018.27.7.456

Crawford JM, Lal BK, Durán WN, Pappas PJ. Pathophysiology of venous ulceration. *J Vasc Surg Venous Lymphat Disord*. 2017;5(4):596-605.

de Carvalho MR. Comparison of outcomes in patients with venous leg ulcers treated with compression therapy alone versus combination of surgery and compression therapy: a systematic review. *J Wound Ostomy Continence Nurs*. 2015;42(1):42-46.

Finlayson K, Edwards H, Courtney M. Relationships between preventive activities, psychosocial factors and recurrence of venous leg ulcers: a prospective study. *J Adv Nurs*. 2011;67(10):2180-2190.

Gould DJ, El-Sabawi B, Goel P, Badash I, Colletti P, Patel KM. Uncovering lymphatic transport abnormalities in patients with primary lipedema. *J Reconstr Microsurg*. 2020;36(2):136-141.

Hedayati N, Carson JG, Chi YW, Link D. Management of mixed arterial venous lower extremity ulceration: a review. *Vasc Med*. 2015;20(5):479-486.

Karges JR, Mark BE, Stikeleather SJ, Worrell TW. Concurrent validity of upper-extremity volume estimates: comparison of calculated volume derived from girth measurements and water displacement volume. *Phys Ther.* 2003;83(2):134-145.

Levenhagen K, Davies C, Perdomo M, Ryans K, Gilchrist L. Diagnosis of upper quadrant lymphedema secondary to cancer: clinical practice guideline from the Oncology Section of the American Physical Therapy Association. *Phys Ther.* 2017;97(7):729-745.

Lloret P, Redondo P, Cabrera J, Sierra A. Treatment of venous leg ulcers with ultrasound-guided foam sclerotherapy: healing, long-term recurrence and quality of life evaluation. *Wound Repair Regen.* 2015;23(3):369-378.

Lurie F, Passman M, Meisner M, et al. The 2020 update of the CEAP classification system and reporting standards [published correction appears in *J Vasc Surg Venous Lymphat Disord.* 2021 Jan;9(1):288]. *J Vasc Surg Venous Lymphat Disord.* 2020;8(3):342-352. doi:10.1016/j.jvsv.2019.12.075

Milic DJ, Zivic SS, Bogdanovic DC, Karanovic ND, Golubovic ZV. Risk factors related to the failure of venous leg ulcers to heal with compression treatment. *J Vasc Surg.* 2009;49(5):1242-1247.

Mutlak O, Aslam M, Standfield NJ. An investigation of skin perfusion in venous leg ulcer after exercise. *Perfusion.* 2018;33(1):25-29.

Mutlak O, Aslam M, Standfield N. The influence of exercise on ulcer healing in patients with chronic venous insufficiency. *Int Angiol.* 2018;37(2):160-168.

Okhovat JP, Alavi A. Lipedema: a review of the literature. *Int J Low Extrem Wounds.* 2015;14(3):262-267.

Raffetto JD. Pathophysiology of chronic venous disease and venous ulcers. *Surg Clin North Am.* 2018; 98(2):337-347.

Silva AK, Chang DW. Vascularized lymph node transfer and lymphovenous bypass: novel treatment strategies for symptomatic lymphedema. *J Surg Oncol.* 2016;113(8):932-939.

Stather PW, Petty C, Howard AQ. Review of adjustable Velcro wrap devices for venous ulceration. *Int Wound J.* 2019;16(4):903-908.

Takahashi PY, Chandra A, Cha SS, Crane SJ. A predictive model for venous ulceration in older adults: results of a retrospective cohort study. *Ostomy Wound Manage.* 2010;56(4):60-66.

Tew GA, Gumber A, McIntosh E, et al. Effects of supervised exercise training on lower-limb cutaneous microvascular reactivity in adults with venous ulcers. *Eur J Appl Physiol.* 2018;118(2):321-329.

Tzani I, Tsichlaki M, Zerva E, Papathanasiou G, Dimakakos E. Physiotherapeutic rehabilitation of lymphedema: state-of-the-art. *Lymphology.* 2018;51(1):1-12.

Zasadzka E, Trzmiel T, Kleczewska M, Pawlaczyk M. Comparison of the effectiveness of complex decongestive therapy and compression bandaging as a method of treatment of lymphedema in the elderly. *Clin Interv Aging.* 2018;13:929-934.

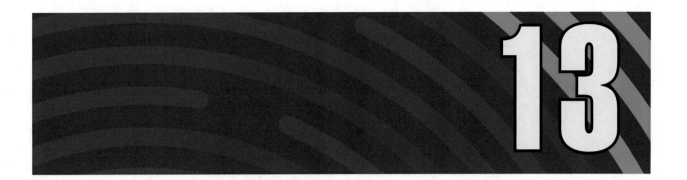

Traumatic and Surgical Wounds

Traumatic and surgical wounds are typically managed initially in the emergency department or by the surgeon creating the wound. Under some circumstances, acute wounds may be seen in other settings for debridement and possibly other interventions due to the wound's nature. Some acute wounds also carry a high risk of complications requiring prolonged intervention. Acute wounds may be referred to other clinicians in the cases of gross contamination requiring cleaning of the wound before closure, a blistered wound such as a second-degree burn over a large area, a third-degree burn over a small area, infection of an acute or surgical wound, the presence of unhealthy tissue within the wound such that primary closure is not feasible, a compromised immune system, dehiscence (defined later), and any other reason for tertiary/delayed primary closure.

Irion GL, Gardner JA, Pignataro RM.
Comprehensive Wound Management, Third Edition (pp 237-254).
© 2024 Taylor and Francis Group.

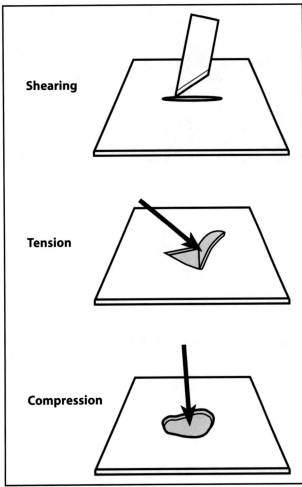

Figure 13-1. Mechanisms of lacerations.

TRAUMATIC WOUNDS

Lacerations

Lacerations are among the most common wounds seen in emergency departments. As occurs with any acute wound, lacerations typically have a high risk of contamination. Frequently, however, they can be cleansed sufficiently to allow primary closure with sutures, glue, staples, or tape. They are caused by 3 basic mechanisms: shearing, tension, and compression (Figure 13-1). A shearing injury is created by a small amount of energy focused on a small area, basically a sharp edge such as a knife or broken glass. These wounds are the equivalent of a surgical incision, except that the injuries are not created with sterile conditions. The tissue is divided, but minimal cell injury occurs beyond the sharp edge. These wounds can be cleaned and repaired with primary intention with a thin scar and little risk of infection.

Striking the body with a blunt object at an angle with high energy creates a tension injury. A triangular flap is created (partial avulsion). The tissue flap is at risk of ischemic

necrosis with the loss of blood supply from the free edges, especially if the flap base is distal rather than proximal. The risk of infection is greater due to the potential for ischemia and greater tissue destruction compared with a shearing type of injury.

A compression injury is caused by a high force striking straight on, especially over superficial bone. The wound will have jagged and even shredded edges, with much greater cell injury than the other 2 types. The injury may extend to subcutaneous tissue, including the bone. These wounds are at much greater risk of infection, requiring extensive cleaning, irrigation, and debridement. Primary repair is very extensive and may result in a cosmetically poor scar. In many cases, primary repair is not achievable because of the extent of cell injury creating tissue loss. The mechanisms leading to the 3 types of lacerations are depicted in Figure 13-1.

Skin Tears

Skin tears are a special type of laceration associated with the removal of adhesives from the skin or other relatively minor trauma such as bumping an extremity against an object (eg, a bed rail or doorframe). These injuries usually, but not always, produce a flap. Although skin tears can occur at any age, they tend to be associated with skin of older adults. Prevention of skin tears requires avoiding or minimizing adhesive use on the skin and meticulous removal of tape to avoid pulling. Younger people may be accustomed to pulling tape off the skin without any injury to the skin. Unfortunately, such hasty tape removal is prone to tear the skin of older individuals, and even young, healthy skin can be torn. Due to the skin's weakness, minor trauma causes the skin of older patients to tear easily. Often this occurs due to the removal of tape used to keep intravenous lines in place. Skin this fragile is typically thin, almost transparent, and demonstrates multiple ecchymoses and purpura (cigarette paper skin as described in Chapter 9). Prevention also requires protecting vulnerable areas of skin from trauma. Various means of protection are available, including tubular bandages and bandage rolls. Rather trivial trauma such as striking the dorsal hand and distal forearm on furniture, drawers, cabinets, and so forth when reaching for objects may also produce skin tears.

Skin Tear Categories

The International Skin Tear Advisory Panel (ISTAP) describes 3 categories of skin tears. Category I describes a skin tear without any tissue loss. Frequently, this occurs from blunt trauma creating a triangular epidermal flap as described for a tension type of laceration. Often the flap can be replaced and covered with an appropriate dressing to protect the wound during re-epithelialization. Partial

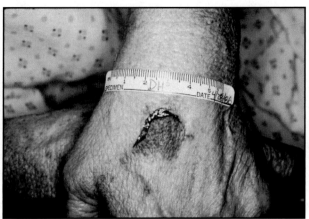

Figure 13-2. Skin tear. This flap is still attached and would receive a class I from ISTAP, 1B from Payne-Martin, and 2B from STAR. The flap is still present but cannot be pulled back into position and has less than 25% tissue loss. The flap is also dusky, leading to the 2B classification from STAR. (The image is a copyrighted product of AAWC [www.aawconline.org] and has been reproduced with permission.)

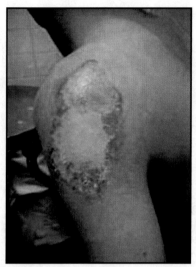

Figure 13-3. Road rash on the left shoulder from falling off a motorcycle. Note the lack of pigmentation of the abraded skin and the darkening of the burned edges of epidermis. The wound is deeper over the acromion process than the surrounding tissue that is able to deform during the injury.

loss of epidermis with the skin tear is a category II. This type of injury is frequently due to the removal of adhesives. The adhesion between tape and the epidermis may be stronger than the cohesion and adherence of the epidermis to the dermis. Category II may also be caused by a combination of tension and compression. Category III is the complete loss of the epidermal flap, either by adhesive removal or blunt trauma to the skin. Categories II and III are also treated with dressings that protect the dermis as re-epithelialization occurs. Steri-strips and similar adhesive materials may be used to secure any of the flap that can be salvaged. Figure 13-2 depicts a category II tear with no skin loss, but the edges do not easily approximate.

The Payne-Martin classification system provides subcategories to the ISTAP classification. Type 1A represents a linear injury, and type 1B describes a flaplike injury. Type 2A is used for 25% or less flap loss, whereas type 2B is used to describe a skin tear with greater than 25% flap loss. Type 3 as in the ISTAP system is complete loss of the flap. Figure 13-2 shows a Payne-Martin type 1B injury.

The Skin Tear Audit Research (STAR) system also includes 3 categories with subtypes. This system emphasizes the ability to easily realign the edges and a visual assessment of the health of the flap. Type 1A is used for a skin tear with edges that realign easily without requiring stretching of the skin and the flap is not pale, dusky, or darkened (ie, appears to be healthy). If the edges realign easily but the flap is pale, dusky, or darkened, type 1B is assigned. Type 2 is used when the edges do not realign easily. The A and B subcategories of type 2 have the same meaning as in type 1. As in the other 2 systems, type 3 is used to communicate the loss of the skin flap. The example of a skin tear shown in Figure 13-2 is classified as 2B in the STAR system.

Abrasions

Abrasions are also common injuries. Their prevalence is difficult to determine because many are self-treated. These wounds are caused by friction and tangential shearing of skin along a rough surface. Because they commonly occur along the road surface during cycling or motorcycle accidents and to ejected unrestrained passengers or pedestrians in motor vehicle accidents, the term *road rash* is often used to describe this injury. Abrasions are superficial wounds and usually only need cleaning and protection. Thorough cleansing is important to remove contaminants for 2 reasons. Microbes must be removed to prevent infection; secondly, contaminants that are not removed may remain permanently in the skin, causing discoloration called *tattooing*. Deeper injuries are produced if abrasion occurs over bony prominences. An example of road rash in shown in Figure 13-3.

Degloving (Avulsion)

A more serious injury in which the skin is pulled from the body is called *degloving*. This term is particularly descriptive for the upper extremity. It is similar to a tension laceration, but no flap remains; the base of what would be a flap is torn. This type of injury is sometimes also called an *avulsion*. The term avulsion refers to tearing of tissue, which could also apply to a tension laceration or a skin tear. Degloving more specifically occurs during motor vehicle or industrial accidents in which skin catches on a sharp edge while the body moves away from the object, resulting in a much greater skin loss. This

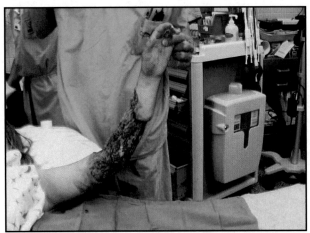

Figure 13-4. Degloving or avulsion. Skin was forcibly torn from the forearm in a motor vehicle accident.

occurs in motor vehicle accidents in which the skin of a driver or passenger becomes caught on torn metal as the person is ejected from the vehicle. The skin is then torn and pulled away from the body. Skin will tear down to an area in which it is attached firmly beneath. For the upper extremity, degloving tends to occur distally to the wrist. Depending on the body part, this injury is covered by either a partial- or full-thickness graft. An example of degloving is shown in Figure 13-4.

Extravasation and Compartment Syndrome

Extravasation implies that fluid intended to be infused into a blood vessel is instead allowed to accumulate in or below the skin. Enormous quantities may be misdirected, creating pressure below the skin and necrosis. Intravenous catheters may either miss or go through a vein into interstitial space and fill it with fluid. Substantial fluid volume may also be pumped into the skin during hemodialysis intended for a rubber tube shunt placed in the arm. Extravasation may produce injuries similar to those created by compartment syndrome.

Compartment syndrome is typically produced by trauma. The trauma may be chronic (eg, running on hard surfaces) or acute (eg, from a musculoskeletal injury causing swelling of a compartment). Frequently, the musculoskeletal injury is a fracture, but severe sprains are capable of causing compartment syndrome. An injury produced by compartment syndrome produces further swelling as cell contents are released into the interstitial space. Permanent injury to peripheral nerves, ischemia within and downstream of the compartment, myonecrosis, and skin necrosis may result. Pressure must be relieved as early as possible by fasciotomy; treatment of inflammation; and, if possible, removal of any causes of edema within the compartment.

Puncture Wounds

Long pointed objects such as ice picks, knives, and animal teeth can produce puncture wounds. Nails and other fasteners may also puncture the feet by stepping on them. The seriousness of puncture wounds is primarily due to the risk of contamination deep into the body, particularly into the bone. A puncture wound scoring system has been developed to assess the risk of a puncture wound and guide treatment. The scale consists of 4 areas of 1 to 3 points and one with 0 to 9 points. The items consist of age of the wound, shape of the wound, depth of the wound, footwear at time of puncture (if in the foot), and radiographic evaluation. For the presence of concomitant disease, add 1 additional point. The scoring system is given in Table 13-1.

A score of 1 to 4 indicates the need for local cleansing; 5 to 8 indicates local cleansing, irrigation and debridement (I&D), exploration, and placement of a drain. Any score greater than 9 indicates the need for lavage, intravenous antibiotics, and hospitalization.

Gunshot Wounds

Pistols, rifles, and shotguns have the potential for the transfer of enormous energy, injuring the body. Wide ranges of projectile velocity and mass exist, ranging from BB guns to large-caliber handguns and high-powered rifles. In addition to the soft tissue wounds along the trajectory of the projectile, gunshot wounds can cause multiple wounds due to their interaction with tissues. In many cases, injuries are immediately lethal or lethal in a short time due to direct and indirect injury to the brain (herniation) and tearing of major blood vessels. Gunshot wounds may also cause limb amputation.

Deformation of a bullet as it passes through tissue causes greater energy loss and, therefore, more transfer of energy to tissues and tissue damage. When a bullet strikes the denser medium of tissue, its flight becomes unstable; the more unstable it becomes, the more energy it transfers into the tissue. The instability can manifest itself as a tumbling or yawing motion, which increases the bullet's surface area, striking the tissue and transferring greater energy into the tissue. Moreover, the irregular movement increases the probability that the bullet may deform or even fragment.

Depending on the tissue's depth struck relative to the velocity of the bullet, different outcomes are possible. Low-velocity bullets and shot may lodge in tissue with an entry wound only, whereas high-velocity bullets produce

TABLE 13-1
Puncture Wound Scoring System

CATEGORY	0	1	2	3	9
Age		< 6 hours	6 to 24 hours	> 24 hours	
Classification		Small, sharp, clean edges; superficial	Ragged, irregular margins; moderate depth	Irregular edges, necrotic tissue, foreign body, and drainage	
Depth		Only epidermis and dermis	Through dermis with no structural involvement	Through dermis with structural involvement	
Footwear		None	Stockings	Stockings and shoes	
Radiographic exam	No evidence of osseous involvement				Osseous involvement

For presence of concomitant disease, add 1 additional point. Data source: Krych and Lavery, 1990.

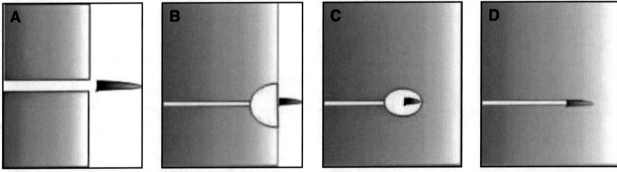

Figure 13-5. Types of wounds created by gunshots. (A) High-velocity bullet through a thin target produces a small entry and exit wound and a narrow tract. (B) Typical wound created by a high-velocity bullet going through an intermediate-thickness target. Cavitation produces a large exit wound. (C) High-velocity bullet entering a thick target producing cavitation but no exit due to dissipation of kinetic energy within the tissue. (D) Low-velocity bullet lodged in thick tissue with narrow entry wound and tract. Note that fragmentation of the missile and wound created with shot can result in substantial scattering of foreign material, including material from clothing.

both an entry and a larger exit wound. High-velocity bullets can also produce devastating cavitation (Figure 13-5). Cavitation is the result of high velocity producing waves of pressure through the tissue. The cyclic expansion and collapse of the track tear tissue; therefore, more cavitation is produced in thicker tissue. A bullet can pass through a relatively thin area of tissue with little cavitation (see Figure 13-5A). Very soft tissues, such as internal organs, suffer greater cavitation than hard tissues, with skeletal muscle having an intermediate susceptibility to cavitation.

The simplest outcome of a gunshot wound is a small linear wound with an entry wound and a small or possibly no exit wound with a narrow tract of tissue damage. This will occur if a high-velocity bullet passes rapidly through a narrow path (see Figure 13-5A). In the case of a thicker area of tissue, the bullet may produce enormous tissue damage by cavitation with an exit wound. The exit wound may

become very large if cavitation occurs maximally at the exit (see Figure 13-5B). In addition to the damage caused by the bullet's tract through tissue, secondary missiles may be produced by fragmentation of either the bullet itself or bone struck by the bullet.

Shotgun shells are available in different sizes and velocity of shot. Shells are classified by the diameter of the shell and the number of shot pellets in the shell. Damage is inflicted by the deceleration of a large number of small lead spheres striking tissue. Although a shot may leave the muzzle at high velocity, individual pellets are poorly aerodynamic and lose velocity rapidly. Additionally, the individual pellets diverge with distance. Therefore, the distance of the body from the shotgun is the chief determinant of the damage inflicted. At very close range, the individual pellets behave like a single large missile.

An additional consideration is the material carried from the surface deep into tissue, including clothing. Gunshot wounds require careful exploration due to the unpredictable path of tissue destruction. In terms of treatment, gunshot wounds are generally not closed and require thorough irrigation and filling of the tracts with nonocclusive materials such as packing strip or, if large enough, a bandage roll. Substantial necrosis of tissue surrounding the tracts is expected, and I&D may need to be carried out for several days. The material used to fill the tracts is frequently soaked in a topical antibiotic solution. Psychosocial issues are common with gunshot wounds. The clinician's ability to handle these issues may influence the patient's adherence to the plan of care.

Fractures

Fractures present 2 sets of potential problems related to wound management—wounds created by open fractures and surgical wounds to repair the fracture. The exception would be a closed fracture managed with closed reduction and immobilization. Wounds are created by bone fragments in open fractures and by surgeons for either open reduction or external fixation. Open fractures are frequently accompanied by skin loss in the area, although some lacerations can be repaired surgically. In other cases, severe avulsion or degloving injuries can cause large skin areas to be torn from the limb. Open reduction wounds will typically be closed surgically, and several incisions may be created depending on the procedure used. In certain types of injuries, fracture blisters may form and cause severe wounds that are often associated with infection. Within this section, care for pins used for skeletal traction following a fracture and external fixation used to manage complex fractures or limb lengthening are addressed, and fracture blisters will also be discussed.

Open Fractures

An open fracture, formerly known as a *compound fracture*, causes tearing of the soft tissues against the sharp edge of the fractured bone. The risk of open fracture depends on several factors, including the injury's mechanism, the type and amount of soft tissue surrounding the bone, and the bone's pliability. Open fractures are more likely to occur with injuries caused by high-energy mechanisms such as car and motorcycle wrecks and falls from great heights. Twisting injuries or blows perpendicular to long bones are also more likely to cause open fractures. A bone stabilized by thick pliable tissues such as the femur of an athlete is less likely to tear through soft tissue than a superficial bone with little support, such as the distal tibia. Brittle bones of older adults are more likely to tear soft tissue than very young children's highly pliable bones.

Open fractures present several serious problems. Bone and soft tissue are exposed to the external environment, and depending on the circumstances, the contamination can be very extensive (eg, a farm implement accident). Contamination of bone with bacteria increases the risk of osteomyelitis, which can be very difficult to clear. Large amounts of necrotic tissue may be present in the wound due to injury from the sharp bone edges. In addition, the border between necrotic and healthy tissue may be difficult to determine early. Failure to remove necrotic tissue from the wound increases the risk of infection. Open fracture wounds need to be probed carefully to find any dead space below the wound surface created by open fractures. Allowing re-epithelialization to occur over an area where dead space has failed to fill with granulation may lead to hematoma and abscess formation in the future.

Neurovascular compromise is always a threat with an open fracture, especially the radial nerve with midshaft humerus fractures and the peroneal nerve with tibial/fibular fractures. However, any peripheral nerve is at risk. Nerve injuries caused by open fractures and, in some cases, even closed fractures or severe sprains can lead to complex regional pain syndrome (CRPS), a condition of persistent pain and autonomic dysfunction requiring protracted physical therapy to manage. CRPS is a term that encompasses the variety of dysfunctions formerly known as *reflex sympathetic dystrophy, shoulder-hand syndrome, minor causalgia, major causalgia,* and others. These conditions are characterized by mechanical allodynia in which normal mechanical stimulation is perceived as pain and is accompanied by swelling and atrophy of the skin and bone. Sensory re-education and desensitization are performed in physical therapy. Autonomic blockade of sympathetic ganglia with local anesthetic is sometimes used but is not successful for many individuals with CRPS.

Fracture Blisters

Generally, fracture blisters occur in a small percentage of fractures but are much more likely to occur in superficial bone areas with tight skin (5% in these areas). They may also occur in other injuries that do not produce fractures (eg, severe ankle sprains) in the ankle, elbow, foot, and distal tibia. In these areas, tissue injury can cause edema between the dermal and epidermal layers of skin. In these areas, the proximity of the involved bone or ligaments and the lack of skin mobility cause separation of the epidermis from the dermis with subsequent necrosis of the epidermis. Fracture blisters are 4 times more likely to occur if surgical stabilization is delayed more than 24 hours. Wound infections, delayed fracture treatment, fracture nonunion, increased hospital stay, and increased costs of care may result from these blisters. A fracture blister's presence causes surgical incisions to be placed in areas that may not be optimal for the surgical procedure due to the risk of spreading infection from the blister. Compression may not help prevent fracture blisters because veins are more superficial in the areas where blisters tend to occur, and compression is likely to impede venous flow.

In contrast, compression tends to aid in deeper venous return. Efforts to prevent fracture blisters include early immobilization; elevation; and surgical repair of twisting injuries of the foot, ankle, elbow, and distal tibia. Rupture of the blister is not recommended, but a dry, absorbent dressing to protect the blister is recommended. Occlusive dressings such as hydrocolloids are recommended once the blister ruptures if the wound is clean. Topical antibiotics are not recommended unless the wound is infected and not healing. Systemic antibiotics are recommended if infection occurs. In this case, occlusive dressings should not be used. Re-epithelialization of fracture blisters is expected in 4 to 21 days depending on individual factors.

Bites

Several vertebrates may inflict humans with bite injuries, ranging from armadillos to zebras as well as humans. Bite wounds typically contain multiple microorganisms. These may include aerobes, anaerobes, and fungi and may originate from the biting animal's oral flora or the person's skin. Bites may be complicated by infection; lymphadenitis; lymphangitis; osteomyelitis; septic arthritis; and, particularly when the hand is involved, tenosynovitis. Infections with severe morbidity and mortality are possible. Examples include rabies from dogs and wild mammals, tularemia from cats hunting wild rabbits, Herpes B virus from monkeys, leptospirosis from rodents and dogs, rat-bite fever (*Streptobacillus moniliformis*), and cat scratch fever (*Bartonella henselae*). Rat-bite fever causes polyarthritis, rash, fever, and headache. It can be fatal due to endocarditis, meningoencephalitis, or septic shock. Cat scratch fever produces pronounced regional lymphadenopathy and signs of systemic inflammation. Tularemia is also known as rabbit fever but affects rodents as well. It is acquired by a tick bite or handling of the infected animal. The bacterium can also be inhaled or ingested.

The majority of human bites result from striking another with a clenched fist. True occlusion bites represent about 40% of these injuries. Clenched fist injuries are particularly problematic because of the involvement of finger tendons from striking another person's teeth. Human bites are likely to lead to infection if untreated and may lead to infection of tendon, joints, and bone with possible loss of tendon function in extreme cases. Hepatitis B and C and human immunodeficiency virus may also be transmitted.

Although several animals commonly bite humans—cats, squirrels, mice, rats, guinea pigs, hamsters, and rabbits—dog bites are particularly likely to cause severe injury. Other animals may be involved depending on occupational or recreational exposure, such as horses, pigs, fish, monkeys, and so on. Most dog bites occur on the lower extremities. However, in children, wounds may also occur on the head, neck, face, and upper extremities. Wound infections are estimated to occur in 5% to 10% of dog bites. Multiple organisms are likely to be obtained; however, intravenous antibiotics are not typically used unless a patient is at high risk for infection. Tetanus shots, however, are given as they would be for puncture wounds in general. Several breeds of dogs can create extensive damage during a bite, causing crush injuries in addition to lacerations and punctures. Crush injuries are more likely to cause tissue necrosis and hematomas that increase the risk of wound infection. Multiple bites during an attack may require thorough debridement of the affected area and grafting. Cat bites are more likely to become infected than dog bites because these injuries are more likely to cause puncture rather than crushing or laceration. Inoculation with bacteria from the cat's mouth can reach deeply in or through the skin. Small rodents kept as pets are more likely to cause thin lacerations with a lower risk of infection than cat or dog bites. Bites from marine animals may transmit *Vibrio vulnificus*, a cause of necrotizing fasciitis, which is discussed later.

Arthropod Bites

Ulcerations caused by chemicals injected by arthropod bites are categorized as toxic ulcerations. Notable among these, in specific areas of the country, is the brown recluse spider's venom. The venom spreads rapidly through fatty tissue and can produce ulcers several centimeters wide and deep. One such example includes a brown recluse injury that created an ulcer 10 cm × 8 cm × 7 cm deep in the buttock of a woman bitten while sitting on a wooden outhouse seat. These wounds can be cleaned and healed but may take several weeks to months depending on the wound's size. As with any wound, the potential for infection exists if the wound is not debrided. With appropriate debridement and dressings, these wounds should heal without complication. Spider bites appear to be extremely overdiagnosed. Skin abscesses due to folliculitis with methicillin-resistant *Staphylococcus aureus* (MRSA) are commonly blamed on spiders without evidence of brown recluse spiders in that geographical region.

TREATMENT OF TRAUMATIC AND ACUTE WOUNDS

The viability of tissue surrounding the wound must also be assessed to determine whether to close a wound. Lacerations, in particular, produce flaps of skin that may lose their blood supply. If this is the case, that part of the wound will need to be left open for 2 important reasons.

First, sutures will not hold in devitalized tissue, and second, any devitalized tissue is likely to become infected. The amount of tissue loss in a wound needs to be determined to develop a closure plan. Some wound areas can be sutured and other areas left to heal by secondary intention or to receive a graft where tissue loss occurs. Determining the amount of tissue loss can be difficult where tissue is elastic and taut. Plastic surgeons can often develop a plan to close a wound entirely, even in the presence of some degree of tissue loss. The depth of injury also affects the plan of care. A small wound can be allowed to re-epithelialize regardless of the wound's depth, whereas a large wound with full-thickness injury will need to be grafted. Acute wounds must be cleaned before closure. The surrounding skin is carefully prepped, usually with an iodophor such as povidone-iodine, and the wound itself is irrigated and debrided.

Simple lacerations with minimal tissue injury usually require only irrigation. More complex wounds and more extensive tissue necrosis will require more extensive I&D. Systemic antibiotics are considered to be of little value in the treatment of acute wounds unless a therapeutic level can be obtained within 4 hours of wounding, and the use of systemic antibiotics after this time may, in some cases, increase infection rate. Systemic antibiotics may be used, however, in the case of spreading cellulitis without purulent drainage.

The cause of the wound will also determine how extensive the I&D needs to be. An untidy wound, such as an industrial accident, farming accident, or bite, will need more extensive care. Heavily contaminated wounds can be cleaned with pulsatile lavage or a syringe with an attached catheter. With cleaning of the wound, any embedded material is removed, and a decision whether debridement is necessary is made. Foreign materials left in the wound will produce inflammation and infection. Long-term consequences include excessive scarring and tattooing. If necrotic tissue or embedded material remains in the wound, debridement becomes necessary. Debridement needs to be done judiciously to minimize the amount of tissue removed from the wound so that the wound can be closed with minimal scarring. Local anesthesia for closure is dependent on the extent of the repair. For simple repairs, either 1% or 2% lidocaine is sufficient. For repairs that may require more than 1 hour, a longer-acting local anesthetic is needed. Bupivacaine may be used, but it takes longer to achieve anesthesia than lidocaine. Most wounds will be infiltrated with epinephrine in combination with lidocaine. Epinephrine acts as a vasoconstrictor, decreasing bleeding during repairs and reducing the vascular washout of lidocaine from the tissue, thereby increasing lidocaine's duration of action.

A variety of suture materials are available, with specific advantages for different situations. Suture material may be either absorbable or nonabsorbable and either monofilament or braided. Absorbable sutures are used subcutaneously or for special conditions in which suture removal is not desired. Polyglycolic acid sutures are braided and degrade by autolytic action rather than phagocytosis, so the risk of tissue reaction is decreased. Nonabsorbable sutures are used for the skin and may be braided or monofilament. The spaces within the braid are a concern for producing tissue reactions or for harboring bacteria. Monofilament sutures, however, are more difficult to tie. Sutures come in different sizes; 6-0 is preferred by many experts for more meticulous work such as the face, whereas 4-0 works well on other parts of the body. Wounds may also be approximated with staples, especially skin grafts. Surgical adhesives are also available, and wounds may also be approximated with tape. Taping reduces the time required for wound closure and the need for local anesthesia but may not produce as precise closure as suturing.

Suturing techniques are critical for a good outcome. Poor technique can lead to excessive scarring or dehiscence (the opening of a closed surgical wound). Deep-layer approximation becomes necessary when an injury involves subcutaneous tissue. Failure to provide deep-layer approximation increases tension on the outer sutures and will leave subcutaneous dead space. Therefore, deep-layer approximation reduces the risk of fluid accumulation and infection below the skin. Suturing the skin can be done in several ways. The critical component is to gain closure of the wound with minimal tension. Following closure, swelling will increase the tension on the sutures. Excessive tension produces circulatory compromise of the edges of the wound and can lead to infection, dehiscence, or both. Sutures can generally be removed in 5 days on the face and 7 days on the trunk. Extremity sutures may be allowed to remain longer than 7 days. Formerly, surgeons were concerned about leaving sutures too long because of inflammation caused by a reaction to the suture material. Newer synthetic materials allow a longer time to ensure adequate wound strength. In some cases, the application of skin tape is performed following suture removal to reduce tension on the immature scar to prevent scar widening or dehiscence. The tape strips are allowed to remain for several days until they loosen and detach on their own.

Pin Care

In fractures requiring external fixation, pin care can be a challenge for both the patient and the caretaker. Pin care addresses 3 issues: compromised circulation, pin reaction, and infection. Compromised circulation is caused by excessive skin tension by the pin leading to necrosis of skin around the pin. Pin reaction is described as inflammation due to tissue reaction to the presence of the pin. Signs of inflammation (redness, swelling, tenderness, and discharge) must be present for more than 72 hours to be considered a reaction, and clear drainage alone is not considered to be a pin reaction. Excessive movement of the pin and blockage of drainage increase the risk of pin reaction. Minor pin reaction refers to a situation in which redness, swelling, tenderness, or clear drainage is present and improves with lancing the skin. A major pin reaction or infection is defined as a condition that does not improve with lancing and results in the need to remove pins due to the risk of osteomyelitis and the difficulty of managing osteomyelitis. Problems include excessive motion and necrotic tissue around the pin, promoting infection and increasing the risk of abscess development around the pin.

Six issues related to pin care include pin care frequency, cleansing solutions, use of ointments at the pin-skin interface, management of crusts on the pins, when to use sterile technique, and the use of dressings. Many experts suggest that keeping pins clean and allowing slow drainage from the tissue onto the pins is the best strategy for avoiding infection. Thus, recommendations aim to promote the free flow of drainage, avoidance of disturbance of the normal balance of skin flora, and avoidance of skin and subcutaneous tissue irritation. The frequency of pin care needs to be individualized. Too frequent pin care causes inflammation, whereas infrequent observation can lead to serious problems. A simple guideline is for pin site care every 8 hours in the presence of drainage and daily with no drainage. Although many individuals commonly use hydrogen peroxide or povidone-iodine, recommendations are for normal saline use only. Normal saline dilutes the bacteria present on the pins, whereas disinfectants have a higher, not lower, infection rate. The recommendation is to clean only the pin with alcohol, whereas skin cleansing should only be done as needed and with normal saline. Cleansing also needs to be performed by sweeping away from the skin and avoiding moving contaminants toward the open wound. Ointment use is discouraged because it can occlude the pinhole and allow an infection to occur.

For the same reason, the recommendation is to remove crusts from the pin-skin interface to allow drainage. Some authors have suggested that crust removal is not necessary for pins used for skeletal traction placed in areas with little soft tissue, but crusts should be removed with external fixators. Gauze dressings are recommended for covering the pin sites to reduce surface contamination and to absorb drainage. Dressings should not hold moisture against the skin, nor should they be cut before placing them over the wounds because frayed ends may irritate the wound. Sterile technique is only recommended during hospitalization due to the presence of multidrug-resistant organisms in hospitals.

INFECTION

Any defect in the skin places an individual at risk of infection, and even in the presence of intact skin, exposure to some microbes can cause infection. Whether infection occurs with exposure will be determined by the combination of which microbes are present, the wound environment, and the patient's immune status. Before surgery, careful skin preparation, thorough cleansing/irrigation, and debridement reduce bacterial counts in and around the wound. These procedures minimize but do not eliminate the risk of infection, even for a person with normal immunity. Even with optimal conditions of a clean wound with minimal necrotic tissue, a person with diminished immunity has a much higher risk of infection than a person with normal immunity who has a contaminated wound.

Risk Factors for Infection

Wound infection is indicated by either localized purulent drainage or surrounding cellulitis and excessive inflammation. Common risk factors for infection are the cleanliness of the wound; the mechanism of injury; age of the wound (how much time has passed since the injury); the extent of the injury; local blood supply; and the presence of necrotic tissue, foreign bodies, hematoma, and dead space.

Several terms have been used to describe the cleanliness of a wound. The terms *tidy* and *untidy* indicate a degree of contamination with foreign materials. *Clean, clean-contaminated,* and *contaminated* have also been used to describe the cleanliness of surgical wounds. A clean or tidy wound has little, if any, foreign material and a low bacterial contamination level. How clean the wound is can often be inferred from the mechanism of the injury. A wound from farming equipment or a bite is likely to have a much greater degree of contamination than one from a piece of glass or kitchen knife. A kitchen accident with broken glass or a knife would be considered to be tidy or clean, although some bacteria will be introduced. An untidy wound or contaminated wound has foreign materials that are likely to produce inflammation and is likely to carry large numbers of viable bacteria and spores. Clean, as it is used in surgical terminology, implies that proper sterile technique was maintained, and no trauma or inflammation that might contaminate the site is present. Clean-contaminated refers to surgical or diagnostic procedures on the gastrointestinal, respiratory, or genitourinary tracts in which no significant contamination occurs (ie, spills from the tracts do not occur). These tracts are exposed to the outside environment and are likely to be contaminated with bacteria. Contaminated is used to describe a situation in which either spillage from a tract or a significant break in sterile technique occurs. *Dirty* implies the presence of frank purulence, inflammation, or necrotic tissue in the surgical site.

The possibility of embedded materials and the amount of tissue necrosis of the wound can be deduced from the mechanism of injury. The age of a wound is important in deciding whether closure or healing by secondary intention is preferable. The longer a wound is left untreated, the greater the risk of infection. However, the local blood supply is also a factor in deciding whether to close a wound. A greater blood supply provides a better immune response. Facial injuries are commonly sutured even after 12 hours. In the past, the concept of a "golden period" dictated that closure must be accomplished within 6 to 12 hours, or the wound should be left open to heal by secondary intention. Modern practice with better debridement and antibiotic coverage allows greater latitude on how long a wound may be left open before surgical closure.

Surgical Site Infection

Surgical wounds present the least potential for complications associated with wounds in general. The skin is prepared with an antiseptic such as povidone-iodine, and the wound is created under sterile conditions. In addition, areas surrounding the sterile field are draped to avoid contamination. Although surgical site infections (SSIs) are not common, they are the most expensive hospital-acquired infection, with an estimated annual cost of $3.3 billion. They are associated with nearly 1 million additional inpatient days. Given the increasing number of surgical procedures performed yearly, approximately 157,500 SSIs are expected annually. In response to this problem, the Centers for Disease Control and Prevention has issued SSI guidelines. Several recommendations to be discussed include avoiding shaving the surgical site, applying antiseptic to an area large enough for any possible incision during the procedure in concentric circles moving peripherally, adequate oxygenation of the patient, smoking cessation, glucose control, and appropriate sterile technique.

Adequate preparation of the skin is critical to prevent surface flora from being carried into the wound. For this reason, shaving of hair is discouraged. Instead, hair should be trimmed sufficiently to prevent loose hairs from entering the sterile field or hairs becoming entangled in the sutures. Shaving is likely to abrade the skin and may transmit surface bacteria into the skin. Preparation of the skin is then done after hairs are trimmed from the area of interest. Circular biopsy punches of the skin may be approximated with sutures to decrease the size of the scar. Alternatively, these wounds could be covered with an occlusive dressing and allowed to heal by secondary intention.

Complications may result from contamination released by surgery on the gastrointestinal tract or undetected bleeding, forming a hematoma. The other major complications are related to suturing technique and excessive tension placed on wounds by movement, coughing, and other maneuvers that increase abdominal pressure, leading to dehiscence. Although the vast majority of surgical wounds heal without complications, many of these wounds will experience complications of infection, dehiscence, or both. Several risk factors for infection were discussed earlier in this chapter and in Chapter 5.

Surgically closed wounds with purulence, peripheral cellulitis, and induration require incision, irrigation, and drainage. Once bacterial burden is below 100,000/g, delayed closure has a 96% success rate. Excessive tension placed on sutures can cause necrosis of the wound margins, leading to infection or dehiscence of the wound. Dehiscence is discussed in greater detail in the following sections. In addition, poor nutrition, corticosteroid use, diabetes mellitus, and smoking are among the potential causes of delayed healing and may prevent healing or lead to necrosis of the wound margins or infection.

Two-thirds of SSIs are due to the incision, whereas one-third of SSIs are due to infection of the space or organ involved in the procedure. Both hematoma and dead space allow bacteria to accumulate under intact skin. Dead space can occur in several ways. During surgery, subcutaneous tissues must be approximated before the skin is closed. Failure to achieve subcutaneous tissue approximation leaves space for bacterial growth to occur. In chronic wounds, dead space occurs when the wound's base fails to completely granulate before re-epithelialization occurs, bridging the dead space. Hematomas may form postoperatively if adequate hemostasis is not attained before surgical closure. Blood may accumulate gradually and go un-noticed until sufficient tension on the suture line allows blood or pus to escape. Hematomas may also result from trauma that injures subcutaneous structures and causes bleeding under intact skin. Generally, these are musculoskeletal injuries, especially muscle tears. Hematomas create an additional risk factor beyond dead space by providing nutrients to bacteria, possibly accelerating their growth beyond the immune system's capacity to destroy them.

Wound Dehiscence

The opening of a surgical wound is termed *dehiscence*. This type of wound is caused by the failure of sutures or staples to maintain the primary closure of a surgical wound. A wound dehisces when the sutures, staples, tape, adhesive, or the skin itself is overcome by pressure or shear. Common causes include excess or improper lifting, necrosis of the wound edges due to vascular compromise or infection, or skin weakness caused by corticosteroids or other causes.

Sternotomy wounds caused by open-heart surgery and other procedures are frequently dehisced by patients who ignore lifting restrictions or are not taught proper transfers and other precautions to reduce sternal stress. These precautions include avoiding shoulder extension, bilateral abduction, and pushing up in bed from long sitting. Instead, the patient needs to be taught to roll into sidelying and drop the legs off the bed as a counterweight to come to sitting. Some patients may prefer to scoot in prone until the legs are cleared from the bed. Patients need to be taught to avoid low furniture with soft cushions and pushing up through the hands to come to standing from sitting. A typical example of ignoring lifting restrictions is one particular person who lifted his bass boat into the water from his trailer. Abdominal surgical wounds may dehisce due to lifting but also due to intra-abdominal pressure or bloating.

Infection can cause a wound on any part of the body to become dehiscent. In many cases, the dehiscent wound becomes so contaminated or the potential for tissue loss or necrosis is so great that primary closure is not attempted again. In this case, the typical approach is lavage, antibiotics, and delayed primary closure when the wound is clean and stable, and sufficient granulation tissue formation has occurred to relieve strain on the apposed edges of delayed primary closure. In other cases, secondary closure is allowed to continue to completion, which may take months for some large abdominal wounds. Infection may cause dehiscence or be a result of dehiscence. Dehiscence may occur due to the pressure caused by the accumulation of purulence beneath the skin. Alternatively, poor healing of a surgical incision site allowing microbes access to subcutaneous tissue and infection may cause dehiscence. Wounds may be closed by gradual third intention in which sutures are placed across the wound and tied as the wound becomes clean and sufficiently filled with granulation tissue to minimize tension on the sutures.

Managing Risk of Dehiscence

Patients at risk for dehiscence should be identified and given particular attention to avoid events that might lead to dehiscence. The patient's history gives some risk factors including smoking, diabetes, obesity, and the use of corticosteroids. Additional risk factors include disorders associated with coughing and large pendulous breasts for sternal wounds and constipation or other conditions associated with the Valsalva maneuver for abdominal wounds. The patient's nutrition and glucose need to be carefully monitored and corrected. Body mechanics during transfers from bed to sitting and from sitting to standing should be taught, monitored, and corrected as needed. Trapeze

bars should be removed from beds, and the use of bed rails or other pulling techniques during transfers must be discouraged.

Inspection of the wound needs to be done regularly. The visual inspection should show epithelialization bridging the incision. The absence of epithelialization, increased separation of the sides of the incision, and continued signs of inflammation or evidence of infection are signs of potential dehiscence. Erythema, edema, pain, and warmth should be decreasing. Increasing signs of inflammation with induration and purulence place the wound at a high risk of dehiscence. Within 5 days, a definite healing ridge should be palpable. The absence of a healing ridge from postoperative days 5 to 9 represents delayed healing and dehiscence risk.

Complications of Specific Types of Surgical Wounds

Certain types of surgical wounds are more prone to complications such as infection and dehiscence. Sternotomy, lower extremity incisions for the harvesting of veins for coronary artery bypass grafting (CABG), incisions for bypass surgery of the lower extremities, fasciotomy, tumor excision, joint replacement surgery, abdominal surgery, panniculectomy, and pilonidal cysts are discussed in the following sections.

Medial Sternotomy

Median sternotomy is the typical access site for open-heart surgery. Perioperative complications occur in a small percentage of cases, including hematoma, infection, and wound dehiscence. Any of these 3 factors may lead to the others. Lack of adequate hemostasis leading to hematoma provides a suitable environment for the rapid proliferation of bacteria. Inadequate primary closure of the soft tissue overlying the sternum can lead to dehiscence. However, dehiscence may occur in the presence of technically adequate wound closure, presumably due to excessive forces placed on the sternum and overlying tissue, particularly in patients who are overweight, have large pendulous breasts, and have diseases that stimulate frequent coughing. Large mechanical stresses are commonly believed to be a risk factor for dehiscence and subsequent infection. Infection of the soft tissue overlying the sternum may then predispose the patient to osteomyelitis of the sternum and mediastinitis, which is associated with a high (~40%) mortality. Osteomyelitis generally requires sternectomy, debridement of necrotic soft tissue, and plastic surgery to close the wound. A dehiscent sternal wound is shown in Figure 13-6.

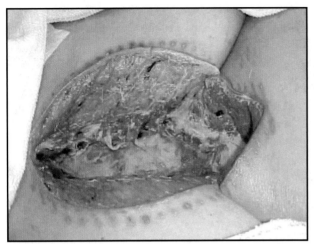

Figure 13-6. Dehiscent sternotomy wound. Note the degree of gapping and the inflammation of the suture wounds.

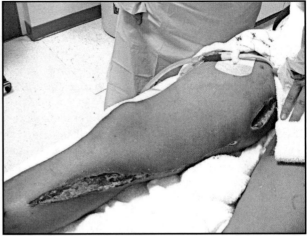

Figure 13-7. Dehiscent saphenous vein harvesting sites on both the leg and thigh. Similar wounds were found on the contralateral limb.

Lower Extremity Incisions for Bypass Surgery and Fasciotomy

Other common postoperative infection sites include lower extremity incisions used to harvest the saphenous vein for CABG. Depending on the quality of vein harvested, multiple incisions may be necessary to retrieve a sufficient length of usable vein. Many patients receiving CABG have other ischemic diseases, including the lower extremities, putting the incisional wounds at risk for infection and dehiscence. Incisional wounds created for bypass surgery of arteries of the lower extremities may have a similar fate. Likewise, flaps and grafts used to cover wounds may fail for the same reasons that the wounds would not close without plastic surgery. An example of dehiscence involving bilateral leg and thigh donor sites for CABG is shown in Figure 13-7.

Fasciotomy wounds are similar to bypass graft donor sites, except the wounds are deeper. These wounds are at risk due to the injury that required the fasciotomy. An additional problem is the potential for premature closure of the skin without complete granulation, leaving a dead space that may lead to abscess formation in the future.

Tumor Excision

Tumor excision wounds may be relatively simple in the cases of squamous cell or basal cell carcinoma of the skin, but excision of melanoma is more complex. The risk of metastasis of melanoma is related to the depth of skin involved. Therefore, the excisional wound may be full thickness, and regional lymph nodes may be removed for diagnostic and therapeutic reasons.

Arthroplasty

Joint replacement surgery is very common, and a small fraction of these surgical wounds will be complicated by infection. Joint infection is seen in approximately 0.3% to 1.7% of all total hip arthroplasties and 0.8% to 1.9% of all total knee arthroplasties. These infections can be quite devastating and may lead to loss of limb mobility, loss of ambulation, and potentially amputation. Once a joint becomes infected, removing the prosthesis and implantation of antibiotic-releasing material are frequently performed to allow for future implantation of a new prosthesis. Prevention of these infections is imperative and frequently done via silver-impregnated dressings that are placed intraoperatively and left intact for 7 to 10 days.

Abdominal Surgery

Abdominal wounds, especially those created for intestinal surgery, are at risk for infection. Bacteria from the inside of the bowel may contaminate the surgical site and incision despite copious irrigation. Edema, pain, induration, and expression of purulence are obvious signs of infection. The complete reopening of the entire wound is usually not necessary for drainage. Frequently, an abscess will be limited to one or more small areas beneath the incision. Careful probing of the wound is necessary to discover any tracking of the wound. Subcutaneous connections between openings are common, requiring irrigation through the tracts and packing to prevent the openings from closing before the tunnels are granulated.

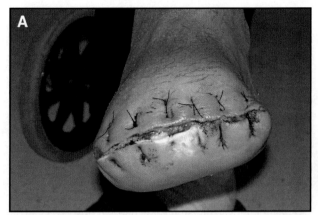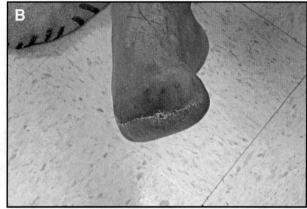

Figure 13-8. (A) The beginning of infection and dehiscence of an amputation wound. This amputation was subsequently revised and healed. (B) The same foot after revision and serial debridement leading to healing of the amputation site.

Panniculectomy

Panniculectomy is the surgical removal of redundant abdominal skin and subcutaneous tissue following extreme weight loss. The panniculus (pannus, "apron") may substantially overlap tissue, producing intertrigo, a condition of maceration, inflammation, and fissuring of the skin. Intertrigo complications include fungal infection, bacterial superinfection, and skin breakdown. Insurance coverage for panniculectomy remains controversial because some payers see this procedure as strictly cosmetic rather than recognizing it as a risk factor for tissue injury and infection.

Pilonidal Cyst

Abscess formation within pilonidal cysts is a common problem. The term *pilonidal* means "nest of hair." Those with pilonidal cysts have a dimple and increased hair growth in the sacrococcygeal area, just superior to the gluteal cleft. Cysts most often become problematic in late teen and early adult years. Although abscesses within these cysts are frequently treated with incision and drainage, they do not heal well, and these infections are notoriously recurrent even after wound closure. Alternatives to incision and drainage are excision of the cyst with primary closure or plastic surgery and excision with healing by secondary intention. Statistically, excision with secondary intention has the best outcome, and I&D has the highest rate of complications and recurrence. Abscessed pilonidal cysts have a great propensity for sinus tract formation, including multiple and long tracts that may extend along the fascia of the posterior thigh. Because of the long tracts, they also tend to close on the surface even as they are still expressing purulence. If allowed to close over purulent dead space, recurrence is very likely. These wounds need to be irrigated frequently and packed to stay open until all tracts have granulated, and the wound bed fills.

Amputation Sites

Depending on the cause and site, amputation wounds may need to be closed in different ways. In general, a suture line is not desired on a weight-bearing surface. To create a suture line on the anterior surface of a residual limb, sufficient viable skin must be left on the extremity's posterior surface to be brought over the weight-bearing surface and sutured or stapled to the anterior surface. Suppose this condition cannot be met because of excessive loss of functional limb length. In that case, equal amounts of skin from the posterior and anterior surface of the limb can be approximated across the weight-bearing surface. However, this approach risks damage and possible dehiscence with early weight-bearing, preventing a common goal of postamputation rehabilitation. Sufficient soft tissue is needed between the skin and the residual bone to prevent injury to the skin making contact with a prosthesis.

Complications of amputation sites may occur shortly after the procedure or years afterward. Acute wounds are generally caused by infection of the surgical site. The wound site may open due to pressure caused by the volume of purulence, but wounds may become infected because the surgical wound opens up due to poor healing. An example of an amputation site requiring intervention due to infection is shown in Figure 13-8. In either case, the dehiscence of an amputation wound requires intervention. Because large pus-filled tracts may occur, careful examination of the wound must be performed. Wounds may be caused years after the amputation due to excessive wear of the prosthesis or an ill-fitting prosthesis. If the patient still has postoperative swelling of the residual limb during prosthetic fitting, the socket may become too large, causing movement inside the socket and damage to the residual limb's skin. Figure 13-9 shows an example of a wound created over the patient's fibular head due to a poorly fit prosthesis.

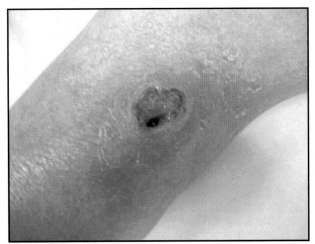

Figure 13-9. Wound over the fibular head secondary to poorly fitting prosthesis.

Skin and Soft Tissue Infections

Skin and soft tissue infections (SSTIs) are increasing in prevalence and may be the most common type of wound seen in some practices. The causative agent is frequently MRSA. Increased incidence is likely due to the development of community-acquired MRSA, whereas MRSA in the past was generally a nosocomial infection. Excessive use of antibiotics and patients' failure to finish courses of antibiotics have been blamed for the increased incidence of MRSA. Approximately 5% of all hospitalized patients in the United States have MRSA either in their nose or on their skin; a common practice in intensive care units now is to swab the patients' nares to determine if they are carriers of MRSA. This helps prevent the spread of MRSA by heightening awareness of the health care providers and rooming patients with MRSA together. With increased vigilance in preventing MRSA's spread, a significant decline occurred in the number of hospital-acquired MRSA cases from 2005 to 2012; however, this number has since plateaued.

SSTIs typically occur in the forms of folliculitis and skin abscesses, either as furuncles or carbuncles. A furuncle is a skin abscess with a limited area, generally surrounding a hair follicle or other opening in the skin. A carbuncle is a coalesced mass of furuncles that typically occur within a fascial plane. Areas of loose skin to fascia attachment, such as the nape of the neck, are particularly prone to carbuncle development. Most skin abscesses tend to occur on the back and between the waist and knee, although they may appear anywhere on the body. Some individuals are prone to recurrent SSTIs. They may develop abscesses on a buttock, then several months later one on the thigh, and then one on the back, or they may develop in similar or the same area. A severe form of SSTI is necrotizing fasciitis.

Hidradenitis Suppurativa

Infection of the apocrine sweat glands, located in the axilla, groin, perineum, perianal area, buttocks, scrotum, and submammary region, is termed *hidradenitis suppurativa*. The process is similar to folliculitis in general, in which keratin comedones occlude the apocrine ducts, promoting inflammation and infection. The rapid proliferation of bacteria leads to abscess formation, chronic infection, and spread through the glandular mass. As the process is allowed to continue, induration and tract formation may occur, allowing infection to spread through the area's apocrine glands. This disease is divided into 3 stages. Stage 1 is characterized by single to multiple abscesses but no sinus tracts or scarring. In stage 2, the patient has recurrent abscess formation, tracts, and scarring. Diffuse involvement with multiple interconnected tracts and abscesses throughout the region of glands is observed in stage 3. Patients may require a large number of small incisions to allow purulence to drain. Due to its recurrent nature, excision of the apocrine sweat gland masses may become necessary in these areas.

Necrotizing Fasciitis

The cause of necrotizing fasciitis has been dubbed "flesh-eating bacteria." It may be linked to traumatic or surgical wounds but frequently occurs idiopathically. A typical patient is a middle-aged man with a secondary immunodeficiency, especially a combination of poorly controlled diabetes and alcoholism. The typical case (type 1) is produced by mixtures of aerobic gram-negative and anaerobic bacteria that act synergistically, eroding fascial planes and necrotizing subcutaneous tissue seemingly overnight. Accumulation of subcutaneous gas usually occurs due to anaerobic, gas-producing microorganisms.

Three categories of necrotizing fasciitis have been described based on the bacteria involved. Type 1 necrotizing fasciitis is a mixture of aerobes and anaerobes. Typical organisms for this type are group A beta-hemolytic *Streptococcus*, *Staphylococcus aureus*, *Escherichia coli*, *Clostridium* species, and *Bacteroides*. Unusual components are group B, C, and G *Streptococcus*; *Haemophilus influenzae* type b; *Pseudomonas aeruginosa*; and *Vibrio vulnificus*. A combination of group A beta-hemolytic Strep and Staph aureus exists in type 2 necrotizing fasciitis. Type 3 is caused by *V. vulnificus*. This type is frequently caused by entry directly into a wound from contaminated seawater (bay or river mouth) or indirectly through a bite from fish or insects. An example of type 3 necrotizing fasciitis due to entering Mobile Bay with an open neuropathic ulcer is shown in Figure 13-10.

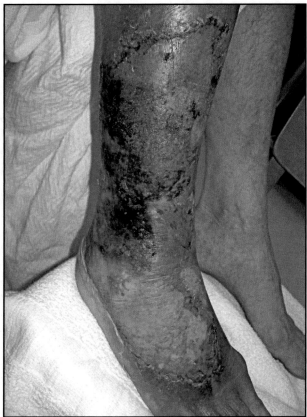

Figure 13-10. Example of type 3 necrotizing fasciitis (*Vibrio vulnificus*) caused by going into seawater barefoot with an open neuropathic ulcer.

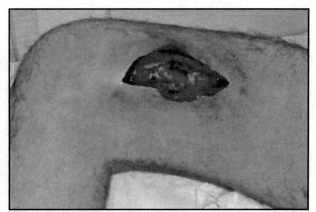

Figure 13-11. I&D wound due to skin abscess with MRSA. The wound required serial debridement and packing to allow drainage to continue. The wound closed without any further complications over the course of 3 weeks.

Overlying skin must commonly be excised to halt the progress of tissue necrosis adequately. Frequently, a combination of excision and I&D must be performed, leaving pockets that benefit from daily irrigation and packing pockets and tracts with a topical antibiotic in addition to systemic antibiotics. Because of the different mixtures of flora in different individuals, the clinical course may vary tremendously. The mortality of necrotizing fasciitis remains high, partly because of compromised immunity that preceded the infection, such as poorly controlled diabetes, cancer, peripheral arterial disease, organ transplants, human immunodeficiency virus, neutropenia, and alcoholism.

Necrotizing fasciitis occurs in hypoxic areas due to hypoxia's effect on neutrophils that allows aerobic bacteria to proliferate. Consumption of oxygen by the aerobes then allows anaerobes to proliferate as well. Patients generally require supplemental oxygen, one or more surgical excisions, and multiple antibiotics to cover the variety of possible bacteria. Hyperbaric oxygen has been shown in multiple studies to decrease mortality tremendously. Usually, group A hemolytic *Streptococcus* or *S. aureus* is the initiator of the process, followed by any of a number of anaerobes. The combination of bacterial toxins can disable multiple parts of the immune system and digest tissue, allowing fascial spread. The patient usually presents with a painful, edematous, and erythematous area with crepitus that progresses to anesthetic and dusky. The spread is dependent on the thickness of subcutaneous tissue. Spread is particularly rapid through the scrotum and penis due to their lack of subcutaneous fat.

Fournier's Gangrene

The term *Fournier's gangrene* is used specifically for necrotizing fasciitis of the perineum/scrotum and often the penis of adults. The scrotum may become several times its normal size. Early diagnosis may allow treatment with I&D, but excision of some or all of the scrotal skin and, on occasion, that of the penis and perineum may become necessary depending on the spread of the infection. Plastic surgery to rebuild the scrotum or create pockets in the thigh to implant the testes is necessary in severe cases. The term *Fournier's gangrene* has been applied to women and children by some sources if necrotizing fasciitis of the perineum is present.

Diagnosis of Skin and Soft Tissue Infections

Generally, SSTIs are easily diagnosed. Commonly, patients report a sudden onset of swelling and pain in the area of the SSTI. Purulence may be expressed spontaneously or from the patient squeezing or picking at the abscess. The volume of purulence can be disturbing to the patient because a great deal of space within a fascial plane may fill seemingly overnight. Palpation of the area demonstrates warmth and induration in addition to the observation of erythema and the complaint of pain from the patient. Figure 13-11 shows an example of the profound edema that can occur with a skin abscess.

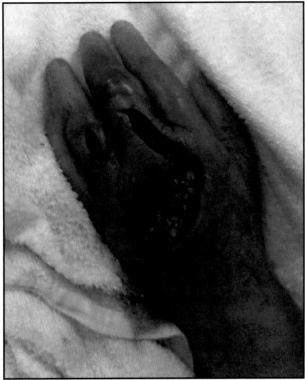

Figure 13-12. Gangrene on the dorsum of the hand secondary to incisions to drain a skin abscess.

Treatment for Skin and Soft Tissue Infections

The standard treatment for SSTIs is I&D in conjunction with systemic antibiotics such as clindamycin, vancomycin, or the combination drug trimethoprim and sulfamethoxazole (Bactrim). One or more incisions are placed in the abscess(es), and purulence is expressed. The open wound created is irrigated and allowed to drain as it closes by secondary intention. Patients may be treated by a physician as an outpatient and given oral antibiotics, or the patient may be admitted to a hospital and placed on intravenous antibiotics. Patients may require more than one I&D procedure. The wound is usually filled with a packing strip—either plain or iodoform to allow the purulence to drain. An alternative to the packing strip is a Penrose drain. A Penrose drain is a length of flat rubber tubing that prevents premature closure of the incision and allows drainage to continue as long as it is deemed necessary. Other types of drains using vacuum bulbs may be used in some cases. The packing strip is changed daily or more often and will generally be coated with thick yellow drainage early for a variable number of days. In some cases, purulence may persist as the wound granulates, and preventing re-epithelialization may become difficult but critically important. Performing an I&D may compromise

the skin's circulation, resulting in the death of skin overlying the abscess being drained as shown in Figure 13-12.

SSTI frequently occurs in diabetic feet. When a deep infection is suspected, I&D is generally indicated. This procedure is also used for infected surgical wounds, osteomyelitis, puncture wounds, tunneling, or sinus tracts. Deeper wounds may require the placement of a drain in addition to packing. In select cases, delayed primary closure may be used rather than secondary intention. Packing a larger wound may be done with saline-moistened gauze sponges or bandage rolls to prevent the wound from filling with granulation tissue if delayed primary closure is desired.

Pulsatile lavage is suitable for this type of wound to remove bacteria and necrotic tissue. Patients who are admitted to a hospital will generally need to continue therapy as outpatients. With the placement of peripherally inserted central lines, patients can continue with intravenous antibiotics either at home or an outpatient intravenous service if oral antibiotics are not appropriate. When the wound is clean and stable, closure may be performed with sutures, staples, or plastic surgery techniques discussed in the following sections. Readmissions occur occasionally. Some patients may be seen cyclically as an inpatient, outpatient, and inpatient again over a period of months to years.

Peritonitis

A life-threatening infection of the abdominal cavity, peritonitis most commonly develops from perforation of the bowels (including the appendix) with the release of bacteria into the peritoneum. The esophagus and stomach may also be the source. Spillage of gastric acid due to a perforated ulcer, bile acids from a perforated gall bladder or lacerated liver, and digestive enzymes from an inflamed pancreas are also potential causes. Infected fallopian tubes or ruptured ovarian cysts are potential causes in women. Disease may be manifested as either generalized inflammation (peritonitis) or intra-abdominal abscess. Like necrotizing fasciitis, peritonitis can spread rapidly. Peritonitis may be divided into primary, secondary, and tertiary. Primary occurs spontaneously (does not involve perforation), whereas secondary peritonitis exists if the cause is either a disease process or iatrogenic. Tertiary peritonitis refers to recurrent disease. Mortality is low if the disease is uncomplicated and treated promptly (5% to 10%) but may reach 70% in cases of massive infection and organ damage.

Primary peritonitis is most commonly caused by chronic liver disease. Many patients with cirrhosis and ascites (~30%) will develop spontaneous bacterial peritonitis. This form is usually due to a single bacterial species, usually gram-negative, and most commonly *E. coli*.

Common causes of secondary peritonitis are appendix rupture, perforated gastric and duodenal ulcers, strangulation of the small bowel, and perforated sigmoid colon secondary to diverticulitis or cancer. This type of peritonitis is usually due to anaerobes that do not cause problems within the gastrointestinal tract but are allowed to proliferate within the peritoneum. Massive fibrosis or abscess formation may occur within the peritoneum, sequestering bacteria and impairing an immune response.

A patient with peritonitis will present with typical signs of systemic inflammation, abdominal pain complaints, and tenderness on palpation and will have abdominal wall muscle rigidity. The onset ranges from acute to insidious, and the clinical presentation may range from limited, mild disease to systemic disease with septic shock. Treatment includes appropriate antibiotics and either percutaneous or open abdominal drainage. Dehiscence of surgical wounds for open drainage of peritonitis is 3 times as likely as abdominal surgery in general.

Another complication of peritonitis is abdominal compartment syndrome (ACS). This syndrome is characterized by intra-abdominal hypertension and multiple organ dysfunction. Excessive intra-abdominal pressure can affect multiple systems, notably pulmonary, cardiovascular, renal, and splanchnic. It may also damage skin and musculoskeletal structures. ACS is most commonly associated with massive hemorrhage, the need for extensive fluid resuscitation, prolonged surgical procedures, and coagulopathies. ACS may develop insidiously or acutely. In either case, the abdominal compartment will eventually lose extensibility, and pressure will rise steeply.

Like compartment syndromes of the extremities, ACS results in compression and then injury to whatever is located in the compartment. Hollow organs collapse; ischemia and metabolic acidosis occur in the abdominal organs; and release of bacteria, histamine, and serotonin into the peritoneum increases fluid accumulation in the peritoneum, furthering ischemia of abdominal organs and impairing the kidneys, central circulation, ventilation, and cerebral perfusion. ACS is increasingly being suspected for acute decompensation in critically injured patients.

ACS is suspected in those with a predisposing injury and distended abdomen and difficulty breathing with wheezes, crackles, and cyanosis. The patient will appear ill (wan appearance), pale, listless, and weary. Surgical drainage and supportive care are required, but mortality is very high. Untreated ACS is considered to have 100% mortality; overall, the mortality of documented ACS cases is approximately 70%.

SUMMARY

Although traumatic wounds and wounds caused by skin infections are typically managed in the emergency room or by a surgeon, physical therapists may receive referrals to treat these wounds once they have been acutely managed. Understanding the causative agent of these wounds is important to be able to treat them appropriately and understand how the trajectory of healing may differ from other, more common wounds.

QUESTIONS

1. Contrast the appearance of a normally closing traumatic or surgical wound to a poorly closing wound.
2. What causes dehiscence? What type of wounds are especially prone to dehiscence?
3. Why are amputation sites at higher risk of infection than other surgical wounds?
4. What is the general treatment strategy for an SSI?
5. What distinguishes a puncture wound from other traumatic wounds?
6. What are the common causes of puncture wounds?
7. What is required for high-risk puncture wounds?
8. Contrast shearing (sharp object), tension (blunt object), and compression types of lacerations.
   a. Causes
   b. Type of closure
9. What typically causes skin tears? Who is particularly at risk? What determines the category of skin tear?
10. What causes road rash? How is it typically treated?
11. What is degloving/skin avulsion? How is it treated? What is the role of the physical therapist?
12. What causes compartment syndrome? How are severe cases treated? Why are physical therapists sometimes consulted?
13. What complicates gunshot wounds? What is the difference between bullets and shot pellets in terms of the injuries produced?
14. What are the roles of physical therapy in the management of open fractures?
15. Describe pin care for external fixation or with patients treated with the Ilizarov apparatus.
16. Why and where do fracture blisters form? How are they managed?
17. Contrast dog and domestic cat bites.
18. What are the problems created by human bites?
19. How are spider bites distinguished from skin abscesses?
20. What is the general strategy for treating traumatic wounds?
21. What are the most common causes of skin abscesses?
22. Contrast the terms *folliculitis*, *furuncle*, and *carbuncle*.
23. What is the standard treatment for furuncles and carbuncles?

24. What is hidradenitis suppurativa? What areas of the body are particularly prone? What is done in severe cases?

25. What is a pilonidal cyst? What is considered best practice for their management?

26. How is necrotizing fasciitis recognized? Is crepitus always present?

27. How is necrotizing fasciitis managed?

28. What can happen in severe cases?

29. What is necrotizing fasciitis of the scrotum and perineum called?

30. What is the range of options for treating Fournier's gangrene?

31. What is the general treatment strategy for wounds secondary to infection?

BIBLIOGRAPHY

Bone RC, Balk RA, Cerra FB, et al. Definitions for sepsis and organ failure and guidelines for the use of innovative therapies in sepsis. The ACCP/SCCM Consensus Conference Committee. American College of Chest Physicians/Society of Critical Care Medicine. *Chest.* 1992;101(6):1644-1655.

Chase CW, Franklin JD, Guest DP, Barker DE. Internal fixation of the sternum in median sternotomy dehiscence. *Plast Reconstr Surg.* 1999;103(6):1667-1673.

Driscoll JA. Integumentary management of the patient with multiple traumatic injuries. *Acute Care Perspectives.* 1999;7(2):1-18.

Finley JM, McConnell RY. *Emergency Wound Repair.* University Park Press; 1984.

Goldstein B, Girior B, Randolph A. International pediatric sepsis consensus conference: definitions for sepsis and organ dysfunction in pediatrics. *Pediatr Crit Care Med.* 2005;6(1):2-8.

Irion GL, Boyer S, McGinnis T, Thomason M, Trippe A. Effect of upper extremity movement on sternal skin stress. *Acute Care Perspectives.* 2006;15(3):1-6.

Irion GL, Boyte B, Ingram J, Kirchem C, Weathers J. Sternal skin stress produced by functional upper extremity movements. *Acute Care Perspectives.* 2007;16(3):1-5.

Kaplan EN, Hentz VR. *Emergency Management of Skin and Soft Tissue Wounds. An Illustrated Guide.* Little, Brown, and Company; 1984.

Krych SM, Lavery LA. Puncture wounds and foreign body reactions. *Clin Podiatr Med Surg.* 1990;7(4):725-731.

Kuo J, Butchart EG. Sternal wound dehiscence. *Care of the Critically Ill.* 1995;11:244-248.

Levy MM, Fink MP, Marshall JC, et al. 2001 SCCM/ESICM/ACCP/ATS/SIS International Sepsis Definitions Conference. *Crit Care Med.* 2003;31(4):1250-1256.

McCallum I, King PM, Bruce J. Healing by primary versus secondary intention after surgical treatment for pilonidal sinus. *Cochrane Database Syst Rev.* 2007;4:CD006213.

McKenzie LL. In search of a standard for pin site care. *Orthop Nurs.* 1999;18:73-78.

Robson MC. Wound infection. A failure of wound healing caused by an imbalance of bacteria. *Surg Clin North Am.* 1997;77:637-650.

Swan KG, Swan RC. Gunshot Wounds. *Pathophysiology and Management.* Year Book Medical Publishers; 1989.

Varela CD, Vaughan TK, Carr JB, Slemmons BK. Fracture blisters: clinical and pathological aspects. *J Orthop Trauma.* 1993;7:417-427.

Veal J, Sellars BB. Reduce sternal dehiscence and infections. *Cardiovasc Dis Manage.* 2002;8(11):6.

Zeitani J, Bertolodo F, Bassano C, et al. Superficial wound dehiscence after median sternotomy: surgical treatment versus secondary wound healing. *Ann Thorac Surg.* 2004;77(2):672-675.

Burn Injuries

OBJECTIVES

- Describe causes of thermal, electrical, chemical, and radiation burns.
- Discuss the advantages and disadvantages of different methods of computing percent body surface area.
- Define the depths of burn injuries using both common systems.
- Discuss the causes and potential outcomes of different depths of burn injuries.
- Describe typical medical management of severe thermal injury.
- Describe types of skin grafting/replacement available.
- Discuss how skin grafting affects exercise programs.
- Discuss appropriate exercise for individuals with thermal injuries.
- Discuss scar management following thermal injury.

BURN INJURIES

A burn is an injury to skin, and potentially deeper tissues, that denatures the proteins, leading to tissue necrosis if the intensity and time of exposure are sufficient. Burn injuries can be reversible or irreversible, and degrees of injuries account for both the depth and reversibility of the injury. Causes of burn injuries are extremes in temperature, electricity, caustic chemicals, friction, and radiation. More than half of the hospitalizations for burn injuries occur in one of more than 120 major burn centers in the United States. Statistics from 2016 show almost one-half million burn injuries annually for which medical attention is sought. A major burn, by definition, involves more than 25% of the body surface area (BSA). Those admitted to burn centers are predominantly male (68%), and the home

Irion GL, Gardner JA, Pignataro RM.
Comprehensive Wound Management, Third Edition (pp 255-272).
© 2024 Taylor and Francis Group.

is the most common site of injury—73% home, 8% occupational, 5% vehicular, 5% recreational/sport, and 9% other. Flames are the most common admission cause, with scalding a close second—43% fire/flame, 34% scald, 9% contact, 4% electrical, 3% chemical, and 7% other.

Burn center referral criteria include partial-thickness burns greater than 10% total BSA; burns involving the face, hands, feet, genitalia, perineum, or major joints; full-thickness injuries in any age group; electrical burns, including lightning; chemical burns; inhalation injury; burn injury in those with pre-existing health problems; burns with concomitant trauma such as fractures in a vehicular incident; burned children in hospitals without qualified personnel or equipment; and burn injury in patients with special social, emotional, or rehabilitative needs.

Heat

Transfer of heat into the body in excess of 44°C causes proteins to denature, leading to the breakdown of skin. Heat may be transferred by contact with hot fluids such as water, cooking oil, steam (scalding), gases (flames, fireballs), and contact with a hot object (contact burn). Prolonged radiation of heat from a source such as a fireplace or space heater can result in burn injuries. In particular, insensate feet placed closer to the source of heat than areas of the body with adequate sensation are at risk of this type of injury. This injury typically occurs to the diabetic individual who props cold feet in front of a fireplace.

The amount of heat transferred is due to the temperature of the object, the mass and heat capacity of the material transferring the heat, and the length of exposure. Flames can have a very high temperature but have very little mass and low heat capacity. Very brief exposure to a flame may produce no injury whatsoever, but prolonged exposure in a house or vehicle fire or exposure to an extremely hot fireball from a gas explosion will produce deep wounds. Scalding injuries are common because water has a high heat capacity, and a body part can be immersed in it, resulting in a substantial injury. In contrast, the splashing of hot water that can drip off the body will not produce much, if any, injury. Oil, used for cooking or other purposes, produces much more severe injuries. Oil can cling to the skin and prolong exposure to heat. In addition, oil can be heated to a much higher temperature. Whereas water boils at 100°C, cooking oil can reach a temperature of 300°C. Although boiling point limits water temperature during conventional cooking, food and liquids heated with a microwave oven can be superheated, reach temperatures higher than boiling, and be ejected at great velocity, resulting in a severe burn injury. Contact burns from hot metal, such as an iron, cookware, or component of an engine's exhaust system, will produce very deep injuries due to the rapid transfer of heat.

Ignition of clothing from flames causes severe injuries that are made worse by clothing made of materials that can melt into the skin. Removal of burned clothing is critical to stop the transfer of heat into the skin.

Cold

Cold-induced tissue damage is termed *frostbite* and is caused by the freezing of tissue. Ice crystal formation leads to loss of cellular water and damage to proteins, cell membranes, and capillaries. Rewarming can lead to additional injury, especially if the tissue freezes again. A less severe form is termed *frostnip*.

Prolonged exposure to subfreezing temperatures produces necrosis that may be similar in appearance to that caused by heat. These injuries typically occur due to being stranded outdoors in cold weather (homeless or outdoor sports related) or due to excessive occupational exposure in a freezer. Mountain frostbite occurs in mountain climbers due to the additive effects of cold and hypoxia. Risk of frostbite is increased by peripheral artery disease, Raynaud's disease or phenomenon, diabetes mellitus and other peripheral neuropathies, smoking, use of beta-blockers, and alcohol consumption. Apical areas of the body are most susceptible to frostbite due to their large surface area relative to mass. As such, the nose, ears, fingers, and toes are most likely to be injured. Amputation of affected areas may be required. Sophisticated plastic surgery techniques are available to reconstruct noses and ears.

Frostbite injury may initially appear pale and feel indurated and cold. The affected area is anesthetic with possible deep, aching pain. However, as the area warms, it may show extreme erythema, and the patient may experience intense pain. If skin freezes, however, the tissue becomes white, no sensation returns, and necrosis occurs. Skin becomes darker, blisters, and then demonstrates wet gangrene with possible injury to deeper structures including bone. In addition to these injuries, a person is likely to experience hypothermia with the risk of injury to internal organs and arrhythmia.

Care includes fluid resuscitation and rapid rewarming with water at 40°C to 42°C for approximately 20 to 40 minutes until flushing of the affected area is noted. Debridement of clear, fluid-filled blisters is recommended but not hemorrhagic blisters due to the risk of infection.

Electrical

Electrical injuries include thermal injury to the skin and the effect of electrical current on subcutaneous structures and blood. The amount of heat dissipated in tissues is determined by I^2R (current squared × resistance) and the exposure time. Dry skin has a higher resistance than moist skin; therefore, more energy is dissipated in the skin. Dry skin, therefore, increases the risk of skin injury but decreases the risk of internal injury. With wet skin, burns of the skin are minimized, but internal injury could become severe. Mucous membranes also have a low resistance, and subcutaneous injury is more likely to result. The size of the injury is also related to the BSA (current density). A given current limited to a small area is more likely to cause injury (eg, biting into an electrical cord).

Household current of 110 V is unlikely to cause injury to intact skin. The 220-V current used in appliances such as ranges, electric dryers, and air-conditioning units is more likely to damage the skin. This voltage is also used for household current in most of the world outside North America and the Caribbean. High-voltage lines of 500 V and greater are very likely to cause skin injuries. Depending on the path of high-voltage current, severe edema and thrombosis of blood vessels in the damaged area can occur. Edema, compartment syndrome, and thrombosis compound the injury caused by electrical exposure by adding a component of ischemic injury. Internal organs and skeletal muscle may also be severely injured. In the case of touching a high-voltage line while standing on a conductive surface such as a metal ladder, shattering of bone and open fractures may result. Cardiorespiratory arrest is possible due to ventricular fibrillation and damage to the brain stem. Amputation may become necessary depending on the severity of tissue injury.

Chemical

A wide variety of chemicals are capable of injuring the skin. Exposure to acidic, alkaline, or other injurious chemicals may rapidly produce skin necrosis, similar to thermal injury. Other chemicals produce erythema, blistering, and more gradual necrosis. Chemical injuries are usually the result of industrial accidents due to the inadvertent release of caustic substances from their containers. The extent of the injury is related to the concentration of the substance and the time of exposure. For this reason, chemicals must be flushed from the skin as quickly as possible, including the removal of clothing and contact lenses.

Radiation

Ionizing radiation damages tissue primarily due to structural damage to DNA. Indirect injury may also occur due to the generation of free radicals by ionizing radiation. Cell death may occur immediately, or cells may not be able to replicate following exposure. Additionally, blood vessel injury may produce ischemic injury to additional tissue. Long-term effects are mainly fibrosis of tissue in the path of the ionizing radiation. Skin loses its rete pegs, elastic fibers are damaged, and the injury induces abnormal fibroblast activity. Because of genetic damage induced by radiation, malignancies and nonhealing wounds may develop over time. The loss of fibroblasts and dysfunction of remaining fibroblasts may require wide excision of the injured tissue and either grafting or a flap to cover the wound. In severe cases, it may require an amputation of an extremity.

Radiation injury may be repaired or cause acute injury, chronic injury, or delayed injury. Injuries can occur in the setting of medical treatment (usually for cancer) or industrial from instruments using radiation. The vast majority result from excessive exposure to radiation therapy. Brachytherapy is delivered locally in the form of "seeds," and other forms use beams of protons, gamma rays, or X-rays. Dry, itching skin is the most common form of injury. Blistering and peeling of skin can occur with greater injury. Late, long-term effects may include cancer. Additional adverse effects are related to the site of radiation treatment such as lung injury, nausea and vomiting, diarrhea, and neuropathy. A skin injury can also be caused by ultraviolet radiation. Gamma radiation can cause deep gamma burns, whereas beta radiation used for superficial cancers can cause very shallow burns. Although alpha particles do not penetrate the skin, they can cause internal damage from inhalation. Radio waves and microwaves are also potential sources of injury. Radio waves are used in the treatment of incompetent communicating veins and catheter ablation in the heart.

Although the application of radiation therapy is designed to minimize injury to the skin and subcutaneous tissue while producing irreversible injury to neoplastic tissue, beams of radiation from sources such as Cobalt-60 are capable of inflicting tremendous genetic injury to healthy tissue between the source of radiation and the tumor. Therefore, multiple beams are aimed from different directions toward the neoplasm to enhance the injury to the tumor and minimize damage to other tissues. However, the accumulation of injury may still result. Short-term complications of radiation therapy are estimated at 5% to 15%. Longer-range complications may be seen in patients irradiated many years prior. However, the actual rate is unknown due to the death of patients before long-term complications can be observed. Patients with fistulas, osteonecrosis, sclerosis of skin, and skeletal structures may be seen in a typical clinic due to remote radiation therapy.

Radiation dermatitis is prevalent (95% of patients). Dermatitis may occur immediately or months after treatment. Transient erythema is the least severe form. Dry desquamation, hair loss, long-lasting erythema, wet desquamation, blistering, and necrosis result from progressively

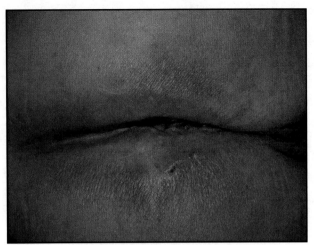

Figure 14-1. Appearance of radiation dermatitis.

higher exposure based on a combination of time of exposure and dose. The term *desquamation* outside the context of radiation exposure is considered a normal process in which keratinocytes are shed after a typical 14-day stay. Pathological desquamation occurs with a superficial partial-thickness burn (first-degree) typical of sunburn. In the context of radiation injury, dry desquamation refers to the shedding of dry, scaly, erythematous, radiation-injured skin. Moist desquamation refers to the blistering of radiation-injured skin with exposure of a moistened dermal surface. An example of radiation dermatitis with xerosis, fibrosis, and induration is depicted in Figure 14-1.

CLASSIFICATION SYSTEMS FOR EXTENT OF INJURY

Means of classifying the extent of burn injury include depth and surface area. Both depth and surface area are classified by 2 systems in common use. Although both depth and surface area are essential in making clinical decisions, additional factors need to be taken into account. These include pre-existing conditions and the presence of other injuries such as musculoskeletal, neuromuscular, and, most importantly, inhalation injuries. Age, resilience/frailty (taking into account the general wellness of a person at a given age), and immune status are also critical components in the outcome of a burn injury. Therefore, neither the depth nor the percentage of BSA alone is entirely predictive of a burn injury's outcome. Computations designed to aid in clinical decisions are presented in the following sections.

Body Surface Area

Of the methods in general use to calculate the total body area affected by a burn, the Lund and Browder method is more accurate, but the Rule of Nines is more rapidly computed. Both are limited by the fact that burn injuries do not stop at the arbitrary border of body parts. Fractions of multiple body parts will generally occur. Moreover, not all individuals have the same proportions of surface area occupying each body part. Because both systems were developed for adults, adjustments are used for children. Although the differences in BSA gradually decrease with age, arbitrary cutoffs are used for adult and child values. Children have a much greater percentage surface area on the head and much less on the lower extremities. Thus, the adjustments for children capture the total BSA less accurately. Although major clinical decisions will not be made based on small differences in BSA estimations, one should not attempt to compare the severity of injury based on a small difference in BSA.

Lund and Browder Method

The older method of Lund and Browder uses charts with percentages of BSA, as shown in Figure 14-2A. One determines which body parts are burned, and if necessary, uses a fraction of a body part, mainly when the burn injury is limited to either the front or back of the body. The percentages read from the chart are summed to determine the total BSA. Simple erythema is not to be included, so early assessment may result in a less accurate estimation of burned surface area due to either the inclusion of surface area with reversible injury or exclusion of surface area that later evolves into an irreversible injury. The adult chart is used for children from 7 years old to adults. The child's version is used for newborns up to the age of 7. Although this method is reasonably accurate and takes into account changes in body proportions with age, the Lund and Browder method takes some time to compute.

Wallace Rule of Nines

Because the Lund and Browder method requires charting and computation, the Rule of Nines is faster to use in a multiple-injury triage situation. The body is divided into parts conveniently valued at 9% or multiples thereof. This system creates 11 potential multiples of 9 for 99%. For convenience, the genitalia/perineum is assigned a value of 1%. In trying to commit this to memory, one needs to keep in mind that (1) the trunk represents about one-third of BSA, and (2) the lower extremities account for about twice as much BSA as the upper extremities. With this in mind, the entire head and the entirety of each upper extremity are assigned 9%. Both the front and the back of the trunk

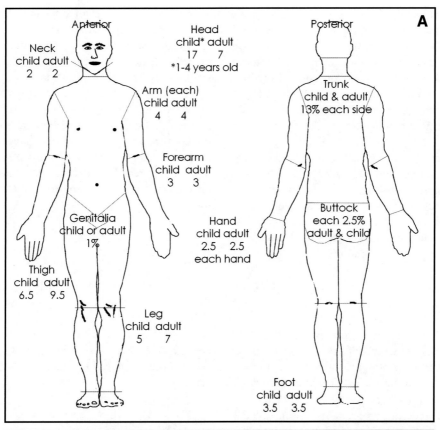

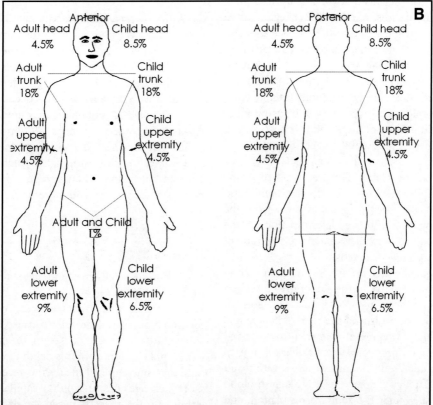

Figure 14-2. Methods of computing BSA. (A) Lund and Browder method. (B) Rule of Nines.

are assigned 2 × 9% = 18% for the front and again for the back (36% total for the trunk). Each lower extremity is also assigned 18% giving a sum of head (1 × 9), upper extremities (2 × 9 total), trunk (4 × 9 total), lower extremities (4 × 9 total) = 11 × 9%. Because one side of the body is often affected without the other, one may use 4.5% for the face or one side of an upper extremity, 9% for one side of a lower extremity, and 18% for one side of the trunk in calculations.

An adaptation of the Rule of Nines has been created for children to account for body proportions with age. Several attempts to devise a system for children have been developed, but the simplicity of the addition of nines becomes lost, and the Lund and Browder system could be used instead. One such system is depicted in Figure 14-2B along with the Rule of Nines for adults.

Depth of Injury

To explain the evaluation of thermal injuries of the skin, a review of several aspects of skin anatomy is necessary. The epidermis is the avascular layer of the skin with 4 strata (5 on the palms and soles). The deepest stratum, the stratum basale, is the regenerative layer. The interface of the dermis and epidermis forms an undulating, wavelike surface; the area of the dermis that extends up into these waves is the papillary dermis, and the thicker region of the dermis beneath this is the reticular dermis. Melanocytes are present in the stratum basale, and necrosis down to this layer carries the risk of pigment loss from the skin. Of the sensory receptors located in the dermis, the Pacinian corpuscle is located most deeply. Hair follicles and other appendages of the epidermis dive deeply into surrounding reticular dermis. Knowledge of these points is necessary to perform an examination to reveal the depth of injury.

Most burn injuries other than superficial thickness will be combinations of depths. The area exposed to the greatest amount of heat will have the deepest injury, and the depth of injury decreases progressing away from the site of greatest injury. Definitive determination of the injury stage may require 3 to 4 days due to the evolution of the wound and the presence of eschar.

A concept frequently used to explain this phenomenon of the depth of injury relative to the site of greatest insult is to classify areas of the injury into 3 zones: the zone of coagulation, the zone of stasis, and the zone of hyperemia. The zone of coagulation represents the area that received the most severe injury, producing irreversible cell injury. The zone of stasis represents an area of less severe insult with reversible cell injury characterized by sluggish blood flow. This region surrounds the zone of coagulation, and cell death may occur in this zone if the tissue is exposed to further insult. Surrounding the zone of stasis is the zone of hyperemia. This area is inflamed but is expected to recover completely. A deep partial-thickness wound is an example of a wound with a zone of coagulation that extends into the reticular dermis. The remainder of the reticular dermis would likely be in the zone of stasis.

Further injury to the reticular dermis would convert the deep partial-thickness injury into a full-thickness injury. Additionally, areas of the body have different skin thicknesses, and skin thickness changes with age. Areas of very thin skin or the skin of infants and older patients will receive greater depths of injury as classified in the following sections for the same amount of heat transferred to the skin.

Degrees

A simplistic, older system is the first-, second-, and third-degree system. This system misses a critical distinction between a full-thickness injury and a deep partial-thickness injury. An additional term, fourth degree, was created to describe a subcutaneous injury. Although this system is inadequate, it is still in common use, even in burn centers.

First Degree

A first-degree burn describes an injury limited to the epidermis. Reversible injury to the dermis causes dermal swelling and itch but not blistering. The skin becomes dry, red, and painful to touch. The epidermis will exfoliate in approximately 1 week. First-degree burns are commonly associated with sunburn but also occur from brief contact with small quantities of moderately hot liquid or mildly hot objects as in cooking mishaps. More prolonged contact or hotter liquids or liquids that adhere to the skin may produce deeper injuries. Although a single episode does not cause any permanent injury, repeated sunburn increases the risk of skin cancer, and more severe sunburn can cause deeper injury.

Second Degree

Blistering, erythema, and pain are characteristic of this level of injury. Greater transfer of heat to the skin than what occurs in a first-degree injury results in sufficient inflammation of the dermis to cause leakage of transudate. Fluid then accumulates in the space between the dermis and epidermis. In this depth of injury, generally, no more than one-third of the dermis receives an irreversible injury. Leakage of fluid from the capillaries of the papillary dermis into the space between the dermis and epidermis can continue for several days, and evolution of the injury

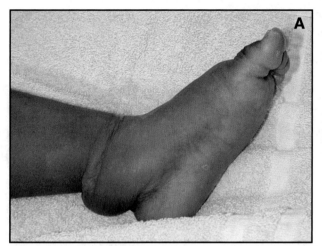
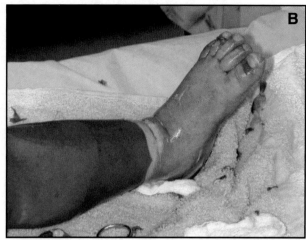

Figure 14-3. Example of second-degree/superficial partial-thickness burn injury. (A) Prior to debridement. (B) After debridement. (Reproduced with permission from Arkansas Children's Hospital, Little Rock, Arkansas.)

from erythema to blistering may occur over 3 to 5 days. In these areas of injury, massive quantities of serous fluid can accumulate, breaking hemidesmosomes between the layers. Pain from this degree of injury is the greatest of any depth of injury due to the intact nociceptors in the skin. Blistering may range from less than 1 cm to several centimeters in diameter and height above the surrounding skin. Exposure of the dermis with rupture of blisters increases the risk of infection. An example is shown in Figure 14-3.

The decision to deliberately rupture blisters remains controversial. The intact but nonviable and stretched epidermal layer prevents contamination of the dermis below and loss of water vapor from the wound that would occur from the exposed dermis. However, these blisters may rupture spontaneously and become contaminated under uncontrolled conditions. Molecules related to the inflammatory process are present within the blister fluid, slowing wound healing. Blisters may be debrided with surrounding necrotic tissue and covered with a broad-spectrum antibiotic such as silver sulfadiazine or polymyxin and bacitracin, which is often used on the face.

Because blisters may continue to evolve within the injured area over 3 to 5 days with new blister formation and increasing size of blisters, one should assume that any erythematous and painful area will develop blisters and treat these areas as if blisters will form. Second-degree injuries are typically caused by scalds, brief contact with hot objects, and brief contact with flame. If the blisters rupture, the wound will appear moist and red. Healing occurs spontaneously within 2 to 3 weeks without scarring. Pigmentation of the injured area will require several days to weeks, and some alterations of normal skin pigmentation may occur with hyper- or hypopigmentation.

Third Degree

A third-degree injury extends through the full thickness of the dermis (Figure 14-4). Cell death through the entire depth of reticular dermis causes anesthesia and coagulation of the blood vessels throughout the skin. The appearance of the skin varies markedly, especially with different causes of the injury. The skin may initially appear to be intact but devoid of coloration due to the cessation of blood flow (eg, due to a scalding injury). Conversely, prolonged contact with an extremely hot object such as a muffler may cause visible charring of skin.

Blood may be trapped in coagulated vessels visible from the skin's surface, but the skin will not blanch and refill. A wound that does not extend through the entire reticular dermis will allow blanching and refill of the skin. In addition, if the deep reticular dermis remains viable, vibration and pressure sensations will be intact from the Pacinian corpuscles located deep in the dermis. Because full-thickness depth of injury destroys all cells capable of regenerating dermis and the sources of epidermal cells from within the wounded area, hairs slide out easily, in contrast to the resistance to pull that occurs with a deep partial-thickness injury. Full-thickness burns are caused by prolonged contact with hot objects, scalding with very hot liquid, and particularly by the ignition of clothing.

Full-thickness injuries require the generation of granulation tissue and epidermal cell migration across the surface from surrounding epidermis and will contract unless extensive scar management is provided (covered in Chapter 17). Although some smaller wounds may close due to granulation tissue and epithelialization from the edges, wound contraction associated with healing by secondary intention of full-thickness wounds more than a few centimeters across is likely to cause functional impairments; therefore, grafting is

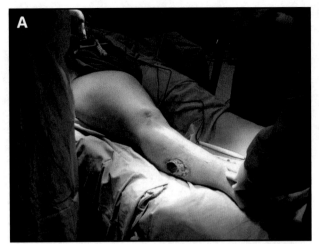 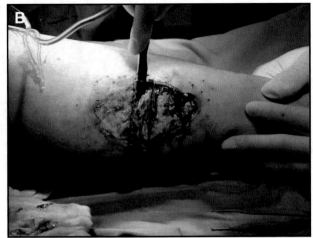

Figure 14-4. Example of a full-thickness burn injury. (A) Prior to debridement. (B) During surgical debridement. (Reproduced with permission from Arkansas Children's Hospital, Little Rock, Arkansas.)

generally done on all full-thickness burn injuries. However, skin grafts may also contract without appropriate intervention. In addition, very deep partial-thickness injuries may not close with enough dermal depth for adequate healing to occur and may also require grafting.

Fourth Degree

Very hot and prolonged contact with heat or cold can result in a depth of injury beyond the skin. Fourth-degree injuries may also be caused by very high voltage or prolonged exposure to chemicals. Tissues with a large surface area relative to their volumes, such as fingers, toes, ears, and nose, are especially at risk of fourth-degree injuries. Amputation of these areas may be required. The nose and ears may be reconstructed. Generally, the skin involved will be charred, and tissue beneath such as bones may be exposed.

Depth of Tissue Nomenclature

The preferred system among health care providers is the depth of tissue involved. A superficial injury affects just the epidermis and is synonymous with first degree. It may also be called an *epidermal burn*. A superficial partial-thickness injury is typically limited to the upper third or papillary dermis. It is characterized by blistering and is synonymous with second degree. It may also be called a *superficial dermal burn*. A full-thickness injury extends the entire depth of dermis and is synonymous with a third-degree burn. A subcutaneous injury is synonymous with a fourth-degree burn. The depth of injury system adds the concept of a deep partial-thickness injury.

Deep Partial-Thickness Injury

A deep partial-thickness injury involves some depth of the reticular dermis. It is the most critical depth in terms of preventing further injury. Additional trauma such as infection or overheating this depth of injury can result in the death of the remaining dermis and conversion to a full-thickness injury. This depth is not described adequately in terms of "degrees." Although some might refer to this depth as a *second-degree burn*, the term is generally reserved for an injury characterized by blistering. This depth may also be termed a *deep dermal burn*. Deep partial-thickness burns (Figure 14-5) are the most difficult to distinguish, especially early on. They may be a variety of colors, ranging from tan to white and red. Severe injury to the papillary dermis that extends partially into the reticular dermis coagulates blood vessels in the papillary dermis but leaves the deepest parts of hair follicles and other appendages that produce epidermal cells intact. Blisters will not be evident even in the presence of severe edema due to the thickness of injured tissue and the adherence of injured tissue.

In a deep partial-thickness injury, blood vessels in the deeper reticular dermis remain viable, but a slow capillary refill will be present compared with more superficial injuries. Sensory testing will reveal the preservation of pressure sensation to a pinprick but not a normal sharp sensation. Because of the depth of the hair follicle within the skin, hair follicles are still viable in deep partial-thickness injuries. Therefore, one may be able to distinguish deep partial-thickness injuries from full-thickness by pulling on available hairs. If flames cause the injury, however, hairs may not be available for the evaluation of the depth. Skin can potentially re-epithelialize and regain nearly normal appearance and function over weeks to months of remodeling of the injured dermis. However, necrosis of more superficial tissue with loss of its barrier function places the reversibly injured deep dermis at risk of irreversible injury and necrosis due to infection, trauma, and other stresses.

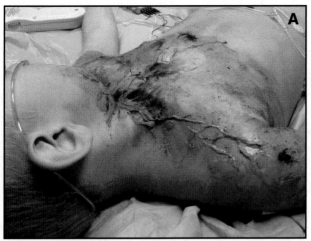
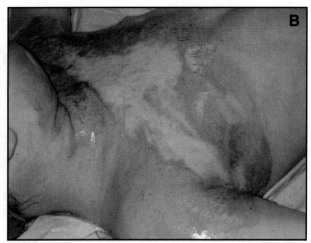

Figure 14-5. Example of deep partial-thickness burn injury. (A) Prior to debridement. (B) After debridement. (Reproduced with permission from Arkansas Children's Hospital, Little Rock, Arkansas.)

In all types of injury, new epithelial cells will be thinly layered and dry and, therefore, easily damaged. Regenerating skin must be protected from mechanical trauma, elevated temperature, and sun exposure. In deep partial-thickness and full-thickness injuries, moisturizers are needed to prevent excess drying secondary to damage to sebaceous glands. Coagulated tissue, even in deep partial-thickness injuries, may form eschar on top of tremendous swelling and produce compartment syndrome with possible vascular and neural compromise. Therefore, capillary refill of distal tissues must be checked. In the case of substantial eschar, especially in circumferential injuries, with swelling in deep partial-thickness and full-thickness burns, an incision through eschar to relieve pressure on subcutaneous tissues, called an *escharotomy*, will need to be performed (Figure 14-6). Characteristics of burn injury depth classes are summarized in Table 14-1.

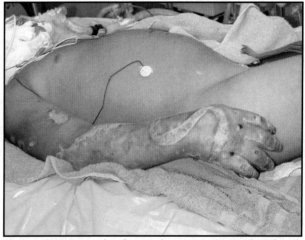

Figure 14-6. Example of an escharotomy. (Reproduced with permission from Arkansas Children's Hospital, Little Rock, Arkansas.)

Other Prognostic Indicators

In addition to the BSA and depth determinations, 2 other systems are used to estimate the severity of burn injuries.

Burn Index

Neither BSA nor depth alone is sufficient to assess the overall severity of the injuries. Burn index was developed in an effort to take both factors into account rapidly. The computation is based on the assumption that a partial-thickness depth injury is only 50% as severe as a full-thickness injury. Burn index is calculated as BI = % full thickness + 0.5 × % partial thickness. This calculation would assume that a full-thickness injury over 10% of BSA is equivalent to a partial-thickness injury over 20% of the BSA.

Baux Score

This score was designed to predict the severity of burn injury outcome based solely on the sum of the percent body surface burned and the patient's age. Originally, a score greater than 140 was considered unsurvivable. The modified version takes into account inhalation injury, which adds 17 points. Therefore, the modified Baux score is computed as % burned BSA + age + 17 points if inhalation injury occurs. With the improvement in burn therapy since the development of the Baux score, approximately 50% of those with a score of between 130 and 140 are expected to survive.

TABLE 14-1
Characteristics of the Different Classes

DEGREE	CAUSE	APPEARANCE	PAIN LEVEL	HEALING TIME
First/superficial	Sunburn, scald, flash flame	Dry, no blisters	Painful	2 to 5 days with peeling, no scarring
Second/superficial partial thickness	Brief contact with hot liquids or solids, flash flame, chemical	Pink to cherry red; moist blisters	Painful	5 to 21 days, no grafting
Deep partial thickness	Similar to above and below with corresponding greater or lesser intensity	Mixed white, waxy, pearly, or deep khaki; blanches with pressure. Dry, leathery; hairs (if any) resist tugging	Some pain	If no infection, then 21 to 35 days. If infected, converts to full-thickness
Third/full thickness	Contact with hot liquids or solids, flame, chemical, or electrical	Mixed white, waxy, pearly, deep khaki, mahogany, or charred. Dry, leathery	No pain in this area but painful in surrounding areas of partial and superficial thickness	Large areas may need months with skin grafting; small areas need weeks with or without grafting

BURN INTERVENTIONS

Treatment of the burned person may include some or all of the following depending on the extent and severity of burns. Medical management includes emergency care, pain management, surgical debridement, and grafting. Physical therapists and other health care providers may be involved in further debridement, dressing changes, exercise, positioning, splinting, and scar management. Persons with small, partial-thickness wounds may require no emergency medical procedures. These individuals may receive only pain medications and either brief inpatient or outpatient care for debridement, dressing changes, exercises, positioning, splinting, and scar management.

Medical Management

Major burns due to a combination of severity and BSA are life-threatening and may have complications requiring emergency care. Life-threatening complications of burn injuries include hypovolemic shock, inhalation injury, and burn infection. Hypovolemic shock is due to the profound loss of fluid through multiple mechanisms. Fluid is lost directly through open wounds by evaporation. Additionally, even greater loss of fluid from cells and blood occurs from the burn injury. Fluid is lost from intracellular to interstitial space due to the osmotic effect of dead tissue. Loss of plasma proteins from damaged blood vessels creates a substantial loss of fluid from the vascular to the interstitial space. This loss of fluid to the interstitium creates substantial swelling, but a rather large volume must be given to prevent hypovolemic shock. Fluid resuscitation is calculated as $4 \text{ mL/kg} \times \% \text{ BSA}$, with half administered over 8 hours. For example, a 70-kg person with 20% BSA burned would receive a total fluid replacement of $4 \text{ mL/} (\text{kg} \times \% \text{ BSA}) \times 70 \text{ kg} \times 20\% \text{ BSA} = 5600 \text{ mL}$.

Lungs can be injured due to both heat and inhaled toxins, which may lead to the development of acute respiratory distress syndrome. Burn infection may be caused by loss of the first barrier to infection, the presence of necrotic tissue, decreased blood flow to the burned area, and immune suppression that occurs with burn injury. Following burn infection, bacteremia, especially if gram-negative organisms are involved, may produce septic shock and death. Burn injuries are also particularly susceptible to fungal infections.

For those admitted to a major burn center, management can be discussed as occurring in 4 phases. Hospitalization is expected to be approximately 1 day for each percent BSA burned plus 5 days for each grafting procedure, barring serious complications. Many individuals are hospitalized for months and may be intubated several times during hospitalization. Wound infections will also add to the length of stay.

The initial phase consists of lifesaving measures lasting 1 to 3 days. Initial evaluation consists of determining the severity of the injury, intravenous access, weighing the patient to monitor fluid intake and output, and fluid resuscitation. In addition, any other injuries that may have occurred and any comorbid conditions are assessed.

The second phase consists of the excision of dead skin and coverage of open wounds. Debridement of a full-thickness injury is demonstrated in Figure 14-4B. At this stage, the wounds are covered by one or a combination of materials such as allografts and xenografts to protect against fluid loss and infection. Full coverage may require multiple operations over several days.

The third phase includes definitive wound closure, typically through autografting, as much as possible. The fourth phase is rehabilitation and reconstruction. Rehabilitation and some reconstruction, such as hands and face, may have occurred during the third phase, but the fourth phase consists of just these elements. Rehabilitation during the third phase may be interrupted to allow time for grafts to take sufficiently. This time can vary significantly among surgeons. Early and high-quality rehabilitation is paramount due to the risk of loss of motion. One study found that even after 17 years, many patients reported joint pain and stiffness, difficulty with mobility, and limited motion, particularly in the neck, axilla, and hands.

Debridement and Cleansing

Debridement and cleansing may be the responsibility of physical therapists, occupational therapists, or burn technicians. The type and extent of debridement or cleansing depend on the severity of the wound in terms of the depth of injury and the percentage of BSA burned. Small, partial-thickness wounds may be cleaned and debrided daily or twice per day. Large, full-thickness wounds may be surgically debrided to the extent possible immediately on arrival in a burn center. During hydrotherapy or another cleansing method, water temperature should not exceed body temperature; excess heat can exacerbate damage to reversibly damaged cells. Preceding dressing changes, some clinics may use either whirlpool or cleansing with a basin and sterile saline to continue debridement and remove topical medications and remaining contaminants. Silver sulfadiazine may be covered with a dressing or left uncovered. A simple bandage roll may suffice to protect the silver sulfadiazine from being removed by normal contact of the extremity during activity. Other options include Sulfamylon (mafenide acetate) and silver dressings. In the case of superficial partial-thickness burns with blisters, fanfolding the bandage roll or placing multiple gauze sponges over the blisters may be necessary to absorb drainage that might occur should the blisters rupture. Once necrotic tissue is debrided, the risk of infection is decreased substantially, as is the need for silver sulfadiazine. Wounds should be evaluated at least briefly whenever dressings are changed as wounds may evolve over 3 to 4 days after the injury.

Grafting

Large full-thickness burns can only regenerate from the edges; therefore, re-epithelialization is usually too slow to be feasible. Moreover, repair by secondary intention is more likely to lead to unacceptable wound contraction and loss of function. Persons with large full-thickness burns will need skin grafts to cover their wounds. An autograft is taken from unburned areas of the patient's skin (donor site). The thighs, buttocks, and trunk are the most common, but the site chosen depends on the size of the wound and what areas are not burned. An allograft is skin derived from another person, usually a cadaver. A xenograft is taken from another species. Artificial skin and cultured skin may be used when there is not enough viable skin available for grafting. Over several weeks, a small area of skin can be grown into a large sheet under culture conditions.

Removal of donor skin is done under anesthesia with a device called a *dermatome*. Either a full-thickness or split-thickness graft may be cut. A full-thickness graft removes the entire thickness of the reticular dermis. It is required for areas such as the face, neck, and flexor surfaces such as the elbow and axilla due to the superior functional and cosmetic results. Split-thickness grafts are cut approximately 0.017 inches in thickness and may be either placed as a sheet or meshed before attaching them. One or more partial-thickness sheets are secured to the recipient site, typically by suture or staple.

The recipient site must be clear of necrotic tissue, and care is taken to avoid the accumulation of blood or serum under the graft. A sheet graft initially adheres to a site by a fibrin clot. Later, blood vessels invade the sheet and either anastomose with existing vessels in the sheet or form new vessels in the sheet. The advantage of a sheet is a cosmetically better result, but the accumulation of fluid under the graft or infection can cause graft failure. A meshed split-thickness graft can be stretched to cover up to 3 times the donor site's size, which increases the efficiency of wound coverage. Applying a split-thickness, meshed graft converts a single large wound into multiple small wounds with a short distance for cells to migrate to fill the wound. In addition to the greater coverage of a meshed graft, fluid will not accumulate beneath, thereby reducing the risk of graft failure. Healed split-thickness grafts usually produce a characteristic diamond pattern on the healed skin (Figure 14-7). Full-thickness donor sites are covered with a split-thickness graft to heal the donor site. Split-thickness grafts can be harvested repeatedly after 10 to 14 days to cover more areas (Figure 14-8). This process allows autografting to cover large areas but requires more time to provide complete coverage.

Skin grafts may fail to take for several reasons. As discussed previously, grafts first adhere to the recipient site by fibrin clot, and within several days blood vessels invade the

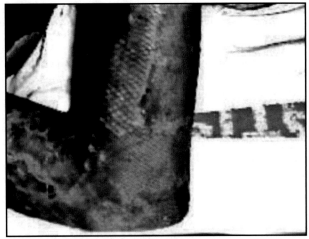

Figure 14-7. Closed split-thickness graft. (Reproduced with permission from Arkansas Children's Hospital, Little Rock, Arkansas.)

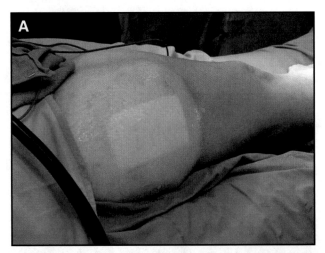

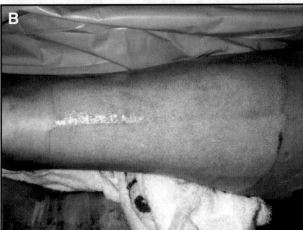

Figure 14-8. Split-thickness donor sites. (A) Buttock. (B) Posterior thigh. (Reproduced with permission from Arkansas Children's Hospital, Little Rock, Arkansas.)

graft and collagen fibers form between the graft and underlying tissue. Inadequate excision or debridement of necrotic tissue on the surface of the recipient site, inadequate contact of the graft due to accumulation of blood or serum, infection, and excessive mobility of the graft on the site are the primary reasons for grafts to fail. In many facilities, stretching and active exercise of the grafted areas are discontinued for 3 to 5 days for upper extremity and trunk grafts and 7 to 10 days for lower extremity grafts. Other facilities allow active movement within the range of motion within the limit of staple pain on the day following grafting.

RANGE OF MOTION, POSITIONING, AND SPLINTING

Exercise, positioning, and splinting are performed to avoid contractures and edema. Patients will generally hold limbs in the position of greatest comfort rather than move through a range of motion. Unwillingness to move a limb or an area of the trunk and neck is a risk for contracture; therefore, when only one side of a limb is burned, the simple solution is to splint or position so that the burned surface is put on a stretch. A second consideration for preventing contractures is knowing the propensity of the given body segments to develop contractures. The most likely areas are the hand, axilla, neck, elbow, and foot. Equinus deformity of the foot can occur even without burn injury in individuals confined to bed, especially when they are incapable or unwilling to perform active movement of the lower extremities. Those using ventilators should be watched to ensure that the ventilator tubing does not pull the neck in one direction and cause a lasting neck rotation limitation.

Contractures on the face may occur at the epicanthus, the commissures of the mouth, and lower lip. Burns to the anterior or lateral neck will cause flexion or lateral deviations of the head. Patients need to be positioned with the neck extended and rotated to the opposite side of any scar formation. This position may be accomplished by the use of 2 mattresses on the bed, with the body supported by the top mattress and the head by the lower. Contracture of the anterior axillary fold will primarily limit shoulder abduction, whereas scarring of the posterior axillary fold will limit shoulder flexion. Patients will need to have the shoulders placed in abduction and/or flexion with burns to these areas to reduce the risk of contractures.

The affected upper extremity may be placed in a tubular stocking and suspended from an overhead frame or intravenous poles to achieve the desired position. Burns involving both the neck and axilla on the same side are particularly troublesome. An involved axilla needs to be put in abduction as much as possible; however, stretching the axilla places the skin of the neck on slack, and stretching the neck requires the axilla to be placed on slack. The patient should not be placed permanently in either position, but a schedule must be developed to accommodate the positioning needs for both body segments. A patient at risk of elbow flexion contracture may need to be statically splinted in extension and alternated with flexion.

The hand is at risk for several deformities. The hand's functional position may be promoted for cases in which it is likely to become contracted. The functional position is considered to be thumb opposition, slight wrist extension, and slight finger flexion to promote grasp and allow the patient to reach the mouth for feeding and grooming. The palm is very adherent and taut, and left untreated, burn injury can produce finger flexion and opposition contractures. A burn of the palm will require a full-thickness graft to decrease the risk of contracture. The skin of the dorsum of the hand can accommodate substantial swelling, which, in turn, can produce a variety of deformities of the fingers. Unresolved swelling of the dorsum of the hand produces a claw hand deformity with metacarpal-phalangeal extension and proximal and distal interphalangeal joint flexion. Injury to the relatively superficial extensor tendons of the hand can also produce boutonniere, swan neck, or mallet finger deformities.

Burns of the lower extremities may produce contractures into hip abduction and flexion and knee flexion, but the foot is at greatest risk of loss of function. The foot can develop either a contracture into dorsiflexion or plantar flexion depending on the surface injured. Plantar flexion contractures are common problems when both sides are involved and the patient is bedbound. The weight of the foot compounded by sheets and blankets over the feet place the foot in a plantarflexed position. Simple low-temperature thermoplastic splints placed on the foot are generally inadequate to overcome the forces of plantar flexion. More sophisticated and expensive devices are needed to prevent loss of dorsiflexion (Figure 14-9). Knee immobilizers and prone positioning are options to decrease the risk of knee and hip contractures; standing erect and ambulation should be used as much as practical to minimize risk.

As a general rule, if a patient is burned on both a flexor and extensor surface, one may choose to splint or position the joint in extension because of the greater ease of stretching tissue back into flexion than stretching back into extension. Frequent range of motion into both directions becomes even more imperative in this situation to minimize shortening in either direction. If possible, one should position the patient's body segments to avoid dependence of burned area and promotion of edema. In addition, skin creases above and below the burned area should be evaluated. As scarring and wound contraction proceed, the reservoir of skin elasticity is taken up in all directions from the site of injury.

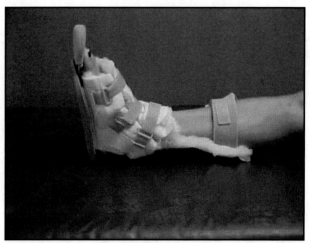

Figure 14-9. Splint used to prevent equinus deformity and protect the foot from bedding.

A potential complication that needs to be addressed in treatment planning is that skin elasticity is not equal in all directions of the body. Langer's lines represent a graphical means of discussing this phenomenon. Along the extremities, the skin is generally more extensible in a proximal-distal direction than in a medial-lateral direction. On the trunk, head, and neck, the skin is more extensible in the cephalic-caudal direction than medially and laterally. Scars oriented vertically on the trunk or extremities have greater tension than those running along Langer's lines (horizontally). Some of the Langer's lines are curved or oblique, especially at the transitions between body segments. Lines in these areas correspond to large muscles below. Over the gluteal, pectoral, and scapular regions, lines run perpendicular to the line of pull of these muscles. A scar forming along the line of pull of these muscles has greater stress on it than one forming perpendicular to the line of pull. Because the skin has more tension along these lines than between them, a round wound preferentially contracts perpendicular to these lines, resulting in an oval scar that is elongated along a Langer's line instead of a round scar. Another manifestation of tapping into the skin's reservoir of elasticity is the loss of extensibility at adjacent skin creases. If a burn occurs over 3 adjacent skin creases such as the wrist, elbow, and shoulder, the middle joint is most affected by the loss of extensibility. In the case in which 2 adjacent surfaces are injured, the more proximal joint is likely to lose extensibility.

Edema may persist following grafting. Compression garments are impractical due to the rapid decreases in swelling, leading to the need for resizing. Elastic tubular bandaging, elastic bandaging, elevation, and massage are strategies that can be customized to the individual.

Exercise

Although the prevention of contracture needs to be the primary goal of therapy, strength and cardiovascular condition need to be maintained as much as possible without compromising range of motion. Adults should have an individualized exercise program for the potential return to work, household, and community activities. Children require developmentally appropriate activities that achieve goals for range of motion, strength, aerobic capacity, and endurance. Many burn centers exist specifically for children, and their therapists should design an exercise program for the child to continue on discharge from the facility. As much as possible, the type of exercise should combine as many aspects of range of motion, strength, and aerobic capacity/endurance as possible. Ambulation for lower extremity burns and upper extremity ergometry can be utilized.

Whirlpool treatments for open wounds have been discouraged and largely replaced by shower-type hydrotherapy when needed. The Choosing Wisely campaign specifically discusses the potential problems with this modality of treatment (https://www.choosingwisely.org/clinician-lists/american-physical-therapy-association-whirlpools-for-wound-management/). Some clinicians may continue to use whirlpool to promote active range of motion exercises. Many patients who otherwise could not tolerate active movement of a hand or other body part can do so in the turbulent water. The patient needs to start moving the affected segment early. As the wound evolves and nerves regenerate, the patient may become increasingly unwilling to move affected parts of the body. Because of the potential for loss of extensibility throughout a limb due to scarring, active range of motion of other joints in the same extremity must also be encouraged despite pain; however, measures to mitigate the pain should be prescribed by the physician. The type of pain management used must be a compromise between reducing pain and allowing the patient to participate in rehabilitation.

The type of exercise used to promote range of motion may range from passive range of motion in which the movement is performed without any effort by the patient to active-assisted range of motion in which the patient's movement is guided and assisted as necessary by another person. Proprioceptive neuromuscular facilitation, better known simply as PNF, patterns and techniques can be used to more efficiently stretch tissue at several joints at once with movement in 3 planes simultaneously. The patient performs active range of motion, but they may receive verbal or tactile cues to guide the motion. An unresponsive person can only receive passive range of motion. However, the force placed on the healing skin cannot be gauged nearly as well by the person performing the passive range of motion, and the movement can be excessive.

Range of Motion

When possible, range of motion exercises are performed coordinated with dressing changes, which allows the therapist to visualize the injured tissue and decrease the risk of applying excessive force to it. Gloves are worn throughout treatment when working with burn injuries. When the patient has dressings over the burned tissue, the same pair of gloves may be used during range of motion activity. However, in the case of touching the patient's skin directly, glove changes may be required to prevent contamination among body parts. For example, a right upper extremity burn injury may be colonized with fungus that we do not wish to spread to the other upper extremity.

During range of motion exercise, the clinician needs to monitor the patient for skin blanching, complaints of pain, excessive force needed to move a body segment, and signs of apprehension from the patient. Generally, these responses will occur at the same point in the stress-strain relationship of the skin when the slack has been taken out of the affected skin, and it is stretched into the linear portion of the stress-strain relationship. The type and location of the pain reported by the patient also guide the force applied. Pain in the area of limited skin movement accompanied by tightness and blanching indicates the need to reduce force. A pain caused by movement, especially compression of the tender skin overlying a moving body segment, is not an indication to stop exercise. Finally, if a patient demonstrates an optimally expected range of motion but the skin over the area blanches, they will continue to need therapy until the body segment can be moved independently through the range of motion without blanching.

Active range of motion exercises are least likely to harm healing tissue and grafts but may be too difficult for a given individual to accomplish, especially if an individual has an altered nutritional status, diminished strength, severe pain, and already limited range of motion. Active-assisted range of motion is often an intermediate step in the progression to active range of motion exercises. When the patient is near the end of a safe range of motion, they will cease moving the limb, letting the clinician or caregiver know that an appropriate range of motion has been achieved. Active range of motion exercises are generally indicated if edema needs to be reduced in a particular body segment, if tendons are exposed, and during the first week after a skin graft. The muscle-pumping effect assists in the removal of excess fluid from the body part. An additional benefit of active rather than passive range of motion, particularly in PNF patterns, is the return to normal neuromusculoskeletal function.

Active-assisted range of motion exercise is typically indicated for a person with sufficient strength and coordination to follow verbal and tactile cues but who already has elevated metabolic demands such that active exercise may increase cardiovascular demands excessively. If existing scar tissue needs to be stretched, or if stretching of an area of an escharotomy or skin graft adherence is needed, the type of motion may need to be increased from active to active-assisted range of motion. Passive range of motion becomes necessary in some rather obvious instances, such as peripheral nerve injury or other loss of motor input to the limb, including the use of general anesthesia. Passive range of motion may also be indicated for areas that need more extensive tissue elongation or an area of escharotomy. In addition, if the patient cannot tolerate active-assisted range of motion due to excess metabolic demands, passive range of motion may be necessary for several days.

Passive range of motion exercises should not be performed in the cases of finger burns with an indeterminate depth due to the risk of tendon injury, in areas of heterotopic ossification, exposed tendons, or in extraordinarily resistive or combative patients. Range of motion exercises may be done while the patient is in full dressings, but performing these exercises during dressing changes has the advantages that the clinician can see the skin's response to the motion, and the patient will have received analgesia for the dressing change. If the burn wounds are covered, active range of motion exercises are preferred to avoid excessive force that cannot be adequately monitored.

More forceful, passive range of motion can be performed more readily while the patient is under anesthesia. Other advantages to range of motion during anesthesia include the ability to accurately determine the available range of motion and identify soft tissue restrictions, rather than limitations due to weakness or pain during active motion. Moreover, because the patient cannot feel the tissue mobilization, more thorough stretching can be performed. Disadvantages of performing passive range of motion during anesthesia include the potential for excessive movement that may result in joint dislocation, fractures, tearing of compromised ligaments and tendons, and tissue separation.

To recover lost range of motion after grafts have taken, prolonged low-load stretch is preferred. This prolonged low-load stretch can be accomplished using a dynamic splint, which uses springs or similar devices to move an extremity toward the desired position or a continuous passive movement machine. Continuous passive movement moves the affected extremity through a range of motion that can be specified in terms of its starting and stopping angle and the speed through which the extremity is moved. Gravity-assisted range of motion can be accomplished by positioning a patient such that gravity pulls the desired body segment in the desired direction. For example, a person with decreased knee extension may lie in prone with a weight attached to the foot. If this type of therapy is used, the clinician needs to monitor for blanching and skin dryness to prevent cracking of the relatively weak and brittle scar tissue of a healed burn injury. Cracking and bleeding of burned skin are common complications of attempts to restore range of motion. Care to prevent these complications should be taken, but they may not be avoidable.

Strengthening

Strength training is needed to avoid loss of lean body mass and negative nitrogen balance. With increased demands for protein and calories to repair a wound, the resultant hypermetabolic state can lead to a wasting of muscles. The patient can be instructed in simple exercises that combine range of motion and strength to provide an anabolic stimulus. Avoid exercises that place frictional or shearing forces on grafted skin and donor sites. Dietary supplementation and anabolic steroids can be prescribed to restore muscle mass.

Cardiovascular

Cardiovascular exercise is needed to maintain or improve cardiopulmonary function. Upright positioning progressing to ambulation and other cardiopulmonary training are needed to improve hematocrit and plasma volume. While working to achieve improved orthostatic tolerance, the clinician should monitor vital signs, especially if the patient experienced extensive burns or has been medically unstable. The patient may not initially be able to tolerate an upright position for ambulation. The clinician may need to wrap the lower extremities in elasticized bandages to maintain central venous pressure in upright positions. The patient may need to start with sitting up, dangling legs, or a tilt table protocol to develop sufficient orthostatic tolerance for cardiopulmonary training. If the patient lacks the mobility to reposition, a tilt table may be necessary to provide upright positioning.

The therapist should be aware of the potential of both equinus deformity and dorsal foot contractures. A patient may not be able to put the heel on the floor with an equinus deformity or put toes on the floor with a dorsal foot contracture. Such patients may be candidates for surgical releases to allow normalized ambulation.

Burns may have destroyed large numbers of sweat glands, diminishing a patient's ability to dissipate heat. During exercise, avoid overheating the patient. Have a fan available, and provide rest and water breaks during the activity. Upper extremity ergometry is particularly useful for burn rehabilitation for several reasons. Movement of the upper extremity ergometer encourages upper extremity range of motion. Because the patient is in a seated position, they can take frequent rest breaks as needed. With the lower extremities wrapped, the patient is better able to tolerate upright positioning in addition to the cardiovascular training that can be provided. The range of motion can also be progressed by moving the seat further from the ergometer.

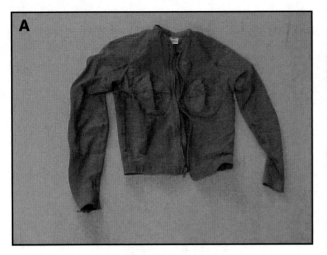

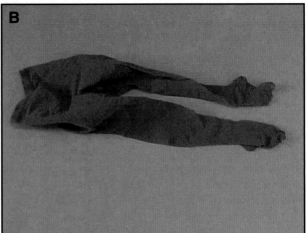

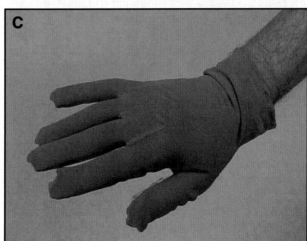

Figure 14-10. (A to C) Examples of pressure garments.

SCAR MANAGEMENT

Burn wounds, more so than other types, are likely to result in proliferative scarring. Pressure garments are typically used to minimize over-repair. Examples of pressure garments are shown in Figure 14-10. Garments are specially measured and custom-made to exert 35 mm Hg pressure equally on recovering skin. Rather than elasticized garments, clear acrylic masks are used to exert pressure on the face to minimize scarring. Patients are encouraged to begin using compression garments within 6 months of injury and to continue to use them up to 2 years to receive better results if the scar is still active in the remodeling stage and highly vascularized. Pressure garments are worn 23 hours/day and only taken off for bathing.

No predictive factors are known for which patients will respond favorably or unfavorably to compression garments. Compression garments can be uncomfortable, and maintaining garments properly can be difficult for some patients. Moreover, given that they are to be worn up to 2 years after the injury, replacing them regularly can become a financial burden. Patients who abandon pressure garments prematurely tend to have a worse outcome than those who continue to wear them for the prescribed duration. Garments are available for any body part with the delivery of a custom garment in 24 to 48 hours. The mechanism by which pressure affects scar formation is not fully understood. Some literature suggests a hypoxic effect on fibroblasts, diminishing collagen formation. Another theory suggests a mechanical effect that prevents the formation of whorls of collagen and promotes flatter ribbons of collagen fibers.

Other treatments proposed to reduce scarring of burn injuries include friction massage and ultrasound to the scars, neither of which is feasible with large areas of burns. Further discussion of scar management is provided in Chapter 17.

SUMMARY

Burns are common injuries, although the vast majority of them are minor and self-treated. Major burns are severe injuries requiring intensive care and rehabilitation. Therapy for burn injuries includes wound debridement, dressing changes, exercise, positioning, and splinting. Technicians in burn centers usually perform debridement and dressing changes for large full-thickness injuries, but less severe injuries may be managed in a physical therapy inpatient or outpatient clinic. Grafting, exercise, positioning, and splinting are performed to minimize the loss of elasticity of the skin. If possible, the injured area is kept on stretch, but both surfaces may be injured, and clinical decisions to minimize loss of function must be made. Critical areas include the neck, axilla, elbow, and foot. The appropriate use of active, active-assisted, and passive range of motion are described. In addition to range of motion, exercises must be directed at maintaining muscle mass and cardiovascular function.

QUESTIONS

1. What are the 2 systems for quantifying the depth of burn injury?

2. What are the advantages and disadvantages of depth names vs degrees?

3. What is the appearance of a superficial burn injury? What is the equivalent in degree? What tissue is irreversibly injured? What tissue is reversibly injured? How does this relate to the appearance?

4. What intervention is required for a first-degree injury? Why might medical attention be required?

5. What characterizes superficial partial-thickness injuries. What is the equivalent in degree? What tissues are irreversibly injured? What tissue is reversibly injured? Why does blistering occur as opposed to a first-degree injury?

6. What is the time frame for the appearance of blistering?

7. What intervention is required for second-degree injuries?

8. What characterizes a deep partial-thickness injury? How can it be distinguished from a full-thickness injury? What is the degree equivalent?

9. What is an escharotomy? Why is it performed in deep burn injuries?

10. What is the primary goal of treating a deep partial-thickness wound?

11. What intervention is required for deep partial-thickness injuries?

12. What happens if a deep partial-thickness injury becomes full-thickness?

13. What constitutes a major burn such that a patient is sent to a major burn center?

14. What is the significance of burn injuries having a combination of depths?

15. What are the implications of the zones of hyperemia, stasis, and coagulation?

16. What is the Rule of Nines method of quantification of BSA?

17. What is the advantage of the Rule of Nines? What is the advantage of the Lund and Browder method?

18. What are the primary differences in quantifying BSA in adults and children?

19. What is the purpose of the burn index? How do you compute it?

20. What causes frostbite? What is frostnip? How is frostbite managed?

21. What are the complications of electrical burns, including high voltage vs lower voltage?

22. Distinguish wet and dry desquamation.

23. What is the purpose of a full-thickness graft? Where are they typically used? What is the limiting factor in full-thickness grafting?

24. What is the purpose of a split-thickness graft? What advantages do they have? What is the primary disadvantage?

25. When might whirlpool be indicated in burn treatment? What is the primary problem with using whirlpools? What has superseded whirlpools in major burn centers?

26. What temperature should be used with hydrotherapy? Why?

27. What is the most critical aspect of physical therapy involvement in burn injuries?

28. Why are gloves changed between different body parts when touching burned areas without bandages?

29. What are the advantages and disadvantages of passive range of motion, active-assisted range of motion, and active range of motion?

30. What options are available to optimize time working on range of motion, strength, and conditioning?

BIBLIOGRAPHY

Abdelbasset WK, Abdelhalim NM. Assessing the effects of 6 weeks of intermittent aerobic exercise on aerobic capacity, muscle fatigability, and quality of life in diabetic burned patients: randomized control study. *Burns.* 2020;46(5):1193-1200.

Ahmed ET, Abdel-aziem AA, Ebid AA. Effect of isokinetic training on quadriceps peak torgue in healthy subjects and patients with burn injury. *J Rehabil Med.* 2011;43(10):930-934.

Björnhagen V, Ekholm KS, Larsen F, Ekholm J. Burn survivors' pulmonary and muscular impairment, exercise tolerance and return-to-work following medical-vocational rehabilitation: a long-term follow-up. *J Rehabil Med.* 2018;50(5):465-471.

Cambiaso-Daniel J, Rivas E, Carson JS, et al. Cardiorespiratory capacity and strength remain attenuated in children with severe burn injuries at over 3 years postburn. *J Pediatr.* 2018;192:152-158.

Chao T, Herndon DN, Porter C, et al. Skeletal muscle protein breakdown remains elevated in pediatric burn survivors up to one-year post-injury. *Shock.* 2015;44(5):397-401.

Chen H, Pan W, Zhang J, Cheng H, Tan Q. The application of W-plasty combined Botox-A injection in treating sunk scar on the face. *Medicine (Baltimore).* 2018;97(30):e11427.

Diego AM, Serghiou M, Padmanabha A, Porro LJ, Herndon DN, Suman OE. Exercise training after burn injury: a survey of practice. *J Burn Care Res.* 2013;34(6):e311-e317.

Donovan ML, Muller MJ, Simpson C, Rudd M, Paratz J. Interim pressure garment therapy (4-6 mmHg) and its effect on donor site healing in burn patients: study protocol for a randomised controlled trial. *Trials.* 2016;17(1):214.

Flores O, Tyack Z, Stockton K, Paratz JD. The use of exercise in burns rehabilitation: a worldwide survey of practice. *Burns.* 2020;46(2):322-332.

Fufa DT, Chuang SS, Yang JY. Prevention and surgical management of postburn contractures of the hand. *Curr Rev Musculoskelet Med.* 2014;7(1):53-59.

Gacto-Sanchez P. Surgical treatment and management of the severely burn patient: review and update. *Med Intensiva.* 2017;41(6):356-364.

Gauffin E, Öster C, Sjöberg F, Gerdin B, Ekselius L. Health-related quality of life (EQ-5D) early after injury predicts long-term pain after burn. *Burns.* 2016;42(8):1781-1788.

Gittings PM, Grisbrook TL, Edgar DW, Wood FM, Wand BM, O'Connell NE. Resistance training for rehabilitation after burn injury: a systematic literature review & meta-analysis. *Burns.* 2018;44(4):731-751.

Hardee JP, Porter C, Sidossis LS, et al. Early rehabilitative exercise training in the recovery from pediatric burn. *Med Sci Sports Exerc.* 2014;46(9):1710-1716.

Jeschke MG, van Baar ME, Choudhry MA, Chung KK, Gibran NS, Logsetty S. Burn injury. *Nat Rev Dis Primers.* 2020;6(1):11.

Karimi H, Mobayen M, Alijanpour A. Management of hypertrophic burn scar: a comparison between the efficacy of exercise-physiotherapy and pressure garment-silicone on hypertrophic scar. *Asian J Sports Med.* 2013;4(1):70-75.

Klein GL. Burn injury and restoration of muscle function. *Bone.* 2020;132:115194.

Klein GL, Herndon DN, Le PT, Andersen CR, Benjamin D, Rosen C. The effect of burn on serum concentrations of sclerostin and FGF23. *Burns.* 2015;41(7):1532-1535.

Klein GL, Xie Y, Qin YX, et al. Preliminary evidence of early bone resorption in a sheep model of acute burn injury: an observational study. *J Bone Miner Metab.* 2014;32(2):136-141.

Klifto KM, Dellon AL, Hultman CS. Risk factors associated with the progression from acute to chronic neuropathic pain after burn-related injuries. *Ann Plast Surg.* 2020;84(6S Suppl 5):S382-S385.

Koller T. Mechanosensitive aspects of cell biology in manual scar therapy for deep dermal defects. *Int J Mol Sci.* 2020;21(6):2055.

Kraft R, Herndon DN, Al-Mousawi AM, Williams FN, Finnerty CC, Jeschke MG. Burn size and survival probability in paediatric patients in modern burn care: a prospective observational cohort study. *Lancet.* 2012;379(9820):1013-1021.

Lensing J, Wibbenmeyer L, Liao J, et al. Demographic and burn injury-specific variables associated with limited joint mobility at discharge in a multicenter study. *J Burn Care Res.* 2020;41(2):363-370.

Levi B, Jayakumar P, Giladi A, et al. Risk factors for the development of heterotopic ossification in seriously burned adults: a National Institute on Disability, Independent Living and Rehabilitation Research burn model system database analysis. *J Trauma Acute Care Surg.* 2015;79(5):870-876.

Muschitz GK, Schwabegger E, Fochtmann A, et al. Long-term effects of severe burn injury on bone turnover and microarchitecture. *J Bone Miner Res.* 2017;32(12):2381-2393.

O'Brien KH. Dimensions of burn survivor distress and its impact on hospital length of stay: a national institute on disability, independent living, and rehabilitation research burn model system study. *Burns.* 2020;46(2):286-292.

Pearson J, Ganio MS, Schlader ZL, et al. Post junctional sudomotor and cutaneous vascular responses in noninjured skin following heat acclimation in burn survivors. *J Burn Care Res.* 2017;38(1):e284-e292.

Pham TN, Goldstein R, Carrougher GJ, et al. The impact of discharge contracture on return to work after burn injury: a Burn Model System investigation. *Burns.* 2020;46(3):539-545.

Polychronopoulou E, Herndon DN, Porter C. The long-term impact of severe burn trauma on musculoskeletal health. *J Burn Care Res.* 2018;39(6):869-880.

Riaz HM, Mehmood Bhatti Z. Quality of life in adults with lower limb burn injury. *J Burn Care Res.* 2020;41(6):1212-1215.

Rivas E, Herndon DN, Beck KC, Suman OE. Children with burn injury have impaired cardiac output during submaximal exercise. *Med Sci Sports Exerc.* 2017;49(10):1993-2000.

Rivas E, Sanchez K, Cambiaso-Daniel J, et al. Burn injury may have age-dependent effects on strength and aerobic exercise capacity in males. *J Burn Care Res.* 2018;39(5):815-822.

Rontoyanni VG, Malagaris I, Herndon DN, et al. Skeletal muscle mitochondrial function is determined by burn severity, sex, and sepsis, and is associated with glucose metabolism and functional capacity in burned children. *Shock.* 2018;50(2):141-148.

Rowan MP, Cancio LC, Elster EA, et al. Burn wound healing and treatment: review and advancements. *Crit Care.* 2015;19:243.

Spronk I, Legemate C, Oen I, van Loey N, Polinder S, van Baar M. Health related quality of life in adults after burn injuries: a systematic review. *PLoS One.* 2018;13(5):e0197507.

Spronk I, Legemate CM, Dokter J, van Loey NEE, van Baar ME, Polinder S. Predictors of health-related quality of life after burn injuries: a systematic review. *Crit Care.* 2018;22(1):160.

Tan J, He W, Luo G, Wu J. iTRAQ-based proteomic profiling reveals different protein expression between normal skin and hypertrophic scar tissue. *Burns Trauma.* 2015;3(1):13.

Toussaint J, Chung WT, Osman N, McClain SA, Raut V, Singer AJ. Topical antibiotic ointment versus silver-containing foam dressing for second-degree burns in swine. *Acad Emerg Med.* 2015;22(8):927-933.

Won YH, Cho YS, Kim DH, Joo SY, Seo CH. Relation between low pulmonary function and skeletal muscle index in burn patients with major burn injury and smoke inhalation: a retrospective study. *J Burn Care Res.* 2020;41(3):695-699.

Zhang B, Yang L, Zeng Z, et al. Leptin potentiates BMP9-induced osteogenic differentiation of mesenchymal stem cells through the activation of JAK/STAT signaling. *Stem Cells Dev.* 2020;29(8):498-510.

Wound Bed Preparation

Irion GL, Gardner JA, Pignataro RM.
Comprehensive Wound Management, Third Edition (pp 273-296).
© 2024 Taylor and Francis Group.

REASONS FOR
WOUND BED PREPARATION

Optimizing wound healing is an appropriate goal for almost any case. Because desiccated tissue acts as a barrier to cell migration, its removal is a clear benefit to patients. However, even moist necrotic tissue is problematic. Slough occupies space within a wound and thereby decreases the ability of cells to migrate. Devitalized tissue and damaged cells release chemical mediators of inflammation, delaying proliferation required to fill a wound and promote epithelialization. Inflammation, in turn, leads to leakage of blood vessels in the wound bed, leading to loss of protein and fluid through open wounds. The leakage of proteins causes additional problems. Loss of protein from the vascular space leads to edema and malnutrition both locally in the dependent areas in which edema occurs and, in general, in the form of protein malnutrition. Fibrinogen leaking onto the surface of the wound is converted into the hard, insoluble protein coat of fibrin on the surface of a wound.

The failure to remove necrotic tissue adequately leads to chronic inflammation. Chronic inflammation can become self-sustaining due to the production of molecules that further slow healing and aging of cells within the wound bed. The other long-term consequence of chronic inflammation is the potential for malignancy. Malignancy, as a result of chronic wounds, is discussed specifically in Chapter 18.

Most critically, necrotic tissue provides an environment conducive to bacterial growth. Although infection is generally considered to be an acute problem, a chronically inflamed wound may become infected even after a long period of stability. Debridement is critical in decreasing the potential for infection. Dead tissue acts as a medium for infection and may hide infection, abscesses, tunnels, and sinus tracts. Rapid debridement can bring a wound into bacterial balance. In one series of patients, pressure injuries that had a bacterial burden of greater than 100,000/g were sharply debrided. Of these, 96% remained at less than 100/g. The ideal environment is one in which the bacteria are in balance—not bacteria free. Low levels of bacteria may accelerate certain aspects of wound healing, but a burden greater than 100,000/g severely retards healing. In particular, bacterial production of proteases capable of breaking down growth factors and the attraction of neutrophils appear to be responsible for delayed healing. The presence of ß-hemolytic streptococci is particularly problematic even in low numbers. Fibrinolysins, leukocidins, hemolysins, and hyaluronidase allow the bacteria to protect themselves from the immune system and spread through tissue. In addition to the benefits of debridement, we must also consider the risks associated with not debriding. These include slow healing, osteomyelitis, the need for amputation of an infected limb, advancing cellulitis, sepsis, and, in extreme cases, death. On these bases, debridement generally meets the definition of medical necessity. Moreover, species capable of generating a biofilm may occupy the wound and create a condition conducive to chronic inflammation.

WOUND CLEANSING

The Agency for Health Care Policy and Research (AHCPR) has recommended wound cleansing during the initial visit and at each dressing change. Prevention of injury during cleansing is emphasized. As such, some authorities recommend against using any direct scrubbing action on the wound. Others have even challenged the notion that wound cleansing must be done with every dressing change. However, the clinician who must assess the wound during a dressing change must cleanse the wound sufficiently to make appropriate decisions for further management. The failure to clear the surface of excessive bacteria may lead to biofilm formation, which may tip the balance of the wound toward chronic inflammation. The AHCPR recommends the use of normal saline or certain types of specialized detergents with a mild irrigation pressure that allows wound cleansing without traumatizing the wound bed or driving bacteria into the wound.

Irrigation

Simple cleansing by irrigation can be performed in several ways. AHCPR guidelines have suggested that irrigation pressure be between 4 and 15 psi. Pressure lower than 4 psi is believed to be ineffective at removing bacteria and debris from a wound bed. Pressures exceeding 20 psi are believed to drive bacteria into the wound. If removal of surface bacteria is the cleansing goal, commercially available irrigation bulbs produce too little pressure. Another option that provides sufficient pressure to remove surface bacteria is using a 19-gauge catheter syringe, as demonstrated in Figure 15-1.

If greater force than simple irrigation is needed to remove surface material, wound cleansing may also be done with a minimal amount of mechanical force with gauze, cloth, sponges, and either normal saline or special detergents. Although antiseptics and disinfectants have historically been used for wound cleansing, the AHCPR recommends that clinicians not use agents such as sodium hypochlorite; Dakin's solution; hydrogen peroxide; iodine; acetic acid; or antiseptics designed for use on intact skin such as Phisohex (Sanofi-Aventis), Phisoderm (Mentholatum Company), Hibiclens (Molnlycke), or povidone-iodine scrub on pressure injuries. Although some of these agents may be appropriate for initial cleansing of acute wounds, the principle for which the AHCPR panel recommended against the use of antiseptic agents on pressure injuries should be extended to other chronic wounds.

Other means of cleansing a wound overlap with debridement. These methods include whirlpool and pulsatile lavage with concurrent suction (pulsed lavage). Devices designed specifically for cleaning teeth and gums have historically been used for irrigation. These devices are not designed to produce appropriate pressure, and splattering cannot be contained. Irrigation devices should have a splash shield and preferably a transparent drape to prevent splattering necrotic tissue and contaminated fluid over the treatment area and aerosolizing bacteria. Several devices have recently been developed incorporating both the irrigation pressure desired and a splash shield. Pulsatile lavage devices deliver appropriate pressure and include splash shields and suction to aid in removing loosened necrotic tissue and to minimize the spray of contaminated fluid in the treatment area. Some pulsed lavage kits include a drape to prevent aerosolization and splashing. When used specifically to remove necrotic tissue, pulsatile lavage is considered a form of debridement rather than wound cleansing. Whirlpool treatment has mostly been supplanted by pulsed lavage and should only be considered for particular cases for which it might be appropriate. Whirlpool treatment has serious issues with infection control, as discussed in Chapter 5, including difficulty in adequate cleaning and disinfection, cross contamination, and aerosolization. Whirlpool can be useful to clean residues of materials such as silver sulfadiazine from full- and partial-thickness burns when simple irrigation is insufficient. Another benefit of using whirlpool for this type of injury is the patient's willingness to perform range of motion exercises in the moving water that would not be tolerated otherwise.

DEBRIDEMENT

Guidelines from organizations such as the American Diabetes Association and the National Pressure Injury Advisory Panel encourage debridement for most cases. Also, insurance providers may deny payment for many adjunct therapies if debridement has not been performed. The AHCPR guidelines call for the removal of any necrotic tissue from the wound, when appropriate, using the method most appropriate to the patient's condition and goals and the need to assess and control pain. Because of the availability of different methods for individuals with

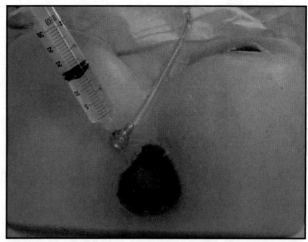

Figure 15-1. Irrigation by syringe and catheter. This type of system provides the optimal irrigation pressure that is effective without driving bacteria into the wound.

different treatment goals and in different settings (eg, inpatient vs home health), the recommendation of AHCPR for debridement of pressure injuries cannot be more specific. These guidelines also state that any one or a combination of sharp, mechanical, enzymatic, or autolytic debridement techniques may be used unless an urgent need for removal of devitalized tissue with sharp debridement arises.

Types of Debridement

Four basic types of debridement are typically described: sharp, mechanical (nonspecific), enzymatic (chemical), and autolytic. A fifth type, biologic or larva therapy, uses sterile medical maggots. The type of debridement suitable for a given wound, as with any intervention, depends on the complete clinical picture including characteristics of the wound, characteristics of the patient, social and work responsibilities, resources available, and the setting in which the patient is being seen. Important factors to consider in deciding which type of debridement to use include the type of wound (etiology); the amount of necrotic tissue, which may not be observable initially; the condition of the patient, including terminal illness; the care setting, which includes time constraints on discharge; and the clinician or caregiver experience. The clinician must examine the wound's depth of necrotic tissue using good lighting and be familiar with different tissue types. The clinician should also consider patient preferences. Issues related to patient preference include the time frame for the plan of care, pain, and psychological issues and who will be available to perform dressing changes.

Mechanical Debridement

To remove necrotic tissue from a wound quickly, mechanical shearing or scrubbing forces can be applied. Most of these techniques cannot selectively remove necrotic tissue and are often discussed as a means of nonspecific debridement. A straightforward technique is scrubbing the necrotic tissue with a saline-moistened gauze or another type of sponge. Rather than using direct scrubbing on the wound, some clinicians will utilize hydrotherapy and irrigation. Hydrotherapy and wound irrigation are useful for softening and mechanical removal of eschar and debris. A recommended method is irrigation through a 19-gauge catheter or equivalent to produce optimal irrigation pressure. Too little pressure is ineffective in removing necrotic tissue, whereas excessive pressure may drive bacteria into the wound and create splattering and aerosolization. When a very rapid debridement of substantial necrotic tissue is required (eg, with advancing infection), nonselective, mechanical debridement should be stopped as sharp debridement is now indicated.

Wet-to-Dry Dressings

The wet-to-dry dressing is largely misused and, as such, is not considered to belong in modern wound management. A moistened gauze sponge (frequently 4 × 4) is placed into the necrotic area and is allowed to dry completely. The adherent necrotic tissue is pulled out of the wound with the 4 × 4 sponge. This procedure can be excruciating and is nonspecific in that healthy tissue may be removed along with the necrotic tissue. Wet-to-dry dressings should be changed every 4 to 6 hours using adequate analgesia. Although sharp debridement is likely to produce a better outcome, wet-to-dry dressing removal done properly can provide rapid debridement to prepare a wound for operative repair or to prepare a patient for discharge to home when the wound is clean and stable.

Clinicians should never place a dry dressing on granulation tissue. Removal of dry dressings from granulation tissue causes bleeding and damages the new tissue. Wet-to-dry dressings are not cost-effective for small wounds or wounds with little necrotic tissue, nor do they have any place in a facility where sharp debridement could be performed. Ethical considerations contraindicate wet-to-dry dressings unless a clear benefit to the patient can be demonstrated. Pain and the loss of healthy tissue must be counterbalanced with an improved outcome such as earlier discharge from the hospital to meet ethical standards. The use of wet-to-dry dressings under circumstances in which a gentler method yields a similar outcome must be considered unethical. The purpose of the wet-to-dry dressing is also undermined when clinicians soak the dressing off the wound. If a referral is received requesting a wet-to-dry dressing and the clinician determines that this approach is inappropriate, the clinician should arrange a discussion with the referring physician explaining the appropriate options. Sharp debridement is more selective and less likely to cause pain and damage to granulation tissue.

Hydrotherapy

As noted in Chapter 14, whirlpool treatments for open wounds have been discouraged as part of the Choosing Wisely campaign (https://www.choosingwisely.org/clinician-lists/american-physical-therapy-association-whirlpools-for-wound-management/). The detrimental effects of whirlpool therapy are also described in the following. A typical hydrotherapy session is carried out in a whirlpool tank (Figure 15-2) for 20 minutes with water at a temperature generally in excess of body temperature. Agitation is directed toward the wound requiring debridement. Several benefits, but also many detrimental effects, have been described for whirlpool treatments. Also, several of the benefits commonly ascribed to whirlpool treatment have no sound physiological basis. Benefits of whirlpool therapy include moisture to soften and agitation to loosen adherent necrotic tissue, increased temperature to increase blood flow, increased metabolic rate, and proliferation of granulation tissue and epithelial cells. However, softening/loosening necrotic tissue may not be necessary with good sharp debridement skills, and wounds on some regions of the body may not be accessible to the agitated water.

Clear detrimental effects include maceration of surrounding skin, dependent position of the lower extremities, potential occlusion of venous and arterial vessels in a limb hung over the edge of a whirlpool tank, increasing the demand for blood flow in a limb with arterial insufficiency, and increased damage to burned tissue by the elevated temperature of a whirlpool. Elevated temperature increases circulation to a limb with normal, healthy blood vessels. Increased temperature raises the metabolic rate, which, in turn, increases blood flow to the area. This effect, however, only occurs in a person with the reserve to dilate blood vessels. In a person with arterial insufficiency, the demand for blood flow is increased with increasing tissue temperature, thereby aggravating the arterial insufficiency. If sufficient body surface area is exposed to a high temperature, hypotension may occur in patients with compromised cardiovascular systems or those taking antihypertensive medications.

Prolonged exposure to water creates maceration, and the removal of oil from the skin may subsequently cause dry, cracked skin. Although tanks and turbines are

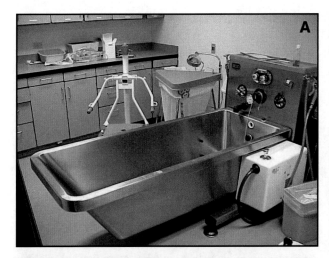

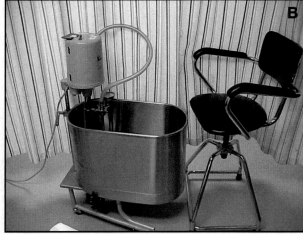

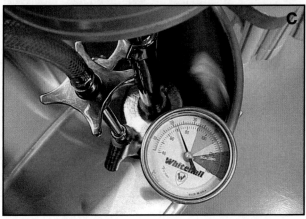

Figure 15-2. (A) Hydrotherapy tank typically used in wound care. The unit has a built-in water jet that allows the entire body to be submerged. (B) Hand/foot tank may be used for wounds on the distal leg and foot or the distal forearm and hand. (C) Close-up view of the air control and thermometer of the hand/foot unit in Figure 15-2B.

disinfected between patients, contamination may occur between disinfection and patient treatment. *Pseudomonas aeruginosa* is particularly problematic with hydrotherapy. The presence of multiple wounds may result in cross contamination. Although whirlpool tanks are cleaned with an abrasive cleanser before disinfection to remove proteinaceous deposits, the drain below the drain cover and inside the turbine cannot be scrubbed prior to disinfection. Moreover, as discussed in Chapter 2, the growth of granulation tissue occurs most rapidly at normal body temperature. The elevated temperature of most whirlpools will not increase tissue growth but is more likely to retard growth. The temperature should be kept in a lower range between 92°F and 96°F (33°C and 35.5°C). Failing to pay attention to water temperature in the whirlpool may also lead to burns in individuals who are insensitive to temperature or cause deeper injury to an area that has been burned. The turbulence of the water in the whirlpool tank can aerosolize microbes and deposit them several feet away from the tank. Additives for infection control discussed in Chapter 5 are frequently cytotoxic and may retard wound healing.

Contraindications and Precautions

Patients with range of motion limitations or who exceed the weight limits of equipment such as lifts or chairs may not be able to get into a whirlpool tank. If any area of the body should not become wet, such as a newly closed surgical incision, colostomy, ileostomy, vascular access, percutaneous instrumentations such as gastrostomy, or the patient has a cast that cannot be protected from the water, an alternative treatment is needed. In addition, patients who are not allowed out of their rooms because of isolation or require a ventilator cannot be transported to a whirlpool tank. Patients may have allergies to additives to the whirlpool. Wounds that are actively bleeding or have proteinaceous exudate will cause large bubbles to form and possibly spill over the edge of the tank. A bottle of lotion or specific defoaming agents should be available during treatment. Because anything that is placed in a whirlpool tub may be deposited in the wound, patients with colostomies, gastrostomies, ileostomies, or incontinence should not be put in a full-body tub. Care must be taken with central lines or other medical devices that pass through the skin. If possible, these areas are left out of the water and placed in a waterproof device such as a shoulder-length glove.

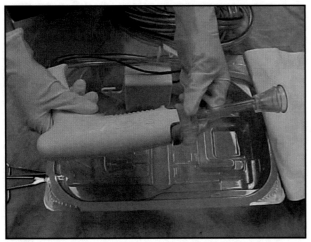

Figure 15-3. Inserting a tip on a pulsatile lavage handpiece.

Otherwise, the patient should not be placed in the whirlpool tub. Even for patients without these issues, fecal material and bacteria and fungi from the rectum and genitalia may be deposited in the wound.

Pulsatile Lavage With Concurrent Suction

Pulsatile lavage devices offer a distinct advantage of portability and improved ability to aim the shearing force of hydrotherapy. Patients in intensive care units, on isolation precaution, and those who are too difficult to move can be treated in their rooms as long as they have solid walls and a door. Due to the potential for aerosolization, pulsatile lavage must be performed in a closed room. Curtained-off areas with multiple patients are not considered appropriate; patients should be transferred to a private room, or the procedure should be performed in a room designated for it. Equipment used and demonstration of their use are shown in Figures 15-3, 15-4, and 15-5.

Pulsatile lavage devices operate under the same concept as carpet cleaners. They simultaneously irrigate with controllable pressure and remove excess fluid from the wound. This technique has become very popular, and in many facilities, pulsatile lavage has totally or nearly supplanted whirlpool treatments. Four basic components exist in all types of pulsatile lavage units—suction, adjustable pump, tip, and handpiece. Suction is provided by either wall suction or a portable pump. In the case of wall suction, a pressure regulator must be placed on the wall outlet. All hospital rooms have wall suction available, and many have pressure regulators available in the rooms. In many outpatient locations, however, wall suction is not available. Portable pumps, such as that depicted in Figure 15-6, may be purchased for approximately $400. Often these are mounted onto a cart ($200), which can also be used to store supplies. A suction canister is placed between the pulsatile lavage unit and either the wall suction pressure regulator or the portable pump. The canisters are designed to collect fluid and prevent the movement of fluid into the suction pump.

Setting up the suction aspect of the device does not require sterile technique and should be done before removing dressings from the patient. Handpieces may have either fixed or variable settings. Placing the device into the variable mode allows the operator to vary the lavage pressure by altering the grip on the handle between high, medium, and low pressures or high and low settings. The fixed mode locks the lavage pressure into the high, medium, or low setting and requires the operator to depress a button to unlock the setting, similar to locking features on power tools such as drills.

As initially developed, all pieces of pulsatile lavage handpieces came directly in contact with either the patient or body fluids. These were designed for disposal with infectious waste. In the case of handheld, battery-operated units, everything used was to be thrown away after treatment. Although disposal of the complete unit was thought to be feasible for trauma surgery, reimbursement for nonsurgical use made the devices cost prohibitive if the handpiece could only be a single-use device. Battery-operated units have been redesigned with the suction tubing built into the disposable tip, rather than running through the handpiece. With this arrangement, the handpiece can be reused on the same patient for multiple uses, while the suction tubing, tip, and canister contents are discarded. Generally, a handpiece is reused until the batteries run down. It is then discarded, and a new handpiece is used for the patient's next visit.

A variety of tips are available. Usually, 2 sizes of tips with splash shields are available as shown in Figures 15-3, 15-4, and 15-5. A long flexible tip with a measuring guide is available for some models to allow lavage and suction of tunnels/tracts (see Figure 15-5). The markings allow measurement of the tract's depth for evaluation purposes and ensure that the tip is placed the correct distance into the defect for appropriate debridement. Splash shields are very flexible, and their contours can be manipulated to approximate the shape of the wound. One hand is generally left on the tip to guide it across the surface of the wound with light pressure and to manipulate the shape of the splash shield to optimize cleansing by approaching the necrotic tissue from different directions/angles. Manipulating the tip shape also minimizes the amount of fluid running out of the wound or being sprayed from the wound into the environment.

In addition to the obvious risk of splattering fluid under pressure, fluid can become aerosolized and carry microbes a short distance. While using pulsatile lavage, personal protective equipment (PPE) should be worn. A

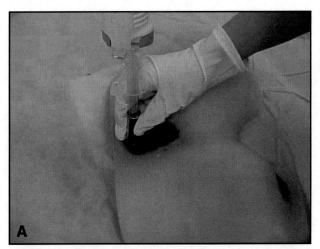
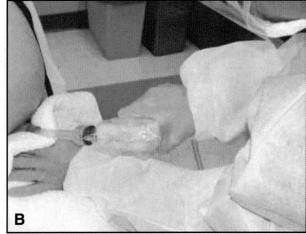

Figure 15-4. (A) Use of a pulsatile lavage unit on a wound model. Note that one hand is used to guide and contour the tip along the surface of the wound. (B) If the wound is larger than the splash shield and the area is too irregular to maintain light contact, towels around the tip may be used to prevent loss of fluid.

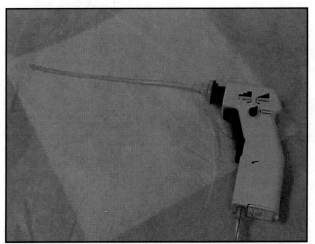
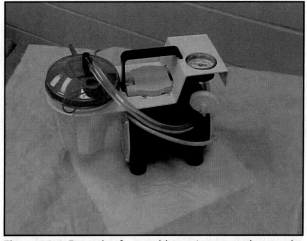

Figure 15-5. Example of a flexible tip used for tunnels/tract. Markings on the tip allow the depth to be determined.

Figure 15-6. Example of a portable suction pump that may be used when wall suction is not available. Note that these pumps can be loud and require disinfection between patients.

full mask or mask with a built-in eye shield is preferred over a separate mask and eye protection. The clinician's clothing needs to be protected to avoid transmitting anything that might be splattered or aerosolized during treatment (see Chapter 5). Several preparatory steps must be carried out before the actual process occurs. The bags of saline need to be warmed to skin temperature by approved methods. Saline bags are most conveniently warmed with microwave ovens. The time required for microwave heating of saline bags varies with the size of the bag and power output of the microwave oven. Heating a 1-L saline bag with a typical small microwave oven is likely to require 1 to 1 1/2 minutes to reach body temperature. A biomedical engineer or technician can measure the temperature of saline bags to find the correct time. Heating with a

microwave oven also confers the benefit of better infection control. The outside wrapper can be left in place as the bag is warmed and removed just before being used.

The patient needs to be draped appropriately, especially if the procedure is performed in their bed. Sufficient clean towels are placed where the fluid is likely to run off the patient, and sterile towels are placed surrounding the wound. When fluid is difficult to contain in the splash shield, towels can be placed around them to prevent leakage, as depicted in Figure 15-4B. Also, check the operation of the vacuum pump. Placing a hand over the end of the lavage tip allows one to feel whether suction is adequate. A plastic drape allowing visualization but capable of containing splashes is supplied with the Davol Simpulse's tips. Some clinicians have developed their own drapes to contain fluid.

TABLE 15-1
Pulsatile Lavage Procedure

- Warm bags of sterile saline.
- Drape patient.
- Attach suction canister to regulator or portable pump.
- Set the suction to desired vacuum and check for normal operation.
- Hang bag(s) of saline.
- Place handpiece and tip on sterile field.
- Attach appropriate tip on handpiece.
- Attach vacuum tubing to vacuum source.
- Spike the bag(s).
- Remove lock pin if applicable.
- Squeeze trigger to fill the incoming line with saline.
- Begin lavage.
- At end of procedure, release trigger.
- Ensure wound is not full of fluid.
- Turn off vacuum source and detach handpiece tubing from vacuum source.
- Discard appropriate items in appropriate biohazard containers.

The procedure should be explained thoroughly to the patient. Procedures for pulsatile lavage are listed in Table 15-1. The carpet cleaner analogy is generally sufficient. Any necessary medications should have been given to the patient in advance so that desired plasma concentrations exist at the time of the procedure. The topical application of local anesthetic may be used as needed by individual patients. The first step is attaching the suction canister to the vacuum source—either wall suction or a portable suction pump—and setting the regulator to the proper negative pressure. The bag(s) of normal saline should be prewarmed to skin temperature and hung on a pole to allow spiking. The handpiece is removed from the package and placed on a sterile field. The appropriate tip is then applied to the handpiece. The tip cannot be inserted incorrectly on the handpiece; it will only fit if the suction and spray are correctly aligned. A different size or shape exists on the vacuum and spray openings.

Identify the suction tubing coming from the handpiece, and attach it to the vacuum canister on the port marked "patient" or "ortho." Another tube is attached between the suction pump and the port marked "suction." Next, the tube running through the handpiece with a spike on its end is identified and inserted into a bag of sterile

saline. Check for a lock pin on the handpiece before starting. The Davol Simpulse uses a black lock pin. Leaving the lock pin in place causes the tubing to fill as soon as the saline bag is spiked. The pin must be removed before saline runs out of the tip. The handpiece trigger can be squeezed as the device is held over a waterproof container until the tubing fills with sterile saline and begins to exit the tip. Care should be taken to prevent overfilling suction canisters. Be sure to select a large enough canister to hold a fixed volume of fluid used to irrigate the wound.

If a wound is smaller than the splash shield, no movement of the tip across the wound is necessary; however, making subtle changes in the direction of the pulsed fluid across the wound by angling the handpiece with respect to the splash shield will enhance the shearing effect compared with holding the tip stationary. During the procedure, follow the contours of the wound carefully to avoid dragging the tip across the wound surface. Keep enough pressure to avoid leaking around the splash shield, but try to avoid hurting the patient by holding down with too much pressure. The tip does not need to be moved briskly across the wound, but all areas that need lavage should be covered. Therefore, the tip may be held in various locations instead of scraping across the surface and inflicting pain. If the wound contour does not allow adequate suctioning, fluid will run out of the wound onto the patient as the towels become overwhelmed with fluid. If fluid leaks from under the splash shield, try to change the shape of the splash shield to prevent leakage. If that approach still causes fluid to leak around the splash shield, holding a towel around it will hold the fluid under it sufficiently to allow suction to carry the fluid out of the wound. This technique is demonstrated in Figure 15-4B. Also, take care to avoid occluding the holes built into the splash shield. These holes allow air to be suctioned into the tip to prevent the collapse of the tip and latching on to the wound, which may cause pain and bleeding. Latching on occurs on loose tissues that can be suctioned into the splash shield and block the holes in it. Two options for preventing latching are maintaining a fingertip under the splash shield so a continuous flow of air into the tip is ensured and stretching the loose tissue to pull it taut under the splash shield.

Flexible tips, as shown in Figure 15-5, are used to irrigate and suction tunnels/tracts. The flexible tip should also be moved within the tunnel/tract to receive the maximum effect rather than irrigating the bottom only. Careful probing of the wound ahead of time will allow the clinician to know how far to insert the tip. On occasion, the tip may not seem to go any farther. Clinicians will know to push the probe more if they already know how far it should go. Not knowing the depth of a tunnel, a clinician may have difficulty getting the tip into a tunnel and assume that it has closed. A flexible tip may need to be manipulated to maintain suction. A sound similar to that caused by a dentist's suction will be heard if suction is working well. The flexible tip can also latch onto the sides of a tunneling wound. If the irrigation solution runs out of the wound and no suctioning sound can be heard, give a gentle twist to permit suction to occur. With either type of tip, stop irrigation until the cause of fluid leakage can be determined.

Two potential issues to troubleshoot are the failure of fluid (effluent) to enter the suction canister and the failure of fluid to be pumped out of the handpiece. Effluent refers to the fluid coming off the wound and captured in the suction canister. If the wound begins to fill with saline, stop the lavage and troubleshoot the lack of suction before excessive fluid spills. Potential problems include not turning on the suction pump, incorrect placement of hoses, malfunction of the pump, and kinking or occlusion of a vacuum line. Suction canisters have a float valve that will seal off the suction source if too much volume enters the canister. The float valve prevents fluid entry into the pump itself. Suction will fail if the canister fills, and the float valve inside the canister shuts off the suction source. This could happen if the canister is too small for the volume of saline used or by forgetting to replace a canister if a second bag of saline is used. Failure to hold the splash shield effectively over the wound can cause fluid to leak despite normal suction. Lack of fluid moving through the handpiece can be caused by twisting of the saline bag where the spike enters. If a bag is spiked by twisting only in one direction, the supply line can recoil, causing the flexible area where the spike enters the bag to then twist and occlude. Lack of irrigation can also happen when one forgets to spike the second bag after the first is depleted, and the suction canister is changed.

Following the procedure, lavage is terminated by releasing the trigger, moving the tip away from the patient in such a way to minimize spilling fluid, and then the suction is discontinued. Do not turn off the suction pump with a glove that was used for the lavage procedure. Any tubing that has carried fluid from the wound must be discarded as well as the tip inserted into the handpiece. Suction canisters and saline bags are single-use items. Regardless of how much saline is used or how much the canister is filled, these are to be discarded. Some suction canisters are permanent with disposable liners as opposed to a disposable canister. In that case, only the liner is discarded. Care should also be taken to avoid spilling the contents of the canister. The fluid within the suction canister is disposed of in a manner consistent with the facility's procedure. The facility's procedure may allow the dumping of the contents in a sink or commode and the disposable canister in a biohazard bag. Another option is solidifying powder that forms a gel when added to the contents of the canister. A glass canister is placed in a container approved for return to central sterile supply after the fluid and liner are discarded.

Quantity of Saline and Number of Tips Used

The amount of saline used depends on the size of the wound and the difficulty in removing necrotic tissue and debris. Although some clinicians might be tempted to use a single bag of saline for each patient, clinical judgment must be exercised and a reasonable quantity determined. In some cases, a full bag should not be used. Once the lavage stops removing necrotic tissue and debris, lavage should continue for a brief time to ensure that nothing else will be removed. For example, a small tract 4 cm deep might have copious purulent drainage, and after 400 mL of lavage, the effluent is clear. Continuing to irrigate under pressure is unlikely to produce any further debridement, but it may instead damage healthy tissue within the wound and promote inflammation. At the other extreme, a person with confluent pressure injuries of the sacrum and bilateral ischial tuberosities may have a wound 20 cm across and ranging from 12 to 8 cm long. The wound bed is 60% covered in adherent yellow slough, and drainage from the wound has been copious and yellow. Lavage with only 1 L saline is unlikely to be as effective as 3 L. In addition, some patients will need lavage with both a splash shield and flexible tip. Patients with abscesses or pressure injuries frequently have both large open areas and tracts. Sufficient saline should be used in both types of wounds, and both tips should be used. Although the flexible tip does not suction well from a tract with a depth of less than 3 cm, a splash shield tip is unlikely to be effective in a tract's debridement.

In some cases, such as dehiscent abdominal wounds, a tract runs between 2 openings of the wound. Lavage, in one direction, will demonstrate fluid running from the other opening. In such wounds, consider lavage from both directions to ensure that debris is not merely being forced to the other opening without being suctioned out of the wound. If one opening is higher than the other, consider lavage from the lower opening and then from the upper opening to drive out any debris that might have lodged in the other end.

Frequency and Duration

With the emphasis on earlier discharge from acute care hospitals, once a patient is referred for pulsatile lavage, they will likely be treated daily until discharge. In a small number of cases, the continued presence of foul odor, copious purulence, or the quality of fluid collected in the canister (effluent) dictates twice daily treatment. Under unusual circumstances that have created a more extended inpatient stay, pulsatile lavage might be discontinued during an inpatient stay. Such possibilities might include a wound that is already rather clean with minimal necrotic tissue or a patient who has a protracted length of stay for complications other than the wound itself that allow the wound to become clean and stable. Another such case would be that of preparing a wound for grafting. Treatment would be discontinued when the wound bed is deemed ready by the surgeon. Good communication between the clinician performing pulsatile lavage and those placing grafts is essential to prevent premature grafting that fails because the wound bed is not ready. Pulsatile lavage may also be discontinued for surgical debridement and might be resumed after surgery. Again, good communication is essential. A surgeon may assume that pulsatile lavage has been resumed when the clinician performing it has not been notified of the surgeon's desire to resume treatment.

For outpatients or those in longer-term care facilities, no hard rule for treatment frequency or duration exists. A patient with a large wound and several complications may need to be seen for several weeks, whereas a patient coming from an extended inpatient stay might need very few treatments. The wound bed and the effluent from the pulsatile lavage should be described in documentation tying together the purpose of the treatment, the patient's condition, and the need for continued treatment. Both persistent purulence and tissue necrosis should be considered. The discovery of a new tract or pocket of purulence should also be documented. Some insurance providers consider pulsatile lavage strictly as an instrument for debridement of necrotic tissue. The risk of not continuing treatment of a wound with persistent purulence must be emphasized. Without adequate documentation of the state of the wound, many treatment visits might be provided without payment.

Although several factors must be considered, a starting point for a plan of care is daily treatment for approximately 1 week and then every other day or longer. Factors to be considered are the amount of necrotic tissue; the amount of purulence; the quality of the effluent; and patient resources such as their ability to care for the wound between treatments, transportation issues, and insurance coverage. Biofilm is often a factor in wounds becoming chronic. Biofilm can re-form over an unstable wound in about 24 hours. Because biofilm cannot be visualized grossly, a wound bed may look good to the unaided eye, but the canister contains tan, opaque effluent indicating a high bacterial burden that creates the risk of spread of infection. Such wounds should be treated at least daily. If a wound has mostly granulation tissue and only cloudy effluent, pulsatile lavage every other day is likely to be sufficient. When a wound is nearly or fully granulated, and effluent is clear, wounds should show a rapid reduction in size. When this occurs, and the patient or caregiver can manage cleansing and dressing changes, the patient should be discharged with instructions for home care. Examples of effluent are shown in Figures 15-7A to 15-7C.

Indications, Precautions, and Contraindications

Pulsatile lavage with suction is a useful method of shearing bacteria and slough from the surface of wounds, including undermined areas and tracts. It is an excellent alternative to avoid the pitfalls of whirlpool treatments noted earlier. Pulsatile lavage can be directed to a specific site; therefore, fluid from one area of the body does not carry material into the wound. Because the devices are portable, they can be taken to patients who cannot be transported. In some facilities, all pulsatile lavage treatments are done at the bedside. Other facilities limit bedside treatment to those who cannot be transported due to the use of a ventilator, isolation, or weight limits.

Pulsatile lavage does not replace sharp debridement but is useful in conjunction with it. Pulsatile lavage is particularly suitable for neuropathic and venous ulcers but is not useful over hard eschar. Abscesses that have been surgically drained, surgical site infections, and dehiscent wounds are good candidates, particularly where tunneling cannot be visualized between surface openings of dehiscent wounds. After surgical debridement of pressure injuries and necrotizing fasciitis, pulsatile lavage can remove necrotic tissue that remains or that develops after surgical debridement.

No specific contraindications for pulsatile lavage have been described in the literature. As noted previously, patients with burns or certain skin diseases over larger surface areas may be treated more effectively with whirlpool therapy instead of pulsatile lavage. Precautions for pulsatile lavage include use near internal organs, superficial nerves and exposed blood vessels, and areas with excessive bleeding. Care must also be taken with patients who have immune deficiencies. Such patients should wear face masks to avoid inhaling aerosolized microbes. Some facilities may require patients to wear face masks or require clinicians to use drapes that contain any aerosolization.

Enzymatic (Chemical) Debridement

Enzymatic debridement occurs naturally but may be rendered less effective by the presence of copious necrotic tissue and chronic inflammation. The process can be enhanced by using an exogenous enzyme, collagenase, produced for this purpose. Enzymatic debridement is indicated as an alternative for a patient who cannot tolerate sharp debridement or for the patient who has no time constraints or risk of infection and wishes an alternative to sharp debridement. This type of debridement may also be used in any setting to complement other types of debridement. Enzymatic debridement works well in long-term facilities, home care, and outpatient settings but only if the ulcer is not infected. Breakdown of tissue within the wound increases the risk of bacteria entering

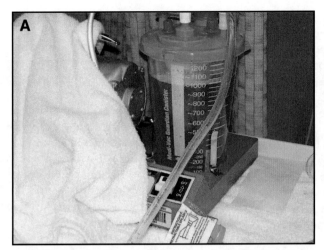

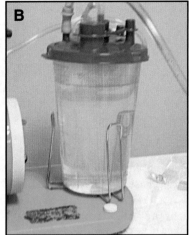

Figure 15-7. (A) Tan, opaque effluent. Effluent of this quality indicates
a need to continue treatment. (B)
Cloudy effluent. Effluent of this quality indicates that the surface has not
been completely cleared of material
and the patient may not be ready for
discharge. (C) Clear effluent suggesting the need to re-evaluate the need
for continued pulsed lavage.

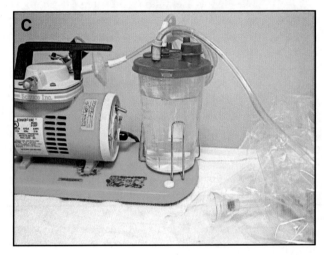

the circulation and causing sepsis, and the clinician needs to monitor for signs of sepsis. More absorbent dressings must be used with enzymatic debridement because of the increased drainage associated with enzymatic debridement caused by solubilized necrotic tissue. However, if moist dressings are left in place too long, they can desiccate and adhere to the wound. If the dressing becomes adherent, gentle irrigation to remove the adherent dressing is reasonable. Some clinicians use petrolatum gauze products such as Adaptic (Johnson & Johnson) or Xeroform (Kendall) over the enzymatic debrider to minimize desiccation and adherence. Enzymatic debriders should be discontinued when the necrotic tissue is cleared from the wound, if signs of sensitivity are present, or the product fails to remove necrotic tissue within a 2-week trial period. Enzymatic debriders should also be discontinued in the presence of bacterial super-growth or tunneling to other body cavities. The use of enzymatic debriders is limited by the need for a physician's order and prescription.

Effective January 1, 2008, the Centers for Medicare & Medicaid Services removed all products without an approved Food and Drug Administration application from the Medicare Formulary Reference File. Collagenase ointment is the only enzymatic debrider that remains available. Collagenase is available in a white petrolatum base as Santyl. The collagenase enzyme is produced by the bacterium *Clostridium histolyticum*. Collagenase may also produce erythema in some patients. Collagenase is indicated for enzymatic debridement in both chronic wounds and burn injuries. Collagenase is effective because collagen makes up such a large proportion (75%) of the dry weight of skin. The breakdown of collagen is generally believed to enhance the migration of cells. Enzymatic debridement will be less effective if applied to wounds indiscriminately. Good results will only be obtained if the enzymatic debrider is used according to the manufacturer's directions. Enzymes of any type are only effective within a specific range of pH and can be inactivated by other chemicals and by a poor wound bed environment. Therefore, a thorough cleansing of wounds should be done before the application of enzymes. Because these proteins are effective only on the surface available to them, the clinician needs to crosshatch eschar to increase surface area. Crosshatching with a scalpel, as demonstrated in Figure 15-10A, increases the number of edges of eschar over which the enzymatic debriders can function. When done correctly, the enzyme converts one large mass of eschar into a large number of small areas of eschar that will lift off the wound or be solubilized. Enzymatic debriders require prescriptions from a physician; therefore, they are unlikely to be available at the first treatment session unless a physician writes a script before referring a patient.

Hydrogen peroxide and heavy metals inactivate the collagenase. Topical medications and dressings containing silver must not be used with collagenase. Because the effectiveness of collagenase is limited to a pH of 6 to 8, acetic acid, Dakin's solution, or anything else with an extreme pH must not be present in the wound. Wounds need to be irrigated copiously to remove any acid or metal that might remain. Cleansing may be done with normal saline.

Autolytic Debridement

As noted in the section on enzymatic (chemical) debridement, autolytic debridement occurs on its own due to the production of enzymes within the wound bed by the inflammatory process. Clinicians can optimize this type of debridement by creating an optimized environment by using occlusive dressings. The term *autolytic debridement* is generally used in the sense that this is the only technique being employed rather than augmenting it with any mechanical means, sharp debridement, or exogenous chemicals. The wound environment is optimized by filling cavities loosely to prevent abscess formation but not tightly to prevent granulation. If the wound is dry, the clinician should hydrate the wound to allow enzymes access throughout the wound bed. For a dry wound, a combination of hydrogel and film may be used as long as the surrounding skin does not become macerated. Foam or hydrocolloid dressings may be used to promote autolytic debridement in cases of greater drainage. Types of dressings are discussed in the following chapter. However, occluding a wound for several days to promote autolytic debridement creates an exudate that others may mistake for pus. Others may need to be shown that the exudate simply rinses away, and no odor remains with irrigation. Autolytic debridement is an alternative for the patient who cannot tolerate sharp debridement or other methods but also has no time constraints or risk of infection. Because the wound must be occluded with a synthetic dressing and occlusion promotes bacterial growth, autolytic debridement is contraindicated in infected ulcers.

Sharp Debridement

Indications for urgent sharp debridement include advancing cellulitis or sepsis. Sharp debridement is the most rapid means of debridement and is the most appropriate for debriding thick, adherent eschar and extensive quantities of necrotic tissue from ulcers. Sharp debridement has the best combination of specificity and speed. Incisional sharp debridement refers to a situation in which instruments are used to cut through healthy tissue and is reserved for physicians. Excisional sharp debridement involves cutting of only devitalized tissue. Further discussion of the distinction between the 2 is described next. Sharp debridement must be done with sterile instruments. A clean, dry dressing should be applied for 8 to 24 hours if bleeding occurs. After bleeding ceases, moist dressings, if appropriate, should be used again. In addition, sharp debridement is reserved for individuals who meet licensing requirements and have demonstrated skill in this technique. Sharp debridement may be used in conjunction with mechanical or enzymatic debridement techniques. One recommendation associated with debridement has remained controversial. Heel ulcers have received special consideration in terms of debridement. AHCPR guidelines state that heel ulcers with dry eschar should not be debrided if they do not have edema, erythema, fluctuance (boggy feel), and drainage. However, the guidelines also state clearly that such wounds should be assessed daily for complications that may require debridement. One source of the controversy is the singling out of heel ulcers. Wounds with dry eschar on other body parts are not explicitly addressed. Another important recommendation is pain management. Clinicians often resign themselves to causing pain during debridement. AHCPR guidelines specifically recommend the prevention or management of pain associated with debridement as needed. Strategies for pain management are addressed specifically in Chapter 6. Arrange for patients to be medicated sufficiently ahead of time to allow maximal plasma concentration of any oral or injected analgesics. Oral medications will take much longer than those administered by intravenous or intramuscular routes.

Sharp debridement is found in 2 places in the Current Procedural Terminology codes. The 11000 series is used for incisional debridement, in which a physician must cut through tissue to remove necrotic tissue, usually with anesthesia. Excisional debridement is covered by the 97597 and 97598 codes. The 97597 code allows health care providers other than physicians to perform sharp debridement limited to cutting of necrotic tissue only. The application of maggots, enzymatic debridement, and nonselective forms of debridement such as wet-to-dry and scrubbing are paid at a lower rate using the Current Procedural Terminology code 97602. The method of choice with a risk of infection or progression of infection is sharp debridement. It may also be the method of choice for removing large quantities of necrotic tissue rapidly. This method may not be suitable for some individuals. In particular, this method needs to be used with caution in patients with bleeding disorders or anticoagulation. Sharp debridement is the most efficient means of removing necrotic tissues. Sharp debridement may not be appropriate in cases in which it does not speed healing and the procedure causes pain or other untoward events. Sickle cell leg ulcers and hospice care are 2 examples for which sharp debridement may not be the best choice.

Clinicians typically allowed to perform sharp debridement include physicians, physician assistants, physical therapists, and advanced practice nurses. These individuals are required to have licenses issued by individual states. In addition, payers may require evidence of advanced training to receive payment for sharp debridement. State practice acts may limit which health care providers are allowed to perform sharp debridement and may list additional requirements. Note that organizations such as the American Physical Therapy Association have issued position statements regarding appropriate clinicians for performing sharp debridement. The American Physical Therapy Association has taken a position that regardless of state practice acts that may allow physical therapist assistants to perform sharp debridement, it is only to be performed by physical therapists and not by physical therapist assistants due to the need for ongoing evaluation during the procedure, which is considered part of the training of physical therapists but not physical therapist assistants.

Surgical Debridement

A physician should debride wounds requiring extensive debridement, cutting through healthy tissue, near organs, or at risk of extensive bleeding in an operating room or special procedures room. More specifically, surgeons working with an anesthesiologist should be involved in cases in which the procedure may cause severe pain, if extensive debridement is required, if the degree of undermining/sinus tract/tunneling is undetermined, if bone must be removed, if debridement must be done near vital organs, or the patient is septic. Surgical debridement should also be considered if the patient is immunosuppressed.

Bedside Debridement

In cases other than those described earlier, surgeons and clinicians other than surgeons may perform the procedure at bedside or in a room designated for wound debridement. Tools typically used include curved scissors; forceps; curettes; scalpels with #11, #15, or #10 blades (Figure 15-8); silver nitrate sticks; and local anesthetic. The

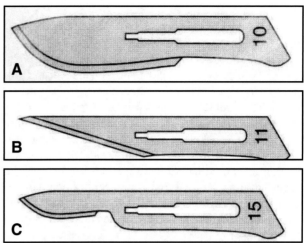

Figure 15-8. Scalpel blades commonly used for sharp debridement. (A) The #10 blade is more versatile than the other types of blades. (B) The #11 blade is useful for sawing type of motion needed to remove eschar parallel to the surface. (C) The #15 blade is useful for tight areas but dulls more quickly due to its small size.

clinician may choose to use either lidocaine or benzocaine spray, lidocaine gel, or eutectic mixture of local anesthetic (EMLA) cream, which consists of 2.5% lidocaine and 2.5% prilocaine. The clinician should create an optimal environment for the procedure, including appropriate lighting, positioning, and infection control. Visibility of the wound is easily taken for granted. A procedure light and magnifiers greatly enhance the ability to discern colors and details in the wound bed. A comfortable position for both the patient and clinician should be assumed to prevent fatigue or other problems in both the patient and the clinician. As such, a high/low table or patient's bed should be adjusted to minimize awkward positioning for the clinician, which can lead to early fatigue and potential errors during the procedure. Because excisional debridement only involves tissue that is already colonized, the level of sterile technique used in an operating room is not required. Principles of sterile technique described in Chapter 5 are used to minimize the risk of contaminating the wound. For example, a second person opens packages, and the person debriding touches only the inside of packages with the gloved hands. However, either sterile or exam gloves may be used depending on facility policy and the patient's immune status. Sterile instruments must be used, and the instruments' tips should not be touched by either exam or sterile gloves. For these reasons, bedside debridement will always be excisional, except for emergency cases. The need for an environment closer to sterile largely eliminates the use of incisional debridement at the bedside.

Frequency and Duration of Sharp Debridement

No simple rules exist for how often or how long a session of sharp debridement should be. Both patient and provider tolerance must be considered, as well as the practical aspect of scheduling other patients. Debridement codes are untimed but are expected to last a minimum of 15 minutes. This time includes examining the wound, evaluating the patient's progress, and providing ongoing education. Cutting for more than 15 to 30 minutes can be very difficult. The provider needs to have proper positioning/body mechanics and lighting to tolerate the procedure. In addition, the patient may not be able to tolerate the necessary positioning or endure any pain for as long as the provider wishes to continue. On occasion, a provider may perform sharp debridement for well beyond 30 minutes. Debriding callus on a foot may require substantial time and does not provide any additional payment. The clinician's ability to focus carefully on the wound and cut without error is generally the limiting factor. Also, the operator may become hot and uncomfortable from wearing PPE.

Therefore, the point of stopping the session of debridement rests on the personal judgment of the provider. The second issue is the frequency of treatment. One must make a judgment based on the patient's tolerance, scheduling limitations, and how quickly necrotic tissue is being removed or is developing from dying tissue in the wound bed. Sharp debridement limits the development of biofilm, which can regenerate in approximately 24 hours. Several studies have shown clearly that frequent debridement is more successful than less frequent, which may be related to minimizing the opportunity for biofilm to be regenerated from planktonic bacteria. In general, one should consider daily sharp debridement until a definite change in the wound's trajectory is noted. This change in the wound's trajectory may require daily debridement for 1 week or longer. The clinic's policy on weekend and holiday provision of services may need to be considered.

Basic Techniques

Sharp debridement requires the use of PPE to protect the clinician from body fluids and to protect the wound from contaminants on the clinician. The face should be protected with either a mask with a built-in eye shield or a face shield. A cap, gown, and gloves are also needed. One may become complacent after debriding many wounds and having never experienced any splash or splatter from a wound. Unfortunately, the cost of one incident of blood splattering in a clinician's eye greatly exceeds any costs of being prepared. In a similar vein, a clinician who has been wearing PPE for pulsatile lavage might be tempted to take off this PPE before performing some minor sharp debridement. The risk of contamination dramatically outweighs any benefit of improving the clinician's comfort by removing PPE.

In all cases, sharp debridement should be considered a highly selective form of debridement. As such, the clinician should endeavor to minimize damage to healthy tissue. Also, bleeding may obscure the clinician's vision. Because of the risk of bleeding during this procedure, the clinician should start debridement at the bottom of the wound and work toward the top. Other considerations include working from the center of the wound where it is less sensitive to pain to its periphery, which is more likely to be sensitive. A general rule to follow is to debride the areas likely to bleed or to be painful last. On occasion, these 2 rules may conflict. If so, consider how repositioning may allow both of these areas to be performed last. These problems can be minimized by using local anesthesia to reduce pain and silver nitrate sticks to stop bleeding.

Another consideration is to stay within a given plane to avoid spreading bacteria into lower layers. If a fascial plane is reached, one must stop and reassess the situation to determine whether deeper debridement is needed. Following sharp debridement with a high risk of bleeding, a dry dressing should be placed on the wound for 8 to 24 hours if significant bleeding occurs during the procedure. The wound may need to be packed (discussed in Chapter 16) more tightly to maintain hemostasis. The dressing may later be changed to an appropriate occlusive dressing (see Chapter 16).

In some cases, a wound may only require a single sharp debridement procedure. However, several procedures may be required for a number of reasons. Stopping may become necessary because of excessive pain or bleeding, the clinician's fatigue, or patient request. Debridement may be continued later, particularly with a large wound, a wound with painful areas, and wounds that bleed.

Moreover, areas that appeared to be viable one day may be necrotic the next day, requiring further debridement. Other forms of debridement may be necessary in addition to sharp debridement to prepare a wound for surgical closure or transfer of the patient's care. Wounds with excessive bioburden but little necrotic tissue may require several days of pulsatile lavage and periods of sharp debridement.

During debridement, care must be taken to avoid cutting into undermined or tunneled areas and areas in which purulent drainage compromises visibility. The clinician should never cut what cannot be seen. Reasons to stop debridement include exposure of tendons, bones, and blood vessels; excessive bleeding; the patient no longer being able to tolerate debridement; and clinician judgment. Because each compartment surrounded by fascia has its own blood supply and because fascia acts as a barrier for bacterial penetration, the clinician must pause and assess whether deeper debridement is warranted if a fascial plane is reached.

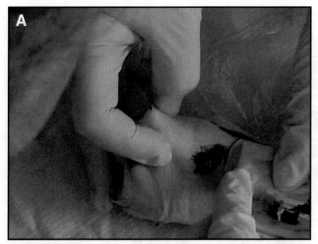
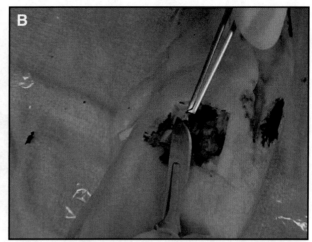

Figure 15-9. Practicing debridement on a pig's foot. (A) Motion used to practice shaving callus. (B) Using forceps and scalpel to cut material from the wound bed.

Cutting can be performed with a scalpel or scissors. Although either instrument carries the risk of inadvertent cutting of nearby tissue, more damage can be done more rapidly with a scalpel. A clinician should develop skill with scissors before using a scalpel for cutting necrotic tissue. Traction using forceps is needed to allow cutting. In many cases, traction alone will result in necrotic tissue tearing at the margin between viable and necrotic tissue. Regardless of whether a pair of scissors or a scalpel is used, cutting, especially for the novice, should be performed parallel to the surface of the wound to avoid accidental cutting with the tips of scissors or slipping of the instrument. Cutting with a scalpel is performed by holding the scalpel in the same manner as a pen. The scalpel is then moved across the tissue to be cut by rolling the curved edge using wrist flexion.

Another form of cutting is sawing eschar off the surface of a wound, holding the scalpel across the crease of palm so that the edge is parallel to the skin's surface. The scalpel is first used to cut under the loosest spot along the edge of the eschar (if one exists). Once an edge is created, it is lifted with forceps, and a sawing motion under the eschar but within necrotic tissue is used to cut the eschar off the wound's surface. Adherent slough not amenable to traction with forceps may be removed with a curette, using a scooping type of motion. Large quantities of necrotic fatty tissue can be removed this way quickly.

In addition to cutting, scalpels are also useful for trimming callus and scoring eschar. An individual should have substantial experience in using a scalpel in a safe setting. Practice on a model such as the pig's foot in Figure 15-9 or fruit with a hard surface, as shown in Figure 15-10, allows one to gain experience using a scalpel for scoring eschar and trimming callus before using a scalpel on a patient. Novices should still be supervised until competence is demonstrated. Cantaloupes are useful for teaching shaving

because the brown outer surface can be shaved down to a green one similar to how the tan callus gives way to light tan and eventually pink as the callus is shaved. Dehydrated pigskin or cantaloupe or other fruit with a hard surface can be used for practicing the scoring of eschar. The technique of scoring eschar involves rolling the length of a scalpel blade with wrist flexion along the hard surface while providing sufficient force until the clinician feels the surface give. Several such incisions are made in parallel 1 to 2 mm apart to cover the eschar in one direction. The process is repeated perpendicularly to the first set of incisions to produce a "checkerboard" appearance, as demonstrated in Figures 15-10A and 15-10B.

Instruments

Forceps and scissors are available in disposable suture removal kits, or good-quality surgical instruments may be obtained (Figures 15-11A to 15-11D). Although the initial cost of good surgical-quality instruments and cost of repeated sterilization following each procedure may influence administrators to choose disposable forceps and scissors, these instruments have such poor quality that they are not suitable for sharp debridement. If quality surgical instruments are used frequently, the initial cost becomes offset to a large degree by their durability. Forceps that will hold tissue securely cost $40 or more and have the added cost of sterilization each time they are used. Forceps should have serrated tips as a minimum. Adson and other types of forceps with teeth (see Figure 15-11C) on the tips will hold tissue better.

Scissors with good-quality cutting edges are even more expensive and can cost $30 for small scissors up to $80 or more. Clinicians use several types of scissors. Scissors may have blunt tips, sharp tips, or one sharp and one blunt tip

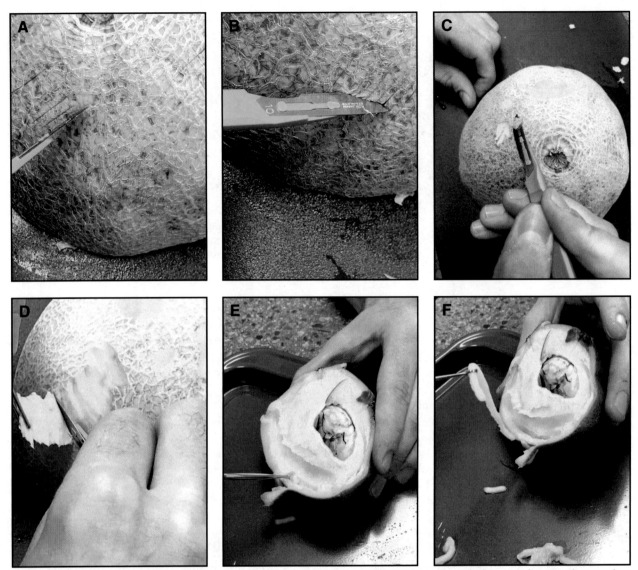

Figure 15-10. Using a cantaloupe and mango for debridement practice. These have the advantages of easier cleanup, less foul odor, and stability compared with pig's feet, which can be greasy, develop a foul odor until they are collected with trash disposal, and can roll during debridement practice. (A) Parallel shallow cuts to practice scoring eschar. (B) Series of cuts perpendicular to the first series of cuts to finish the scoring. Scoring is used in conjunction with enzymatic debridement. With practice, one can feel the give of eschar with appropriate depth of cutting. (C) Practice shaving callus. A change in color from tan to lighter tan to pink occurs on the foot. With the cantaloupe, one attempts to remove the brown and expose the green beneath. (D) Practice sawing eschar from a wound's surface. One attempts to minimize the amount of yellow material on the underside of the removed material. A #11 scalpel blade is used to create a corner, which is grasped with the forceps and pulled away as cutting continues beneath. (E) Practicing removal of slough using a curette on a mango. This can be done with any pulpy fruit, including cantaloupe. (F) The creation of a "mango worm." The ability to cut slough from a wound bed is simulated by creating a continuous cut with the curette.

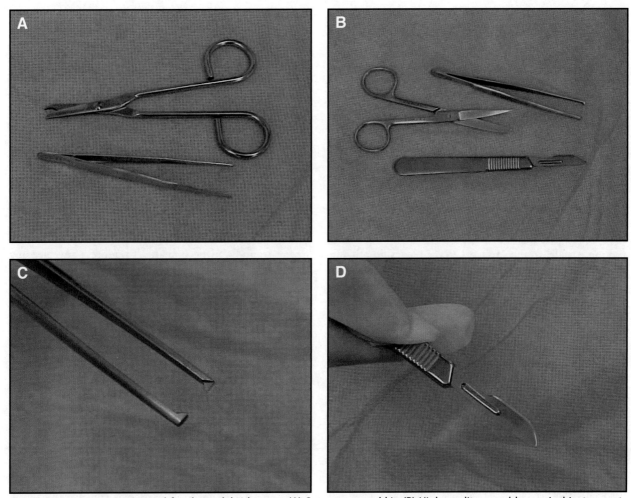

Figure 15-11. Instruments used for sharp debridement. (A) Suture removal kit. (B) High-quality reusable surgical instruments suitable for sharp debridement. (C) Close-up of toothed tissue forceps. The teeth improve the handling of necrotic tissue. (D) Close-up of a #10 scalpel blade on a #3 handle, showing proper handling.

(blunt/blunt, sharp/sharp, or blunt/sharp, respectively). Curved scissors are preferred to flat scissors for 2 reasons. Cutting with the tips of curved scissors up reduces the risk of accidental injury. Conversely, cutting can be performed in a tighter area with the tips down. Although the novice may wish to start with a pair of blunt/blunt curved scissors because of the safety issue, more experienced clinicians may prefer curved sharp/sharp iris scissors. Because iris scissors are smaller, the clinician can reach into tighter areas of the wound.

A safer alternative to using iris scissors in tight locations is a curette. A curette can scoop underneath adherent necrotic tissue, avoiding the awkward manipulation of scissors and forceps in a tight area, or trying to pick up adherent necrotic tissue with forceps and cut under it with scissors. Curettes come in a variety of sizes and compositions. Sterilizable metal curettes have better cutting properties. Cheap dermal curettes with a plastic handle and metal loop do not cut as well as more expensive versions. The curette works well with a technique similar to making melon balls. Holding the curette as a pencil, supination of the forearm cuts under adherent necrotic tissue.

Scalpel blades, like scissors, are available in several different types, and operator preference plays a large role in the type used. A number identifies the type of blade. Blades may have curved or straight cutting edges and are available in different sizes. Blade type may be selected based on particular tasks. In addition, different number blades fit onto different types of handles (also identified by number). Both the number 3 and number 7 handles fit a series of useful blades for working in tight areas—the smaller #10, #11, and #15 blades. The number 3 handle is familiar to most people. It is shaped to fit in the palm as well as being held with a pencil-like grip and has a serrated portion to aid grip with the thumb and index finger. The number 7 handle also fits these blades, but it has a thinner handle and may not be as easy to grasp for the novice. The number 4 handle fits the larger #20, #21, #22, and #23 blades. The #10 blade and #20 blade are versatile with a rounded cutting edge. This edge is designed to work with wrist flexion and use the entire length of the cutting surface. The #11 blade has a triangular blade with a straight cutting edge and narrow tip. The #15 blade is quite versatile due to its small size. It has a curved cutting edge similar to a #10 but is much smaller. It can fit into tighter areas but will dull faster.

Any of the blades can be used for the basic sharp debridement techniques of scoring, shaving, and cutting, but some blades are better suited for specific tasks. The #11 blade with its straight cutting edge can be more challenging to handle for scoring or other cuts perpendicular to the surface. In contrast, the #10, #20, or #15 blade allows a more natural wrist and finger flexion motion for scoring. A #11 blade can be used effectively for the sawing type of motion parallel to the surface. Curved blades do not supply as much cutting edge for this maneuver. For fine work, a #15 blade works nicely. However, because of its size, it is not suitable for the removal of a large amount of easily accessible necrotic tissue because it has a short cutting edge and dulls rapidly. Eventually, most clinicians will likely develop a personal preference for specific blades. Just like scissors and forceps, scalpels may be either disposable or reusable. In either case, the blades are discarded after each use. Disposable scalpels come with blades already attached, and both the handle and blade are discarded together without removing the blade, thereby reducing the risk of injury by removing blades. Moreover, disposable scalpels are very cost-effective and have a low purchase price, avoiding the cost and inconvenience of sterilizing the handles. The risk associated with changing blades is reduced by changing the blade with either hemostats or, preferably, a scalpel blade remover available from surgical instrument suppliers. Because sterile technique is followed during sharp debridement, scalpel packages will need to be opened ahead of time or by another individual not involved in the sterile technique.

Bleeding

Bleeding is mostly unavoidable if sharp debridement is to be accomplished effectively. Although necrotic tissue does not bleed, small viable blood vessels may still carry blood through necrotic tissue. Creating bleeding is not a requirement for good sharp debridement. However, if no bleeding occurs, some necrotic tissue will likely be left in the wound. With careful debridement, bleeding usually stops readily. Hemostasis is only problematic when healthy tissue is cut, the patient is using anticoagulants, or the patient has a bleeding disorder. Sharp debridement may be done on patients at risk for excessive bleeding. Regardless of the reason, all bleeding during sharp debridement will stop eventually. With appropriate hemostatic measures, the amount of bleeding is usually insignificant from a

hemodynamic standpoint. Several means are available to promote hemostasis. Silver nitrate sticks appear similar to cotton-tipped applicators, with a small amount of silver nitrate on their tip rather than cotton. They need to be touched briefly to small bleeds and should be moistened slightly with saline. Flushing the rest of the wound with saline minimizes the silver nitrate's damage to other areas of the wound. Hemostasis may also be promoted by applying pressure with a small piece of alginate dressing. For larger bleeds, pressure may need to be applied for several minutes with 4×4 cotton gauze sponges. Copious bleeding may occur during the first visit of an inpatient after surgery. Blood-soaked dressings should cue the clinician that bleeding may still be occurring or may be easily initiated. In such cases, one should carefully remove any packing in the wound and be prepared to address any bleeding. Irrigate the wound bed with normal saline, if necessary, to prevent tearing the wound bed with an adherent dressing and causing more bleeding. If needed, surgical hemostatic agents may be obtained. These agents typically contain collagen, a natural hemostatic. Surgicel and gelfoam are 2 well-known hemostatic agents.

Anatomical Considerations

Although debridement may be required on any body part, it tends to be needed more commonly in a few locations. These locations include common areas for pressure injuries, such as the sacrum, ischial tuberosity, greater trochanter, and sites common for neuropathic ulcers such as the metatarsal heads. A particular concern is avoiding damage to flexor tendons of the foot. Knowledge gained from a cadaver-based anatomy course equips the clinician to navigate among important structures located in any region of the body. The clinician will be able to envision the location of arteries, veins, nerves, tendons, ligaments, and fascial boundaries. Knowledge of fascial compartments is vital in locating likely areas for tracts to form and where to direct pulsatile lavage to clear these tracts.

Low-Frequency Ultrasonic Debridement

Low-frequency ultrasound devices utilize ultrasound in the kilohertz range. Devices may be contact or no-contact types. The low frequency employed allows energy to be focused on a small depth of tissue. Contact devices allow nonviable tissue to be destroyed with no apparent injury to healthy tissue. An example of contact low frequency is the Söring Sonoca. This device transmits ultrasound by near contact with a probe that constantly drips saline. The saline acts as the conductive medium for the ultrasound. Contact devices operate on the principle of cavitation created by the ultrasound. Cavitation destroys bacteria and fibrin deposits while penetrating fissures within the wound bed. A variety of tips are available to suit the shape of the wound. The handpieces are interchangeable and may be autoclaved after use. No consumable supplies are used other than normal saline; however, the device is costly (about $30,000). The Sonoca operates at 25 kHz. Intensity is adjustable, but the frequency is not. The increased efficiency of debridement may offset the cost. Söring terms this technology "Ultrasonic-Assisted Wound Treatment." The device has 3 modes. As the name implies, the contact mode involves touching the wound with the tip to provide more energy. The noncontact mode is designed for more sensitive tissues. The dipped mode is used for wounds that can be filled with fluid, such as deep wounds and subcutaneous defects that can be filled with fluid. The ultrasonic energy is transmitted through the fluid. The Qoustic Curette (Arobella Medical) transmits low-frequency ultrasound that supplements the use of the curette to debride sharply.

Low-frequency, noncontact ultrasound such as MIST (Celleration) is not marketed explicitly as debridement at the gross level. The fluid is driven through the device onto the wound bed as a mist that vibrates at the frequency determined by the device, promoting wound healing while removing bacteria, fibrin, and slough. Although the Sonoca and Qoustic Curette devices are considered to be high-intensity, low-frequency, contact ultrasound, MIST is considered to be low-intensity, low-frequency, noncontact ultrasound.

WHEN NOT TO DEBRIDE

Not all necrotic tissue needs to be debrided. Specific examples include stable heel wounds and severe arterial insufficiency. In addition, technical issues need to be considered. General guidelines for not debriding heel wounds include eschar that is firmly adherent, lack of inflammation of surrounding tissue, lack of drainage from below the eschar, and eschar that does not feel soft or boggy. Small wounds a few millimeters to centimeters with eschar may heal just as rapidly without debridement. Necrotic tissue caused by arterial insufficiency should not be debrided. In these wounds, a lack of blood flow not only retards healing but prevents the immune system's handling of bacteria that may enter the wound. Moreover, exposure of necrotic tissue to surface bacteria presents the risk of potentially serious infection. As a general rule, the clinician should never debride what cannot be seen. As tempting as rapidly removing what is believed to be necrotic tissue may be, the clinician risks damaging healthy tissue and introducing bacteria into the blood.

LARVA THERAPY

Larva therapy is the most specific form of debridement. Maggots only digest devitalized tissues. The use of maggots (fly larvae) for tissue debridement has been traced to the Civil War. At that time, wound infection was a major cause of mortality. Wounds infested with maggots appeared to have a lower rate of infection and mortality than those that did not. Larva therapy declined with the introduction of antibiotics but has survived and enjoyed a recent resurgence. Maggots used for wound debridement are sterile larvae of blowflies obtained from specialized laboratories. Appropriate wounds include any chronic wound that does not require surgical intervention for debridement. Any wound for which autolytic or enzymatic debridement is suitable may be treated with maggots. Maggots perform highly selective debridement of necrotic tissue and maintain a suitable level of bacteria in the wound.

A number of protocols for using maggots have been developed. The maggots may be contained over the wound or allowed to migrate (free range). They are typically left in place for 48 to 72 hours. Two approaches are available to constrain maggots. One approach is to use maggots contained in a mesh bag. The other method requires 2 hydrocolloid sheets. A hole approximating the size of the wound is cut in the first hydrocolloid sheet and applied around the wound. The bottle of maggots is applied to the wound and covered with a mesh material. A second hydrocolloid sheet, also with a hole in it, is placed over the first to secure the mesh in place. The top hydrocolloid sheet is removed and discarded with the maggots and mesh between layers. The bottom hydrocolloid sheet is left. The procedure is repeated up to twice per week until the wound bed is completely debrided. Two to 6 applications may be necessary. A summary of the advantages and disadvantages of different types of debridement are given in Table 15-2.

SUMMARY

The debridement process is preceded by the development of a plan of care addressing why debridement is necessary and which method is most suited to reach the outcomes outlined. Examples of wounds requiring debridement are shown in Figures 15-12A to 15-12M. Four types of debridement are described. Sharp, mechanical, enzymatic (chemical), and autolytic debridement are options determined based on the characteristics of the wound, characteristics of the patient and the facility, and time constraints placed on wound debridement. In many cases, sharp debridement is preferred to manage the risk of infection. Sharp debridement requires sharp instruments to cut along the border between viable and necrotic tissue and a high skill level. Mechanical means of debridement

		TABLE 15-2	
		Types of Debridement	
METHOD	**DESCRIPTION**	**ADVANTAGES**	**DISADVANTAGES**
Incisional	Removal or cutting into viable tissue as well as removing nonviable tissue	Rapid removal of necrotic tissue Ability to control bleeding rapidly No pain during procedure	Surgical procedure Makes wound larger May have substantial postoperative pain Need for general anesthesia or block Operating room Expense
Excisional	Removal of visible nonviable tissue only	Can be provided by nonsurgeon Can be provided bedside Relatively inexpensive Can be combined with pulsed lavage or other procedures May not require much pain management	Cannot access hidden necrotic tissue Limited by tolerance of patient and provider More difficult to stop bleeding Need physician to arrange pain management
Mechanical	Use of nonspecific means such as pulsed lavage, wet-to-dry, whirlpool, scrubbing	Less skill required Relatively inexpensive	Less specific Pulsed lavage is much more specific than the other forms Wet-to-dry painful and can damage granulation
Autolytic	Allows body's enzymes to degrade necrotic tissue using occlusive dressings	Does not inflict pain, suitable for many sickle cell or other painful ulcers Cost of dressing changes only	Slow Risk of infection if not monitored adequately
Enzymatic	Supplements body's enzymes with collagenase	Cost of application and dressing change minimal Faster than autolytic Can supplement serial debridement	Cost of collagenase Slower than forms of sharp debridement
Larva therapy (biologic, maggots)	Sterile maggots placed on wound for one or more episodes as needed	Very selective Pain free	May not be acceptable to the patient Expense

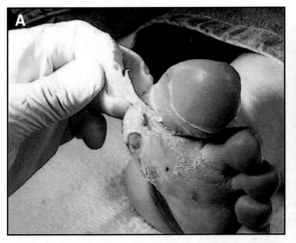

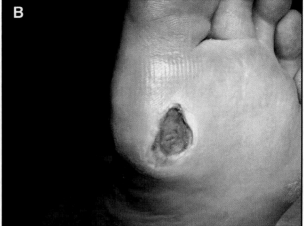

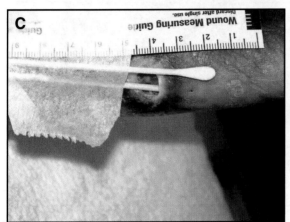

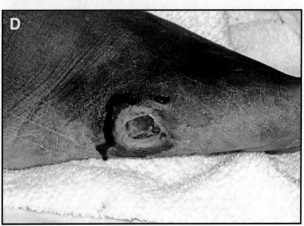

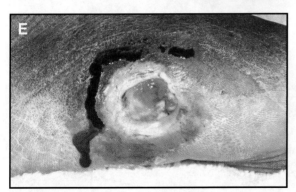

Figure 15-12. Examples of wounds requiring debridement. (A) Extensive callus on plantar surface of diabetic foot. A combination of peeling and shaving was used to remove callus. (B) Foot debrided of callus after multiple visits. (C) Pocketing with nonviable tissue over pocketed area. All tissue overlying cotton-tipped applicator required debridement. (D) Foot following debridement of waxy, necrotic tissue from foot in Figure 15-12C. Debridement was performed by shaving waxy tissue with scalpel. Edges of viable tissue beveled. (E) Close-up of same foot as in Figures 15-12C and 15-12D. Note bleeding from edges of viable tissue. *(continued)*

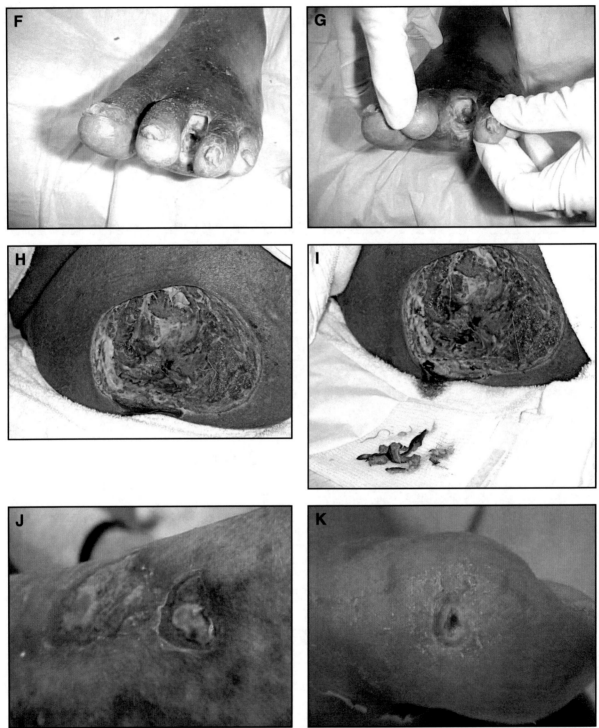

Figure 15-12 (continued). (F) Necrotic tissue appearing in third ray amputation. Although all apparent necrotic tissue is removed in surgery, tissue unable to survive following surgery appears as in photo and requires further debridement. (G) Same wound as in Figure 15-12F following sharp debridement of necrotic tissue. Wound needs to be examined the following day for the appearance of further necrotic tissue requiring debridement. (H) Pressure injury over right greater trochanter. Yellow slough present at 12:00, 3:00, and scattered throughout; black eschar at 9:00; note necrosis of greater trochanter surface. (I) Same wound as in Figure 15-12H following one episode of sharp debridement. Eschar and slough removed with scissors are shown in foreground. (J) Slough from leg wound removed by combination of pulsatile lavage and sharp debridement with forceps, scissors, and curette. (K) Callus around wound on great toe, which was removed by peeling using forceps. *(continued)*

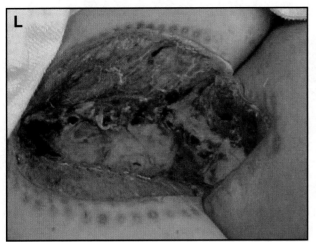 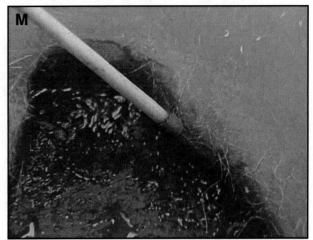

Figure 15-12 (continued). (L) Adherent yellow slough in dehiscent sternal wound. Slough removed by pulsed lavage, sharp debridement, and hydration of wound bed. (M) Silver nitrate stick used in debridement and hemostasis. Tip is wet with normal saline and touched to area requiring debridement or hemostasis. Wound is then flushed with normal saline to remove residual silver nitrate.

include the use of hydrotherapy, scrubbing, and irrigation. Autolytic debridement allows the wound to clean itself with endogenous enzymes under an occlusive dressing. Enzymatic debridement involves the use of commercially produced enzymes requiring a physician's prescription to degrade necrotic tissue. Autolytic and enzymatic debridement are useful when time constraints and infection are not issues. Debridement is not performed on dry gangrene caused by arterial insufficiency and may not be necessary for stable heel ulcers. Sharp debridement is the preferred method for rapidly removing necrotic tissue, especially in cases of a high risk of infection or neuropathic ulcers. Cutting is performed along the margins between necrotic and viable tissue, and bleeding is likely to occur. Bleeding may need to be controlled by silver nitrate sticks, alginate, or gauze. Dry dressings are placed on bleeding wounds for several hours to prevent hematoma formation.

QUESTIONS

1. How does debridement differ from cleaning a wound?
2. Should physical therapists be routinely cleaning wounds?
3. Contrast excision debridement from surgical debridement.
4. Who is allowed to perform surgical debridement?
5. Why is debridement performed?
6. What are the benefits of sharp debridement?
7. Contrast the appearance of viable and nonviable tissue.
8. Is bleeding alone sufficient to determine viability?
9. When are simple irrigation and scrubbing appropriate?

10. Do these qualify for payment as "Active Wound Management" Current Procedural Terminology code 97597?
11. What is payment when surface area debrided exceeds 20 cm²?
12. Does the surface area debrided correlate with the work involved?
13. What is meant by wet-to-dry dressings? Why are they used? Why should they not be used?
14. How effective is whirlpool as a debriding modality?
15. What are the problems associated with using whirlpool with open wounds?
16. When is whirlpool a good choice?
17. What are the advantages of pulsed lavage over whirlpool?
18. What are the problems associated with pulsed lavage?
19. How are these problems mitigated?
20. What PPE is needed for pulsed lavage?
21. What are the basic tips used in pulsed lavage?
22. What is effluent?
23. What does the quality of the effluent tell you?
24. How much saline should be used during pulsed lavage?
25. What is autolytic debridement?
26. What is the primary indication for autolytic debridement?
27. What type of dressing is needed to enhance autolytic debridement?
28. What are the contraindications for autolytic debridement?
29. What chemical debrider is still available for use?

30. What are the indications for chemical debridement?

31. What can be done to enhance the effectiveness of chemical debridement?

32. When should chemical debridement be the sole method of debridement?

33. What are the contraindications for chemical debridement?

34. Why should sharp debridement be the primary method used by a physical therapist?

35. What are the 3 primary cutting instruments in sharp debridement?

36. Why are forceps necessary? What characteristics should your forceps have?

37. When does debridement need to be referred to a surgeon instead of a physical therapist?

38. What are the primary precautions for sharp debridement?

39. Why does callus need to be debrided and beveled?

40. What is the payment for callus removal when the patient is referred for debridement of a foot ulcer?

41. Who can be paid for callus removal?

42. What are the rules for handling scalpels and scissors?

43. How is a curette handled?

44. What is available to stop excessive bleeding?

45. What should you do when bleeding does not stop?

46. What is low-frequency contact ultrasound? How does it produce debridement?

47. What is larva therapy? What are the indications and contraindications?

BIBLIOGRAPHY

Ahluwalia R, Vainieri E, Tam J, et al. Surgical diabetic foot debridement: improving training and practice utilizing the traffic light principle. *Int J Low Extrem Wounds*. 2019;18(3):279-286.

Anvar B, Okonkwo H. Serial surgical debridement of common pressure injuries in the nursing home setting: outcomes and findings. *Wounds*. 2017;29(7):215-221.

Elraiyah T, Domecq JP, Prutsky G, et al. A systematic review and meta-analysis of débridement methods for chronic diabetic foot ulcers. *J Vasc Surg*. 2016;63(2 Suppl):37S-45S.e1-2.

Faschingbauer M, Boettner F, Bieger R, Weiner C, Reichel H, Kappe T. Outcome of irrigation and debridement after failed two-stage reimplantation for periprosthetic joint infection. *Biomed Res Int*. 2018;2018:2875018.

Gethin G, Cowman S, Kolbach DN. Debridement for venous leg ulcers. *Cochrane Database Syst Rev*. 2015;2015(9):CD008599.

Huett E, Bartley W, Morris D, Reasbeck D, McKitrick-Bandy B, Yates C. Collagenase for wound debridement in the neonatal intensive care unit: a retrospective case series. *Pediatr Dermatol*. 2017;34(3):277-281.

Kim PJ, Attinger CE, Bigham T, et al. Clinic-based debridement of chronic ulcers has minimal impact on bacteria. *Wounds*. 2018;30(5):114-119.

Lavery L, Niederauer MQ, Papas KK, Armstrong DG. Does debridement improve clinical outcomes in people with diabetic foot ulcers treated with continuous diffusion of oxygen? *Wounds*. 2019;31(10):246-251.

Linger RJ, Belikoff EJ, Yan Y, et al. Towards next generation maggot debridement therapy: transgenic Lucilia sericata larvae that produce and secrete a human growth factor. *BMC Biotechnol*. 2016;16:30.

Mancini S, Cuomo R, Poggialini M, D'Aniello C, Botta G. Autolytic debridement and management of bacterial load with an occlusive hydroactive dressing impregnated with polyhexamethylene biguanide. *Acta Biomed*. 2018;88(4):409-413.

Michailidis L, Bergin SM, Haines TP, Williams CM. A systematic review to compare the effect of low-frequency ultrasonic versus nonsurgical sharp debridement on the healing rate of chronic diabetes-related foot ulcers. *Ostomy Wound Manage*. 2018;64(9):39-46.

Michailidis L, Bergin SM, Haines TP, Williams CM. Healing rates in diabetes-related foot ulcers using low frequency ultrasonic debridement versus non-surgical sharps debridement: a randomised controlled trial. *BMC Res Notes*. 2018;11(1):732.

Raizman R, Dunham D, Lindvere-Teene L, et al. Use of a bacterial fluorescence imaging device: wound measurement, bacterial detection and targeted debridement. *J Wound Care*. 2019;28(12):824-834.

Reyzelman AM, Vartivarian M. Evidence of intensive autolytic debridement with a self-adaptive wound dressing. *Wounds*. 2015;27(8):229-235.

Roberts PA, Huebinger RM, Keen E, Krachler AM, Jabbari S. Mathematical model predicts anti-adhesion-antibiotic-debridement combination therapies can clear an antibiotic resistant infection. *PLoS Comput Biol*. 2019;15(7):e1007211.

Scalise A, Campitiello F, Della Corte A, et al. Enzymatic debridement: is HA-collagenase the right synergy? Randomized double-blind controlled clinical trial in venous leg ulcers. *Eur Rev Med Pharmacol Sci*. 2017;21(6):1421-1431.

Schoeb DS, Klodmann J, Schlager D, Müller PF, Miernik A, Bahls T. Robotic waterjet wound debridement—workflow adaption for clinical application and systematic evaluation of a novel technology. *PLoS One*. 2018;13(9):e0204315.

Schultz GS, Sibbald RG, Falanga V, et al. Wound bed preparation: a systematic approach to wound management. *Wound Repair Regen*. 2003;11(Suppl 1):S1-S28. doi:10.1046/j.1524-475x.11.s2.1.x

Sheets AR, Demidova-Rice TN, Shi L, Ronfard V, Grover KV, Herman IM. Identification and characterization of novel matrix-derived bioactive peptides: a role for collagenase from Santyl® ointment in post-debridement wound healing. *PLoS One*. 2016;11(7):e0159598.

Tewarie L, Chernigov N, Goetzenich A, Moza A, Autschbach R, Zayat R. The effect of ultrasound-assisted debridement combined with vacuum pump therapy in deep sternal wound infections. *Ann Thorac Cardiovasc Surg*. 2018;24(3):139-146.

Wu L, Chung KC, Waljee JF, Momoh AO, Zhong L, Sears ED. A national study of the impact of initial débridement timing on outcomes for patients with deep sternal wound infection. *Plast Reconstr Surg*. 2016;137(2):414e-423e.

Selection and Application of Dressings

Clinicians are expected to make decisions concerning the optimal dressing for each patient. Each decision made in choosing a wound dressing must be based on a combination of the following factors: pathophysiology of the wound, ease of use by patients, amount and quality of drainage, presence or absence of infection, depth, social and economic issues, and the properties of the dressing. This chapter aims to develop a decision-making process

Irion GL, Gardner JA, Pignataro RM.
Comprehensive Wound Management, Third Edition (pp 297-328).
© 2024 Taylor and Francis Group.

by which a wound dressing may be chosen. More importantly, the process includes deciding when to use a different dressing type as the wound and other factors may change. Four categories of products must be considered for their appropriateness on any given wound: dressings that cover wounds, dressings that fill wounds, products to protect the surrounding skin, and secondary dressings to hold dressings in place.

FILLING VS COVERING AND PRIMARY VS SECONDARY DRESSINGS

Some wounds will be sufficiently shallow that no material needs to be placed in the wound, just over it. This type would be considered a covering type of dressing. A filling type of dressing is used when a wound has substantial depth. If a wound with substantial depth is only covered and not filled, drainage or blood can accumulate and create infection risk. A filling type of dressing should be restricted to the wound bed to prevent wicking of fluid onto the surrounding skin and damaging it.

A dressing placed directly on or in a wound is called a *primary dressing*. It can be the only dressing on a shallow or surgically closed wound. In some cases, more dressing material needs to be placed over the primary dressing. This may be to hold a dressing in place or to absorb any drainage that the primary dressing cannot handle.

A covering type of dressing is often simply the primary dressing over a superficial wound. However, a covering type of dressing can be used as a secondary dressing over a filling type of dressing. A filling type of dressing is always a primary dressing and will require a covering type of dressing as a secondary dressing. In some unusual instances, a secondary dressing could be covered by a tertiary dressing. One example is the use of antibiotic cream as a primary dressing, gauze sponges as a secondary dressing, and a bandage roll as a tertiary dressing. Examples of primary vs secondary and filling vs covering dressings are demonstrated in Figure 16-1.

PURPOSES OF WOUND DRESSINGS

Armed with an understanding of the cause of the wound and possible complicating factors, we can begin the process of selecting a wound dressing. The next step is to understand the purposes, first of dressings in general, and then the properties and purposes of specific classes of dressings. As discussed in the following text, even within a class of dressings, substantial differences in properties

may make one brand of dressing more appropriate than another.

Starting with the simplest purpose, dressings serve to physically protect the wound from the external environment and prevent contamination. Dressing selection usually differs between acute and chronic wounds. With acute wounds, the greatest concerns are infection and hematoma formation, which are tremendous risk factors for infection. In contrast, chronic wounds are usually colonized, although contamination with microbes new to the wound increases infection risk. The major concern with chronic wounds is optimizing the wound's microenvironment without compromising the surrounding skin's integrity.

A second purpose for dressings is promoting breakdown and removal of necrotic tissue. A third purpose is filling dead space in a wound to prevent the formation of hematomas, abscesses, tunnels, and sinus tracts. Managing drainage, whether purulent exudate or serous transudate, is the fourth purpose. Dressings that hold fluid within wounds (occlusive and semiocclusive dressings) promote healing by maintaining moisture, retaining growth factors and enzymes, and allowing autolytic debridement. Purposes for dressings are listed in Table 16-1.

CLASSIFICATIONS OF DRESSINGS

Dressings may be classified by the way they are used to manage drainage. Categories of dressings recognized by the Centers for Medicare & Medicaid Services (CMS) are listed in Table 16-2. A dry-to-dry dressing is placed on a wound dry and removed when it is dry. These are used to absorb very light drainage and promote hemostasis in acute wounds. These dressings are commonly used to cover acute wounds closed by primary intention and may also be used for small acute wounds. This type of dressing is usually not employed for large or chronic wounds.

A wet-to-wet dressing is moistened, usually with either normal saline or an antiseptic solution such as triple antibiotic, to soften eschar or treat an infected wound (Figure 16-2). They are also commonly used when wounds need frequent inspection and debridement (daily or more often). A third type is the wet-to-dry dressing, which is used for nonselective debridement of wounds with either large amounts of necrotic tissue or wounds that must be debrided rapidly. Debridement with wet-to-dry dressings, discussed in the previous chapter, is highly discouraged.

Microenvironmental (occlusive and semiocclusive) dressings are designed to optimize the wound environment to promote healing. The term *occlusiveness* is quantified by the water vapor transmission rate (WVTR). Occlusive dressings do not allow anything to cross them in either direction. A truly occlusive dressing would have a WVTR of zero. Semiocclusive dressings allow some water vapor

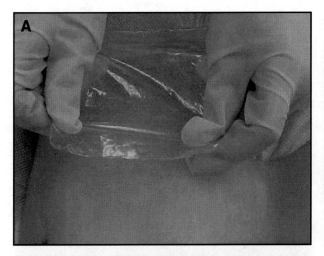

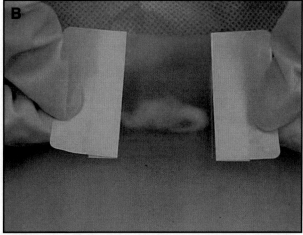

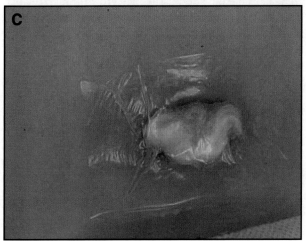

Figure 16-1. Primary and secondary filling and covering dressings. (A) A hydrogel sheet being applied directly to a wound bed without any measurable depth is an example of a covering dressing being used as a primary dressing. (B) A wound with substantial depth is first filled with an alginate dressing. This is the primary dressing and a filler. A semipermeable film is being placed over the alginate dressing. The semipermeable film is a secondary dressing and a cover. (C) The covering of the filler is completed.

TABLE 16-1
Purposes of Dressings

- Physical protection of wound, prevention of contamination
- Promote autolytic debridement
- Retain warmth, moisture, cells, enzymes, and growth factors in wound bed
- Fill dead space to prevent formation of hematomas, abscesses, tunnels, and sinus tracts
- Management of drainage by absorption, evaporation, or occlusion

and other gases across them; therefore, they have a measurable WVTR. Occlusiveness exists on a continuum and is only one factor in choosing a dressing. In some cases, the occlusiveness of a dressing is obvious; in other cases, some dressings termed *microenvironmental dressings* may not be any more occlusive than nonmicroenvironmental dressings. Occlusiveness of different dressing types is discussed with each type of dressing. Several subtypes of microenvironmental dressings are discussed next. In addition to differences in the ability to retain moisture, other characteristics to consider are the ability to absorb drainage and maintain the wound bed's temperature.

NONOCCLUSIVE DRESSINGS

Products in this category are typically constructed of cotton gauze and rayon. Gauze sponges have a long history in wound care, and many individuals who do not stay current with appropriate care may consider saline-moistened gauze to be a standard of care. Gauze products are readily permeable to bacteria, gas, and fluid and are, therefore, considered nonocclusive. They handle heavy drainage primarily by absorption by multiple layers of material. They are indicated for protecting acute wounds closed

TABLE 16-2
Categories of Dressings Recognized by CMS

- Hydrogels: sheets
- Biologicals and synthetic membranes
- Impregnated
- Collagens
- Silicone gel sheets
- Contact layers
- Silver technology
- Elastic gauzes
- Transparent films
- Wound fillers
- Gauzes and nonwoven dressings
- Liquid skin protectants
- Hydrocolloids
- Moisture barriers
- Hydrogels: amorphous
- Therapeutic moisturizers
- Hydrogels: impregnated dressings
- Skin substitutes
- Oxygen-reconstituted cellulose

by primary intent, absorption of copious drainage, and bleeding to prevent a hematoma. Nonocclusive dressings are also indicated for infected wounds and as a wet-to-dry dressing when rapid debridement is necessary. Products include Telfa pads (Covidien), gauze sponges, and bandage rolls. Cotton gauze is reasonably absorbent and can be layered to provide sufficient absorption of copious exudate. Layers of dry gauze perform acceptably well as a bacterial barrier when wounds are not draining. They lose their effectiveness as they soak through with drainage. Wet gauze is not a good bacterial barrier because it can transmit bacteria through moisture into a wound. Gauze also permits uncontrolled evaporation of fluid from a wound as it wicks fluid, leading to desiccation of wound beds if drainage is not heavy enough to keep them wet. This often leads to the additional problem of dressings adhering to desiccated, proteinaceous exudate. Removal of adherent dressings is also associated with the release of bacteria into the air causing infection control issues. Evaporation of fluid as it is wicked from the wound reduces its temperature, which will decrease the production of granulation tissue and the effectiveness of immune cells. Lowering the temperature of a wound has been shown to increase the risk of infection.

Because gauze dressings will adhere to desiccated fluid in wounds, Telfa and related products have been designed to act as nonstick layers between the wound surface and the absorbent material. Unfortunately, these "nonstick" materials frequently fail to perform as advertised. Exudate is absorbed across the nonstick surface, dries across the pores, and adheres to the wound bed. Other nonstick options include dressings coated with a petrolatum product. Vaseline gauze (Covidien) or Adaptic (Johnson & Johnson) consists of white petrolatum coating a synthetic mesh. Xeroform (Covidien) has a yellow color due to bismuth tribromophenate, an antimicrobial in a petrolatum base applied to a fine mesh cloth. Although the petrolatum coating decreases adhesion risk, drainage can also dry across these perforations in the same manner described for Telfa pads. Granulation tissue may grow through the perforations, causing adherence and bleeding during dressing removal. Examples of petrolatum-impregnated gauze are shown in Figure 16-3.

Another possible nonstick dressing is a contact layer. These are designed to allow water and electrolytes to cross the dressing but not cells and proteins responsible for the adherence of dressings to wound beds. Contact layer dressings and composites (dressings with multiple material types) with contact layers are made of nonstick material similar to Telfa but with much smaller perforations that allow some evaporation of excessive moisture while minimizing the risk of adherence. Some products (eg, Exu-Dry [Smith & Nephew]; Figure 16-4) combine a contact layer with a layer of highly absorbent material. This type of dressing has characteristics suitable for acute or infected wounds without the drawbacks associated with gauze, Telfa, and petrolatum dressings. A final nonadherent dressing to consider is silicone dressings. They gently stick to the wound to protect it but easily come off without causing trauma to the wound or surrounding skin. Silicone is generally reserved for more expensive microenvironmental dressings. An example of a silicone dressing is shown in Figure 16-5.

Cotton gauze material is woven, and, based on the quality of its production, stray pieces of material can be shed from them into the wound bed. Contamination of the wound bed with small cotton pieces shed from the dressing can promote chronic inflammation and stimulate copious drainage from the wound. The continual use of gauze in wounds can promote a vicious cycle of inflammation, copious drainage, and the use of a dressing material that promotes more inflammation. Cotton gauze can be useful as a dressing when ointments are used directly on wounds requiring frequent dressing changes (eg, over silver sulfadiazine or over enzymatic debriding agents to minimize desiccation).

Petrolatum gauze (see Figure 16-3) may help protect a wound from outside contamination, retain moisture in

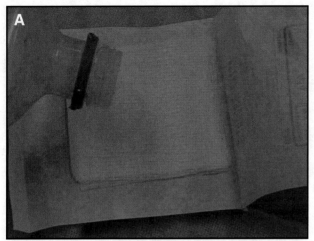
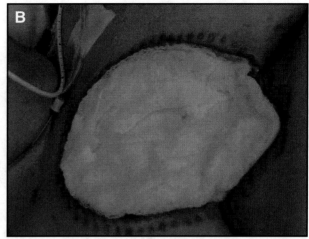

Figure 16-2. Saline-moistened gauze dressing. (A) Wetting a sterile 4 × 4 with sterile normal saline. (B) Bandage roll moistened with normal saline in a dehiscent sternal wound being used as a primary and filling type of dressing in a large, dry wound still requiring substantial debridement.

a wound, and reduce the risk for adherence. Because cotton fibers are not directly in contact with the wound bed, irritation and drainage will be reduced compared with cotton gauze. However, petrolatum-coated materials lack absorbency and require frequent dressing changes. These dressings are more occlusive than gauze sponges, so using them on infected wounds must be done with caution.

MICROENVIRONMENTAL (OCCLUSIVE AND SEMIOCCLUSIVE) DRESSINGS

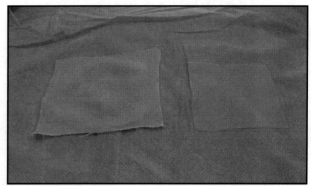

Figure 16-3. Examples of petrolatum-impregnated gauze—Xeroform (yellow) and Adaptic (clear).

Occlusive and semiocclusive dressings offer several advantages for the wound, the patient, and the clinician. These dressings are designed based on the principle that healing is the most effective if the wound microenvironment is optimized. Optimization of the wound microenvironment includes maintaining an appropriate moisture level and temperature, availability of macromolecules of healing (glycosaminoglycans, proteoglycans, and collagen), availability of growth factors (macrophage and platelet derived), acceptable levels of nonpathogenic microflora, and protection of the environment from pathogens.

Wound moisture is critical for the migration of epithelial cells, movement of enzymes, growth factors, and structural molecules. An appropriate occlusive dressing maintains wound bed moisture while preventing excessive moisture accumulation that can damage the surrounding skin. An appropriate microenvironmental dressing also prevents desiccation that leads to scab formation. Desiccated fibrin and blood may act as a dressing to retain moisture below and keep out pathogens but slows epithelial cell migration as cells are forced below to resurface a wound.

Promoting autolytic debridement is an important indication for microenvironmental dressings. Autolytic debridement can proceed under these dressings due to the retention of fluid and enzymes under them. Although the properties of microenvironmental dressings are useful for chronic wounds, they may be harmful to infected wounds for the same reason that they promote autolytic debridement. Occlusive dressings should not be used over infected wounds because they will promote the growth of microbes with the potential spread of infection. Some occlusive and semiocclusive dressings are useful for acute wounds that have little necrotic tissue or drainage, and they may be left in place for several days at a time. Many times, wounds will be closed when the occlusive dressing is removed. Another advantage of occlusive dressings is the decreased handling of the wound. Decreased handling minimizes inflammation, which, in turn, decreases drainage from the wound. Although some microenvironmental dressings are nonadherent, others are very adherent to the surrounding skin. Very adherent dressings should be reserved for wounds

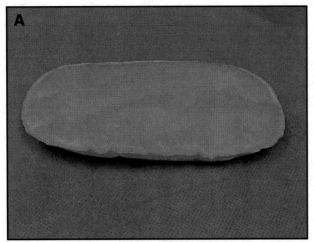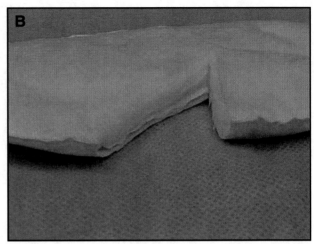

Figure 16-4. Composite dressing. (A) Intact Exu-Dry dressing. (B) Exu-Dry dressing cut in a cross section to reveal layers. Contact layer is on top. Such dressings can combine features of primary and secondary dressings with protection of the wound bed, absorption of drainage, and prevention of desiccation from uncontrolled evaporation.

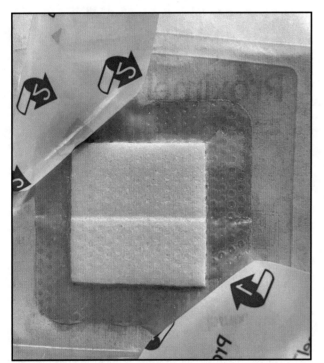

Figure 16-5. Example of a silicone dressing designed specifically to adhere with minimal skin injury.

that may be covered safely for several days to minimize trauma. Certain microenvironmental dressings, especially hydrogels, are soothing to irritated wounds, especially thermal, chemical, and radiation burns. Among the microenvironmental dressings, only alginates and their synthetic equivalents are not contraindicated for infected wounds.

Semipermeable Film Dressings

Many brands of semipermeable polyurethane films are now available. Film dressings have an acrylic adhesive that allows them to adhere to skin but not to wound beds. An example is shown in Figure 16-1. These dressings are semiocclusive and allow some evaporation of fluid. However, they cannot absorb any drainage and will allow excessive drainage to accumulate under them. Therefore, they are only indicated for minimal drainage because they cannot handle moderate or maximum drainage levels. Should drainage become too great, the dressing will loosen and leak. Film dressings are particularly useful for superficial wounds or partial-thickness wounds with minimal drainage. They are useful as secondary dressings to hold a more absorbent material in the wound. Film dressings have a low coefficient of friction and can protect skin against friction injury. However, friction on the edges of a film dressing may dislodge it.

When applying film dressings, a margin of more than 1 inch (3 to 4 cm) of healthy surrounding skin should be covered. Because this type of dressing is quite adherent, frequent, repeated removal will damage a patient's skin. A skin protectant should be applied to the surrounding skin. Skin protectants are discussed later in this chapter. Skin protectants improve the adhesion of these dressings and decrease the probability of edges rolling up while protecting the skin from direct contact with the adhesive. Depending on the dressing location, films may need to be taped to prevent the rolling up of edges. These dressings should not be used on infants and small children too young to understand the dressing's purpose. Because these are made of polyurethane with an adhesive backing, they may be deliberately or accidentally removed and become a choking hazard.

To prevent skin injury, proper technique must be used when removing semipermeable films, especially with older individuals' skin. If pulled directly from the wound, the skin may adhere more strongly to the film dressing than to itself, causing the skin to tear, especially in older patients or others with fragile skin. The skin should be stabilized when using an adhesive dressing to prevent excessive pulling on it. The proper technique to remove a film is to lift a corner and stretch the semipermeable film tangentially to the wound, causing the dressing to stretch and loosen. Pulling a film dressing back over itself with a long lever can result in skin tears and denudation of the skin surrounding a wound. As the dressing is removed, fingers are moved closer to where the dressing is still adherent to prevent this long lever.

Semipermeable films, in particular, and any dressing should be applied with care to avoid restricting adjacent parts of the body, particularly with sacral and coccygeal wounds. Care must be taken not to bridge the gluteal cleft with these dressings. If a semipermeable film is to be used in this area, several alternatives may be used. First, the dressing may be turned such that a corner of it is placed in the cleft, between fingers or toes, or other areas. A second option is to cut a dressing into a valentine/heart shape and apply it with the point in the cleft. Placing 2 dressings with one on either side and overlapping in the middle to cover the entirety of the wound is another option. If placing a single piece of dressing material across an area such as the gluteal cleft cannot be avoided, start with the dressing folded and place it in the center and delicately smooth outwardly so that full mobility is unimpeded. This process is depicted using abdominal pads in Figure 16-6. Abdominal pads are common secondary dressings over acute wounds with substantial drainage, particularly in the acute care setting with moist gauze sponges as the primary/filling dressing. They are available in 2 basic sizes of 5×7 and 8×10. They can be layered and overlapped as needed based on the clinician's creativity to absorb drainage and maintain patient mobility.

Hydrogels

Hydrogels are available in 2 basic forms: sheets and amorphous. Examples of hydrogels are shown in Figures 16-1 and 16-7. Hydrogels are not generally used to

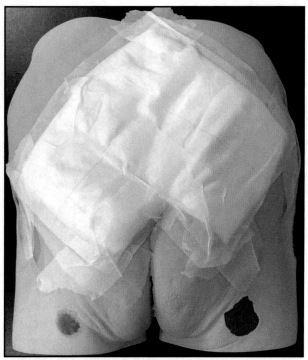

Figure 16-6. Using overlapping abdominal pads as a secondary dressing over a sacral wound. The overlapping allows substantial movement of each side of the buttocks despite tape being used to secure the pads. Clinicians must be aware of any movement restrictions that dressings may impose on the patient.

manage drainage, but they provide some occlusion, absorption, and evaporation. The primary purpose of hydrogel is hydrating dry wounds. In addition, hydrogel can be very soothing on wounds, especially abrasions, burns, and radiation burns. Hydrogel sheets may also be used on partial-thickness or full-thickness wounds. Sheets are also available over the counter in nonsterile form, which are very popular for cyclists and other athletes prone to abrasions. Due to their high water content, hydrogel sheets adhere to wounds without adhesives and are removed without trauma. However, they can slide off the wound, potentially requiring taping to keep them in place. The sheets come with polyethylene film on both sides. The inner film is always removed, and the outer film may be removed to increase the evaporative loss of fluid from the wound.

Amorphous gel is available in tubes and other squeezable containers for use in wounds with subcutaneous involvement. Amorphous gel is well suited for hydrating dry wounds. It is especially useful for protecting tendons, ligaments, nerves, and blood vessels from desiccation. A thin layer of amorphous gel may also be used to line cavities; Medicare specifically states that hydrogel should only be used to coat and not to fill a wound. In addition to hydrating a wound, hydrogel may soften and loosen slough.

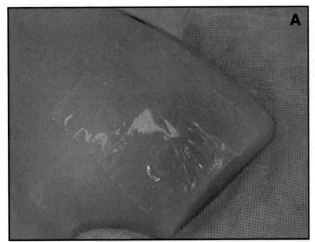
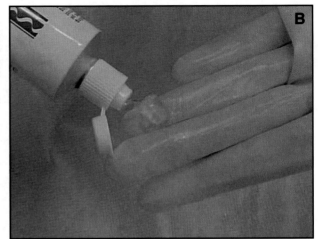

Figure 16-7. Examples of hydrogel dressings. (A) Hydrogel sheet. (B) Amorphous hydrogel used to moisten a dry wound bed.

If the wound must be held open, another form of filler can be used on top of hydrogel. Hydrogel-impregnated gauze sponges are available as electrodes for electrical stimulation as a means of increasing wound healing. Metronidazole gel is available for treating wounds infected with gram-negative bacteria. Amorphous hydrogel and hydrogel sheets can also be used as an interface for therapeutic ultrasound (see Chapter 17).

Hydrocolloids

A material easily distinguished by its appearance, hydrocolloids are the most occlusive of the microenvironmental dressings. Many brands and types are available (Figure 16-8). They have a characteristic appearance with a distinctive tan color. This material comes in a variety of thicknesses. The thicker varieties are opaque and a deeper tan. Thin hydrocolloid sheets are a lighter tan color and allow limited visualization of the wound. This material is also capable of absorbing moderate drainage in addition to occluding the wound. As hydrocolloid absorbs water, it becomes lighter in color and softer and should be changed when it becomes soft and white. These dressings are very adhesive and designed to be worn for several days, which leads to several precautions. First, these dressings should never be used on infected wounds. They are also not recommended for wounds with subcutaneous defects, including undermining, tracts, and tunnels. The outer surface is impermeable to water; therefore, hydrocolloid dressings can be worn in the shower if prolonged contact or soaking can be avoided.

Because of the adhesion of hydrocolloid sheets necessary to allow the dressing to stay in place for several days between dressing changes, hydrocolloids should only be used if the clinician is comfortable allowing the wound to stay covered for 5 days or longer. Like semipermeable films, hydrocolloid dressings should have a margin of 2 to 3 cm of healthy skin beneath them coated with skin protectant. When hydrocolloid dressings are removed, the product of several days' worth of autolytic debridement trapped under them will have a mild odor and superficially resemble purulence. However, when the drainage is cleansed from the wound, the odor and soupy drainage will be gone, indicating that the wound is not infected. Hydrocolloids also have a low coefficient of friction, which minimizes friction injury to the wound area. The edges of hydrocolloid sheets will frequently roll up, especially when placed in locations where shearing forces are present with bed mobility. In these cases, clinicians frequently tape the edges of hydrocolloid sheets.

Application of skin protectant beneath hydrocolloid sheets prevents rolling the edges of hydrocolloid sheets and skin injury during hydrocolloid dressing removal. Hydrocolloids are also available for filling cavities and managing drainage. They can be formulated in pastes, granules, and spiral-cut sheets to fill a wound. These absorption products require a secondary dressing to hold them in the wound. The secondary dressing could be a hydrocolloid sheet or something simpler such as a film or gauze. These fillers will allow the absorption of greater drainage and will reduce the need for dressing changes. Decreasing the frequency of dressing changes increases patient comfort and patient adherence to the plan of care and decreases the opportunity for contamination and chronic inflammation caused by rough handling. Like semipermeable films, hydrocolloid sheets must also be removed carefully to prevent injury to the wound's surrounding skin, and a skin protectant is used to protect the skin from injury. Like film dressings, hydrocolloids can be cut in creative ways to make them fit over specific parts of the body, such as the sacrum and toes. Cutting hydrocolloid dressings to allow dressings to conform well is shown in Figure 16-8.

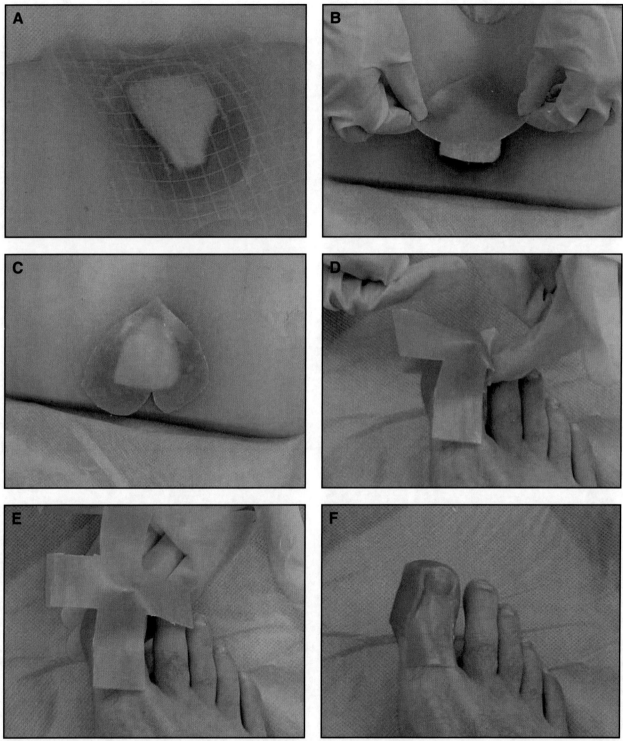

Figure 16-8. Hydrocolloid dressings. (A) Thin hydrocolloid sheet used as a secondary dressing over alginate. (B) Thicker hydrocolloid sheet cut in a valentine shape to cover an alginate primary dressing of a sacral ulcer. This shape is used specifically to prevent adhesion of the dressing across 2 sides of the buttocks, allowing free movement. (C) Same dressing adhered to periwound skin. The notch at the top is also designed to allow movement. (D) Using a hydrocolloid sheet around a digit. The sheet is cut in a cross shape to allow tabs to be folded over 4 surfaces of the digit. (E) Folding the tabs into place. (F) Completed application of hydrocolloid over the end of a great toe. Holding a hand over the hydrocolloid sheet to warm it increases the conformability and adherence of the dressing to provide a good fit of the irregular shape of the toe.

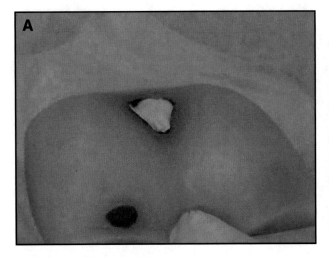

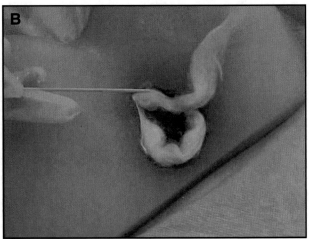

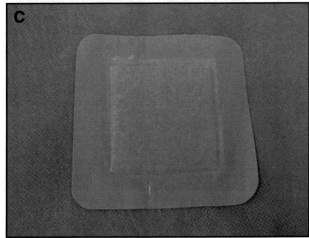

Figure 16-9. Alginate and hydrofiber dressings. (A) Hydrofiber sheet used as a primary/filling dressing in a sacral ulcer model. The sheet can be cut to size and manipulated to fit the wound bed without the dressing touching the surrounding skin. (B) Alginate rope used for the same purpose. The rope type can be more useful for irregular sites, especially undermined areas. (C) Example of a composite dressing combining hydrofiber with foam.

Alginates and Hydrofibers

The most versatile microenvironmental dressings, alginates, are derived from long-chain sugars obtained from seaweed and have the property of changing from a fiber to a gel as they absorb fluid. Alginate dressings can hold up to 20 times their weight in water and may desiccate wounds with little drainage. Hydrofibers are synthetic improvements on the older-generation alginate products. Examples are shown in Figures 16-1B and 16-1C and Figure 16-9. A composite dressing of alginate with polyurethane foam is shown in Figure 16-9C. With an appropriate secondary dressing, alginates and hydrofibers can be used with maximum drainage. This material has sufficient tensile strength that the gel formed by absorbing water is removed easily from the wound bed as a single piece. Following removal of the gelled alginate, flushing the wound with normal saline should remove any residue. Although some clinicians like to pre-moisten alginates to fill desiccated wounds, alginates were designed to absorb drainage, not hydrate wounds. A simpler and more cost-effective approach to wound hydration is coating the wound with amorphous hydrogel. Alginates and hydrofibers should not be used on dry wounds, hard eschar, or third-degree burns. If a wound bed begins to dry, cease alginate/hydrofiber use and switch to a less absorbent dressing.

The secondary dressing used over alginate or hydrofiber can be selected based on the drainage. A semipermeable film can be used with minimum drainage (see Figures 16-1B and 16-1C), whereas foam or absorbent secondary dressings may be used for copious drainage. If a hydrocolloid is used as the secondary dressing (see Figure 16-8A), the clinician must be willing to leave the dressing in place for several days. Alginates come in the forms of sheets and ribbons, have remarkable tensile strength, and can be placed into undermined and irregularly shaped areas (see Figure 16-9). Although alginate and hydrofiber dressings are more forgiving with respect to wicking fluid onto surrounding skin, they should be manipulated to keep them in the wound bed. Some clinicians have a habit of fluffing the alginate sheets before filling a cavity, but this practice is un-necessary. Instead, they can be cut, torn, or folded into appropriate shape so they can remain in the wound, off the surrounding skin. Alginate can be combined with collagen. As the alginate absorbs drainage, collagen is absorbed into the wound to promote healing.

Semipermeable Foams

These semiocclusive dressings manage drainage by absorption, evaporation, and occlusion. An example is shown in Figure 16-10 and as a composite with hydrofiber in Figure 16-9C. They are the most absorbent of the microenvironmental dressings. A variety of foam thickness is available to manage a wide range of drainage. Foam dressings will retain large quantities of fluid in the wound, absorb excessive drainage, and some brands allow substantial evaporation to occur as well. They are not as permeable to gas and water vapor as films but are less occlusive than hydrogels or hydrocolloids. The major advantages of foams, in addition to their absorbency, are the physical cushioning of wounds and thermal insulation to maintain the temperature of the wound closer to the optimal temperature for the growth of fibroblasts and epithelial cells. Foam dressings are often used in an effort to prevent pressure injuries and are often placed under medical devices to prevent medical device–related pressure injuries. Manufacturers have constructed these dressings with additives, including surfactants and detergents, to help clean wounds and charcoal to absorb odor. Charcoal can also be built into foam-based composite dressings.

Superabsorbent Dressings/ Specialty Absorbents

Frequently, wounds, especially large wounds or venous ulcers, have excessive drainage that cannot be effectively managed by an alginate/hydrofiber or foam dressing. This is where the use of a superabsorbent or specialty absorbent dressing is useful. These are made to absorb moderate to copious amounts of drainage and can absorb 4 to 5 times their weight in drainage. Some superabsorbent dressings have "diaper technology" that gels when it comes in contact with drainage, such as Xtrasorb (Patterson Medical Holdings, Inc) or Sorbion (BSN Medical). Others have multiple layers that wick the fluid away from the wound and to the dressing's outer core, such as Drawtex (SteadMed Medical) and Cutisorb (BSN Medical). These superabsorbent dressings require a secondary dressing and can be used under compression. While initially appearing more expensive than other types of dressings, they are more cost-effective because they do not need to be changed as often, thus saving resources such as manpower and secondary dressings.

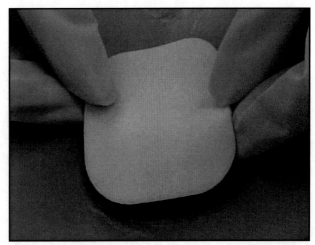

Figure 16-10. Example of a foam dressing being used as a primary dressing and cover.

ANTIBIOTIC CREAMS AND OINTMENTS

Antibiotic creams and ointments can be used as primary dressings. They generally require a secondary dressing, which, in addition to covering the antibiotic, is needed to absorb drainage from necrotic tissue and blisters and to protect the tissue below. Although antibiotic creams/ointments are generally associated with burn injuries, they can be used for other wounds. Silver-containing creams are very expensive; therefore, other types of antibiotic creams or ointments are frequently used for wounds other than burns.

Silver Sulfadiazine

In the form of thick, soothing cream, this antibiotic may be considered a dressing. It is used primarily on burns with or without gauze to protect wounds but can be applied to some types of acute wounds. Silver, whether in this form or as liquid silver nitrate, or silver salt is a broad-spectrum antimicrobial. However, silver impairs fibroblasts and epithelial cells. Despite this, silver may lead to more rapid healing by avoiding chronic inflammation that might occur with high levels of bacteria or fungi on burns or other acute wounds. Silver sulfadiazine should be applied under clean conditions, with a thickness of 1/16 inch after hydrotherapy and debridement (Figure 16-11). It also needs to be reapplied to areas from which it has been removed by

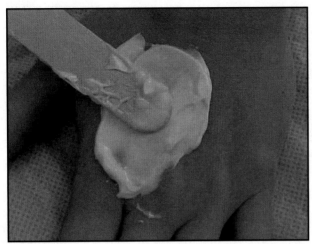

Figure 16-11. Application of silver sulfadiazine with a tongue depressor.

patient activity. The cream is to be left in place for 24 hours. Silver sulfadiazine is contraindicated for pregnant women, infants before the age of 2 months, or premature infants because of the risk of kernicterus (ie, brain damage caused by bilirubinemia). Although frequently used for many days, it should be discontinued when the infection risk has passed, usually when debridement is complete.

Mafenide Acetate

Mafenide acetate is provided as a 50-g packet of white, crystalline powder and as a cream. It is best known as Sulfamylon. According to manufacturer instructions, the powder packet is mixed with 1 L sterile water or normal saline to produce a 5% topical solution. The solution is stored at room temperature and used within 48 hours after mixing. Mafenide acetate is also available as an 11% cream applied similarly to silver sulfadiazine. The primary use of Sulfamylon is on burn injuries as an alternative to silver sulfadiazine. A discussion of the uses of these 2 agents is found in Chapter 14 on burn injuries. Burn dressings are soaked with Sulfamylon to the saturation point and then covered with another layer of dressings. The primary dressing is to be kept wet. The manufacturer suggests using a bulb syringe or irrigation tubing to moisten the primary dressing every 4 hours. Dressings are to be left over grafts up to 5 days, at which time the graft should have taken. Patients may have allergic reactions or develop acidosis during Sulfamylon treatment. Sulfamylon is to be discontinued if an allergic response occurs. With acidosis, the treatment may be discontinued for 24 to 48 hours and possibly restarted.

Neosporin and Polysporin

Both of these are supplied in a petrolatum-based ointment. Although generic equivalents are available, the ingredients may vary among manufacturers. Neosporin consists of 3 antimicrobial agents, whereas Polysporin contains 2. Both contain polymyxin B and bacitracin. Neosporin contains neomycin in addition to the antibiotics in Polysporin. These combinations provide broad-spectrum coverage but are too toxic, especially nephrotoxic and ototoxic, to be used in any manner other than topical. Bacitracin is a cell wall–active agent effective against gram-positive organisms. Polymyxin B damages cell membranes of gram-negative organisms. Polysporin is claimed to be effective against *Staphylococcus aureus*, Streptococcus species, *Escherichia coli, Hemophilus influenzae, Klebsiella* and *Enterobacter* species, *Neisseria* species, and *Pseudomonas aeruginosa*, but the manufacturer states that it is not effective against *Serratia marcesens*. As an ointment, it is used topically on minor wounds, particularly on the face and eye, where Neosporin use is not recommended due to the possibility of allergic reactions to neomycin. Polysporin is also available as a powder, which has been recommended for use with collagenase.

Neosporin, with the additional component of neomycin, gives broader coverage. Neomycin is an aminoglycoside that impairs bacteria protein synthesis. It provides excellent coverage against gram-negative organisms and weak coverage against gram-positive organisms. Other formulations of Neosporin are available. The pain relief variety has pramoxine, a local anesthetic, but does not include bacitracin due to the mixture's chemical properties. Neosporin has been promoted as a means of causing wounds to heal faster; however, the comparison has been done against wounds that did not use Neosporin and not against the petrolatum base without the antimicrobials. Both Polysporin and Neosporin are useful for patients to use at home. Patients need to be told to read the instructions and be specifically warned against any allergic reactions.

OTHER ANTIMICROBIAL DRESSINGS
Cadexomer Iodine

Although iodine-containing antiseptics are not approved for use in wounds, cadexomer iodine has been designed specifically for wounds. Cadexomer iodine provides sustained release iodine rather than the large amount released from povidone-iodine. It can be applied directly to wounds in the form of an ointment or a sheet to be placed in wounds. As the material absorbs drainage, it forms a gel and releases iodine into the wound. Cadexomer iodine is indicated for wounds with heavy drainage, heavily contaminated wounds, and second-degree burns due to its ability to absorb drainage. Its absorptive nature is also useful in controlling odor and protecting surrounding skin from drainage. By maintaining a moist wound bed, cadexomer iodine promotes autolytic debridement. The gel can also conform to the shape of the wound, which also assists in retaining fluid in the wound bed and off the surrounding skin. The ointment form has a brown color and requires a secondary dressing. The gel needs to be replaced when it becomes a yellow or gray color.

Some potential issues with cadexomer iodine exist. The darkly pigmented gel obscures the wound bed, and the color may alarm those who are not familiar with this product (Figure 16-12). Removing the gel from a wound may be uncomfortable for a patient. Cadexomer iodine must not be used on anyone with a known allergy to iodine. According to the manufacturer, the level of sustained release of iodine from cadexomer iodine does not lead to the cytotoxicity associated with povidone-iodine. Cadexomer iodine's uses include chronic wounds and infected wounds. The iodine component does not change the requirement of any systemic antibiotics.

Silver-Containing Dressings

Technology to vaporize silver salts and deposit nanocrystalline silver on materials has allowed silver options for alginates/hydrofibers, foam, and contact layers; their grayish hue makes them readily identifiable as containing silver. The nanocrystalline form of silver produces the sustained release of silver on the wound bed. Contact layer types of silver dressings are wet with water, not with saline; dressings may need to be remoistened with water before they are changed. Silver dressings should not be used with enzymatic debriders; therefore, the clinician must decide which is more important because silver inactivates enzymatic debriders. Silverlon (Argentum Medical) is essentially a contact layer made with nylon mesh. Acticoat (Smith & Nephew) is indicated for burns, graft, and donor sites. It consists of a silver coating on a polyethylene mesh with an inner core of rayon and polyester for absorption. A newer version, Acticoat 7, is designed to be effective for up to 7 days; the original was approved for 3-day wear. Silver alginates and hydrofibers are changed as needed but must be changed daily if the wound is infected. Other uses for silver dressings suggested by manufacturers include venous ulcers and use under negative pressure wound therapy (Chapter 17). Although the materials used in silver dressings appear to be effective bactericides in vitro, they have not been shown to produce more rapid healing than similar dressings without the silver component. In reimbursement

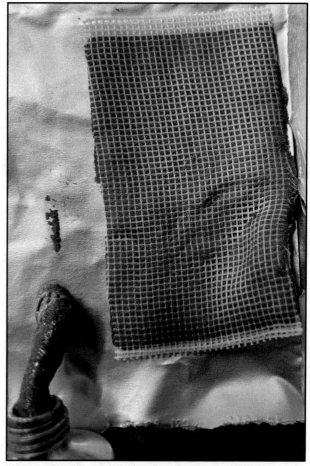

Figure 16-12. Examples of cadexomer iodine.

situations that do not allow for the recovery of dressing material cost, the clinician must consider the greater cost and use them judiciously. An example of a silver-containing dressing is shown in Figure 16-13.

Honey Dressings

Honey dressings are made from specific honey found in New Zealand called *Manuka honey*. Honey dressings come in many delivery systems such as gel, alginate, and hydrocolloid. They are used to help fight bacteria and control odor and aid in autolytic debridement. The way honey dressings work is by osmosis, which changes the wound's pH to improve healing. One benefit of honey dressings important to patients is that they can help decrease pain and speed healing. Examples of honey dressings are shown in Figure 16-14.

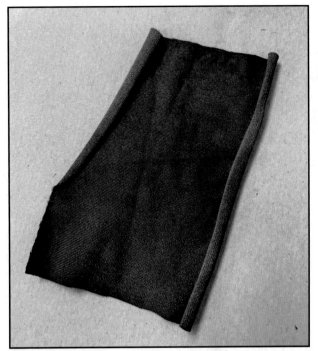

Figure 16-13. Example of silver-containing dressing.

Gentian Violet and Methylene Blue

Multiple types of gentian violet/methylene blue (GV/MB) dressings are available. Depending on their formulations, they may be bacteriostatic, slowing the multiplication of bacteria, or bactericidal. Some types must be hydrated with saline if the wound does not have much drainage. The combination of GV/MB is primarily directed toward managing biofilm. An example of a GV/MB dressing is shown in Figure 16-15.

OXYGEN RECONSTITUTED CELLULOSE

A common problem plaguing chronic wounds is the excessive level of matrix metalloproteinases (MMPs). MMPs are part of the normal response to acute wounds and dissipate as the inflammatory phase of healing occurs. MMPs are a family of 26, possibly more, zinc-dependent proteolytic enzymes produced by multiple cells, including neutrophils, macrophages, fibroblasts, and endothelial cells. These enzymes degrade proteins, including collagen and growth factors. In chronic wounds, the level of MMPs exceeds that of acute wounds, and they persist, creating a vicious cycle of tissue breakdown and chronic inflammation. Part of the regulation of MMPs is the production of tissue inhibitors of metalloproteinases (TIMPs). At least 4 types of TIMPs have been identified, most importantly

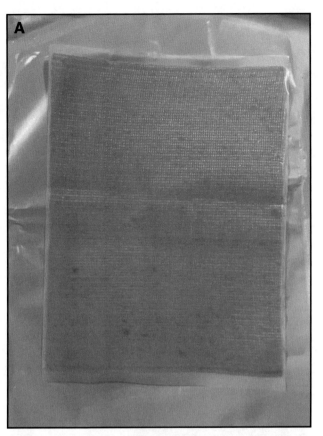

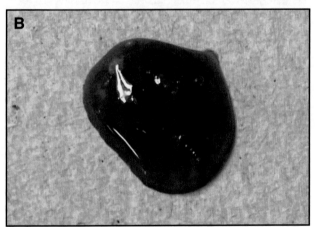

Figure 16-14. Examples of honey-containing dressings. (A) Sheet. (B) Gel.

TIMP1 and 2. These are insufficient in many chronic wounds, thus necessitating the development of dressings made of a material that controls MMP levels in wounds. In addition to controlling MMP levels, these dressings also contribute collagen to the wound.

Oxygen-reconstituted cellulose binds MMPs and forms a gel as it absorbs wound exudate. Promogran (Systagenix) is a freeze-dried matrix of bovine collagen and oxygen-reconstituted cellulose placed in a wound as a thin hexagonal wafer. Promogran Prisma performs similarly, except it has a silver component that protects from infection and can treat low infection levels already in the wound. Endoform is ovine collagen with an intact extracellular matrix that is also used to control MMP levels and provide collagen for granulation tissue growth.

COLLAGEN DRESSINGS

As discussed in previous chapters, collagen is the most abundant protein in the body and acts as a building block or scaffolding for granulation tissue to grow on. In chronic wounds, there is usually not enough collagen available. Thus, these dressings contribute the necessary collagen.

HYALURONIC ACID

Hyaluronic acid is also used as a wound dressing in Hyalofill (Convatec). This material comes in sheets and ribbons similar in appearance to alginate. It is composed of a polymer that releases hyaluronic acid as it absorbs fluid and becomes a gel. Hyaluronic acid is believed to be released for 2 to 3 days into wounds. The manufacturer recommends it for neuropathic ulcers, pressure injuries, and traumatic and surgical wounds.

HYPERTONIC SALINE

Dressings with hypertonic saline absorb exudate, bacteria, and solubilized necrotic tissue. Mesalt is a dressing composed of sodium chloride bound to a synthetic gauze pad. It is simply placed into a wound, where it releases hypertonic saline into the wound. Drainage, bacteria, and other materials are then absorbed into the pad. This dressing is designed specifically for heavily draining wounds. It should not be used on clean wounds with minimal drainage that could be injured by the hypertonicity produced by the release of sodium chloride in a small fluid volume.

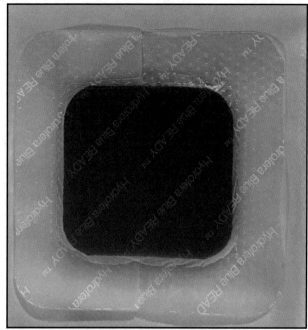

Figure 16-15. Example of GV/MB foam dressing.

TENDERWET

Tenderwet dressings (Medline) promote a moist healing environment by rinsing and debriding wounds. They are soaked with lactated Ringer's solution and allow for high fluid retention. One downfall is Tenderwet dressings require a daily dressing change with an occlusive dressing, but they are good for all types of wounds except infected wounds and those wounds with high potential for infection.

USING DRESSINGS

A few general points about using dressings need to be addressed. The first important point is organization. Organizing the dressing change in advance is key to minimizing contamination of the wound. The clinician should gather all dressing materials and anything else that might be needed to evaluate the wound, especially if cleansing and debridement precede the dressing change. Although a sterile field is not an absolute requirement (see Chapter 5), following the basic principles of maintaining a sterile field in a reasonable manner is good practice to prevent contamination of the wound. The time that packages are left open before being used should be minimized as much as possible. This can be achieved by having an

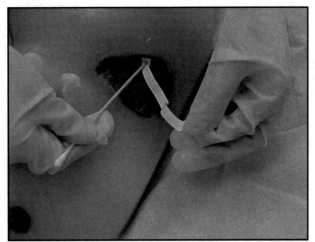

Figure 16-16. The procedure for placing a packing strip into a tract.

assistant available, allowing the patient to be the assistant, or organizing the dressing change as carefully as possible. Sterile dressings must be used on acute surgical wounds, whereas clean dressings are allowable on chronic wounds. However, dressings are generally obtained in sterile packaging. Regardless of the requirement, as much care should be taken to meet sterile technique and maintain a clean environment for wound treatments.

Management of Cavities

Wounds with substantial subcutaneous involvement may require either packing or filling to optimize healing. The term *packing* is frequently used incorrectly to describe a process of placing dressing materials into a wound. Packing refers to a specific type of wound filling used to promote hemostasis and prevent hematoma formation or keep a wound open as it is prepared for delayed primary closure (tertiary closure). Removing postoperative packing can be painful for the patient. The wound is packed under general anesthesia but is usually removed when the patient is conscious. Moreover, the wound is packed more tightly than could be achieved in a conscious patient. When removing packing, carefully determine the best direction to remove the packing material. On occasion, a surgeon may have changed directions while packing a wound, resulting in a knot formation. These are very difficult to remove, requiring patience and possibly cutting pieces from the packing material, whether a packing strip or bandage rolls are used.

Packing prevents the wound from filling with granulation tissue and re-epithelializing, so tertiary closure can be performed once the wound is clean and stable. Incision and drainage wounds created due to osteomyelitis are the usual

type requiring packing. In contrast, filling is used strictly to allow dead spaces to heal from the wound bed, preventing premature closure of the wound surface over a dead space. Dead spaces such as this create an unacceptably high risk for forming a new abscess. Filling is done loosely to promote healing from inside out and manage drainage in wounds with undermined or tunneled wounds or those with sinus tracts; packing such wounds will delay healing. However, inadequate filling of tracts may also allow the tract to close over a dead space. Therefore, filling tracts/ tunnels requires a good feel for the bottom of a tract and pushing the material to the bottom first. Novices may be unwilling to push the packing strip deeply enough due to patient reaction and must learn to focus on the important task of not allowing dead space beyond the packing strip.

The selection of materials used for filling or packing wounds is largely determined by whether the wound is infected and the wound's quantity of drainage. Packing strips can be used for filling wounds as well as packing tracts, tunnels, and other areas within a wound of substantial depth. In addition to physically filling cavities, packing strip wicks moisture and bacteria from the wound. A plain packing strip is dry woven cotton with great tensile strength with no possibility of breaking inside the wound or shedding stray fibers. A continuous 15-feet length is supplied in each bottle of packing strip. This material is available in various sizes such as 1/4 inch, 1/2 inch, 1 inch, and 2 inches. A popular option for infected wounds is Iodoform, which is simply a packing strip moistened with an iodine solution. Iodoform is available in the same sizes. A plain packing strip is commonly moistened before placing it into a wound. Normal saline or antibiotic solution might be used.

The procedure for placing a packing strip into a tract is shown in Figure 16-16. Typical tracts are filled with a 1/4-inch strip, but larger sizes may be used for larger defects. For a typical tract, a packing strip can be lifted straight up from its bottle with cotton-tipped applicators in a chopstick technique; forceps may be used instead. Having removed a previous piece of packing strip from a wound allows the clinician to estimate the length required for a dressing change. If precutting the length of a packing strip, be sure to cut a greater length than necessary. Excess packing strip can be cut off, but being left with a too-short piece requires removing the packing strip and starting anew with a longer piece. This length is cut with scissors that are either sterile or have been cleaned and subjected to high-level disinfection. A cheaper option is the use of a scalpel blade.

The length of the packing strip to be used is held in the nondominant hand, and an end of the strip is held over the tract to be filled. A cotton-tipped applicator is used to push a folded-over end of the strip to the tract's bottom. The stick end is commonly used to push the strip unless the opening is large enough to accommodate the enlarged cotton tip. For a much larger opening, a tongue depressor or gloved finger may be used instead. When using a cotton-tipped applicator, the applicator must be withdrawn carefully to avoid pulling the strip back out of the wound. A twisting motion may be needed to push in the strip and withdraw the stick in a narrow tract. After withdrawing the stick end, the strip is folded over the stick's end, and the strip is again pushed to the bottom. Repeat as many times as needed to fill the tract. By folding the strip over the end of the stick with each push, the strip becomes pleated within the tract, taking up the space of the tract's width. When the tract is filled, cut the strip to leave 1/2 inch or 1 cm protruding to allow it to be removed at the next dressing change. Making certain that the strip is long enough to fill the wound allows the excess to be simply cut. If the strip is too short, it will need to be removed and the process repeated with a longer piece of strip. Never place a second piece on top of the one already in the tract. It might not be found and removed during the next dressing change. An alternative technique is filling tracts directly from the packing strip bottle without cutting until the tract is filled. The problem with this technique is the potential for contaminating the strip as it is pulled from the bottle.

When wide tracts or other areas require filling, a larger-width strip may be used, or a bandage roll may be substituted. A range of 1-inch lightweight bandage rolls through 4-inch bulky bandage rolls may be used depending on the width to be filled. Examples of a bulky 4-inch and a 3-inch lightweight bandage roll are shown in Figure 16-17. Although these may fill the area required, be aware that they are not designed specifically for this purpose. Packing strips are made specifically to prevent the loss of fibers in wounds, whereas bandage rolls may leave fibers. Undermined areas and open areas of the wound may be filled with a greater-width packing strip, bandage roll, or gauze sponges (2 × 2 or 4 × 4) depending on the wound's configuration. The use of multiple gauze sponges in undermined areas creates the possibility of leaving one or more in the wound with the next dressing change and, as such, is not recommended. Using a single piece guarantees that no materials will be left in the wound. If a patient has multiple tracts, be particularly careful to leave the packing strip's ends where they cannot be missed, and document the number carefully in case someone else will be removing them. Plain packing strips, gauze sponges, and bandage rolls are generally moistened with saline or an antibiotic solution rather than placing dry materials into the wound. They should also be placed loosely into an infected undermined or open area but are packed into a wound that is to be kept open for delayed primary closure. Always fill in one direction; choose

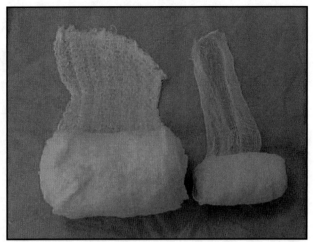

Figure 16-17. Bandage rolls. Bulky 4-inch bandage on left and lightweight 3-inch bandage on right.

one area to fill first, and move consistently across the defect. Going back to an area that has already been filled may create a knot that will be difficult to remove later. Also, keep moist materials within the wound, avoiding the surrounding skin. Prolonged moisture on the surrounding skin is likely to cause maceration and delay re-epithelialization.

Gauze sponges and packing strips will need to be changed daily and possibly twice or more each day to remove infectious material. An alternative to gauze materials is alginate sheets or ropes (see Figure 16-9). Alginate and hydrofiber have greater biocompatibility than gauze packing strips or sponges; therefore, they do not promote inflammation and prolonged heavy drainage. They are also removed easily from a wound, decreasing pain to the patient and trauma to the wound bed. An additional benefit is that alginates and hydrofibers will not wick fluid onto the surrounding skin, which is a common problem with gauze leading to maceration. These materials may be used in infected wounds, but they must be changed at least daily. Also, try to minimize the number of pieces of alginate/hydrofiber placed in the wound. If possible, use one piece to avoid leaving any behind with the next dressing change. Collagen sheets and ropes have the added advantage of the collagen being absorbed into the wound and possibly enhancing the healing rate. Gauze should be avoided on granulation tissue. Clean wet wounds can be filled loosely with alginate or hydrofiber ribbon or sheet, hydrocolloid fillers, or dextranomers. Dextranomers are described in Chapter 15. Wounds with dry wound beds can be lined with hydrogel to provide moisture to assist healing. Strategies for selecting wound dressings to meet goals for treatment are listed in Table 16-3.

TABLE 16-3
Dressing Decision Chart Based on Characteristics of Wound*

TYPE	CHARACTERISTICS	POTENTIAL PROBLEMS	GOALS	DRESSING
Venous insufficiency	Shallow, granulating, moderate-heavy drainage	Maceration, lack epithelialization, edema of wound	Absorb drainage, reduce edema	Alginate/hydrofiber, foam or hydrocolloid, preferred: contact layer under multilayer compression bandaging
Neuropathic	Varied drainage depending on coexisting arterial disease and infection	Continued mechanical damage, possible concomitant arterial insufficiency, potential for infection	Prevent or manage infection, manage drainage, protect from trauma, debridement	Sharp debridement until necrotic tissue and infection cleared; determine dressing-based characteristics
Dry shallow	Formation of scab	Lack of proliferation and autolytic debridement	Moisten	Hydrogel with transparent film
Moist shallow	Signs of chronic inflammation	Maceration of surrounding skin	Absorb drainage	Hydrocolloid or foam
Dry deep	Induration, erythema of surrounding skin	Lack of proliferation and autolytic debridement, dead space	Fill dead space, moisten	Hydrogel with transparent film
Moist deep	Copious exudate, maceration of surrounding skin	Maceration, lack of healing due to edema and damage to epidermis	Absorb drainage, fill dead space	Hydrofiber/alginate filler covered with hydrocolloid or foam
Deep infected	Odor, drainage, necrotic tissue	Spread of infection, lack of healing	Remove necrotic tissue, fill dead space	Sharp debridement covered with moist gauze; brief trial of topical antibiotic
Deep, filled with necrotic tissue	Mild odor, yellow	Potential for infection, slow healing	Remove necrotic tissue, fill dead space	Debridement with dry dressing, enzymatic debrider with moistened gauze
Covered with eschar	Black or yellow covering, base of wound not seen	Potential for infection, slow healing	Remove eschar	Sharp debridement or crosshatch with enzymatic debrider; determined by depth and drainage

*This table is meant as a guideline only and serves as a starting point for a plan of care. Actual plans must take other factors into consideration such as the patient's resources and preferences. Plan of care should change as characteristics of the wound change.

SECONDARY DRESSINGS AND BANDAGING TECHNIQUES

Secondary bandages may have multiple purposes. They are used to hold the primary dressing in place, increase absorption, provide compression when needed, provide warmth and comfort to the area, and physically protect or pad the wound's area. Secondary dressings may consist of adhesive bandages; composite dressings; bandage rolls; gauze sponges (commonly 4 × 4) taped over the primary dressing; or one of several elasticized materials such as Flexinet (Derma Sciences), Tubigrip (Molnlycke), ACE bandages (3M), or certain compression bandages. A tertiary dressing would be placed over a secondary dressing.

Composite dressings can be a primary or secondary dressing. They usually have 3 layers (from inside to out): a nonadherent layer that protects the wound, an absorbent layer that absorbs drainage and protects periwound from maceration, and a bacterial barrier usually made of semipermeable film that protects the wound from the outside environment.

Bandage rolls are convenient to meet most needs of secondary dressings. They come in various widths, although 4-inch bandages appear to be most commonly used. The width of the bandage used varies with the diameter of the body part being wrapped. In applications with smaller or large area diameter, sizes ranging from 1 inch to 6 inches may be used. A 1-inch bandage roll may be used on a finger or toe; a 2-inch bandage roll on a small hand; and a 3-inch on a larger hand, a forearm, or distal leg. Four-inch bandages are generally used on feet, legs, or arms. Six-inch bandage rolls may be used on thighs, trunks, or unusually large distal extremities. The weave of the bandage roll determines many of its properties. A thinly layered interlocking weave provides elasticity to the bandage roll, whereas a loose, bulky bandage provides more absorption and insulation. Lightweight cotton bandages, such as Kling (Johnson & Johnson) or Conform (Kendall), allow mobility. However, they are less absorbent than soft bulky bandage rolls such as Kerlix (Cardinal Health), which are more absorbent and provide better padding but less mobility. Soft bulky bandage rolls may be used for the specific purpose of limiting mobility on occasion. Bulky bandage rolls such as Kerlix absorb, cushion, retain warmth, and can be used to immobilize a body part. Examples of bulky and lightweight bandage rolls are shown in Figure 16-17.

Three basic techniques for applying bandage rolls are commonly used. For all of these techniques, bandage rolls should always be rolled on the patient's body from the bottom (Figure 16-18A). Rolling from the top causes bandage rolls to catch on themselves, causing uneven bandaging and possibly dropping the bandage roll. A simple half-overlapping spiral is used to hold dressings in place and cover wounds (Figure 16-18B). A figure 8 method has several purposes. It can be used to increase the amount of pressure under the bandage or may be used to allow more mobility at a joint. Wrapping around a knee or elbow in a figure 8 with a lightweight bandage roll allows flexion to occur more readily. A half-overlapping spiral with a bulky bandage roll can be used to inhibit movement at a joint. Another advantage of applying a bandage roll in a figure 8 is that it is less likely to collapse with gravity on an extremity than a half-overlapping spiral. A figure 8 wrapping should be attempted first rather than taping the top and bottom of bandages to a patient's skin. Bandages can also be fanfolded (Figure 16-18C) by folding it back over itself. Fanfolding is used to increase absorption and provide padding. Rather than use multiple gauze sponges and only part of a bandage roll, more efficient use of materials is accomplished by fanfolding the bandage roll over the area requiring greater absorption or padding.

When using a bandage roll on the hand or foot, create a lock by making at least one turn (Figure 16-18D) around the wrist or ankle. In general, we wish to keep the thumb separate from the other fingers to allow grasp (Figure 16-18E). Humidity can increase to a damaging level under bandage rolls. If a bandage roll covers toes or fingers, place 2 × 2s between toes or 4 × 4s between fingers to prevent maceration (Figure 16-18F). Bandage rolls and other secondary dressings may be dislodged easily between dressing changes. A plan for securing the secondary dressing should be considered before applying them. Strategies include placing a piece of tape on the bandage roll above the heel or on the wrist just proximal to the hand to prevent loosening and migration of the bandage off the hand or foot (Figure 16-18G) and placing short pieces of tape perpendicular to the turns of the bandage to maintain the spatial relationship among these turns. On conical segments such as the thigh, leg, and forearm, the bandage's turns may simply collapse with gravity loosening the bandage roll and causing it to fall off the body part. A combination of figure 8 wrapping and strategic taping can prevent the bandage roll from collapsing and unraveling. Figure 8 bandaging is shown in Figure 16-18H. Taping over either a primary dressing or a secondary dressing, including bandage rolls, should never be done circumferentially—one end of a piece of tape should never be arranged so it adheres to the other end. If swelling occurs, circumferential taping may lead to limb-threatening ischemia. A safe alternative is placing tape in a spiral such that the ends are still free to move relative to each other. Avoid finishing a bandage roll or leaving any folds under the foot where injury could occur. Ensure that a person has footwear that will accommodate bandaging around the foot.

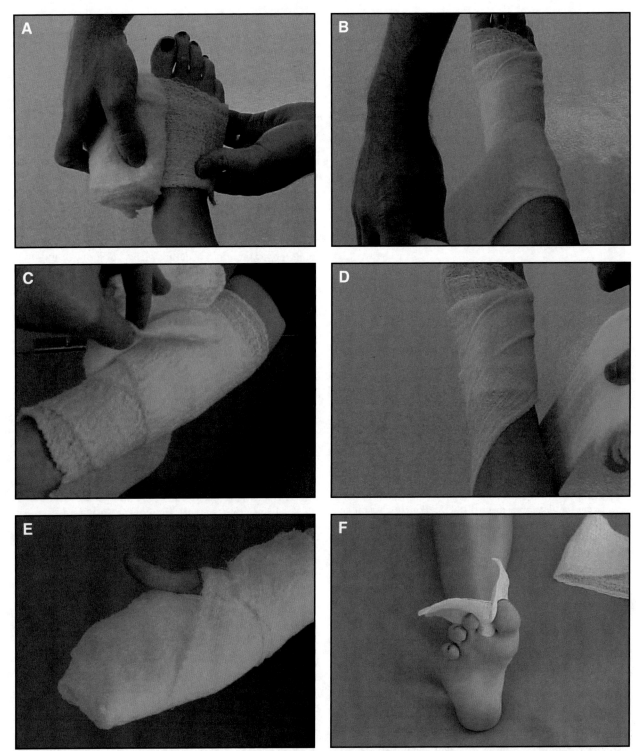

Figure 16-18. Bandaging as a secondary or tertiary dressing. (A) Proper technique involves rolling the bandage from the bottom. (B) Half-overlapping spiral technique. (C) Fanfolding to increase the layering, cushioning, and absorbency in the cubital fossa. (D) Turning the bandage roll around the ankle to anchor it. (E) Proper bandaging of the hand to allow free movement of an uninvolved thumb. (F) Placing a 2 × 2 inch gauze sponge between toes to prevent maceration. Note this technique allows all 4 web spaces to be managed with only 2 gauze sponges. *(continued)*

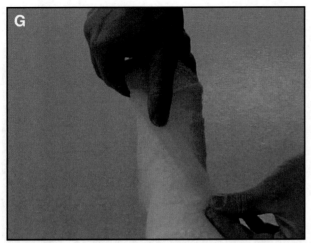

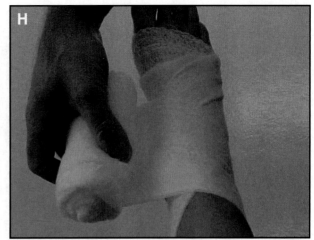

Figure 16-18 (continued). (G) Placing tape across turns of the bandage roll to prevent the bandage from loosening and falling onto the foot. (H) Using the bandage roll in figure 8 wrapping.

Taping

Four basic types of tape are used in wound care (Figure 16-19). They are discussed in order of harshness to the skin. Silk tape, such as Durapore (3M), is the most adhesive of the 4 types. Although it may cause minimal damage when used carefully and occasionally on young, healthy skin, it will tear weak, older skin and damage healthy skin with repeated use. It should be avoided for wound dressings because of cost and adhesiveness; unfortunately, you may find that others may redress a wound on your patient using silk tape. Plastic tape, such as the 3M brand Transpore, is still too adhesive and harsh for skin at risk for damage. It is convenient for use because it tears easily in both directions. Appropriate uses include taping secondary dressings to surfaces other than skin and anchoring a secondary dressing to itself, especially to make "racing stripes" (see Figure 16-18G) on a bandage roll to prevent unraveling. Paper tape, including Micropore (3M), has low adhesion and is hypoallergenic. As such, it is usually gentle enough for repeated applications to healthy skin or occasional application to at-risk skin. It is a lower-cost tape but comes off skin easily. However, the use of skin protectant under paper tape greatly improves its adhesion. Appropriate uses include taping a primary or secondary dressing directly to the skin. The best type of tape to place directly on the skin is an elastic foam tape such as Microfoam (3M). This type of tape has low but adequate adhesion. It is gentle enough for daily or twice a day changes on at-risk skin and is comfortable and water resistant. Due to its elasticity, it conforms to irregular surfaces and stretches with swelling. However, it should not be stretched as it is placed on the skin. The recoil of the elastic tape causes shearing and damage to the skin. This type of tape is expensive and loses adhesion when repositioned. Its uses include taping a primary or secondary dressing directly to skin, especially at-risk skin or those receiving frequent dressing changes.

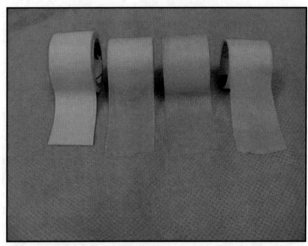

Figure 16-19. Types of adhesive tape. Left to right: foam, paper, plastic, and silk.

TOLERANCE FOR ADHESIVES

Many individuals cannot tolerate the adhesives used in wound care products. One problem is the adhesive strength relative to the cohesiveness of the person's skin, especially older individuals. Younger clinicians with strong, supple skin may not foresee the damage that adhesive may have on older, drier, weaker skin. Many individuals also have immune reactions to adhesives (Figure 16-20A). Wound dressings that are particularly problematic are semipermeable films and hydrocolloids, although other dressings may include adhesives. Semipermeable films are particularly problematic because they tend to be changed more frequently than other microenvironmental dressings. Even dressings that do not contain adhesives can cause problems because of the need to tape them in place or use secondary dressings with adhesives. Several solutions are available. To protect skin from the mechanical aspects of aggressive adhesives, skin

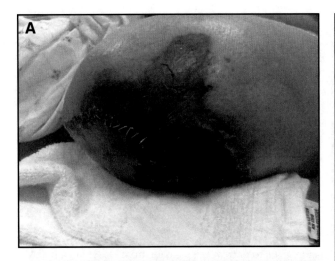

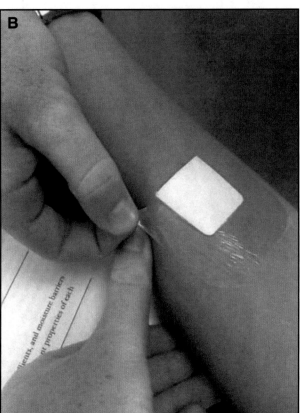

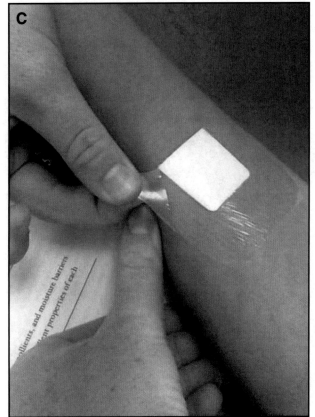

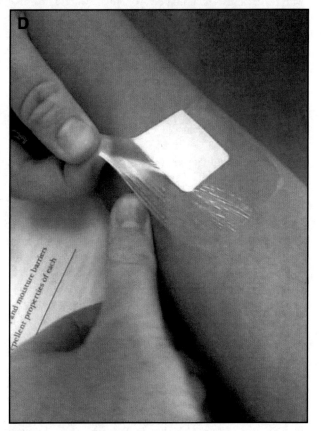

Figure 16-20. (A) Skin reaction caused by the use of tape on a patient's skin. (B to G) Students practicing the sequence for the removal of semipermeable film. A corner is lifted and the material is gradually stretched to reduce the adherence of the dressing, while the skin beneath is stabilized to prevent injury. Clinicians are expected to wear gloves during this procedure. *(continued)*

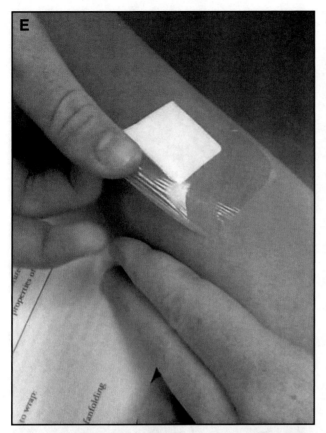

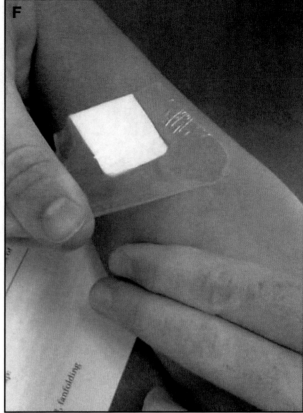

Figure 16-20 (continued).

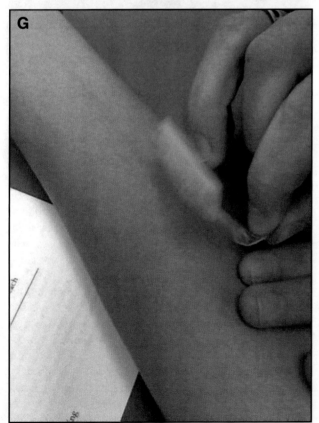

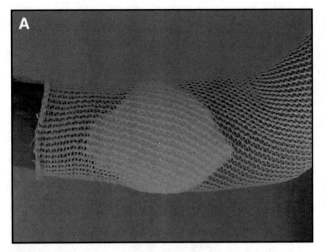

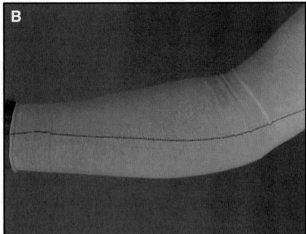

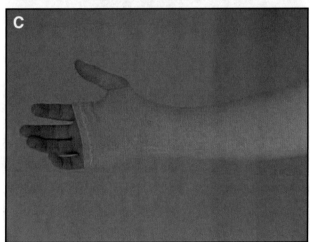

Figure 16-21. Nonadhesive alternative for secondary/tertiary dressings. (A) Stretch netting. (B) Tubular bandage. (C) Elasticized tubular bandage designed specifically for the hand and forearm.

protectants can be used; these are discussed in the next section. Careful removal of the semipermeable film by stretching as described earlier and leaving hydrocolloids in place as long as possible and then carefully removing them from the surrounding skin will minimize trauma (Figures 16-20B to 16-20G). Alternatively, nonadherent dressings may need to be substituted for films and hydrocolloids. For dressings that require taping to hold them in place, a foam tape is the most appropriate, as long as the tape is not stretched as it is applied. Because foam tape is not as adherent as other types, a 2-inch width is usually necessary. Other options include the use of either bulky or elasticized bandage rolls, tubular bandages, or net bandages (Figure 16-21). These may work well on areas of the body not subject to weight shifting and moving, but on highly mobile areas, the nonadherent dressing below is likely to shift.

SKIN CARE

Many skin care products have been designed to promote proper skin moisture levels by adding moisture to the skin, retaining moisture in the wound, or protecting the skin from exposure to excessive moisture or aggressive adhesives used on some dressings. Three categories of skin products are classified by the CMS. These skin products are not used directly on wounds but protect skin at risk for injury or protect the surrounding skin from damage from excessive wound drainage or adhesives used for dressings. The categories are therapeutic moisturizers, moisture barriers, and liquid skin protectants. Other ingredients that may be present in skin care products include antimicrobials, detergents, humectants, preservatives, and surfactants.

Several lay terms may be used for skin care products. An emollient, by definition, is used to soften skin. *Emollient* typically refers to lotions used to moisturize dry skin, but in some cases, a product called an emollient could also be used as a moisture barrier. *Humectants*, such as glycerin, are designed to protect skin integrity by

TABLE 16-4
Categories and Ingredients of Skin Care Products

CATEGORY	TYPICAL INGREDIENTS
Emollient	Aloe vera, glyceryl stearate, lanolin, mineral oil
Humectant	Propylene glycol, glycerin
Preservative	Methylparaben, quaternium-15, propylparaben
Skin protectant	Allantoin, calamine, cocoa butter, dimethicone, glycerin, kaolin, white petrolatum, zinc oxide

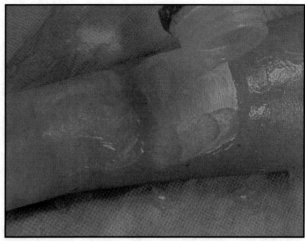

Figure 16-22. Examples of skin care products from left to right: moisturizing cream, protective cream, and protective ointment.

maintaining normal skin moisture. These agents could also be considered a type of skin protectant.

Skin care products are also classified by the terms *lotion*, *cream*, and *ointment*. This classification is determined chiefly by the concentration of solids and the fraction of water within the product. A lotion has high water content and a low concentration of solids. A product classified as a lotion is designed primarily for moisturizing skin that has lost moisture due to dry air or frequent handwashing. Lotion is important for both health care workers and at-risk patients to prevent cracking of the skin. Typical ingredients in lotions are water, mineral oil, stearic acid, glycerin, petrolatum, triethanolamine, magnesium aluminum silicate, glyceryl stearate, dimethicone, carbomer, methylparaben, DMDM hydantoin, aloe vera, and tetrasodium EDTA. In particular, aloe vera has been suggested to promote wound healing. Aloe vera gel is available commercially but is not currently recommended by any wound guidelines. Aloe vera gel has also been shown to reverse the retardation of healing caused by the antiseptic mafenide acetate.

Creams are thicker in consistency with less water than lotions and are frequently combined with zinc oxide solids. *Ointments* consist of substances that repel water and adhere to the skin. Common ingredients of ointments include petrolatum, mineral oil, lanolin, dimethicone, zinc oxide, and glycerin. Ointments and creams are used as moisture barriers for protecting the skin around a draining wound or protecting the perineum of individuals with urinary or fecal incontinence. Common skin care products and their typical ingredients are listed in Table 16-4.

The characteristics of various lotions, creams, and ointments can be tested easily by rubbing a small quantity on your own hand and dropping water on them. An ointment that will function well as a moisture barrier causes water to bead and run off the skin. In contrast, lotions designed as therapeutic moisturizers will allow water to

remain on surfaces. Depending on the purpose of the substance, characteristics of the patient, and cost, different brands of ointments, creams, or lotions may be better suited for a particular patient. Various products may have ingredients better suited for a therapeutic moisturizer or a moisture barrier. Some have a combination of both properties, and these substances have a wide price range.

Optimizing healing of wounds includes maintenance of an optimal level of wound moisture. Wound moisture is necessary for the migration of epithelial cells, movement of enzymes, growth factors, and structural molecules. However, excessive moisture damages the surrounding skin. Maceration may be prevented by less frequent and gentler dressing changes and wound treatment to decrease inflammation. However, less frequent dressing changes allow more drainage to accumulate beneath the dressing. A dressing and wound filler must be selected to allow an optimal combination of dressing wear time, gentle handling of the wound, and protecting the surrounding skin from excessive moisture.

In many cases, the clinician is faced with the choice of more frequent dressing change and promoting inflammation or leaving a dressing in place and causing maceration. An option to lengthen dressing wear time without increasing the risk of maceration is applying a moisture barrier or skin protectant to the surrounding skin and a dressing capable of retaining drainage within the wound. Several products are available for this purpose. An ointment with a substantial petrolatum, dimethicone, or zinc oxide component is useful as a barrier to water, causing beading and runoff necessary to keep fluid off the skin. Examples of skin care products are shown in Figure 16-22.

Liquid skin protectants, also known as *skin sealants* and *skin protectors*, have 2 purposes. Specifically, they are designed to protect skin from adhesives used for wound dressings. Second, they do not allow fluid from the wound

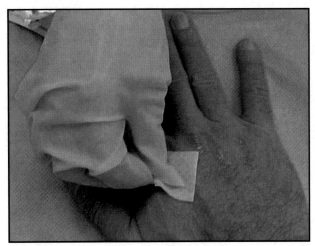

Figure 16-23. Application of skin protectant.

to accumulate on the skin. They consist of molecules (butyl ester of polyvinyl methyl ether/maleic acid copolymer) in a liquid vehicle that polymerizes when exposed to air. The application of skin protectant is shown in Figure 16-23. Isopropyl alcohol is commonly used in skin protectants, causing pain if it gets into the wound or cracks in the surrounding skin. Nonsting formulations that do not use alcohol are also available. With a skin protectant in place, the adhesive of dressings does not contact the skin directly. When the adherent dressing is removed, the skin is less likely to be damaged. In addition, the polymer retains moisture in the skin and keeps moisture off the skin. Skin protectants should always be used under any self-adherent dressings or tape to prevent damage during removal, especially transparent films and hydrocolloid dressings because of the stronger adhesive used on them. Using skin protectants, the problem of protecting the skin from moisture leaking from the wound onto the surrounding skin and protecting the skin from aggressive adhesives can be accomplished simply with a single product.

Common skin protectants include Skin-Prep (Smith & Nephew), Allkare (Convatec), Sween Prep (Coloplast), and 3M No Sting Barrier Film. Skin protectants come in swabs, wipes, and squeeze containers. Regardless of the type of applicator, the material must be allowed to dry before a dressing is applied. Although adhesive removers are available, the removal of skin protectants is not necessary with each dressing change. They should simply be reapplied as necessary. Adhesive removers are made of SD alcohol, propylene glycol monomethyl ether, decahydronaphthalene, ethyl acetate, and stearic acid. Frequent use of these can dry and damage the skin. The use of a skin protectant can reduce the need for adhesive removers. Adhesive removers are typically used for removing dressings with aggressive adhesives. The use of a skin protectant under the adhesive allows the dressing to be removed without adhesive

remover by gently lifting a corner and stretching the dressing material parallel to the skin surface.

Because therapeutic moisturizers and moisture barriers prevent dressings from adhering to skin, special measures need to be used if placed on the skin surrounding a wound when a self-adherent dressing is used. Several means are available for securing dressings in these cases. A simple approach is to extend the dressing beyond the skin protected by these moisture barriers. This approach requires that the moisture barrier be extended no farther than the beginning of the adhesive border of the dressing or skin that can tolerate the increased moisture that may reach beyond the moisture barrier. A second approach uses a sufficiently absorbent dressing or a dressing supplemented with another absorbent material (eg, alginate beneath a hydrocolloid dressing to prevent moisture from reaching the unprotected surrounding skin). A third approach is to secure a nonadherent dressing with an elasticized netting or tubing. The clinician needs to exercise judgment as to the appropriate body part and person. For example, using this approach on the heel or elbow of a person who shifts position in bed frequently is likely to allow the dressing to shift off the wound.

In contrast, this approach would work well on a non–weight-bearing surface, away from joints, or in a person with limited mobility. A fourth approach uses either an elasticized bandage, a lightweight bandage roll, or a bulky bandage roll to secure a nonadherent dressing. Elasticized bandages or bandage rolls have the advantage of also managing edema but may cause excessive pressure and limit the ability to monitor the wound. Bulky bandage rolls have the advantage of absorbing drainage that may leak from under the dressing to protect the surrounding skin. Elasticized netting, tubing, and bandages come in various sizes to allow wounds on any body part to be managed this way. A fifth approach uses a liquid skin protectant as described previously to protect the skin from both moisture and aggressive adhesives. The strategy used will depend on several factors, such as body part, characteristics and availability of different dressing types, patient preference and mobility, and numerous others. Strategies to prevent maceration of surrounding skin are listed in Table 16-5.

WOUND CLEANSERS

The Agency for Health Care Policy and Research guidelines include cleansing of wounds with each dressing change. Two competing goals must be reconciled in deciding whether to cleanse the wound. For the clinician to perform a limited evaluation with each dressing change, the wound bed must be clearly visible. On the other hand, cleansing with each dressing change may cause tissue trauma and promote chronic inflammation. Because each

TABLE 16-5
Strategies for Preventing Maceration
• Apply moisture barrier extending only to adhesive border of dressings or tape.
• Fill wound with more absorbent material that does not wick onto skin.
• Apply moisture barrier and use nonadhesive dressing with stretch tubing or netting.
• Apply moisture barrier and use nonadhesive dressing with bandage roll.
• Apply skin protectant on skin where drainage may accumulate.

TABLE 16-6	
Ingredients of Wound and Skin Cleansers	
CATEGORY	INGREDIENT
Antimicrobial	Benzalkonium chloride, benzethonium chloride, benzoic acid, hexylresorcinol, malic acid, methylbenzethonium chloride
Chelators	Disodium EDTA
Detergents	Ammonium lauryl sulfate, sodium lauryl sulfate
Surfactant	Poloxymer, polysorbate 20

patient presents with a different set of priorities, and priorities are likely to change through the healing process, the clinician should carefully assess the need for cleansing. A reasonable philosophy to follow is that a dressing should be chosen to minimize dressing change frequency. However, with each dressing change, the wound bed should be visualized to determine whether any changes in the plan of care are necessary. Cleansing may become necessary if the clinician cannot make a judgment due to a lack of wound bed visibility. If possible, the dressing should be chosen to fit the number of days before the next evaluation, or the patient or caregiver will be required to change a dressing and monitor the progress of the wound.

Several products are available for cleansing wounds. Many forms of debridement also cleanse wounds (eg, whirlpool, irrigation, and pulsatile lavage). The use of these is discussed in Chapter 15. Cleansers are designed to remove materials other than adherent necrotic tissue, including drainage, desiccated tissue, blood, adherent macromolecules, and foreign materials. Cleansers range from normal saline to complex mixtures of detergents, chelators, surfactants, and preservatives, including poloxamer, hydroxypropyl methylcellulose, potassium sorbate, DMDM hydantoin, methylparaben, D-panthenol, zinc gluconate, magnesium gluconate, and malic acid. Normal saline is least likely to cause tissue trauma and inflammation. Application of saline as a cleanser may be done by simply pouring normal saline over the wound or using low-pressure means such as an irrigation bulb. Higher-pressure irrigation can be performed with a saline-filled syringe with a small catheter attached. Another option is squeezing a bag of normal saline after removing one of the plugs from the bag's bottom. Some studies have indicated that simple tap water is just as safe and effective as sterile normal saline on chronic wounds. Although some individuals use

hydrogen peroxide as a cleansing agent because the effervescence may lift materials from the wound's surface, this approach is not recommended because of the cytotoxicity of hydrogen peroxide. Ingredients found commonly in wound and skin cleansers are listed in Table 16-6.

Commercially available cleansers have a range of tissue toxicity; many of these agents are listed in the Agency for Health Care Policy and Research guidelines for the treatment of pressure injuries. Soaps and detergents dissolve in both water and lipid-containing substances such as cell membranes. Therefore, no soap or detergent is completely safe on wounds. In Chapter 5, soaps and detergents are discussed as antimicrobial methods. By interrupting the surface tension created by hydrogen bonds of water molecules, surfactants allow soaps and detergents to bind to molecules in the wound. Chelators such as EDTA bind metal ions to remove them from the fluid, which softens hard water and improves the effectiveness of soaps and detergents. Combining detergents, chelators, and surfactants makes specialized wound cleansers more effective than normal saline, but these chemicals may injure cells in the wound. Some dressings have these ingredients built into them in an attempt to accelerate the healing process by removing foreign and degraded materials from the wound fluid.

SKIN CLEANSERS

Skin cleansers are designed for use on at-risk skin and are often promoted as complementary products with skin protectants or therapeutic moisturizers. They are designed to be more gentle and effective than typical skin soaps and detergents. In particular, they are used for individuals with fecal and urinary incontinence. Both urine and feces are acidic, and fecal material is often very adherent to the skin. Frequent episodes of fecal incontinence throughout the day can lead to a rapid breakdown of the perineal skin. Unfortunately, frequent cleansing with bath soap and scrubbing with rough washcloths or towels to loosen fecal material can worsen skin damage. Skin cleansers, as described for wound cleansers, contain detergents, surfactants, and chelators. They are also designed to neutralize the acid pH of urine and feces to reduce damage to the perineum.

ECONOMICS OF DRESSING CHANGES

One drawback of occlusive dressings is their cost. However, if we account for the faster healing under occlusive dressings and the greater frequency of nonocclusive dressing changes ($5 to $8 for a 4- to 7-day application) compared with the cost of gauze, the economic picture becomes quite different. The greatest cost of dressing changes does not come from the dressing itself but rather the time for the dressing change to be performed. Materials for a nonocclusive dressing change may cost $3.00 or more depending on the number of gauze layers and their sizes. Moreover, the dressing change may be done twice each day at the cost of up to $6.00 in materials each day compared with $5.00 to $8.00 for the entire 5 days that a microenvironmental dressing is worn. An occlusive dressing left in place for several days decreases costs related to clinician time and may decrease material costs.

For patients covered by Medicare Part B, additional reimbursement issues may need to be considered. Medicare Part B will reimburse only primary and secondary dressings for wounds caused by a surgical procedure, treated by a surgical procedure, or that require debridement. Debridement must be performed by a licensed physician or health care professional as permitted by state law. Debridement may include any of those described in Chapter 15. Medicare will not reimburse for dressings used on skin conditions treated with topical medications; draining cutaneous fistulas; dressings used to protect a healed wound by reducing friction, shear, or moisture; or dressings over catheter insertion points, first-degree burns, skin tears, abrasion, venipuncture, or arterial puncture sites. For reimbursement, a physician, nurse practitioner, clinical nurse specialist, certified nurse-midwife, or physician assistant must order dressings within state regulations. In addition, dressings will be covered only as long as medically necessary.

When procedures requiring the removal of a dressing are billed to Medicare, the cost of applying the dressing is considered incident to the charge and cannot be billed separately. Dressings ordered for home use by the patient for home dressing changes can be billed through the Durable Medical Equipment Regional Carrier (DMERC) based on a fee schedule established for each state by using the Healthcare Common Procedure Coding System code.

No more than 1 month's supply may be ordered at a time. For these dressings, Medicare pays 80% of the fee schedule amount or the actual charge if lower. For dressings with adhesive borders, no payment for other dressings or tape is allowed. The use of more than one type of wound filler or more than one type of wound cover is not allowed. A combination of hydrating dressing with an absorptive dressing on the same wound at the same time is not allowed. Dressing size should be based on the size of the wound. Medicare suggests that the wound cover size be about 2 inches greater than the actual dimensions of the wound. Also, Medicare does not cover skin sealants or barriers, wound cleansers or irrigating solutions, solutions used to moisten gauze, topical antiseptics, topical antibiotics, gauze and dressings used to cleanse or debride a wound but not left on a wound, elastic stockings, support hose, foot coverings, and leotards. Most of the unallowable items are either incident to other charges such as debridement or treatment of venous ulcers. For the most part, these regulations represent good clinical practice. However, note that at this time, dressings cannot be ordered by a physical therapist or occupational therapist. For optimal reimbursement, documentation of wound characteristics must be congruent with the treatment plan. The DMERC will review the documentation accompanying claims to determine medical necessity. Receiving reimbursement is likely to depend on the ability to document any specific or unique condition of the patient that requires an unusual product or combination of products. A letter of medical necessity from the ordering physician or other eligible clinicians and the expected outcome of using the product are also necessary for reimbursement.

Characteristics, problems, and dressing decisions are expected to change through the course of healing. When wound characteristics change, the goals and dressing decisions should change. Note the DMERC guidelines for dressing changes in Table 16-7. This table should guide dressing choice and frequency of dressing changes. Dressing decisions also need to be based on the patient's preferences, financial considerations, and the caregiver's ability to apply the dressing appropriately.

DEVICES FOR SKIN APPROXIMATION

Clinicians may encounter additional means of approximating wound edges. In addition to sutures and staples, Montgomery straps, abdominal binders, and retention sutures may be used for dehiscent wounds or wounds at risk of dehiscence. Montgomery straps and retention sutures are described next, along with techniques for removing sutures and staples.

TABLE 16-7
DMERC Surgical Dressing Utilization Schedule

TYPE OF DRESSING	DRAINAGE/STAGE	ALLOWABLE UTILIZATION
Alginate wound cover	Moderate-high, full-thickness, stage 3 or 4; not allowed for dry wounds or wounds covered with eschar	1 per day
Alginate wound filler	Same as above	12 inches per day
Collagen dressing	Full-thickness wounds (eg, stage 3 or 4 ulcers), wounds with light to moderate exudate, or wounds that have stalled or have not progressed toward a healing goal	They can stay in place up to 7 days; not covered for wounds with heavy exudate, third-degree burns, or when active vasculitis is present
Composite dressing	Moderately to highly exudative wounds	3 per week
Contact layer	Used to line the entire wound	1 per week
Foam	As primary on full-thickness wounds and stage 3 or 4 pressure injuries; as secondary for wounds with heavy drainage	3 per week
Gauze (nonimpregnated)	None listed	6 pads per day without border or 1 per day with border
Gauze (impregnated with other than water or saline)	None listed	1 per day
Gauze (impregnated with water or saline)	None listed	Not covered; reimbursed at gauze rate
Hydrocolloid sheet	Light to moderate drainage	3 per week
Hydrogel sheet	Full-thickness wound with minimum or no drainage stage 3 or 4; not medically necessary for stage 2	1 per day without border; 3 per week for adhesive border
Hydrogel wound filler	Full-thickness wounds with minimum or no drainage stage 3 or 4; not medically necessary for stage 2	Amount not to exceed amount needed to line the wound; additional amounts to fill a cavity are not medically necessary; 3 ounces per wound per month
Specialty absorptive dressing	Moderate to high drainage stage 3 or 4	1 per day without border; 1 every other day for adhesive border
Transparent film	Open partial-thickness; minimal drainage	3 per week

Data source: Centers for Medicare & Medicaid Services.

Montgomery Straps

Montgomery straps are commonly used for dehiscent abdominal wounds and may also be used for sternal dehiscence. Montgomery straps protect the healing wound from trauma caused by patient movement in bed, coughing, sneezing, and similar movement. They can be made with 2-inch silk tape laced with umbilical tape or 1-inch packing strip or Kling. The construction of Montgomery straps is demonstrated in Figures 16-24A and 16-24B. A dehiscent sternal wound is shown in Figure 16-24C, with completed Montgomery straps shown in Figure 16-24D. The skin can be protected by applying the tape onto hydrocolloid sheets placed on both sides of the wound rather than directly on the skin. Montgomery straps are also available premade but are rather expensive. Usually, an abdominal pad is the secondary dressing with either a saline-moistened gauze or alginate primary dressing depending on the dehiscent

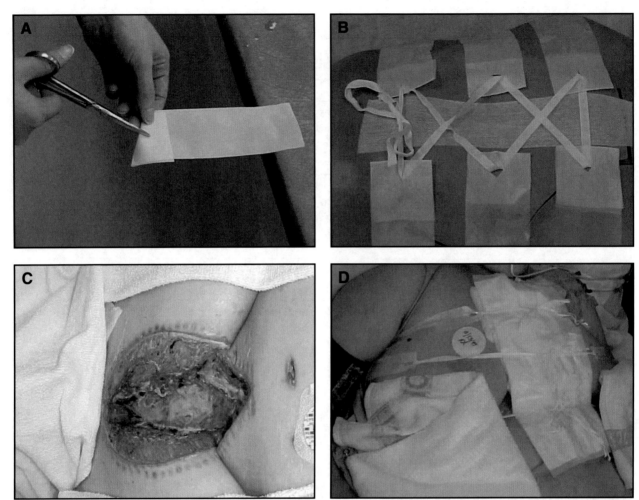

Figure 16-24. Montgomery straps. (A) Preparing an individual strap from 2-inch silk tape doubled over at one end to increase its strength and an opening cut for lacing the reinforced end. (B) Completed Montgomery straps made of 2-inch silk tape and 1/2-inch umbilical tape. (C) Dehiscent sternal wound requiring Montgomery straps. (D) Dressings in place over wound in Figure 16-24C with Montgomery straps attached.

wound's state. Abdominal binders may be used in place of, or in conjunction with, Montgomery straps as a means of preventing abdominal wound dehiscence.

Retention Sutures

A related intervention is the placement of retention sutures (Figure 16-25). Retention sutures are also designed to reduce stress on the edges of wounds. These are made of heavy material and are placed deeply within muscle or fascia, primarily in the abdominal wall. Indications for retention sutures are risk of dehiscence due to a high probability of poor wound healing (malnutrition, immune deficiency, and use of corticosteroids) and increased intra-abdominal pressure from obesity or chronic coughing. They also may be used to assist healing by delayed primary intention. If used to prevent dehiscence, retention sutures are placed

before regular sutures and then passed through a piece of tubing and tied after all appropriate layers are sutured (eg, peritoneum, muscle, fascia, subcutaneous tissue, and skin) and left in place for up to 14 days. When retention sutures are placed around dehiscent wounds, they will be tightened by a surgeon to approximate clean edges as granulation proceeds. The process may advance from both ends of a wound toward the middle.

Staples and Sutures

In some practices, clinicians other than physicians may be requested to remove sutures or staples. These are typically removed after 7 to 10 days depending on the stress placed on the skin and the healing rate at a particular site. Before removing them, one must determine whether sufficient healing has taken place. A tight healing ridge with minimal erythema should be evident. Obvious gaps and leaking of fluid contraindicate removal at that time. Signs of infection or nonhealing should be reported immediately to the referring physician. Slight erythema (1 to 2 mm) on the healing ridge and around each staple or suture is appropriate. A crust or scab on the surface may be cleansed with normal saline or tap water to determine whether sufficient healing has occurred.

Necessary materials are available in a disposable suture removal kit. The scissors in these kits have a hooked tip on one side designed to slip beneath sutures. The kit contains an alcohol skin wipe and a 2 × 2 for skin antisepsis before pulling sutures. Each suture is cut and pulled in the direction that maintains any knots above the surface. They should slide out readily with minimal pulling using the forceps in the kit. Sutures left in the skin too long may have substantial epithelialization that impairs suture removal. Some resistance also may be felt if crusts and scabs are not removed.

Staples are much easier to apply than skin sutures and will be used frequently by surgeons. The stapler bends the legs of the staple inward as it is pushed through the skin. These are easily detached with a surgical staple remover. Two prongs of the remover are inserted under the staple. When the handle is squeezed, the staple's center is pushed down into a V shape, which straightens the legs of the staple. As the tool is lifted from the skin, the staple's legs slide out of the skin. The staple is ejected from the tool, and the process is repeated until all appropriate staples are removed. Removal with hemostats can be performed but requires greater skill than using a tool specifically designed to remove staples.

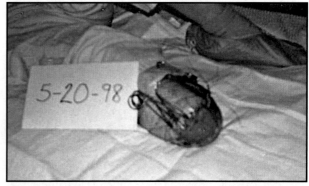

Figure 16-25. Retention sutures used on a dehiscent amputation wound. Sutures are drawn tight as edges become clean and granulated.

Wound fillers are needed to occupy dead space in the wound. Alginates and hydrofibers are very absorbent and biocompatible and suitable for wounds with heavy drainage. Hydrogels are useful for coating dry wounds. Moisture barriers and skin protectants help protect the surrounding skin from excessive moisture and the adhesion of wound dressings. Most types of tape are too harsh for frequent use on skin, especially that of older patients. Foam tape is preferred for direct skin contact. Silk tape is too harsh even for single use on healthy, young skin. Harsh tape can cause skin tears of skin of older patients. Secondary dressings are used in combination with primary dressings to meet the goals of the dressing. They range from simple bandage rolls to occlusive dressings. The proper combination of wound dressing materials cannot be dictated from a chart or company representative but comes from considering all of the pertinent factors gleaned from a thorough history and physical examination.

SUMMARY

Several decisions must be made regarding what dressing is appropriate for a given wound on a given person. A thorough history and physical examination, including issues that may dictate the need for more or less frequent dressing change and the ability to perform dressing changes, must be done. With each dressing change, the appropriateness needs to be reassessed. The clinician must decide on the need for 4 products: wound dressings, wound fillers, skin moisturizers/protectants, and secondary dressings. Nonocclusive dressings are appropriate for acute wounds, infected wounds, and wounds requiring rapid debridement or frequent inspection. Occlusive dressings are suitable for clean, stable wounds or wounds requiring autolytic debridement. Occlusive dressings range in properties from semipermeable films that retain fluid and allow some evaporation, foams that absorb large quantities of fluid, hydrogels that hydrate dry wounds, and hydrocolloids that absorb some drainage but mainly hold drainage in place.

QUESTIONS

1. What are the 3 primary purposes of dressings?
2. Contrast covering vs filling types of dressings.
3. Which types of materials can be used for either covering or filling wounds or both?
4. What is the difference between a primary and secondary dressing?
5. When can a cover type of dressing also be a primary dressing?
6. What is the distinction between an occlusive and nonocclusive dressing?
7. What is the purpose of an occlusive dressing?
8. When are occlusive dressings indicated?
9. When are occlusive dressings contraindicated?
10. When are nonocclusive dressings indicated?

11. Contrast dry-to-dry, wet-to-dry, and wet-to-wet dressings.

12. What is a contact layer? What is its purpose?

13. What is a composite dressing? What is the purpose of a composite?

14. What are the primary indications for petrolatum gauze dressings?

15. Contrast Xeroform and Adaptic/Vaseline gauze.

16. What is implied by the term *microenvironmental dressing*?

17. What are the properties of semipermeable films?

18. When are semipermeable films indicated? When are they contraindicated?

19. What are the advantages of foam dressings?

20. When are foam dressings contraindicated?

21. Contrast amorphous hydrogel and hydrogel sheets.

22. When is amorphous hydrogel indicated? When is it contraindicated?

23. What is hydrocolloid?

24. What is the appearance of dry vs wet hydrocolloid?

25. When is hydrocolloid indicated? When is it contraindicated?

26. How long should strongly adhesive dressings such as films and hydrocolloids be left in place?

27. What can you use instead of strongly adhesive dressings if the wearing time needs to be shorter?

28. What is the purpose of alginate/hydrofiber dressings?

29. When are alginate/hydrofiber dressings indicated? When are they contraindicated?

30. What common antibiotic dressings are available?

31. What role do antibiotic dressings play in wound management?

32. When should antibiotic dressings not be used?

33. Contrast Polysporin and Neosporin. When is Polysporin preferred?

34. What is the purpose of a packing strip? How is it used?

35. What should you do if your piece of packing strip is too short for the depth of the wound?

36. Why must you leave 1/2 inch/1 cm sticking out of the tract/tunnel?

37. When is adhesive tape indicated in securing dressings?

38. What alternatives to adhesive tape are available?

39. What should you do when a patient consistently returns with moisture on the outside of a dressing?

40. What is the purpose of Montgomery straps?

BIBLIOGRAPHY

Ascherman JA, Jones VA, Knowles SL. The histologic effects of retention sutures on wound healing in the rat. *Eur J Surg.* 2000;166(12):932-937.

Atkin L. Chronic wounds: the challenges of appropriate management. *Br J Community Nurs.* 2019;24(Suppl 9):S26-S32. doi:10.12968/bjcn.2019.24.Sup9.S26

Broussard KC, Powers JG. Wound dressings: selecting the most appropriate type. *Am J Clin Dermatol.* 2013;14(6):449-459. doi:10.1007/s40257-013-0046-4

Hess TC. When to use transparent films. *Adv Skin Wound Care.* 2000;13:202.

Hodde JP, Ernst DMJ, Hiles MC. An investigation of the long-term bioactivity of endogenous growth factor in OASIS Wound Matrix. *J Wound Care.* 2005;14(1):23-25.

Hodde JP, Hiles MC. Bioactive FGF-2 in sterilized extracellular matrix. *Wounds.* 2001;13(5):195-201.

Molan P, Rhodes T. Honey: a biologic wound dressing. *Wounds.* 2015;27(6):141-151.

Norman G, Dumville JC, Moore ZEH, Tanner J, Christie J, Goto S. Antibiotics and antiseptics for pressure ulcers. *Cochrane Database Syst Rev.* 2016;4(4):CD011586. doi:10.1002/14651858.CD011586.pub2

Obagi Z, Damiani G, Grada A, Falanga V. Principles of wound dressings: a review. *Surg Technol Int.* 2019;35:50-57.

Parulkar BG, Sobti MK, Pardanani DS. Dextranomer dressing in the treatment of infected wounds and cutaneous ulcers. *J Postgrad Med.* 1985;31(1):28-33.

Rando T, Kang AC, Guerin M, Boylan J, Dyer A. Simplifying wound dressing selection for residential aged care. *J Wound Care.* 2018;27(8):504-511. doi:10.12968/jowc.2018.27.8.504

Rink AD, Goldschmidt D, Dietrich J, Nagelschmidt M, Vestweber KH. Negative side-effects of retention sutures for abdominal wound closure. A prospective randomised study. *Eur J Surg.* 2000;166(12):932-937.

Rippon M, Davies P, White R. Taking the trauma out of wound care: the importance of undisturbed healing. *J Wound Care.* 2012;21(8):359-368. doi:10.12968/jowc.2012.21.8.359

Vazquez JR, Short B, Findlow AH, Nixon BP, Boulton AJM, Armstrong DG. Outcomes of hyaluronan therapy in diabetic foot wounds. *Diabetes Res Clin Pract.* 2003;59(2):123-127.

Veves A, Sheehan P, Pham HT. A randomized, controlled trial of Promogran (a collagen/oxidized regenerated cellulose dressing) vs standard treatment in the management of diabetic foot ulcers. *Arch Surg.* 2002;137(7):822-827.

Wasiak J, Cleland H, Campbell F, Spinks A. Dressings for superficial and partial thickness burns. *Cochrane Database Syst Rev.* 2013;2013(3):CD002106. doi:10.1002/14651858.CD002106.pub4

Winter GD. Effect of air exposure and occlusion on experimental human skin wounds. *Nature.* 1963;200:378-379.

Woo KY, Heil J. A prospective evaluation of methylene blue and gentian violet dressing for management of chronic wounds with local infection. *Int Wound J.* 2017;14(6):1029-1035. doi:10.1111/iwj.12753

17

Adjunct Interventions and Scar Management

OBJECTIVES

- Discuss the use of endogenous and exogenous growth factors to accelerate wound healing.
- Discuss differences between types of cellular and/or tissue-based products, including allografts and xenografts.
- Discuss indications, contraindications, and parameters for the use of electrical stimulation with high-voltage pulsed current and pulsed electromagnetic field.
- Describe the use of diathermy in wound healing.
- Discuss the use of ultraviolet C in wound management.
- Discuss the indications for negative pressure wound therapy.
- Discuss the theory and uses of hyperbaric oxygen therapy.
- Discuss the theory of using therapeutic ultrasound and parameters for wound healing.
- Compare and contrast the types of scars encountered in practice.
- Discuss how abnormal scarring affects function.
- Discuss the role of Langer's lines in the development of scars.
- Describe surgical and physical therapy treatment for dysfunctional scarring.

Irion GL, Gardner JA, Pignataro RM.
Comprehensive Wound Management, Third Edition (pp 329-344).
© 2024 Taylor and Francis Group.

Debridement, dressing changes, patient education, and means to address the underlying cause of wounds are considered the primary wound care components. Additional interventions may be appropriate on a case-by-case basis. These interventions constitute adjuncts to wound care. Adjuncts that are discussed in this chapter are growth factors, cellular and/or tissue-based products, and biophysical agents. Although many adjuncts are available, they are not substitutes for good wound management through debridement, appropriate dressing selection, off-loading, compression therapy, and other means of addressing the underlying cause. A clinician should reassess the treatment plan before arbitrarily employing adjuncts.

GROWTH FACTORS

As of this writing, one form of growth factor has both Food and Drug Administration (FDA) approval and coverage by the Centers for Medicare & Medicaid Services (CMS). According to the manufacturer, 99% of insurance plans cover it. Regranex (Ortho-McNeil) is a 1% becaplermin gel, the trade name for platelet-derived growth factor (PDGF). The PDGF is generated by recombinant DNA technology in which the B chain of PDGF has been inserted in yeast, *Saccharomyces cerevisiae*.

Regranex has been approved for neuropathic ulcers with good circulation. This indication is based on research performed years ago, showing that PDGF factor is deficient in poorly controlled diabetes mellitus. Replacement of endogenous PDGF promotes wound healing in individuals with diabetes mellitus but becomes less effective if they also have peripheral arterial disease. Regranex is provided in a gel to be applied in a thin film once daily and covered with a moist dressing. Because a thicker coating provides no increased benefit and is very expensive, it should be applied carefully. It must be refrigerated between uses. The effectiveness of PDGF is dependent on thorough debridement. It is ineffective if placed on necrotic tissue.

In 2008, the US FDA required a boxed warning on the label of Regranex related to the increased risk of cancer mortality in patients who have used 3 or more tubes of it. The use of Regranex was not associated with an increase in cancer incidence, but those who used 3 tubes or more had a 5-fold increase in cancer mortality. According to the manufacturer, it is not to be used in any area with a malignancy. However, in 2018, the manufacturers of Regranex successfully petitioned the FDA to remove the label, citing several studies that indicated no increase in the risk of cancer from the use of Regranex. In clinical studies, 2% developed an erythematous rash near the wound to the gel base of Regranex. An alternative to Regranex is the on-site production of platelet-rich concentrate from a patient's blood. Several companies make devices to create it. Research is continuing on other growth factors and cytokines to facilitate healing.

CELLULAR AND/OR TISSUE-BASED PRODUCTS

While healing by secondary intention is the ultimate goal, some patients cannot fully close wounds on their own. Although split-thickness skin grafts, as discussed in Chapter 2, can allow a wound to be closed quickly, some patients are not candidates for the harvesting of these skin grafts. This is where cellular and/or tissue-based products (CTPs) can be very beneficial for wound healing. Additionally, CTPs can help prepare a wound for a split-thickness skin graft by increasing granulation and filling the wound. Many products are on the market today, such as Apligraf (Organogenesis) and Integra (Integra LifeSciences). While a split-thickness skin graft is an autograft, those discussed here are either allografts, which means they come from human tissue, or xenografts, coming from other species, such as bovine or porcine. We only discuss a few of these because the application of CTPs is currently considered a "surgical procedure" and thus must be performed by a physician for reimbursement. These products work similarly, producing natural growth factors while protecting the wound and allowing native cells to reproduce and cover the wounded area.

Allografts

Several products from human tissue are currently on the market. Some are actual dermal products, whereas others are amniotic or placental. Alloderm (LifeCell) is an acellular dermal matrix frequently used for breast reconstruction, but it can be used in all wounds. It is processed from cadaver tissue and is placed in a wound, providing a scaffold for the patient's own tissue to grow on. DermaPure (TRx BioSurgery) is also harvested from cadaver tissue and uses dCell technology, which renders the tissue over 99% DNA free. DermaPure is decellularized, leaving behind an intact extracellular matrix. The tissue is terminally irradiated to ensure it is sterile, minimizing the risk of infection or tissue rejection. It consists of the basement membrane and papillary dermis and has intact vascular channels, thus allowing angiogenesis. DermaPure is histologically very much like living human tissue, and it is difficult to distinguish it from living tissue under a microscope. DermaPure may be used anywhere in the body and can be used by orthopedic surgeons to strengthen tendon repairs. Amniotic products come from placental membranes; are often dehydrated; and are used for the proteins, growth factors, and cytokines that are maintained after processing. One example is EpiFix (MiMedx). Placental products also come from placental membranes but are used mostly for the mesenchymal stem cells, collagen matrix, and growth factors they possess and are cryopreserved. An example is Grafix (Osiris Therapeutics).

Xenografts

Apligraf is a material marketed as "living bilayer, cell therapy." It consists of human keratinocytes and fibroblasts in addition to bovine type I collagen. It is not considered a graft but a temporary covering that allows the recipient to eventually replace the applied product with their own skin. This product contains matrix, cytokines, and growth factors normally found in human skin. The presence of growth factors and cytokines is believed to be responsible for the patient's ability to regenerate new skin to replace the product gradually. However, Apligraf does not contain any melanocytes, immune cells, blood vessels, nerves, or accessory structures (sweat glands, hair follicles, or sebaceous glands). Apligraf is currently approved for venous and neuropathic/diabetic foot ulcers. Apligraf is packaged as a disk 75 mm in diameter and 0.75 mm thick.

When applied, Apligraf can be fenestrated ("windows" cut into it) or meshed to avoid fluid buildup under the product to improve its adhesion to granulation tissue. It can be affixed with tape, sutures, staples, Steri-Strips (3M), or skin adhesive. A secondary dressing and compression are applied. The patient is to avoid activities that lead to edema in the area or shear the material from the wound. Dressings directly in contact with Apligraf need to be left in place for at least 5 to 7 days to avoid damaging the material. Outer dressings may be changed more frequently as needed (every 3 to 5 days).

Integra is several different products, but the bilayer matrix wound dressing is most commonly used. It is composed of 2 layers, the bottom layer being a porous matrix of cross-linked type I bovine tendon collagen and glycosaminoglycan from shark cartilage and the top layer being a semipermeable silicone layer. The bottom layer provides a scaffold for cellular matrix and capillary growth, whereas the silicone layer controls water vapor loss, provides a flexible adherent covering for the wound surface, and adds increased tensile strength to the product. It is placed by the surgeon and left in place for 3 weeks. At that time, the surgeon will remove the silicone layer and then decide if another application is needed.

Another cellular/tissue-based product is Oasis (Smith & Nephew). It is produced from porcine small intestine submucosa. This material can be implanted or applied topically. It provides both scaffolding for cell migration and release of growth factors that stimulate angiogenesis, granulation, and re-epithelialization. The porcine intestinal submucosa reduces matrix metalloproteinases, mediators of inflammation, and proteolytic enzymes of chronic wounds, creating an environment closer to that of an acute wound.

BIOPHYSICAL AGENTS

Therapeutic modalities using temperature, light, and other electromagnetic fields have been in use for more than 100 years and some for centuries. Physical therapists are trained and licensed to apply these physical agents for a variety of indications. Nearly every possible modality available has been used in an attempt to facilitate wound healing. Cryotherapy is used for acute injuries to reduce pain and edema. Infrared light has been used in the past to dry wounds in an effort to prevent infection. This may have been useful in military situations in which triaging required some means of caring for wounds that were not considered as serious as those that required immediate attention; however, this is no longer a meaningful therapy. Diathermy and therapeutic ultrasound (eg, 1 MHz, 3 MHz) have not received approval by the FDA to treat wounds, and CMS does not cover these modalities. The forms discussed in the following sections include ultraviolet C (UVC); low-frequency, noncontact ultrasound; electrical stimulation; and pulsed electromagnetic field. Other adjuncts to wound care that are discussed are hyperbaric oxygen (HBO) therapy, negative pressure wound therapy (NPWT), and the application of leeches.

Ultraviolet C

UVC from cold quartz lamps has a long history of topical use for its fungicidal effect. Current recommendations for generating a bactericidal effect for cold quartz lamps are exposure for 72 to 180 seconds with the lamp 1 inch from the wound surface. Instructions provided by manufacturers for specific devices should be followed. The FDA has approved newer forms for bactericidal use on open wounds. UVC has a wavelength between 200 and 290 nm.

In contrast to ultraviolet A, which is used to activate chemicals in the skin such as psoralens for treating conditions such as psoriasis, and ultraviolet B used to activate melanocytes, UVC is directly toxic to susceptible bacteria. Wavelengths between 250 and 270 nm have the greatest bactericidal effect with a peak effect at the wavelength of 266 nm. The new UVC devices have guide bars so the wand can be rested over the wound, rather than requiring the operator to hold the lamp a given distance from the wound. UVC is particularly effective against methicillin-resistant *Staphylococcus aureus* and vancomycin-resistant *Enterococcus faecalis* (VRE) with a 99.9% kill rate using an 8-second exposure of UVC at a wavelength of 254 nm, an output of 15.54 mW/cm, and a distance of 1 inch. VRE was reduced to 99.9% with only 5 seconds of exposure. Exposure for 90 seconds and 45 seconds was required for 100% kill of methicillin-resistant *Staphylococcus aureus* and VRE, respectively.

MIST Therapy

As previously discussed in Chapter 15, MIST Therapy (Celleration), a low-frequency, noncontact therapeutic ultrasound, is used not only for debridement but also for active wound healing. This is done through cell stimulation while also removing bacteria. MIST Therapy is also effective for pain management and works well for patients who cannot tolerate other pain control methods.

Electric Stimulation

High-voltage pulsed current (HPVC), formerly known as *high-voltage pulsed galvanic*, is the only type of stimulation presently available that has been consistently shown to improve wound healing. Some early studies support low-intensity direct current; however, devices of this type are not generally available. On the other hand, microcurrent types of devices, which generate intensities in the micro-amperage range and various waveforms have been shown to be ineffective in promoting wound healing.

Several parameters must be used to describe a treatment protocol. Intensity may be quantified either in units of current (milliamps) or the electromotive force, causing charge to flow (volts). For most devices, intensity refers to current in milliamps, but HVPC devices are set in volts. Some devices will only have a knob or other adjustment marked current or intensity with a relative scale. If these devices are used, the intensity is adjusted to create a response determined by what the clinician observes, such as a minimally observable contraction, or to the patient's subjective response.

Intensity determines the type of neuron recruited by the current. Although transcutaneous current recruits neurons based on diameter, the neuron's distance from the source of current is also important. The first neurons recruited by transcutaneous current would be the motor neurons signaling muscles to contract based on size alone. The next group of neurons recruited would be sensory neurons indicating mechanical stimulation of the skin. Small sensory neurons carrying information about pain, temperature, and crude touch would be recruited last. However,

because motor neurons are located subfascially, and many sensory neurons are located suprafascially, information carried by large sensory neurons is perceived at a lower intensity than that required to produce a motor response. The intensity required to recruit small sensory neurons in the skin may overlap with motor neurons so that a strong motor response may recruit an intolerable number of nociceptors. In contrast, a milder motor response is generally tolerable. As a general rule, the typical recruitment pattern produced by transcutaneous current is (1) the larger mechanoreceptive neurons located within the skin, (2) the large motor neurons beneath the skin, and (3) nociceptive neurons in the skin. These 3 levels of intensity are termed *sensory*, *motor*, and *noxious*, respectively. Although the patient's perception tends to be dominated by the type of neuron newly recruited at each intensity level, these levels are cumulative and overlap.

The second parameter is the frequency of pulsed current. Frequency of pulsed current is usually given in hertz (cycles per second). The frequency of pulsed current determines the quality of muscle contraction. Low frequencies create single twitches. Intermediate frequencies create undulating contractions called *unfused tetanic contractions* in which a slight relaxation occurs between stimuli. High frequencies produce tetanic contractions. The need to use the relative terms *low*, *intermediate*, and *high frequency* is due to different muscles' properties. For example, hand and forearm muscles may tetanize at 15 Hz, whereas quadriceps may require 50 Hz for a tetanic contraction. For the purposes of wound healing, the frequency is generally much in excess of that needed for a tetanic contraction. A continual tetanic contraction would be very uncomfortable for the patient; therefore, electrodes are placed, if possible, away from muscles, and intensity is adjusted to a value that does not exceed a minimally visible muscle contraction.

The third parameter is the pulse duration or width. In general, increasing pulse width produces the same effect as increasing pulse intensity. Compared with devices used for neuromuscular electrical stimulation and transcutaneous electrical nerve stimulation, the pulses used for wound repair are very short, but the intensity is very high.

Waveform describes the combined effects of intensity, duration, and rise and fall times of pulses. The waveform of HVPC is generally described as *triangular*, although this term imprecisely describes the waveform. The pulses have a rapid rise and a slower decay and are paired. This waveform is often termed *twin peaks*. The rapid presentation of the second peak causes the 2 spikes to behave as a single electrical event. Therefore, in HVPC terminology, each set of 2 spikes is considered as a pulse with 2 phases. The timing between the 2 phases is adjustable on some devices as either the interphase or intrapulse interval. A shorter intrapulse interval increases the effectiveness of the pulses but can be more uncomfortable for the patient.

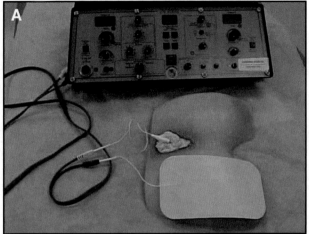

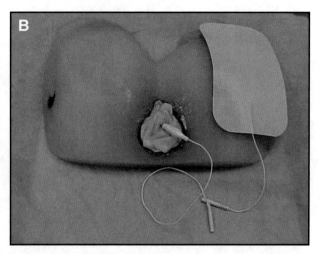

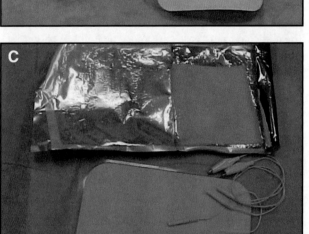

Figure 17-1. (A) Setup of HVPC on a wound model. (B) Close-up of electrode placement. (C) Close-up of electrodes.

Polarity describes the direction that ions or electrons travel relative to electrodes. A cathode attracts positive ions or repels electrons. Anodes attract electrons and negative ions and repel positive ions. For historical reasons, the anode is termed the positive electrode because of its effect of driving positively charged particles away from it, and the cathode is termed the negative electrode. Several studies have been performed with either positive or negative polarities for the electrodes attached to the wound. Other clinicians have started with a positive electrode over the wound and switch to a negative polarity based on a number of criteria. Other parameters include the duration of individual treatment sessions, the frequency of treatments, and the number of treatments given.

General Technique

A typical HVPC device is depicted in Figure 17-1A. Twin-peak pulses are used at an amplitude and frequency of approximately 100 V and 100 Hz, with a pulse duration of approximately 50 microseconds. However, the pulse duration and the interphase (or intrapulse) interval are fixed on many devices. A variety of means for setting up the patient have been described. A typical setup is shown in Figure 17-1B. The positive electrode is placed over the wound with the negative electrode attached to the patient distally. Usually, the electrode that is not over the wound has a larger surface area to minimize current density and, therefore, any electrical effects in the area used to complete the electrical circuit. A typical protocol for using electrical stimulation to augment wound healing is provided in Box 17-1.

Electrodes

Several types of electrodes have been described. One approach to a wound with subcutaneous tissue loss is to place saline- or hydrogel-moistened gauze into the wound and attach the lead wire with an alligator clip. Several manufacturers distribute hydrogel-impregnated gauze for this purpose (Figure 17-1C). The other lead wire is attached to a larger electrode. If this second electrode

BOX 17-1
Typical Protocol for Electrical Stimulation for Wound Healing

- Polarity: initially positive; switch to negative when necrosis gone
  - Switch to negative if healing reaches plateau
- Pulse rate: 100 Hz (some protocols are as low as 30 Hz)
- Amplitude: several volts below contraction
  - Expected to be in range of 100 to 200 V
  - Depends on nature of tissue beneath electrode
  - May be less than 100 V depending on patient tolerance
- Waveform: twin-peak
- Location
  - Bipolar: one electrode on either side of wound
  - Monopolar: active (negative) in wound, large dispersive distant on intact skin

is large enough, one may consider it to be the indifferent electrode. Note the large indifferent electrode in use in Figures 17-1B and 17-1C. A typical protocol is to use a positive electrode in the wound for 1 hour, either daily or 3 times per week, depending on the patient's circumstances. When the wound does not continue to close at the accelerated rate, the polarity of the electrodes is switched to negative. The reversal of electrode polarity continues until the wound is either healed or progressing and stable enough to allow care to be completed by the patient at home. The size and distance between electrodes are adjusted based on the depth of the current desired. Superficial wounds should be treated with smaller electrodes placed close to each other. In a deep wound, larger electrodes placed farther apart are used to drive current more deeply through the tissue of interest.

Electrode arrangements can be monopolar, bipolar, or multipolar. Due to the nature of electricity, any current will be bipolar (ie, electricity will flow from one area to another). The simple bipolar arrangement consists of 2 equally sized electrodes that will produce an equal flow of charge per surface area (current density) at both electrodes. Monopolar electrode arrangement is not truly monopolar but behaves as if only one electrode is active. The monopolar effect is generated by creating a much greater current density at the electrode of interest. The indifferent

electrode's current density is reduced by using a much larger electrode, as shown in Figures 17-1B and 17-1C. The current is dispersed over a greater surface area; therefore, the indifferent electrode is also commonly called a *dispersive electrode*. A multipolar arrangement is produced by arranging multiple electrodes for each polarity; this may be done using a bifurcated lead or a multichannel device.

The impedance of tissue beneath each electrode may vary tremendously from one place on the body to another. Certain areas will cause discomfort or will diminish current. In general, the clinician should avoid dry skin, callused areas, bony prominences, and motor points. Placement of electrodes over these areas or breaks in the skin either will cause patient discomfort and cause the clinician to reduce current to suboptimal levels or will force the clinician to increase current to the point of patient discomfort. No conclusive data exist on optimal locations of electrodes. Several researchers have suggested that the dispersive electrode should be placed proximal to the wound.

Pulsed Electromagnetic Field

An alternative to HVPC is pulsed electromagnetic field (PEMF). PEMF is generated in the same manner as diathermy but at a much lower frequency that does not produce heat. The optimal frequency for wound healing appears to be 15 to 20 Hz. Rather than placing electrodes in or around a wound, PEMF generates a current within tissue by alternating an electromagnetic field around the wound. A great advantage of PEMF over typical neuromuscular electrical stimulators is that PEMF does not require electrodes and can be used over clothing, bandages, casts, and so forth. PEMF has been used as a replacement for bone stimulators with implanted wires and has now been approved for the same purpose as HVPC for open wounds.

Several studies have shown an increased rate of angiogenesis and wound healing, increased tensile strength of closed wounds, and increased release of fibroblast growth factor beta-2 (FGF-2) with PEMF. The use of FGF-2 neutralizing antibody negates the effect of PEMF, suggesting the major effect is mediated through FGF-2. Changes in other angiogenic growth factors also occur with PEMF. Effects other than these growth factors and angiogenesis may be responsible for some aspects of faster and strong wound healing.

PEMF is applied through 1 of 3 basic mechanisms. A ring that encircles a body part would only be used in a clinic and not for home use. Handheld devices can be either held for the prescribed time or strapped on a part of the body. Suggested use for handheld devices is holding the device over the area for 30 to 45 minutes 1 to 3 times per day. Specific home use devices are made with an enclosed coil and battery attached over the body area of interest with a strap or bandage roll. These devices may be left running until the battery fails. PEMF and other radiofrequency devices are not to be used on patients with pacemakers, implanted defibrillators, or similar implanted electronic devices.

Hyperbaric Oxygen

Oxygen is a required nutrient for the survival of most tissues over an extended time. Specific to wound healing, oxygen is necessary for collagen production, neutrophil function to reduce the risk of infection, and macrophage function in autolytic debridement. Moreover, high oxygen levels destroy anaerobic bacteria. On the other hand, high oxygen levels slow the formation of new capillaries, cause arteriolar constriction, and may cause oxygen toxicity. The basic concept of HBO is to increase the oxygen available for wound healing. Claims made for HBO include increased antibiotic efficacy, fibroblast proliferation, collagen production and strength, production of growth factors, growth factor receptor sites, and elevated tissue partial pressure of oxygen. HBO has been demonstrated as an effective treatment for many conditions, including decompression sickness, gas embolism, gas gangrene (clostridial myonecrosis), and carbon monoxide and cyanide poisoning.

Two types of HBO have been described. Systemic administration requires placing the patient in a chamber to accommodate the entire body. The gas composition inside the chamber is changed to 100% oxygen and is pressurized to further increase the amount of oxygen within the chamber. The effect of the oxygen is via inhalation and thus more oxygen being in the arterial blood and then ultimately reaching the wound to affect healing. A second type of HBO called *topical HBO* is administered by using a plastic bag or other device attached to the skin over a wound. Whole-body HBO is still recommended by those in this field instead of topical HBO performed with extremity chambers or spot chambers for areas such as the sacrum. Many case studies have been published, but randomized clinical trials showing the efficacy of topical HBO are lacking, suggesting that true effects of HBO are via inhalation of 100% oxygen and not just by exposing the tissue to 100% oxygen.

Increases in PO_2 of inspired air at normal atmospheric pressure have a negligible effect on the amount of oxygen carried by the blood due to hemoglobin saturation. Under normal circumstances, nearly 100% of the oxygen carried by the blood is bound to hemoglobin. Once hemoglobin is saturated with oxygen, very little additional oxygen can be added to the blood. However, the administration of 100% oxygen under 2 to 3 atmospheres of pressure can produce such a tremendous increase in arterial PO_2 that oxygen can diffuse a much greater distance from capillaries, which should be beneficial in any disease process in which diffusion of oxygen from capillaries is compromised.

Different types of systemic HBO chambers are available in different facilities. The type generally used for wound management consists of a clear tube accommodating one individual or a monoplace chamber. Large chambers, or multiplace chambers, accommodate multiple individuals and are often used for underwater physiology or treatment of decompression sickness (the bends or caisson disease) from too rapid ascent during deep-sea diving or excessive exposure to hyperbaric environments. Typical systemic HBO treatments consist of 100% oxygen pressured to 2.0 to 2.5 atm (2-2.5 times atmospheric pressure) for 2 hours daily or twice a day. The normal partial pressure of oxygen in the environment is approximately 760×0.21, or 160 mm Hg. The partial pressure of oxygen in a whole-body chamber may be as high as 1500 to 2000 mm Hg. However, exposure to such high partial pressure of oxygen can cause oxygen toxicity, which needs to be monitored. Protocols may vary among facilities and types of wounds.

Specific types of wounds appear to respond well to HBO. Crush injuries incurred within a few hours may benefit from the combination of pressure to reduce edema in the enriched oxygen environment and decreased leukocyte adherence. Similarly, skin flaps and grafts compromised by neutrophil accumulation during ischemia may benefit from this treatment. HBO has also been suggested for the treatment of radiation necrosis and refractory ischemic ulcers. Wounds covered by CMS include necrotizing fasciitis, osteomyelitis, and crush injuries. CMS has agreed to cover HBO for diabetic wounds of the lower extremities. Coverage requires that the patient have a Wagner grade III or higher and failure to progress during 30 days of standard wound care. CMS coverage also requires the use of an FDA-approved HBO chamber for treatment. Coverage is ceased if wounds fail to improve within 30 days of HBO treatment. Although CMS recognizes that HBO treatment may require several months, the average treatment time is expected to be 2 to 4 weeks. Unfortunately, the failure of wounds to heal is generally more complex than insufficient oxygen delivery to tissues, which makes the indiscriminate application of HBO to ischemic ulcers suspect. Moreover, the amount of time that can be spent in a hyperbaric chamber is limited. The effectiveness of HBO depends on proper patient selection. Poor delivery of oxygen to tissues is generally caused by arterial disease, which may be improved by surgery rather than intermittent exposure to a source of enriched oxygen.

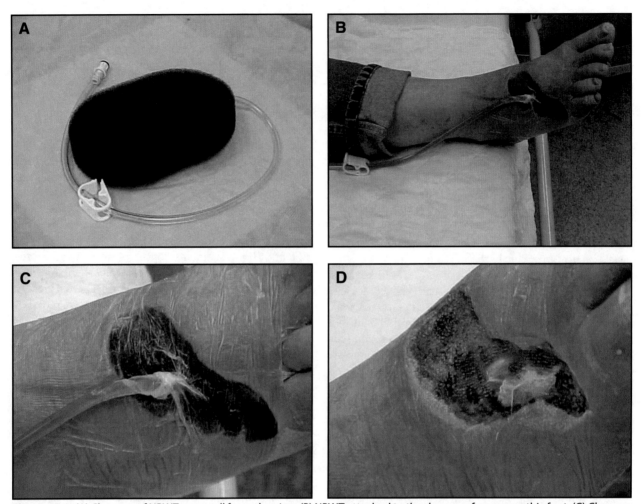

Figure 17-2. (A) Close-up of NPWT open cell foam dressing. (B) NPWT attached to the dorsum of a neuropathic foot. (C) Close-up of negative pressure wound therapy showing the evacuation of fluid from the wound. (D) The same wound as in 17-2B following successful treatment.

Negative Pressure Wound Therapy

In many deep wounds, edema and accumulation of drainage within the wound slow the delivery of nutrients necessary for healing. A constant, negative pressure device applied to the wound with a drainage system can be used to enhance the wound environment by removing excessive fluid. Devices consist of a pump, tubing, reservoir, and special foam type of dressing (Figure 17-2A). The dressing is cut to fit the wound and is placed into a wound with a film cover to seal the vacuum created by the pump (Figures 17-2B and 17-2C). Constant suction is applied to the wound until its dimensions decrease sufficiently that the foam dressing can no longer fit in the wound. A smaller piece of foam may then be used to continue therapy. The appearance of a wound following NPWT is shown in Figure 17-2D.

CMS covers NPWT in either the home or an inpatient facility. For home care, chronic stage 3 or 4 pressure injuries,

neuropathic ulcers, venous or arterial insufficiency ulcers, or chronic (defined by CMS as being present for at least 30 days) ulcers of mixed etiology may be covered. Coverage requires evaluation, care, and wound measurements by a licensed medical professional; application of dressings to maintain a moist wound environment; debridement of necrotic tissue, if present; and evaluation of and provision for adequate nutritional status. Requirements also include attempts to use standard treatment, or they must be ruled out for medical reasons. Specifically for pressure injuries, the patient must have been appropriately turned and positioned, the patient must have used a group 2 or 3 support surface (low air loss or air fluidized) for pressure injuries on the posterior trunk or pelvis (not required if the ulcer is not on the trunk or pelvis), and the patient's moisture and incontinence must have been appropriately managed. Requirements for coverage for neuropathic ulcers are evidence that the patient participated in a comprehensive diabetic management program, and off-loading the foot has been done. For venous insufficiency ulcers, compression bandages or garments must have been consistently applied, and leg elevation and ambulation must have been encouraged. Inadequate documentation that wounds have failed to respond to standard care for the etiology will cause payment denial.

Coverage for inpatient NPWT requires that treatments listed in the previous paragraph were either tried or ruled out for medical reasons, and NPWT, in the treating physician's judgment, is the best available treatment option. Coverage for inpatients includes complications of a surgical (primarily dehiscence) or traumatic wound such as the need for preoperative flap or graft and medical necessity for the accelerated formation of granulation tissue that cannot be achieved by other available treatments. For these approved inpatient conditions, coverage may be continued in the home.

Documentation, evaluation, and care must be performed by a licensed health care professional; this may be a physician, physician assistant, registered nurse, licensed practical nurse, or physical therapist. Denial may occur if debridement of necrotic tissue is not attempted, untreated osteomyelitis is present in the vicinity of the wound, cancer is present in the wound, or if a fistula to an organ or body cavity is present in the vicinity of the wound. For continued coverage, changes in the ulcer's dimensions and characteristics must be documented on at least a monthly basis. Medical necessity can no longer be shown in the absence of any reduction in wound size in terms of either depth or surface area of the wound after 4 months of treatment. Coverage is limited to a maximum of 15 dressing kits and 10 canister sets per month unless documentation that a large volume of drainage, defined as greater than 90 mL/day, is provided.

Application of Negative Pressure Wound Therapy

The negative pressure therapy system consists of a pump, which is durable equipment, and the foam dressing and canister, which are considered consumable supplies. Some newer disposable units are also available. The application should be done following standard infection control procedures. The wound should be cleansed or debrided as needed prior to application; NPWT is contraindicated for necrotic wounds with eschar. The surrounding skin is also cleaned thoroughly, so the semipermeable dressing used in the NPWT application will adhere to the skin surrounding the wound. The procedure should be explained thoroughly to the patient and the patient positioned so the dressing can be placed in the wound without risk of it falling out during application. The patient should also be made as comfortable as possible, and lighting should be adequate.

Once the patient is in position, a new canister is placed in the NPWT pump, and the open-cell foam dressing is cut with the aseptic technique to a size slightly smaller than the wound. The foam dressing is then placed in the wound, and the evacuation tube is connected to the dressing.

When a good seal appears to be in place, the evacuation tube is connected to the canister in the NPWT pump. The power is then turned on, and diagnostics are run automatically by the device. A typical setup generates a negative pressure of 125 mm Hg. NPWT is delivered for 48 hours continuously; then the dressing is removed, and the wound is cleansed and re-evaluated. As needed, NPWT is continued. The canister may be used for up to 1 week or until full. NPWT is discontinued when the goals set for NPWT are reached. Goals may include wound closure, sufficient cleanliness of the wound, or reduced wound size to allow delayed closure. NPWT is generally stopped if no positive results are demonstrated in 1 to 2 weeks despite optimal care.

Types of Foam Used for Negative Pressure Wound Therapy

Two basic types of foam dressing materials are available for use. Also, the foam used for NPWT may be obtained preshaped for specific areas such as the abdomen, hand, and heel. The original black polyurethane foam has large pores, allowing negative pressure to be distributed throughout a covered wound site, even allowing multiple pieces to be linked within or between wounds. The polyurethane foam is flexible and easily trimmed to fit, but small particles of this foam can detach during trimming. This foam should never be cut over a wound, and any cut edges should be rubbed to remove any loose pieces that might come off while in the wound. The large pores reduce the tensile strength, so placing it into a tunnel creates the risk of breaking in the tunnel and leaving the material behind. Polyurethane foam is also available with silver, eliminating the need for a separate silver dressing to be used. Polyvinyl alcohol foam is white, has a greater density than polyurethane foam, and has smaller pores. The greater tensile strength of white polyvinyl alcohol foam allows the filling of tunnels and undermined areas without fear of the foam tearing or breaking and being left in the wound. A new type of reticulated foam (foam with openings in it) has been suggested to provide a debriding effect.

LEECHES

The application of leeches for medicinal purposes originated more than 500 years ago. Although the original goal was to restore health by bringing the body's

4 humors back into balance, the current use is directed at overcoming venous congestion following reattachment surgery. Repair of injuries that involve reattachment of blood vessels such as gunshot wounds of the foot and crush injuries may also be indications for leech therapy. The leech used in current practice is *Hirudo medicinalis*. These leeches can be ordered from a small number of suppliers for overnight delivery and kept for several weeks in a ventilated refrigerator until needed. The saliva of leeches also has anticoagulant properties, which may diminish the risk of thrombosis of reattached digits, ears, and skin flaps. Although some patients may not relish the idea of leeches being attached to them, the leech bites are usually painless but may leave a characteristic "Y"-shaped scar. Because leeches may attempt to migrate to other areas, a protective barrier must be applied around the area of interest. A small risk of infection or allergy also exists.

As needed, leeches are removed from the refrigerator, and the skin is cleaned thoroughly with normal saline. A barrier is made from a 4 × 4 gauze sponge with a hole cut in the center and reinforcement with a towel. The leech should be transferred to the area of interest with forceps and guided as needed to the correct area. If the leech does not show interest, the skin may need to be pricked to draw a drop of blood to the area. The leech will feed for about 20 minutes and perhaps longer. The leech should be allowed to release the skin and should not be forcefully removed. When full, the leech will detach, but if pulled, the leech's mouthparts may be left in the wound and cause infection. The detached leech is then placed in a cup, covered in alcohol, and discarded in an appropriate biohazard container.

The application of leeches may be difficult for the clinician. Because patients may be reluctant to agree to leech therapy, an unsteady or squeamish clinician may cause the patient to refuse an important therapy. Hematocrit and appearance of the site should be monitored regularly to ensure that excessive blood is not lost, and the reattached body part is maintaining good circulation.

TYPES OF SCAR PROBLEMS

Any type of scarring will result in some degree of loss of the skin's normal function and appearance. Elasticity, waterproofing/lubrication, sensation, and sweating will be impaired to some degree. Larger wounds such as burns can result in large inelastic skin areas that limit function, dry and crack, and fail to participate in cooling the body through sweating. Pigmentation, hair, and contour changes can lead to substantial cosmetic problems that can also lead to psychosocial problems for a given individual.

Three major types of scars were described in Chapter 3. Each type forms due to the overexpression of different growth factors. All 3 produce scars that are initially red, raised, and rigid. Although hypertrophic scars may temporarily have these characteristics, they generally regress and become white, flat, and avascular. Keloids occur much more frequently (about 15-fold) in the skin of those of sub-Saharan African descent and less frequently in people of Asian, Latin, or Hispanic descent; keloids extend beyond the site of incision or trauma, sometimes many centimeters distant, and recur if excised. Burn scars are characterized by bridging and pulling across structures. They tend to lose their hypervascularity, but the effect on skin function frequently requires multiple surgical procedures to achieve acceptable function.

Even with seemingly normal scars, adhesions to subcutaneous structures can develop and limit skin and even joint movement. Strategies for preventing and releasing adhesions are described later in the chapter.

Healed vs Closed

Additionally, healing does not always result in sufficient skin repair. For laypeople, closed is frequently thought to be healed. However, healing of the skin should be understood as producing a scar that allows the skin surrounding it to provide good function. As a rule of thumb, a scar produces 10% of normal skin tensile strength at closure and 80% at the end of optimal remodeling. Remodeling improves elasticity and thickness such that skin can glide easily over subcutaneous structures, including bony prominences and allowing tendons to glide easily under the skin. Unfortunately, stresses placed on the skin may prevent it from remodeling appropriately, resulting in tight or thin skin that either does not allow structures to move independently of skin or skin that tears easily. Such an example of under-repaired skin is shown in Figure 17-3.

Areas of skin subject to under-repair are typically located over large bony prominences and superficial tendons or are subjected to other stresses. Certain areas are notorious for under-repair. The olecranon and ulnar crest, tibial crest, patellae, and malleoli are stretched over superficial bony prominences. The dorsum of the hands and feet are located over large, superficial tendons, and the skin is subjected to the additional stress of wrist and ankle movements.

Langer's lines, as described previously, were developed to minimize scarring for surgery. As much as reasonable, surgeons will follow such lines. Some types of surgical procedures are not amenable to following such lines. The incision of abscesses and trauma may result in injuries that do not allow the lines to be followed. For example, a routine cesarean delivery will use the "bikini cut" that follows the Langer's line of the low abdomen. In contrast, an emergency delivery will use a vertical incision to improve the speed of the delivery. The bikini cut places less stress on the incision line than a vertical incision. Scars such as vertical abdominal ones are more likely to create a weak scar and produce adhesions.

Other factors promoting adhesions are poor hemostasis and diabetes. Blood within the incision promotes greater collagen formation through the wound's depth, allowing subcutaneous structures to adhere to the skin. Diabetes mellitus is associated with abnormal healing, including a greater risk of frozen joints and scar adhesions.

Splinting and Positioning

To prevent poor scar development, splinting can be used to position a body part and immobilize it in such a way that skin is not stressed. However, maintaining a static position can promote the adhesion of the developing scar to tissue below. The decision to use a splinting strategy must account for the need to prevent scar adhesion. Techniques for preventing adhesion are discussed later in the chapter. Abdominal adhesions can lead to loss of trunk extension and rotation and potentially loss of upper and lower extremity function. In addition to their effects on joints, upper or lower extremity adhesions may lead to compensations in motor patterns that lead to new injuries.

Surgical Interventions for Problem Scars

Three basic interventions available are excision of the problem tissue with new closure, graft/flap replacement of the tissue removed, and Z-plasty.

In some cases, scar tissue does not form well, but excision with new closure and splinting can result in satisfactory scarring from the second attempt. If substantial tissue is removed, incision and pulling the tissue back together are less likely to succeed. In these cases, a graft or flap can be placed in the area to provide sufficient tissue for closure to occur. The third strategy is a plastic surgery technique in which skin length is taken from one plane to add length to the perpendicular plane. As depicted in Figure 17-4, a Z-shaped incision is created, producing 2 triangular flaps of skin. The apices of the triangles are rotated on the bases such that the "top" and "bottom" of the Z become adjacent. The tissue in the shortened area is now lengthened, and the shortened normal skin can elongate and restore skin function.

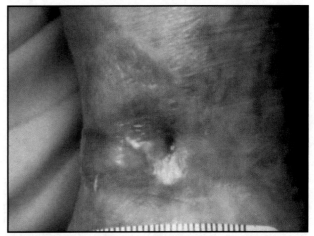

Figure 17-3. Example of a wound with under-repair.

Nonsurgical Interventions

Silicone sheets and onion extract can modify some scars sufficiently for adequate function and cosmesis. Silicone sheets are effective in reducing unwanted characteristics. They are available over the counter. They are still expensive but are reusable for several days depending on how well their adhesiveness is maintained. An example of a silicone sheet over a wound is shown in Figure 17-5. It can be removed for bathing and reapplied to clean dry skin. Shearing from the movement of the body part or clothing over the sheet and repeated reapplication shortens the sheet's life span. These sheets can produce a softer, lower, lighter scar that is less likely to adhere to tissue below. Other types of sheets and other forms of silicone have not been found to be as effective as silicone sheets.

Onion extract is also available over the counter. It improves the cosmetic result of scarring but does not improve the pliability, height, pain, or itch of scars. Onion extract, combined with silicone sheets, provides the benefits of each but does not provide any greater effect.

OUTCOME MEASURES

Standard measures for scar function and appearance are the Scar Mobility Score and the Vancouver Scar Scale (Table 17-1). The Vancouver Scar Scale consists of scores assigned for 4 properties: vascularity, pigmentation, pliability, and height. Vascularity is scored 0, 1, 2, and 3, respectively, for normal pigmentation, pink, red, and purple. Pigmentation scores are 0, 1, and 2 for normal, hypopigmented, and hyperpigmented skin. Pliability is scored 0 to 5, respectively, for normal, supple, yielding, firm, ropes, and contracture. The fourth characteristic is the height with scores of 0 to 3 for flat, < 2 mm, 2 to 5 mm, and > 5 mm. The only property that we can directly change is pliability.

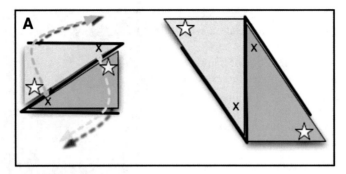

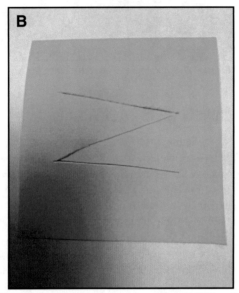

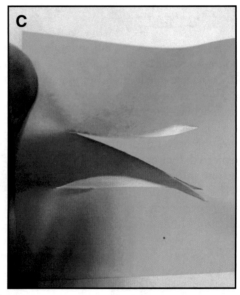

Figure 17-4. (A to C) Model of Z-plasty using a Post-it (3M) note.

Vascularity and pigmentation may change over time but are not impacted directly by treatment. Normal and supple skin generally do not require intervention. Yielding implies a slight limitation that should be easily corrected with the methods in the text following. Rope implies complete immobility in one plane, and contracture is complete immobility in both planes. Ropes are easily seen by pulling along the length of a scar. Adjacent skin moves easily, but the scar becomes taut and indents the skin. In terms of the Vancouver Scar Scale, contracture produces a similar phenomenon but in both planes, such that an area becomes taut and depresses relative to unscarred skin.

The Scar Mobility Score assesses the movement of the scar relative to the tissue below. When inspecting a scar, one should look for areas of puckering. Puckering indicates that the skin surface is being pulled toward subcutaneous tissue and is likely to be adherent. A closed scar should be moved along its length in both directions and perpendicular to its length in both directions. The scar should move in all 4 directions as much as adjacent, nonscarred tissue. If normal movement is detected, a score of 3 is assigned.

A score of 2/3 indicates that movement is minimally limited. This implies that movement in 1 of the 4 directions is limited. A score of 1/3 is moderately limited. This could mean that the scar does not move at all in one plane or has limited movement in more than 2 of 4 directions. A score of 0 means the scar is immobile in both planes. Immobility is not absolute but indicates that the tissue only moves with substantial force within the length of a scar's elasticity. Limited mobility allows a few millimeters of movement, whereas immobility leads to bunching of the scar along its length or puckering when movement perpendicular to the scar is attempted.

As a scar is mobilized, one should feel elasticity in it, and the scar will return to its same position with repeated mobilization. With repeated attempts to mobilize the scar, one should feel a change from elastic to plastic. When the scar progresses from elastic to plastic, it can be mobilized a greater distance than it could be previously. Further mobilization will result in reaching the failure state, which is palpable and will restore the skin's movement over the tissue below. Once a scar reaches failure, the patient must

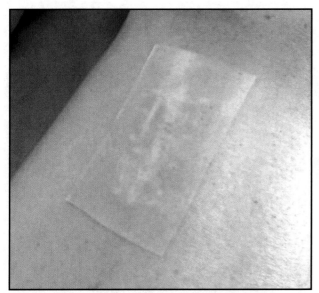

Figure 17-5. Silicone sheet used for scar modification.

TABLE 17-1 Vancouver Scar Scale		
PROPERTY	**CHARACTERISTIC**	**SCORE**
Vascularity	Normal	0
	Pink	1
	Red	2
	Purple	3
Pigmentation	Normal	0
	Hypopigmented	1
	Hyperpigmented	2
Pliability	Normal	0
	Supple	1
	Yielding	2
	Firm	3
	Ropes	4
	Contracture	5
Height	Flat	0
	< 2 mm	1
	2-5 mm	2
	> 5 mm	3
Total		
Data source: Sullivan et al, 1990.		

continue to move through a normal range of motion to prevent new adhesions. Methods for mobilizing mature adherent scars and preventing adhesions follow.

SCAR MOBILIZATION

The management of scars can be divided into prevention and restoration techniques. Within these categories, we have the techniques of desensitization, massage, plucking, and rolling. Desensitization and massage can begin early after surgery, as soon as access to the incision is available. Plucking and rolling are used for adherent scars. They are deeper, more aggressive, and painful techniques that should not be used unless the scar is mature and adherent.

Prevention

Desensitization begins with light massage with a hand. This can be a therapist, family member, or the patient. The scar can be rubbed with a soft texture such as a cotton ball. As the patient tolerates, the texture used becomes progressively rougher such as a washcloth. Massage begins gently up to 1 to 2 inches (2.5 to 5 cm) from the scars until scabs are shed. Once scabs are gone, massage becomes deeper and more aggressive. Early massage, especially while scabs are still intact, should be done by holding the 2 sides of the scar together, between 2 fingers, to avoid pulling the edges apart, as shown in Figure 17-6A. The scar should be moved in all directions. It can be linear such as along the scar and perpendicular to the scar and progress to circular

or other motions. Some directions may be more limited than others and, therefore, require more time massaging into those directions. The intensity of massage should be to patient tolerance, blanching, and change in feel to avoid dehiscence. Do not push beyond the blanching of the skin, and be careful that the 2 edges move together and do not pull apart.

Restoration of Skin Movement

Plucking and rolling are used to restore skin movement following the development of adhesions. Plucking is used specifically for addressing mobility perpendicular to the length of a scar and is demonstrated in Figure 17-6B. Much as a string of an instrument is fixed at 2 points and can be plucked, the scar is held with 2 fingers of one hand, and between the 2 fingers is pulled with a finger of the other hand perpendicular to the scar's length in both directions. More time and intensity are used if one direction has less mobility. One should be feeling for

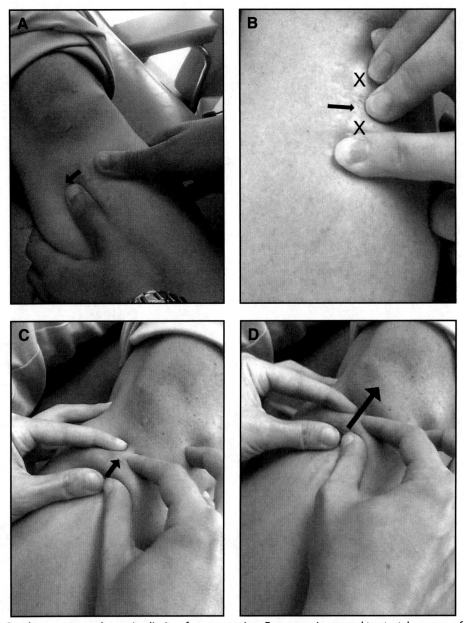

Figure 17-6. (A) Gentle massage to determine limits of scar excursion. Forces are increased to stretch scar as a form of massage. (B) Plucking an adherent scar. Two ends are fixed, and the center (or other places as needed) is moved laterally to stretch adherent areas. (C) Rolling an adherent scar. The scar is overlapped on itself while moving the fingers along the scar's length. (D) A continuation of rolling the scar. In this case, the scar is being mobilized from distal to proximal.

changes from elasticity to plasticity to failure. Multiple treatment sessions may be needed to progress into plasticity. Dimpling beyond the scar is commonly seen as the skin on either side of the adhesion moves freely, but the adhesion constrains the center. Once plasticity is reached, greater intensity can rapidly result in failure. The patient should be told explicitly that these techniques for restoring skin mobility could become quite painful. In addition, blanching and patient tolerance should be used as a guide to force because excessive force in less mature scars could potentially lead to dehiscence.

Rolling is a much more aggressive form of mobilization. It is directed toward improving the scar's longitudinal mobility, but lateral mobility is also improved as adhesions break. The rolling technique is demonstrated in Figures 17-6C and 17-6D. This technique requires using the thumb and index finger of each hand on each side of the scar. A length of the scar is pinched up away from the body as the skin rolls in a wave along the scar. This action lifts the skin's surface away from subcutaneous tissue and is more effective than plucking but is also much more painful. Generally, one should begin with a desensitization protocol, work on plucking, and, if necessary, progress to rolling. As the adhesions become plastic, the pinch of skin that is rolled along the skin becomes larger. Doing so places more stretch on the adhesion. A series of rolls from the bottom to the top of a scar is performed to patient tolerance. Letting the patient know that a scar is about to "break free" can motivate them to tolerate the procedure. As with plucking, multiple sessions may be necessary to move from elastic to plastic, but once plastic is reached, more aggressive rolling will soon lead to adhesion release. The patient should continue efforts to improve the range of motion of any involved joints and desensitization. A comparison of early, more gentle rolling to more aggressive rolling associated with adhesion release can be seen in the difference between Figures 17-6C and 17-6D.

SUMMARY

Topical agents other than debridement and antiseptics are discussed in this chapter. Currently, one form of growth factor is available. Regranex is indicated for slow-healing neuropathic ulcers in the presence of adequate blood flow and debridement. It contains PDGF, which is deficient in diabetes mellitus. Also used in wounds that have failed with conservative efforts are CTPs. They can be used in place of split-thickness skin grafts or as an adjunct to split-thickness skin graft, preparing the wound for better take of the split-thickness skin graft by promoting granulation.

Several adjunctive therapies have been promoted to aid wound healing. Good evidence for the use of electrical stimulation and pulsed electromagnetic field exists, and these are reimbursable through CMS. The evidence for diathermy and ultrasound is not as good, and these carry a risk of injury to the patient. Ultraviolet radiation may be a useful alternative to antiseptics for controlling the growth of bacteria on the surface of wounds. HBO may be useful for wounds such as neuropathic ulcers, but the evidence is lacking to support HBO for indiscriminate treatment of chronic wounds. NPWT can be useful, especially for large dehiscent wounds, and can be used for other wound types to stimulate granulation tissue production.

Scarring is expected with full-thickness injuries, including surgical incisions and grafting. Most scars are not problematic, but many produce a localized limitation of skin motion. Some scars will limit movement of musculoskeletal structures and produce abnormal stresses that may lead to additional injuries. Preventative measures of scar desensitization and massage may reduce the risk of adherent scars. Lengthy immobilization and excessive motion or stresses on the skin around bony prominences and large tendons can lead to adhesions requiring scar mobilization techniques of plucking and rolling to release them. The Scar Mobility Scale and Vancouver Scar Scale can be used for outcome measures.

QUESTIONS

1. What is the purpose of using PDGF for neuropathic wounds? Why is it not indicated for other types of wounds?

2. What is the difference between allografts and xenografts? Why would they be used instead of or in addition to split-thickness skin grafts?

3. What is the primary benefit of using UVC in wound management?

4. How does low-frequency, noncontact ultrasound differ from low-frequency, contact ultrasound used for debridement and high-frequency ultrasound used for tissue mobility?

5. Which adjunctive therapies have received support from CMS?

6. Contrast HVPC and pulsed electromagnetic field therapy.

7. For what types of wounds would leeches be appropriate?

8. Contrast the purposes of systemic and topical HBO therapy.

9. What potential benefits may be derived from HBO? What are some of the possible drawbacks?

10. What wounds can be treated with NPWT? What are some contraindications to using NPWT?

11. Why must we make a distinction between a closed wound and a healed wound?

12. What are the purposes of the Scar Mobility Scale and Vancouver Scar Scale?

BIBLIOGRAPHY

Al-Kurdi D, Bell-Syer SEM, Flemming K. Therapeutic ultrasound for venous leg ulcers. *Cochrane Database Syst Rev.* 2008;1:CD001180.

Callaghan MJ, Chang EI, Seiser N, et al. Pulsed electromagnetic fields accelerate normal and diabetic wound healing by increasing endogenous FGF-2 release. *Plast Reconstr Surg.* 2008;121(1):130-141.

Crow L. New wound therapy offers treatment advantages for PTs. *Acute Care Perspect.* 1999;7(2):10-11.

Feigal DW Jr. Public health notification: diathermy interactions with implanted leads and implanted systems with leads. *J Ir Dent Assoc.* 2003;49(1):26-27.

Heggers JP, Kucukcelebi A, Listengarten D, et al. Beneficial effect of aloe on wound healing in an excisional wound model. *J Altern Complement Med.* 1996;2(2):271-277.

Hudson M. What's old is new again. Leech and maggot therapy: wound care in the 90's. *Acute Care Perspect.* 1999;7(2):15-17.

Kalliainen LK, Gordillo GM, Schlanger R, Sen CK. Topical oxygen as an adjunct to wound healing: a clinical case series. *Pathophysiology.* 2003;9(2):81-87.

Medical Coverage Policies. Blue Cross/Blue Shield of Rhode Island. Accessed November 25, 2022. https://www.cms.gov/medicare-coverage-database/view/article.aspx?articleid=52511#:~:text=Negative%20pressure%20wound%20therapy%20equipment%20is%20covered%20under,related%20Local%20Coverage%20Determination%20%28LCD%29%20must%20be%20met

Medicare Coverage Issues. Transmittal 129. Accessed September 20, 2022. https://www.cms.gov/Regulations-and-Guidance/Guidance/Transmittals/Downloads/R129CIM.pdf

Rossi F, Elsinger E. Topical hyperbaric oxygen therapy for lower extremity wound care: an overview. *Podiatry Manage.* 1997;November:110-111.

Sheffield PJ. Tissue oxygen measurements with respect to soft tissue wound healing with normobaric and hyperbaric oxygen. *HBO Rev.* 1985;6:18-43.

Smith PD, Kuhn MA, Franz MG, Wachtel TL, Wright TE, Robson MC. Initiating the inflammatory phase of incisional healing prior to tissue injury. *J Surg Res.* 2000;92(1):11-17.

Strauch B, Patel MK, Navarro JA, Berdichevsky M, Yu HL, Pilla AA. Pulsed magnetic fields accelerate cutaneous wound healing in rats. *Plast Reconstr Surg.* 2007;120(2):425-430.

Sullivan T, Smith J, Kermode J, McIver E, Courtemanche DJ. Rating the burn scar. *J Burn Care Rehabil.* 1990;11(3):256-260. doi:10.1097/00004630-199005000-00014

Tepper OM, Callaghan MJ, Change EI, et al. Electromagnetic fields increase in vitro and in vivo angiogenesis through endothelial release of FGF-2. *FASEB J.* 2004;18(11):1231-1233.

Wieman TJ, Smiell JM, Su Y. Efficacy and safety of a topical gel formulation of recombinant human platelet-derived growth factor-BB (becaplermin) in patients with chronic neuropathic diabetic ulcers. A phase III randomized placebo-controlled double-blind study. *Diabetes Care.* 1998;21(5):822-827.

Young SR, Dyson M. Effect of therapeutic ultrasound on the healing of full-thickness excised skin lesions. *Ultrasonics.* 1990;28(3):175-180.

Special Cases

Irion GL, Gardner JA, Pignataro RM.
Comprehensive Wound Management, Third Edition (pp 345-363).
© 2024 Taylor and Francis Group.

OBJECTIVES

- Identify atypical wounds.
- List characteristics of Marjolin's ulcer.
- List characteristics of sickle cell ulcers.
- List characteristics of pyoderma gangrenosum.
- Describe cutaneous complications of kidney failure.
- Discuss skin injury risks associated with obesity, intensive care, neonates, and older adults.
- Discuss the decision-making processes involved in palliative care.

ATYPICAL WOUNDS

"Typical" wounds include pressure, neuropathic, venous, arterial, trauma (including burns), and infection either in the form of a skin and soft tissue infection or a surgical site infection. The general category of vascular should not be considered within the usual wounds because some vascular wounds are considered to be atypical and will be discussed in this chapter. In general, the appearance, location, and history of usual wounds are straightforward. A difference in any of those 3 characteristics should prompt the clinician to consider the possibility that the wound has an unusual cause.

Atypical wounds consist of a large number of conditions. Some of these conditions may be fairly common but do not create wounds. Others create wounds but are much less common than the usual wounds. Many clinicians may never see some usual wounds personally. Clinicians in full-time practice, especially those who receive referrals of patients with problematic healing, are much more likely

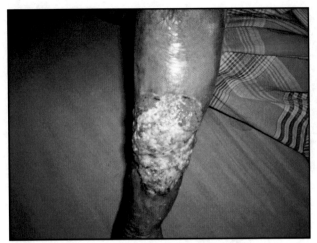

Figure 18-1. Typical appearance of Marjolin's ulcer.

to encounter atypical wounds. As a general rule, atypical wounds do not fit normal diagnostic criteria and do not improve with what seems to be appropriate care. Although biopsy sometimes reveals the cause of the wound, many such wounds are diagnosed by exclusion and whether they respond to a particular type of treatment. In other cases, clinicians with previous experience with a particular type of wound may immediately recognize its appearance. Atypical wounds, for the purpose of this chapter, will be divided into neoplastic disease, autoimmune disease, vaso-occlusive disease, and those caused by anticoagulant therapy and kidney failure.

NEOPLASTIC DISEASE

Skin lesions produced by neoplastic disease include basal cell carcinoma (BCC), squamous cell carcinoma (SCC), melanoma, Kaposi's sarcoma, and cutaneous T-cell lymphoma. Cancer resulting from chronic wounds, commonly SCC, is termed *Marjolin's ulcer*.

In addition to an unusual appearance, location, or history, atypical wounds caused by neoplastic disease commonly feature excessive granulation, described as a fungating appearance; failure to re-epithelialize; pruritus (itching); an unexplained increase in size; and an unexplained change in bleeding, drainage, odor, and pain. The irregular piling of granulation tissue above the surface of the skin (fungating appearance) of a long-standing wound combined with pruritus and unusual odor should prompt a biopsy for potential cancer. The term *fungating appearance* refers to the mixture of granulation and necrotic tissue. Overgrowth of granulation with necrosis produces fissuring/crevices in the surface resembling cauliflower or fungus growth, although it is not caused by fungus. Because the tissue does not have

normal characteristics of granulation and necroses due to the instability of cells, it does not readily allow coverage with epithelial cells, as depicted in Figure 18-1.

Basal Cell Carcinoma

BCC is the most common form of skin cancer, with approximately 1 million new cases per year in the United States. It is frequently described as having a pearly appearance. Raised, translucent lesions with fine, visible blood vessels are common, but BCC may present as a nonspecific lesion on sun-exposed skin. Other presentations include an open wound that bleeds and crusts but does not heal; a reddish patch that itches or crusts; a pearly appearance with darker pigmentation; a pinkish neoplasm with an elevated, rolled border and crusted central indentation and possible surface blood vessels; and a hypopigmented patch that has the appearance of a healed scar.

Common areas include the sun-exposed skin of the face, particularly ears, nose, and lips; the dorsum of the hand; and posterior cervical area. Although BCC is rarely metastatic, it can be highly invasive and erode a large area of continuous skin if untreated. Lesions with unusual characteristics observed on typical areas of excessive exposure to sunlight should be referred for a biopsy to determine whether the cause is BCC. Treatment by excision is generally curative.

Squamous Cell Carcinoma

SCC is the second most common form of skin cancer. Its etiology is similar to that of BCC. SCC also generally occurs on sun-damaged skin. A precancerous lesion called *actinic keratosis* may precede the development of SCC. Additionally, SCC may occur years later in skin damaged by exposure to sunlight or ionizing radiation and skin that has recovered from a burn injury. Like BCC, SCC on sun-damaged skin is rarely metastatic, but the rate of metastasis is much greater on skin injured by ionizing radiation or burns. Risk of SCC is also increased by immunosuppression. Metastasis is also more likely to occur on modified skin such as lips and areolae (20% to 30% as opposed to 0.5%). The treatment of SCC is also simple excision. More invasive treatment including chemotherapy may be necessary if metastasis occurs.

The usual appearance of SCC is a crusted/scaled patch with an inflamed base. However, the appearance might also appear to be a simple bite reaction, scaling, or other trauma (Figure 18-2). The lesion in Figure 18-2 was initially diagnosed as an insect bite but was later confirmed as SCC following biopsy. As with BCC, the unusual characteristics and presence on sun-damaged, radiation-damaged, or healed areas of burned skin should increase the suspicion of SCC. In both BCC and SCC, wounds will not heal and may increase in size.

Actinic Keratosis

Actinic keratosis is the result of sun damage, particularly on fair-skinned individuals. Scaling appears on typical sites of sun injury due to dysplastic cell proliferation in the dermis. These lesions are excised either sharply or by cryosurgical removal. Fair-skinned individuals with a long history of sun exposure may require annual inspection of sun-exposed skin and excision of multiple actinic keratoses.

Melanoma

Although not as common as BCC and SCC, melanoma is more likely to metastasize; mortality increases as vertical growth toward the dermis occurs. As a tumor of melanocytes, melanoma begins in the epidermis and proliferates into the dermis. It spreads to other parts of the body, especially the liver, brain, and lung, by entering the lymphatic system. Intracutaneous metastasis producing satellite tumors indicates a very poor prognosis. Melanoma is excised and regional lymph nodes may be removed as well, leaving wounds in both areas.

Melanoma has a variety of presentations. In contrast to common moles (nevi), melanoma has unusual characteristics. It may be much larger, more irregular, have variegated coloration, be more elevated above the skin, ulcerate, and bleed. The color can range from a tan to almost black with a surrounding halo of hypopigmented skin. The appearance of a new mole on an adult that has some of the characteristics listed earlier should raise suspicion of melanoma. Early excision before the tumor invades the dermis and cells gain access to the lymphatic system is critical.

Marjolin's Ulcer

Chronic wounds from venous disease, thermal and radiation burn injuries, and drainage from osteomyelitis can transform the open wound to SCC. Rather than seek definitive treatment of open wounds, some patients may simply bandage open wounds and allow them to drain for years. DNA damage from radiation injury or chronic exposure to cytokines and growth factors may cause cells within the wound to lose control of normal growth and become malignant. This wound containing malignant cells is termed *Marjolin's ulcer*.

The typical Marjolin's ulcer is found on a lower extremity of a man between the ages of 40 and 70, and the wound has been present from 20 to 50 years. Fungating appearance,

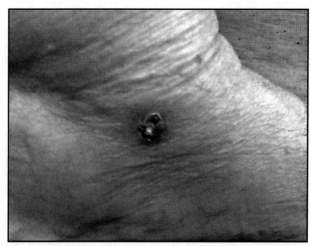

Figure 18-2. Ulcer caused by SCC in an unusual location, near the medial malleolus.

as described previously, and the odor of dimethyl trisulfide are indications of malignancy. Dimethyl trisulfide has a foul odor and is associated with broccoli and cabbage, as well as decomposition of human tissue. Although the cancerous tissue may remain localized, the metastatic rate for Marjolin's ulcer (30%) is much greater than that of squamous cell cancer in general. These wounds should be suspected by both the appearance and duration of the wound. A biopsy is done to confirm the suspicion. Wide excision may be curative, but amputation may be required in some cases. The underlying cause of the ulcer must also be addressed, generally by debridement or amputation of the infected bone.

GENETIC DISORDERS

Two major genetic diseases are associated with atypical wounds. The blistering disorder, epidermolysis is a collection of diseases of both recessive and dominant inheritance. Sickle cell disease frequently produces leg ulcers that may not be diagnosed properly. Because sickle cell disease leads to vaso-occlusive disease, it is described after vaso-occlusive disorders.

Epidermolysis Bullosa Simplex

Epidermolysis bullosa (EB) is not a singular disease but a collection of genetic diseases leading to bulla formation secondary to defects in the basement membrane zone. The disorders are usually diagnosed at or shortly after birth. They are mostly autosomal dominant and have a range of severity. Autosomal recessive types of EB tend to be more serious than dominant.

The vast majority of cases (92%) are the mildest form, termed *epidermolysis bullosa simplex* (EBS). EBS is an autosomal dominant disorder with several subtypes of varying severity depending on the mutation of specific keratin subtypes. The mildest forms affect the skin only with intraepidermal blistering and healing without scarring. Mild EBS may not be diagnosed until adulthood, and in some cases, it is not diagnosed in a parent until a child is diagnosed with EBS. Other forms of EB produce skin separation in different structures. Forms other than EBS are more severe and may include organ involvement. Separation occurs in the lamina lucida of the basement membrane in junctional EB, in the lamina densa in dystrophic EB, and through hemidesmosomes in hemidesmosomal EB. Specific molecular defects have been isolated in these disorders with research ongoing to replace defective genes.

Any form of EB places infants at risk for infection and possible sepsis and death. Metastatic SCC may be lethal in those with the autosomal recessive dystrophic EB during late teens through early adulthood. EBS, the autosomal dominant form of dystrophic EB, and milder forms of junctional EB may not shorten life span if sepsis is avoided.

Wound healing is impaired to varying extents in different types of EB. Loss of barrier function and the presence of serum on the skin place the skin at risk of infection. Some subtypes of EB have immunologic and gastrointestinal defects that increase susceptibility to infection and impair nutritional status. Cleansing of denuded areas with the application of topical antimicrobials and occlusive dressings are typically required. The application of adhesives should be strictly avoided.

SCC may develop in areas of chronic denudation of those with dystrophic EB. Although SCC generally occurs in sun-exposed areas of fair-skinned individuals, those with dystrophic EB may develop tumors on any area, not necessarily those with sun exposure. This malignancy has a peak incidence in the 20s through 30s, which is earlier than SCC usually appears in the general population.

AUTOIMMUNE DISEASES

Diseases affecting the skin may be due to autoimmune disorders that affect specific components of the skin. A large number of vasculitides may produce ulcerations of the skin. Other diseases including pyoderma gangrenosum (PG) appear to have immune components, but their mechanisms remain elusive.

Vasculitis

As autoimmune disorders, vasculitides tend to cause systemic signs of inflammation such as joint and muscle pains, lymphadenitis, fever, and malaise. Many vasculitides have been described in the literature. A number of them have skin involvement and may present as skin lesions/rashes that do not respond to normal treatment. In general, treatments for vasculitides involve immune suppression. Diagnosis generally requires biopsy. Those vasculitides that are more likely to affect the skin include hypersensitivity vasculitis, microscopic polyangiitis, polyarteritis nodosa, rheumatoid vasculitis (associated with rheumatoid arthritis), Churg Strauss vasculitis, Wegener's granulomatosis, cryoglobulinemia, and Henoch-Schönlein purpura. Buerger's disease (thromboangiitis obliterans) is discussed under vaso-occlusive disorders. Behcet's syndrome is discussed next.

Behcet's Syndrome

Behcet's syndrome is a rare disease primarily affecting young adults (20s to 30s). Signs include mouth sores, skin rashes and lesions, and genital sores. The distribution and severity of these lesions vary from person to person, and signs may remit and recur. Oral ulcers begin as raised lesions and ulcerate. They may occur on the lips, gums, and tongue as well. Skin lesions vary from acnelike to red, raised, tender nodules. Similar ulcers may occur on the vulva and penis. These ulcers heal in 7 to 10 days, but recurrence is common. An additional sign of Behcet's syndrome is uveitis. Although uveitis occurs with many other diseases, the combination with skin and oral ulcers should raise the suspicion of Behcet's syndrome. Joint pain, particularly the knee, is another indication of Behcet's. Arthralgia is remitting and recurring. This disease can also cause aneurysm or thrombosis of blood vessels, digestive, and nervous system complications. In addition to the typical signs of Behcet's syndrome, a positive pathergy test assists in the diagnosis. To conduct this test, an injury to the skin is created with a sterile needle. A skin lesion such as a reddened nodule 2 days later constitutes a positive pathergy test. Like other vasculitides, Behcet's syndrome is treated with corticosteroids or immunosuppressant drugs. An additional drug that may be used is interferon-α, which suppresses excessive immune response.

Pyoderma Gangrenosum

PG is a disorder of unknown etiology characterized by the development of skin ulcerations unrelated to any known cause. Patients may describe a small wound that becomes attributed to a spider bite or trauma that has progressed to a large, deep ulcer. Ulcers produced by PG have a characteristic appearance with violaceous, undermined borders (Figure 18-3). Any wound with this appearance should raise a high level of suspicion of PG. In addition, the skin surrounding wounds associated with PG often demonstrate pustules, scabs, and scars from old wounds. PG is a rare disorder with an incidence of about 1 in 100,000 per year. The mortality of PG is very low; however, death might occur due to complications of treatment or an underlying disease associated with PG.

A history of autoimmune disorders is associated with PG in about 50% of cases. In addition to complaints of pain from the ulcer, the patient may experience arthralgia and malaise. Associated systemic diseases include inflammatory bowel diseases, rheumatoid arthritis, and hematologic diseases such as leukemias. Another important characteristic of PG is pathergy. Pathergy in PG specifically refers to the characteristic worsening or development of new wounds with skin trauma. Efforts to debride, forcefully clean, or graft the area are likely to cause the wound to worsen. Grafting is likely to cause the wound to increase in size and may cause PG at the donor site. No laboratory testing is available to diagnose PG, and no characteristic histology can be seen through examination of biopsies. Biopsy is useful only for ruling out other possible disorders. Diagnosis of PG requires a high level of suspicion due to the appearance of the wound and the exclusion of any other causes, particularly malignancies of the skin.

Treatment of PG includes protection of the wound while treating the underlying autoimmune disorder. Medical therapy involves systemic immunosuppression, which might include cyclosporine, oral corticosteroids, and infliximab (Remicade). Infliximab and related drugs inhibit tumor necrosis factor. This drug is currently indicated for use in rheumatoid arthritis and Crohn's disease. Topical and injected corticosteroids might also be used in the treatment of PG. During wound healing, aggressive debridement is contraindicated.

VASO-OCCLUSIVE DISORDERS

A large number of diseases may produce ischemia of the limbs. Atherosclerosis, discussed in Chapter 12, is the most common. Occlusive disease caused by autoimmune vasculitis was discussed earlier in this chapter; distal peripheral microembolism, thromboangiitis obliterans, and sickle cell disease are discussed next.

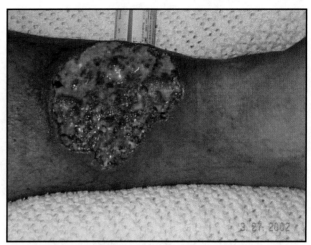

Figure 18-3. Typical appearance of PG with undermined violaceous edges and mixed granulation and slough.

Distal Peripheral Microembolism

Distal peripheral microembolism (blue toe syndrome/trash foot) is not a disease but a phenomenon caused by embolization of atherosclerotic debris into small arteries and arterioles. By definition, microemboli are pieces of atheromas less than 1 mm in diameter. The release of atherosclerotic particles into the blood may occur spontaneously, but most cases of this syndrome are believed to be iatrogenic caused by endovascular approaches to revascularization of the lower extremities. This syndrome has a wide range of morbidity with ischemia and infarction of a limited number of small areas but can also result in widespread embolism resulting in multisystem organ failure. The degree of injury produced by microembolism depends on both the quantity and composition of the emboli. Small emboli consisting of platelets and fibrin can be lysed with only reversible cell injury to distal tissues, whereas a large cholesterol embolus is more likely to cause irreversible injury with tissue necrosis.

In particular, microembolism originating from the aortoiliac arteries produces what is known as *blue toe syndrome* or *trash foot*. The term *blue toe syndrome* is due to cyanosis that may develop in the most distal vessels, which can be occluded by multiple emboli. Showers of atherosclerotic debris may produce tender, mottled areas of cyanotic and cool areas of various sizes and sluggish capillary refill in the foot as well as toes. With accumulation of ischemic injury, tissue necrosis may occur, producing ulcerations. The term *trash foot* is frequently applied to feet displaying this necrosis.

The treatment of distal peripheral microembolization has been compared with frostbite with delayed debridement and amputation only after clear demarcation between viable and necrotic tissue. In both frostbite and distal peripheral microembolization, arterial inflow to the tissue and perfusion to surrounding tissue is adequate, but areas fed by localized branches of the microcirculation are occluded, leading to direct necrosis and later reperfusion injury if the embolus is broken down, restoring blood flow. If possible, the source of microemboli is removed and heparin administered to stabilize plaque instability. Patients may be treated with aspirin and dipyridamole, but warfarin appears to cause increased risk of microembolism in a large percentage of patients at risk.

Buerger's Disease (Thromboangiitis Obliterans)

Thromboangiitis obliterans is a vaso-occlusive, non-atherosclerotic disease primarily of middle-aged male tobacco smokers. Buerger's disease is uncommon, with a prevalence of about 15 cases per 100,000 population. Although mortality due to Buerger's disease is unusual, gangrene of extremities requiring amputation occurs in almost half of those diagnosed. Mortality and severe morbidity may result from sepsis caused by infection of gangrenous extremities. The disease is believed to be caused by a combination of genetic predisposition from inheritance of specific types of antigens and exposure to cigarette smoke.

In Buerger's disease, patients will begin to display signs of peripheral arterial disease such as paresthesia, cold extremities, and weak pulses. Ulcerations of the digits are another sign of vaso-occlusive disorder, but they are not exclusive to Buerger's disease. These also occur in Raynaud's disease, scleroderma, and lupus. Migratory, superficial venous thrombosis occurs in approximately 50% of those with this disorder. Involvement of arterial vessels of organs may occur in a small number of those affected. Buerger's disease is more likely to be suspected if an onset of arterial disease is seen in men younger than 45, the patient smokes, and they display Raynaud's phenomenon. This disease is more common in men, but the difference in prevalence may simply reflect a lower prevalence of smoking in women.

No specific laboratory tests are currently available for Buerger's disease, but tests are likely to be performed to rule out other vaso-occlusive disorders such as one of the vasculitic disorders. To rule out lower extremity atherosclerosis in patients with physical signs of lower extremity ischemia, the Allen test can be performed. The diagnosis of Buerger's disease is more likely with a positive Allen test in addition to a history of smoking and the presence of lower

extremity arterial ulcers. In the Allen test, the patient flexes the fingers into a fist to evacuate blood from the hand. A clinician occludes the radial and ulnar arteries simultaneously with their thumbs. When the arteries to the hand are occluded, the patient relaxes the hand and the clinician releases the ulnar artery while continuing to compress the radial artery. Delayed refill of the hand indicates occlusive disease of the ulnar artery. The procedure is then repeated but with release of the radial artery while maintaining compression of the ulnar artery as a test for the radial artery's patency.

Acute Buerger's disease is characterized by inflammation and thrombosis of small- and medium-diameter arteries. Often the inflammation and injury spread to adjacent veins and nerves. As the disease progresses to the subacute phase, organization of thrombi occurs. Blood vessels may be totally occluded, but some will regain partial arterial flow due to canalization of thrombi. In end-stage disease, blood vessels are fibrosed, with no possibility of ever conducting blood again. As more vessels undergo this process, the patient develops signs of arterial disease such as claudication during exercise. With progression of the disease, pain at rest, skin changes, and skin and soft tissue ulceration requiring amputation of the affected limb will occur in a large fraction of patients.

At this time, no pharmacologic treatments have been found effective despite research into seemingly every possible mechanism of maintaining blood flow. Surgical revascularization is unlikely to be successful given the diffuse effects of the disease. Surgical intervention is only practical in cases in which bypassing discrete focal lesions can restore blood flow. The only treatment known to be effective is smoking cessation. Smoking cessation is imperative but can be difficult. Of those who can successfully cease smoking, 94% avoid amputation, and all of those who cease before any gangrene develops appear to avert amputation. In comparison, 43% of those who continue to smoke will require an amputation within 8 years of symptoms. Risk of amputation exists even in those who switch to chewing tobacco or nicotine replacement therapies. Many of those who eventually require an amputation will progress to multiple amputations including bilateral upper- and lower extremity amputations. Part of patient education is that amputation may be avoided if tobacco use is ceased. In addition, patients must avoid secondhand smoke. Smoking cessation by social contacts and family members may be necessary for multiple reasons, including avoidance of secondhand smoke, avoiding temptation to resume, and having a social support system. Although amputation may be avoided with complete smoking cessation, Raynaud's phenomenon and intermittent claudication may persist.

Digital Ischemia Secondary to Vasopressor Administration

In cases of circulatory shock, adequate blood pressure for survival may require administration of vasopressors that result in severe vasoconstriction of small arteries of the distal areas of the extremities. If the patient survives, varying degrees of ischemic injury may occur, which may require amputation of gangrenous fingers, toes, or more proximal areas. An example of digital gangrene secondary to pressor administration for septic shock is shown in Figure 18-4.

Sickle Cell Disease

Sickle cell disease, formerly known as sickle cell anemia, results from homozygous inheritance of hemoglobin S (HbS), a defective form of hemoglobin. The defect is the result of a single amino acid substitution that reduces the solubility of hemoglobin. The presence of large numbers of malformed (sickle-shaped) red cells leads to obstruction of small vessels with the potential for thrombosis and ischemic injury downstream of occlusions. The shortened life span of abnormal cells produces hemolytic anemia. The sickling process that frequently occurs with sickle cell anemia may be precipitated by multiple factors, particularly events that produce dehydration and acidosis such as viral illness, vomiting, and insufficient hydration when working outdoors. Other stressors such as fatigue, exposure to cold, and psychological stress may precipitate a crisis.

Approximately 0.15% of Black individuals are homozygous for HbS, resulting in sickle cell disease; approximately 8% are heterozygous carriers. Heterozygous individuals have about 30% to 40% of HbS and are usually not affected with the significant morbidity associated with homozygosity. A heterozygous individual is said to have sickle cell trait. Morbidity can occur under severe conditions such as high-altitude flight without adequate pressurization of the cabin. Sickle cell disease has variable morbidity and mortality. Although sickle cell disease is a chronic disorder, morbidity is associated with injuries accumulated by multiple exacerbations or sickle cell crises. Life expectancy is approximately 60 years, with mortality due to several causes. About 30% die during an acute crisis despite the lack of known organ damage. Infection causes most of the mortality in young children, whereas stroke, trauma, acute chest syndrome (see following), splenic sequestration crisis, and aplastic crisis cause mortality in teens and young adults.

Differing types of sickle cell crises tend to occur at different ages. The most common type is vaso-occlusive, which is very painful and may require strong analgesics. Vaso-occlusive injury is particularly severe in bone marrow. Infants are most prone to occlusions in the small bones of

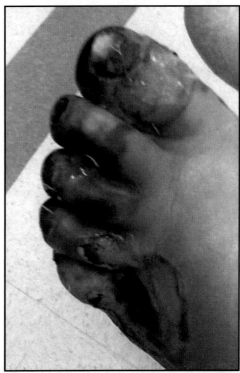

Figure 18-4. Appearance of toes with gangrene secondary to administration of vasoconstrictor drugs during septic shock.

the hands and feet, producing pain and edema. Older children may have more joint pain. Older patients may develop acute chest syndrome characterized by fever, chest pain, dyspnea, and coughing. Acute chest syndrome appears to be caused by a combination of pneumonia and vaso-occlusive disease affecting the lungs. Acute chest syndrome leads to hypoxia and is a life-threatening situation. Abdominal pain similar to acute abdomen with pain, distention, and abdominal rigidity is caused by occlusion and infarction of abdominal organs and the mesentery. Splenic sequestration crisis is a consequence of vaso-occlusive disorder affecting the spleen. Occlusion of splenic sinusoids results in trapping of blood within the spleen. This syndrome may progress slowly, with complaints of fatigue and left-sided abdominal pain. Progression of the crisis can result in infarction of the spleen and hypovolemic shock. Similarly, priapism can result from occlusion of venous sinuses. Left untreated, thrombosis and necrosis may occur. Occlusion of cerebral vessels leads to neurologic symptoms related to the vessels affected, ranging from temporary focal defects to life-threatening stroke. Aplastic anemia crisis is more common among infants and children. Anemia can become severe with reticulocytopenia and very little production of red cells. Patients become severely ill, developing tachycardia and pallor. Crises are frequently due to parvovirus B19, the cause of "fifth disease" in children.

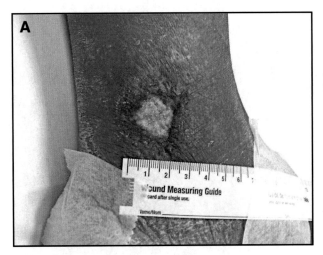

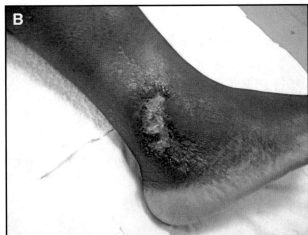

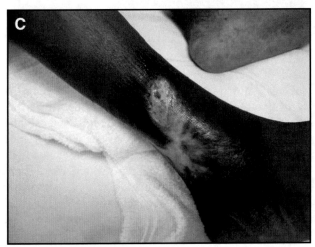

Figure 18-5. Typical appearance and most common location for sickle cell ulcers. (A) Hyperpigmented edges, mixed slough, and granulation are common. (B) Common location near the lateral malleolus. (C) Presence of multiple healed sickle cell ulcers in addition to the current ulcer.

Sickle Cell Disease–Related Leg Ulcers

Ulcers of the lower extremities are common in adolescents and young adults with sickle cell disease. The most common location is proximal to the lateral malleolus. Individuals may have a number of ulcers at various stages of healing located on both lower extremities. These ulcers appear to be the result of vaso-occlusive disease, but the reason for their location is not readily explained. Sickle cell ulcers are shallow, with adherent yellow slough mixed with small areas of granulation tissue. The periwound skin is noticeably darker than the surrounding skin. Many patients have been self-managing these ulcers for months or years before closure of these wounds. Examples of a leg ulcer associated with sickle cell disease are shown in Figures 18-5A and 18-5B.

Aggressive debridement of these ulcers can be difficult due to the intensity of pain experienced by many patients, especially if treatment is occurring during hospitalization for a crisis. Pulsatile lavage may also be poorly tolerated. Either enzymatic or autolytic debridement is more likely to be accepted as a treatment. A dressing that does not adhere to the wound bed is important with this type of ulcer.

While the wound is covered with slough and receiving collagenase debridement, normal saline-moistened 2 × 2s may be used. As slough is debrided, granulation tissue must be protected. The dressing change and interval of changes must be chosen to minimize trauma to the wound bed. Even hydrogel and xeroform may adhere to granulation tissue between dressing changes. In some cases, patients may benefit from compression bandaging or an Unna's boot if significant edema is present. Follow-up visits to ensure effective home care of the clean stable wound should be scheduled if possible. Patients may experience regression of the wound with suboptimal care. Many individuals may be seen repeatedly as inpatients due to recurrent sickle cell crises and may demonstrate regression of a wound.

ANTICOAGULANTS

Both heparin and warfarin are known to cause skin necrosis in rare cases. Both cause subcutaneous bleeding and blistering. A history will indicate which anticoagulant is responsible for the skin injury. Warfarin-induced skin necrosis is rare, occurring in 0.01% to 0.1% of those receiving warfarin anticoagulation treatment, usually women with obesity. Shortly after the initiation of anticoagulation with warfarin, hemorrhagic blisters evolve into large open wounds involving the full thickness of the skin and subcutaneous fat. Tissue injury can occur in other tissues but is generally less severe.

In some cases, patients may have received multiple courses of warfarin before the condition develops. The wounds appear primarily in fatty areas such as the breast, buttocks, and thighs, often in a bilaterally symmetrical pattern. Wounds occur due to a hypercoagulable state in susceptible patients (genetic deficiencies of protein C, protein S, antithrombin, or the presence of lupus anticoagulant). A large loading dose of warfarin in such patients deactivates natural anticoagulants, upsetting the natural balance of coagulants and anticoagulants and leading to a transient hypercoagulable state and thrombosis, especially in fatty tissues. A rapid decline in factor VIII and protein C upsets the balance of coagulation and anticoagulation, leading to transient hypercoagulability and thrombosis of fatty tissues in particular. Wounds may appear similar to necrotizing fasciitis or pressure injuries, but a history of recent initiation of oral anticoagulation and biopsy should lead to a diagnosis of warfarin-induced skin necrosis. Reversal of warfarin with the administration of vitamin K combined with anticoagulation with heparin may limit the amount of skin necrosis. Wounds may be several centimeters in diameter and depth. Similar to other wounds associated with vascular occlusion, they are very painful, rendering bedside debridement extremely difficult without adequate pain management. Patients usually recover, requiring debridement and skin grafts, but some cases of mortality have been reported.

Heparin-induced skin necrosis is similar but appears to have a different mechanism that is related to heparin-induced thrombocytopenia type II. Heparin-induced thrombocytopenia occurs in about 1% of those receiving heparin, but only one-third of those develop thrombosis. In some cases, however, the protein C and S mechanism seen with warfarin may be responsible. Those with a history of heparin-induced thrombocytopenia and thrombosis syndrome are at a higher risk of warfarin-induced skin necrosis. In either case, the offending agent is discontinued, and debridement of large quantities of necrotic fatty tissue is required.

EXTRAVASATION NECROSIS

This form of skin necrosis results from the extravasation of intravenous fluid. Extravasation is the escape of fluids into surrounding tissue by leakage or accidental injection of fluid into tissue surrounding a vein. Extravasation is estimated to occur in 0.1% to 6% of patients receiving intravenous lines. Fluids that cause pain in patients with normal cognitive function are unlikely to create serious damage because patients will complain of pain and the problem will be corrected quickly. Therefore, patients with diminished level of consciousness or cognitive status are at greater risk for extravasation necrosis. Both the volume of intravenous fluid allowed to run into the interstitial space and the physicochemical composition of the fluid determine the degree of injury. Skin necrosis may occur within hours or be delayed several days depending on the nature of what is extravasated.

Normal saline and other isotonic fluids produce little or no injury unless a massive quantity of fluid is extravasated. Solutions that can cause tissue injury due to their physicochemical properties are termed *vesicant drugs* or *solutions*. This term's origin is "blistering," as in vesicles. Hypertonic glucose solutions, calcium chloride/gluconate solutions, sodium bicarbonate solutions, and chemotherapeutic drugs are the most likely substances to cause severe skin necrosis. Hypertonic fluids move more fluid into the interstitial space than isotonic fluids due to a direct osmotic effect and then indirectly due to the osmotic effect of cell death. Movement of hypertonic fluid into the interstitial space may create positive feedback in terms of osmotic effect, fluid movement into the interstitial space, pressure, and cell death within the compartment. Some cancer chemotherapeutic drugs act as irritants, but many cause cell death directly. Tissue necrosis accelerates if thrombosis of vessels occurs within the compartment. Skin necrosis may be severe even with salvage of the remainder of the limb. The range of injury may be limited to edema, erythema, pain, and burning sensation. Dry desquamation and blistering may occur with greater injury, especially with chemotherapeutic agents. Full-thickness wounds with eschar formation and absence of granulation tissue will occur with greater injury. More severe injury may be accompanied by additional complications of compartment syndrome such as paralysis, sensory loss, and amputation.

KIDNEY FAILURE

Several aspects of kidney failure impact the health of the skin. Pruritus caused by accumulation of nitrogen compounds in the blood can result in secondary injury from scratching. Patients should be instructed to pat areas of skin that itch to avoid injury. Skin is also weakened from the xerosis (drying) and scaling (ichthyosis) that often occur, which, when combined, is termed *ichthyosiform appearance*. The presence of uremic frost and the odor of urea on the skin, in addition to pruritus, xerosis, and ichthyosis, are clear indicators of poorly controlled kidney failure. Patients will be receiving hemodialysis and may be awaiting kidney transplants. A more serious consequence described later in this chapter is calciphylaxis, a

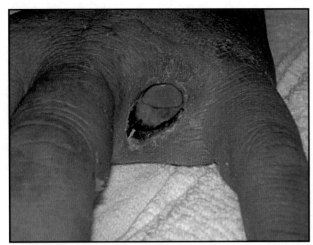

Figure 18-6. Amputation wound secondary to steal syndrome in patient following placement of dialysis shunt (see also Figure 2-10C).

complication occurring in a small number of those receiving dialysis for end-stage kidney disease. Uremic frost is the crystallization of urea on the skin. Areas of a few millimeters to centimeters of white, frostlike patches occur on the skin due to the evaporation of sweat with a high urea concentration.

Hemodialysis is performed either through a large-bore catheter, often inserted in a jugular vein, or a shunt is created in the forearm to attach the arterial and venous access needed for dialysis. Either an arteriovenous fistula or arteriovenous graft may be used. The fistula is created surgically by anastomosing a forearm artery and vein. Alternatively, a length of grafting material may be used to connect an artery and vein for the hemodialysis access. Potential complications include overloading of the venous vessel, resulting in venous hypertension in the upper extremity, the development of an aneurysm as the vein is dilated by the arterial pressure, or the leakage of blood coagulating under the skin, creating a pseudoaneurysm.

More critically, the shunt decreases the arterial inflow reserve to the hand. Pre-existing atherosclerosis of the upper extremity combined with either an arteriovenous shunt or graft can lead to ischemia of the hand, producing what is termed *steal syndrome*. Blood that should be nourishing the hand is "stolen" by the shunt, producing ischemia of the hand. This can lead to ischemia or even gangrene of digits. Complaints of pain; signs of decreased blood flow to the hand including loss of hair; and thin, glossy, atrophied skin on the affected hand should be reported to the patient's nephrologist before gangrene occurs. Patients should be asked whether they experience any unusual fatigue or pain of the hand with prolonged use. Worsening of the steal syndrome may result in pain at rest and gangrenous changes of the hand, resulting in amputation as shown in Figure 18-6.

CALCIFICATION DISORDERS

The 2 main disorders of calcification are calcinosis cutis and the complication of hemodialysis known as *calciphylaxis*.

Calcinosis Cutis

Calcinosis cutis is a term representing a number of disorders characterized by deposits of calcium in the skin. Four classes of calcinosis cutis have been described: dystrophic, metastatic, iatrogenic, and idiopathic. The dystrophic form is secondary to another injury, leading to calcium deposits in the injured tissue. Tissue trauma may result from any of a large number of causes, including neoplastic disease, acne, insect bites, varicose veins, autoimmune disorders, burn, or mechanical trauma. Injured tissue promotes binding of phosphate to denatured proteins, followed by binding of calcium to phosphate and precipitation of crystals. Metastatic calcinosis cutis is caused by metabolic disorders, principally parathyroid, resulting in hypercalcemia, hyperphosphatemia, or both. The high concentration allows calcium phosphate crystals to precipitate in body fluids as hydroxyapatite or amorphous calcium phosphate.

Although calcinosis cutis is a benign process, patients may develop painful lesions, and, depending on the location of lesions, joint mobility or compression of neurons may produce additional pain. Lesions may ulcerate and become infected. In metastatic calcinosis, the underlying disorder such as chronic renal failure or parathyroid disease may cause substantial morbidity. Usually calcinosis lesions have a gradual onset and are asymptomatic. A pre-existing injury may be associated with a dystrophic lesion. Idiopathic calcinosis cutis is not associated with tissue injury or metabolic disease producing elevated calcium or phosphate concentration. Iatrogenic calcinosis cutis is produced by treatment for another condition.

Diagnosis of calcinosis cutis is generally straightforward with the clinical presentation and a biopsy of a lesion displaying calcium deposits. Lesions may be located dermally or subcutaneously but are readily accessible for biopsy. Lesions of calcinosis cutis vary with the etiology. Patients generally present with multiple firm papules or nodules distributed in areas typical for the etiology. Some types produce palpable crystalline material on the lesion's surface. An example is shown in Figure 18-7A. Lesions may ulcerate, and chalky crystal accumulation can be observed within the ulcerated lesion. Lesions of this appearance are also characteristic of gout. Severe calcinosis can affect blood vessels, leading to ischemia and gangrene. Dystrophic lesions are limited to specific, localized area of tissue injury. Metastatic lesions tend to be large and

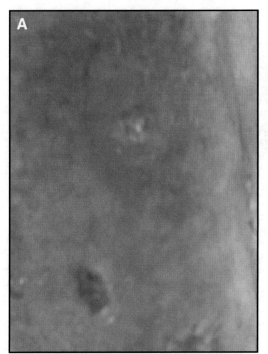 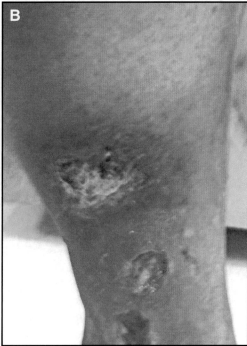

Figure 18-7. Ulcers caused by deranged calcium homeostasis. (A) Calcinosis cutis. (B) Calciphylaxis.

symmetrically distributed. They are commonly located in the areas of larger joints, especially knees, elbow, and shoulders. If dystrophic cutaneous calcinosis is present, visceral and blood vessel deposits are very likely present and will lead to significant morbidity and mortality if the underlying cause is not adequately treated. Idiopathic calcinosis cutis may occur anywhere but is usually limited to one area. Iatrogenic calcinosis cutis is essentially the same process as dystrophic, but the skin trauma is caused by treatment for another disorder.

Treatment for calcinosis cutis is frequently of little value. Treatment is directed toward the underlying cause if it can be identified. Injection of corticosteroids into lesions may produce some benefit. Surgical excision of lesions may be indicated if they lead to excessive pain, recurrent ulceration and infection, or some functional impairment. However, recurrence frequently occurs following excision, and excision may stimulate further calcinosis, exacerbating the problem. Localized wound care of open lesions to prevent or clear infection may become necessary.

Calciphylaxis

Calciphylaxis is a specific type of calcinosis associated with dialysis and end-stage renal failure. Calcification of blood vessels and subcutaneous tissue produces significant lesions that erode the skin, revealing large chalky subcutaneous deposits several centimeters across (Figure 18-7B). The lesions of calciphylaxis are frequently bilateral and fairly symmetrical. Lesions seem to develop suddenly, and skin necrosis may proceed rapidly over the course of several days. The wound bed changes over the course of several days from yellow to brown and black with desiccation of necrotic tissue. Disease characterized by lesions located on the lower extremities has a much lower mortality than disease producing lesions on the trunk. Mortality is high with distal involvement (45%) and approaches 100% with trunk involvement. Because of the intense pain of the lesions and the high mortality, aggressive debridement and dressing changes in an effort to produce a clean, stable wound bed appropriate for healing is generally not a reasonable goal, particularly for lesions on the trunk.

The mechanism of calciphylaxis remains a mystery. Components of the disorder include chronic kidney failure, hypercalcemia, hyperphosphatemia, excessive calcium phosphate product, and secondary hyperparathyroidism. These problems of calcium and phosphate metabolism are common in end-stage renal failure, but only a small fraction (1% to 4%) of those with end-stage disease develop calciphylaxis. Additional factors that might trigger calciphylaxis in end-stage renal failure such as inherited immune components or comorbidity have not yet been identified. Mortality is associated with sepsis due to both infected skin lesions and organ failure. Calciphylaxis is more common in women (3:1) than in men and mostly in middle age. Longer-term dialysis appears to increase risk. Calciphylaxis may appear despite a patient receiving a renal transplant.

Medical care for calciphylaxis is primarily support-ive. Treatment may include efforts to improve control of calcium and phosphate homeostasis and elimination of any of the trigger factors just listed. Administration of intravenous sodium thiosulfate may help by increasing the solubility of calcium deposits in tissues to allow excretion of excessive calcium. Another potential strategy is infusion of low-dose tissue plasminogen activator.

If aggressive debridement becomes necessary to avoid sepsis, debridement under general anesthesia is recom-mended due to the extensive and painful nature of the lesions. Negative pressure wound therapy following thor-ough debridement may be followed by grafting in select cases.

BARIATRICS

The topic of bariatrics in wound management becomes more important as obesity has become more prevalent. Estimates have been given as two-thirds of the population is overweight and one-half of the population is considered obese by Centers for Disease Control and Prevention standards. According to the Centers for Disease Control and Prevention, overweight for an adult is defined as a body mass index (BMI) between 25 and 29.9, and obese is defined as a BMI greater than or equal to 30. BMI is computed as weight in kilograms divided by the square of height in meters (kg/m^2). For example, a person who is 100 kg and 2 m tall has a BMI of 25 (220 pounds and 6 feet 7 inches). Increasing body weight carries the risk of comorbidity associated with wounds. These include type 2 diabetes mellitus, cardiovascular disease in general, lipid disorders, coronary artery disease, and hypertension. Additionally, being overweight requires a greater cardiac output to supply increased body mass, may obstruct venous and lymphatic vessels of the extremities, and compromises the ability to determine blood pressure by sphygmoma-nometry. The inability to produce sufficient diaphragmatic excursion due to obesity leads to chronic hypoventila-tion, which is termed *obesity hypoventilation syndrome* or *Pickwickian syndrome*. Obesity is also associated with obstructive sleep apnea, which can produce severe hypox-emia during sleep and arrhythmias. Orthopnea may also develop for the same reasons as Pickwickian syndrome and obstructive sleep apnea. Following surgery, the obese individual may experience prolonged recovery from gen-eral anesthesia. Chemicals used for general anesthesia are highly lipid soluble. Greater fat mass yields a large reservoir of general anesthetic that can impair the patient's ability to achieve full arousal, and an obese individual can remain groggy for an extended period after surgery. This condi-tion is known as *resedation phenomenon* and may lead to extended periods of immobility and increased risk of peri-operative pressure injuries.

Perineal skin is placed at risk due to the greater effects of incontinence. Cleaning the perineal area is more dif-ficult due to obesity, and decreased mobility secondary to the combination of illness or injury with increased weight may lead to *functional incontinence*, a term describ-ing insufficient mobility to reach appropriate toileting facilities.

Other issues associated with obesity are the greater prevalence of type 2 diabetes mellitus, gall bladder disease, and gastroesophageal reflux disease. Nutritional deficits are common due to an unbalanced diet or episodes of severe caloric restriction. Although weight loss may be an appropriate long-term goal, an individual with obesity is susceptible to protein malnutrition when illness or injury is experienced. Negative nitrogen balance can occur even with an abundant supply of adipose tissue under these conditions. Consultation with a clinical dietitian is necessary to ensure proper dietary therapy. During recovery from an illness or injury, recovery of mobility and exercise tolerance may be very slow because of the greater body mass in the face of a period of inactivity and loss of muscular strength. Obesity is often associated with emotional and financial stressors that may impair efforts to provide optimal wound care.

Skin Changes With Obesity

Tension placed on skin due to obesity increases the risk of skin tears. Other skin changes that may be related to tension placed on the skin include benign neoplasms called *acrochordons* (skin tags); acanthosis nigricans; hyperkera-tosis; xerosis (excessive skin dryness); skin infections with *Staphylococcus*, *Streptococcus*, and *Candida* species; and intertrigo. Acanthosis nigricans is a hyperpigmented, vel-vety-textured area of skin commonly located on skin flex-ures, especially the nape of the neck and axillae. Acanthosis nigricans is also associated with diabetes mellitus and certain forms of cancer. It is believed to be caused by exces-sive serum insulin that stimulates abnormal skin growth secondary to insulin resistance. Acanthosis nigricans may be hereditary, idiopathic, or associated with gastric cancer or polycystic ovary syndrome.

Skin tags have many similarities to acanthosis nigri-cans. They are distributed on the neck, axillae, and groin. They are also commonly found on eyelids. They may also be called *pedunculated papillomas* or *fibroepithelial polyps*. Because they are innervated, anesthesia is required for their excision. In addition to their association with obesity, skin tags are associated with pregnancy and polycystic ovary syndrome.

Xerosis associated with obesity leads to easy fissuring and portals of entry for bacteria and fungus. Bunching of skin results in skinfolds that accumulate warmth and mois-ture, creating an environment suitable for bacterial and fungal growth. Intertrigo is the rashlike injury to such skin.

The skin deep within folds can be extremely erythematous and malodorous. Skin under breasts and pannus are particularly prone to intertrigo. Pannus is the skinfold of the abdomen that may cover the pubic, inguinal, and anterior thigh skin. Zinc oxide or other skin protectants used for incontinence may be used in these areas. Topical antibacterial or antifungal medications may also be used. Silver-containing alginate dressings have also been proposed as a means of controlling intertrigo.

Although the presence of subcutaneous adipose tissue between skin and bony prominences provides cushioning and theoretically reduces the risk of pressure injuries, severe obesity can create so much skin tension that the benefit of subcutaneous cushioning is lost. Instead, the skin is pulled so taut that pressure below it is actually increased. Massive pressure injuries on areas such as the low back/upper gluteal, sacral, and ischial tuberosities may occur when a tremendously obese individual loses mobility for an extended period. Wounds greater than 10 to 15 cm (4 to 6 inches) deep may occur at the low back in very large, immobile individuals. Other sites at risk include anywhere medical devices, tubes, and lines are left under the skin. Skin over the greater trochanters may also be injured by sitting in wheelchairs that are too narrow. Placing the person in a reclined position is an even greater risk for the obese person because shearing on the skin becomes greater due to the increased body mass. Skin is also at risk due to difficulty in repositioning a heavy person. Skin of an obese person is subjected to greater friction during repositioning, and the effectiveness of repositioning may be compromised by the inability to visualize what area of skin is supporting body weight. Although areas of contact with the support surface might appear to be moved, the same bony prominences and skin may remain in contact with the support surface. The inability to see where the patient is in contact with the mattress and the movement of large amounts of tissue above the surface can be deceptive to the uninitiated person. To be certain that the person has actually been repositioned, a person may need to be pulled across the bed with a device specifically designed for repositioning obese individuals.

Surgical intervention such as gastric bypass, gastric banding, or similar procedures may be used to induce malabsorption as a means of reducing body weight. Although many patients who undergo these procedures have no postoperative morbidity, many will have difficulty with healing of surgical incisions, infection, and dehiscence of surgical wounds. Successful weight loss may exacerbate or induce intertrigo as subcutaneous fat is lost and skinfolds overlap more than they did preoperatively. Removal of pannus (panniculectomy) may be considered cosmetic and not covered by insurance, although the presence of pannus remains a risk to skin integrity.

CRITICAL CARE

Another area of concern is intensive care units (ICUs). Patients in ICUs have approximately double the risk of pressure injuries of other patients in a given facility. Skin is at greater risk due to decreased health in general, relative malnutrition created by increased metabolic demand, decreased mobility, and the presence of multiple medical devices attached to the patient. The patient's diminished health and nutrition reduce the skin's tolerance for unrelieved pressure and shear as well as adhesives used to secure devices. Medical device positioning is a particular area of concern because 50% of hospital-acquired pressure injuries are caused by medical devices such as Foley catheters and intravenous lines. Friction from passive repositioning and shearing from the patient being placed in a reclining position for cardiovascular conditioning also increase the risk of pressure injuries. As patients become very ill and develop organ failure, skin injury becomes more likely. Low blood pressure and cardiac output reduce perfusion of skin. Higher extraction of oxygen secondary to low cardiac output leads to hypoxia of the blood perfusing the skin. Venous return from the lower extremities is compromised from compression of blood vessels exacerbating problems with oxygen delivery exacerbated by low cardiac output, which can produce edema of the extremities with further compromise of the nutrition of the skin.

Interventions for patients in the ICU include providing more frequent and meticulous skin examination. Appropriate cleaning after episodes of incontinence and use of skin protectants can reduce the risk of injury. Foley catheters and rectal tubes or pouches may be necessary to prevent injury to the perineal skin. Positioning a person in bed requires greater care to avoid injuries to the skin. Following repositioning, the linens under the patient should be checked to avoid wrinkles and bunching of the sheets, blankets, and underpads. Underpads should also be changed frequently to prevent the retention of fluid against the skin along with inspection of the bed itself for any foreign objects. Caps from medical devices, eating utensils, pieces of food, and cellular telephones have been found under patients turned to receive wound care.

LIFE SPAN

Both older patients with compromised general health and newborns, especially those born prematurely, are at greater risk of skin injury.

Aging Skin

A number of aspects of the gross morphology of aging skin are clearly evident. These include decreased moisture content manifested as greater roughness and scaliness of the skin, decreased elasticity manifested as wrinkling and laxity, the accumulation of benign neoplasms, and increased risk of malignant neoplasms. Some of these effects, however, do not simply appear to be the effect of aging but are due to the accumulation of sun damage. At the microscopic level, flattening of the dermal-epidermal junction can be observed with effacement of dermal papillae. The height of dermal papillae decreases 55% from the third to the ninth decade. As this change occurs, the surface between the vascularized dermis and the epidermis decreases. Several changes observed in the skin of older patients result from the decreased contact between these layers. The area available for nutrient transfer, the number of actively reproducing keratinocytes within the stratum basale, and decreased resistance to shearing result from this loss of contact surface between the dermis and epidermis. Skin changes described with arterial disease such as "cigarette paper" skin with visible blood vessels are also common in the skin of older individuals.

Aging Epidermis

The thickness of the stratum corneum remains unchanged with aging, but increased size and variability of cells are observed. In addition, the number of melanocytes decreases at a rate of about 10% to 20% per decade. As a result of the decline in the number of melanocytes, the skin has a progressively decreased protection from ultraviolet light. In addition, the resident macrophages of the epidermis, the Langerhans cells, experience a 20% to 50% decrease.

Aging Dermis

As opposed to the epidermis, the dermis experiences a significant decrease in its thickness, averaging about 20%. This decrease in thickness produces the transparent appearance of older skin. Due to a 30% decrease in mast cells, less inflammation results from ultraviolet exposure. In addition, regression of the dermal vascular bed and decreased blood flow to appendages lead to gradual atrophy and fibrosis of appendages. Remodeling of elastic fibers into thicker, disorganized elastic fibers causes diminished elasticity and increased risk of tearing.

Functional Changes in the Skin

A 30% to 50% decrease in epidermal turnover has been described from the third to the eighth decade. In addition, a decreased repair rate has been quantified as both decreased wound tensile strength and collagen deposition. Dry, inelastic skin with larger, more irregular epidermal cells leads to decreased barrier function. Moreover, decreased sensory perception increases the risk of injury to skin by mechanical forces such as pressure. Decreased sebum, estimated to decline by 23% per decade, allows the skin to become dry. Due to decreased numbers of Langerhans cells, immunity within the skin declines, putting the skin at higher risk of infection. Due to the more rigid, less elastic, drier nature of older skin with decreased contact area between the dermis and epidermis, the skin of older individuals tears and bleeds easily. Skin tears and multiple ecchymoses are commonplace in the skin of older individuals, especially those with multiple intravenous lines, and with the use of tape to hold intravenous lines in place.

Modifications for the Care of Aging Skin

Foremost, the choice of wound products to be used on the skin of older patients must take into account the fragile nature of the skin. Moreover, because of decreased inflammation and greater risk of malnutrition and dehydration, the clinician must assume a longer period for healing. Therefore, dressings that need to be changed frequently or have strong adhesive need to be used with caution or avoided. Tape of any kind must be used judiciously. In particular, silk and plastic tape should not be used. Alternatives such as stretch netting should be considered. When occlusive dressings are chosen, hydrocolloids and semipermeable films should be used only if other types are not practical. Dressings with silicone adhesives are less likely to damage skin but are more expensive. If films or hydrocolloid sheets are to be used, skin protectant needs to be placed on the surrounding skin. In addition, the absorbency of the dressing needs to be optimized. Although thin hydrocolloid sheets permit better visualization of the wound, thicker hydrocolloid sheets may be necessary to prolong time between changes. Filling the wound with an absorbent material such as alginate or hydrofiber can also prolong wearing time of hydrocolloid and semipermeable film dressings. When these dressings are removed, care must be taken to avoid injury to the skin. The skin should not be pulled with the dressing as it is removed. Gentle peeling of hydrocolloid sheets or stretching of a semipermeable film tangentially to the skin surface as the skin is held in place may reduce the risk of injury.

Cleansing of wounds needs to be done as gently as possible. Pulsatile lavage with suction may be done at a lower impact pressure or replaced by gentle irrigation as necessary. Mechanical damage and maceration can result from vigorous whirlpool therapy for cleansing or nonselective debridement. In the case of many older patients, the clinician must consider the risks and benefits of different types of debridement. Frequently, orders are received for whirlpool and wet-to-dry dressings on the wounds of older patients. Additives to the whirlpools or topical agents placed on the wound may cause severe injury to the wound or surrounding skin. Older patients with wounds who are in the terminal stage of an illness may not benefit from the full range of options available from the clinician. The clinician must ask themselves what benefits the patient will receive from any given intervention. In many cases, wound healing is not achievable due to the nutritional or cardiopulmonary status of the patient, and goals are limited to reducing the risk of infection and managing drainage and odor of the wound. In these cases, treatment consisting of optimizing autolytic debridement is appropriate unless the wound is infected or infection is imminent.

Prevention of Skin Injury in Older Patients

In addition to selecting wound care products carefully, a number of other forms of skin protection should be considered. The skin of older adults tends to become dry and brittle and may fissure and tear with minor trauma. Therapeutic moisturizers may be necessary, especially during the winter or in low-humidity environments. Bed frames and rails should be inspected for sharp edges and padded as needed.

Children

In general, wound healing is more rapid in children than in adults. However, younger children present challenges to wound management. Permission to evaluate and treat children must be obtained from an appropriate adult, usually a parent. Children may not fully understand the interventions and may be fearful and reluctant to receive interventions, particularly pulsatile lavage, sharp debridement, and packing/unpacking wounds. The presence of parents to calm children needs to be assessed on a case-by-case basis. Although some parents may be able to calm a child sufficiently for interventions to be provided, some parents may create a negative environment by being too permissive and allowing tantrums or by being too harsh and increasing the child's anxiety. Children may be more

cooperative if they have the opportunity to inspect or playact any interventions ahead of time with appropriate considerations for infection control. Children should never be left alone in a treatment room because they may become curious and either hurt themselves or contaminate equipment and supplies.

Any parent/guardian in the treatment area will require face masks for protection from airborne microbes along with the patient. Other personal protective equipment will depend on the possibility of secondary contamination. In general, clothing worn by the patient's parent can be treated as the clothing from the patient. If another person with compromised immunity may be exposed to the clothing of the parent, the parent should either wear personal protective equipment or change clothing before encountering anyone with compromised immunity.

Very young children, such as infants, may be difficult to manage because nothing can be explained to them. Infants may also be more susceptible to infection than older children. Clinicians with any signs of respiratory disease should avoid treating infants, children with decreased immunity, or children with sickle cell disease. Rooms used with children should be thoroughly disinfected before and after treatments, especially when hydrotherapy from either whirlpools or pulsatile lavage is used.

Dressings chosen for a child, as those chosen for older patients, should minimize frequency of changes and trauma. However, another consideration may be the durability of dressings for highly active children. Children may be encouraged to avoid physical activity that may disturb wound dressings, but the frequent reality is that this advice will be ignored. Dressings that can stand up to potential physical activity should be chosen. In addition, parents should be instructed early in reinforcing or changing dressings, including principles of sterile technique, disinfection of any scissors or other instruments, and contingencies for changes in the wound's status.

Neonates

Premature neonates have a thinner stratum corneum that allows more evaporation with the potential for dry skin and greater susceptibility to injury. Vernix is a "cheesy" covering of premature neonatal skin that provides protection against evaporation and trauma. A well-intentioned person may attempt to clean vernix from the skin, putting the neonate's skin at risk. Other risk factors for skin injury include the lack of subcutaneous fat to cushion and protect against medical device–related pressure injury. The sheer number of devices and difficulty in tracking all of them also place the skin at risk. Epidermal tears, blisters, and abrasion are more common with prematurity.

TABLE 18-1
Elements of Braden Q

Mobility	1. Completely immobile	2. Very limited	3. Slightly limited	4. No limitation
Activity	1. Bedfast	2. Chair fast	3. Walks occasionally	4. Too young to walk or walks frequently
Sensory perception	1. Completely limited	2. Very limited	3. Slightly limited	4. No impairment
Moisture	1. Constantly moist	2. Very moist	3. Occasionally moist	4. Rarely moist
Friction—shear	1. Significant problem	2. Problem	3. Potential problem	4. No apparent problem
Nutrition	1. Very poor	2. Inadequate	3. Adequate	4. Excellent
Tissue perfusion and oxygenation	1. Extremely compromised	2. Compromised	3. Adequate	4. Excellent

Points are added for each category. The top 3 categories are under the heading of "Intensity and Duration of Pressure" in the full score sheet. The bottom 4 categories are under the heading of *Tolerance of the Skin and Supporting Structure* in the full score sheet. See Noonan C, Quigley S, Curley MAQ. Using the Braden Q scale to predict pressure ulcer risk in pediatric patients. *J Pediatr Nurs.* 2011;26(6):566-575 for full chart.

Risk factors for injury include the presence of adhesives and medical devices; chemical burns from products not designed for neonatal skin; intravenous infiltration due to difficulty in placing intravenous lines in such small veins; birthing injuries from forceps and suction; diaper dermatitis; and injuries from lines used for high-frequency ventilation, extracorporeal membrane oxygenation, and nasal continuous positive airway pressure. Hypotension and hypoperfusion of the skin are additional risk factors, particularly in premature neonates in a critical care unit.

The Braden scale has been adapted to children (Table 18-1), called the Braden Q score. Another assessment tool is the Neonatal Skin Condition Score (Table 18-2).

PREVENTIVE MEASURES

As much as possible, nonadhesive dressings and devices for supporting equipment should be used. If adhesives must be used, long-wearing silicone-based adhesives should be used and foam dressings placed under lines where pressure could be transmitted to the skin. Use of positioning aids may decrease the need for adhesives. Moisture barriers on the perineum and buttocks containing zinc oxide, petrolatum, or dimethicone may be used to reduce the risk of diaper dermatitis and potential skin breakdown.

END OF LIFE

When discussing skin and wound care at the end of life, the focus changes from restorative to palliative care. In the common situation of restorative care, focus is placed on the return to the former level of function including closure and healing of wounds. However, in palliative care, the focus is the support of patients and caregivers and providing comfort rather than cure.

Pressure Injury Risk Factors at End of Life

With terminal disease, as well as any condition resulting in diminished mobility, several risk factors for pressure injuries increase. Patients may develop hip and knee contractures, becoming contracted in the fetal position. When this occurs, the only turning surfaces available expose the sacral and greater trochanter areas to even greater risk. The lack of alternative turning surfaces may lead to the inevitable development of pressure injuries in these 3 sites. Pressure injuries may develop in other susceptible locations in the sidelying or Fowler's position (recumbent with hips and knees flexed). Heart failure, end-stage kidney disease, hypoventilation, acidosis, malnutrition, and a generalized compromise of homeostatic mechanisms result in compromise to the skin's nutrient supply and waste

TABLE 18-2
Elements of Neonatal Skin Condition Score

SKIN CONDITION SCORE					
Dryness	1.	Normal	2.	Dry skin	3. Very dry skin
Erythema	1.	None	2.	< 50% BSA	3. > 50% BSA
Breakdown	1.	None	2.	Small local	3. Extensive
SCORE SUM OF DRYNESS + ERYTHEMA + BREAKDOWN					
SEPARATE SCORE FOR ERYTHEMA OF PERINEAL AREA					

0. None	1. Slight	2. Moderate	3. Strong	4. Nonintact

See Lund CH, Osborne JW. Validity and reliability of the neonatal skin condition score. *J Obstet Gynecol Neonatal Nurs.* 2004;33(3):320-327 for complete scoring.

removal. Risk of skin injury is increased with urinary and fecal incontinence that frequently occurs in association with immobility and loss of homeostasis.

Definition of Skin Failure

Skin failure may be considered part of multisystem organ failure. As the body's largest organ, the skin becomes susceptible to failure for several reasons. Acute failure may result from a medical crisis leading to a lack of perfusion in conditions such as hypotension or compartment syndrome. Acute illness resulting in anemia, malnutrition, or immobilization also may place skin at risk. Skin injury due to chronic disease may result from prolonged immobilization, decreased skin perfusion due to chronic heart failure, and malnutrition due to disease involving the alimentary tract. Chronic illnesses may accumulate (eg, congestive heart failure, kidney failure, anemia, immobility, incontinence, and other diseases that predispose one to skin injury). Most commonly, acute illness superimposed on chronic disease is likely to lead to skin injury. For example, a person with poorly controlled diabetes mellitus may fracture a hip; develop an infection; or experience lower extremity clotting, pulmonary embolus, and multiple other problems resulting in a downward spiral of health that might not have occurred but for the underlying chronic disease of diabetes mellitus.

Kennedy Terminal Ulcer

The classic sign of skin failure occurs in the sacrococcygeal area and has been dubbed the "Kennedy terminal ulcer." Like many stage 4 pressure injuries, the resulting skin failure seems to occur suddenly due to necrosis occurring deeply at first. In most cases, the skin in the sacrococcygeal area becomes red, purple, and then black within

hours and results in a pear-shaped ulcer. This ulcer, indicative of the skin failure component of multisystem failure, is often observed within 24 hours of death. Evidence for this specific type of ulcer has been challenged recently, and efforts have been made to cease the use of this term. The phenomenon described by Kennedy from her small number of cases has not been duplicated and would appear to be a case of selection bias rather than a systematic effect. More recent studies have suggested describing such cases simply as skin failure rather than a Kennedy terminal ulcer.

Palliative Care

Palliative care is provided to individuals known to have a terminal condition. Under Medicare hospice rules, time of death is expected to be within 6 months as certified by a physician. Many individuals may exceed the expected life span or may decline more rapidly. Hospice care paid by Medicare may be provided through either home or inpatient care. Under hospice, patients may not receive treatments specific to the cure of a condition but may receive services that provide improved quality of life by increasing patient comfort and pain relief.

Healing of ulcers already present may not be a reasonable expectation depending on the underlying disease. If a patient has a condition decreasing perfusion to the area of a skin injury due to peripheral arterial disease, low cardiac output, or hematocrit, healing is not expected. If the patient does not have skin injury already, measures to decrease the risk of pressure injuries are in order. The patient's sensation; mobility; and skin condition, including moisture, friction, and shear, need to be assessed. The level of activity in bed (or out of bed if possible) and nutrition, hydration, and body weight should be part of the examination as well.

After physical examination and discussion of patient and caregiver needs and abilities, appropriate goals for palliative wound care may be determined. The most common goals include preventing deterioration and infection of the wound and minimizing the risk of skin injury elsewhere. Because healing may not be a reasonable goal, clinical decisions should be weighted toward patient comfort and minimizing pain. For example, aggressive sharp debridement and frequent dressing changes may not be in the patient's best interest. If a wound is deteriorating and infection is likely to spread, however, aggressive debridement may be necessary. Managing odor and drainage take greater precedence for reasons of the patient's psychosocial well-being. Preventing the loss of social support system due to odor or unpleasant appearance of wound drainage should be addressed in the plan of care.

Dressings used in palliative care should be chosen to minimize the number of changes and pain during changes. Dressings that reduce odor and more effectively manage drainage may also be chosen. However, dressings must be chosen also to minimize the risk of infection. Decreased immunity may be associated with terminal conditions. Several strategies for odor control are available. Because decreasing the risk of infection takes precedence over healing in this state, using cytotoxic agents such as acetic acid or Dakin's solution can be appropriate. Other choices include silver and other antimicrobial dressings. Even in the case of a noninfected wound, the accumulation of drainage under an occlusive dressing may produce an unpleasant odor. Several dressings are available with charcoal to absorb odor and allow dressing changes to be done less frequently. Some compromise between pain management and pain may become necessary when debridement or cleansing the wound are the only means available to control odor and infection. Another solution to odor control is the placement of charcoal or cat litter designed to absorb odors under the patient's bed.

SUMMARY

Atypical wounds are those not associated with those described in previous chapters. Their appearance, location, and history vary from venous, arterial, pressure, and other types covered previously. A lack of response to therapy, unusual odor, bleeding, and itching are other clues of atypical wounds.

Obesity and extremes in life span increase the risk of skin injury, particularly due to pressure. Being proactive and treating these individuals as being at high risk of injury is necessary as well as using products that are gentler to the skin.

Multiorgan system failure may include skin failure. In palliative care, one must determine the needs and priorities of both patients and caregivers. The need for aggressive debridement must be weighed against patient discomfort. Dressings should be chosen that minimize trauma but do not promote pain, leakage, or odor. Cues for atypical wounds include an appearance or location that is out of the ordinary, failure to heal or worsens over time, and abnormal-appearing granulation tissue. In these cases, a biopsy should be performed by an appropriate clinician to rule out neoplastic, infectious, or inflammatory disease.

QUESTIONS

1. What are considered to be the 6 "typical" types of wounds?
2. What else defines a wound as atypical?
3. Do biopsies and lab tests always identify atypical wounds?
4. What is the presumed cause of a fungating wound?
5. What are the 2 general causes of fungating wounds?
6. Where are sickle cell ulcers most commonly found?
7. What is the typical appearance of sickle cell ulcers?
8. What is the preferred form of debridement for sickle cell ulcers?
9. What is Marjolin's ulcer?
10. What is the typical appearance?
11. How is it diagnosed conclusively?
12. What is the underlying cause of pyoderma gangrenosum?
13. What is the typical appearance?
14. How is pyoderma gangrenosum diagnosed?
15. How is pyoderma gangrenosum treated?
16. Why are debridement and grafting not initially performed?
17. What is pathergy?
18. What are the 2 types of wounds associated with pathergy?
19. What is trash foot?
20. Does this phenomenon occur only in the foot?
21. What is the typical appearance of trash foot?
22. How does Buerger's disease lead to open wounds?
23. What is the underlying cause?
24. Why does venous hypertension occur in some patients with shunts for dialysis? How does the appearance of the skin compare with ambulatory venous hypertension due to venous disease of legs?
25. What happens to the skin in severe kidney disease?

26. What is steal syndrome? What are the consequences?

27. What should you tell such a patient to avoid injury from scratching?

28. Why are patients with obesity prone to postoperative pressure injuries?

29. Why is repositioning a patient with obesity so difficult?

30. What is intertrigo? What causes it?

31. Why are the low back and buttocks particularly susceptible to pressure injuries?

32. Why are patients in the ICU at greater risk of pressure injures than others?

33. What specific differences in aging skin require different strategies in using adhesives?

34. What else can be done to protect the skin of older patients?

35. What changes in the plan of care are needed when a patient is a child?

36. Compare the stratum corneum of the premature newborn to older children and adults.

37. What is often present at birth that protects the skin of premature infants?

38. What are the consequences of the lack of fat and immature epidermis in premature infants?

39. What are the consequences of trying to remove vernix from neonates?

40. Why are premature neonates at increased risk of pressure and related skin injuries?

41. What types of dressings are recommended for neonates?

42. What can be applied to protect the perineum and neighboring skin from feces and urine?

43. What can be applied to the skin to minimize pressure injuries at specific places on the neonate's body?

44. How are outcomes different in palliative care?

45. What can be done to reduce odor of wounds?

46. When should aggressive debridement be performed in a palliative care situation?

BIBLIOGRAPHY

Anderson J, Hanson D, Langemo D, Hunter S, Thompson P. Atypical wounds: recognizing and treating the uncommon. *Adv Skin Wound Care.* 2005;18(9):466-470. doi:10.1097/00129334-200511000-00007

Bazaliński D, Przybek-Mita J, Barańska B, Więch P. Marjolin's ulcer in chronic wounds—review of available literature. *Contemp Oncol (Pozn).* 2017;21(3):197-202. doi:10.5114/wo.2017.70109

Brunssen A, Waldmann A, Eisemann N, Katalinic A. Impact of skin cancer screening and secondary prevention campaigns on skin cancer incidence and mortality: a systematic review. *J Am Acad Dermatol.* 2017;76(1):129-139.e10. doi:10.1016/j.jaad.2016.07.045

Chang JJ. Calciphylaxis: diagnosis, pathogenesis, and treatment. *Adv Skin Wound Care.* 2019;32(5):205-215. doi:10.1097/01.ASW.0000554443.14002.13

Dargon PT, Landry GJ. Buerger's disease. *Ann Vasc Surg.* 2012;26(6):871-880. doi:10.1016/j.avsg.2011.11.005

Fawaz B, Candelario NM, Rochet N, Tran C, Brau C. Warfarin-induced skin necrosis following heparin-induced thrombocytopenia. *Proc (Bayl Univ Med Cent).* 2016;29(1):60-61. doi:10.1080/08998280.2016.11929362

Isoherranen K, O'Brien JJ, Barker J, et al. Atypical wounds. Best clinical practice and challenges. *J Wound Care.* 2019;28(Suppl 6):S1-S92. doi:10.12968/jowc.2019.28.Sup6.S1

Kato GJ, Steinberg MH, Gladwin MT. Intravascular hemolysis and the pathophysiology of sickle cell disease. *J Clin Invest.* 2017;127(3):750-760. doi:10.1172/JCI89741

Lund CH, Osborne JW. Validity and reliability of the neonatal skin condition score. *J Obstet Gynecol Neonatal Nurs.* 2004;33(3):320-327. doi:10.1177/0884217504265174

Noonan C, Quigley S, Curley MAQ. Using the Braden Q scale to predict pressure ulcer risk in pediatric patients. *J Pediatr Nurs.* 2011;26(6):566-575. doi:10.1016/j.pedn.2010.07.006

Pozez AL, Aboutanos SZ, Lucas VS. Diagnosis and treatment of uncommon wounds. *Clin Plast Surg.* 2007;34(4):749-764. doi:10.1016/j.cps.2007.08.012

Simmons J. Getting ready for wound certification: assessment and management of atypical wounds. *J Wound Ostomy Continence Nurs.* 2018;45(5):474-476. doi:10.1097/WON.0000000000000464

19

Documentation

OBJECTIVES

- Describe elements of the medical, family medical, social, work, and home history to document in an initial evaluation.
- Discuss the use of photography for documenting wound management.
- Discuss potential problems that substandard documentation may cause.
- List the 4 necessary components for proving a civil court action.
- Discuss how proper documentation can minimize the risks of denial of payments and lawsuits.

THE NEED FOR DOCUMENTATION

The old axiom has been "If it hasn't been documented, it wasn't done." We have now evolved to optimizing documentation of patient care to maximize reimbursement. Increasingly, we also need to document carefully to avoid legal pitfalls. Regardless of the motivation for documentation, the underlying reason for documentation is to provide a clear road map of where we expect patient care to go, any detours, and the final destination. This is true whether one clinician is in a position to provide care through discharge or multiple clinicians must be involved. The plan of care is developed from a simple flow of thought from what has already been documented.

Many facilities use forms for documenting wound management. Some are universal forms; others use forms specific for wound etiology (eg, thermal injuries, another for pressure injuries, and another for venous ulcers). The advantage of etiology-specific forms is that they can be more efficient and readable because they contain only

Irion GL, Gardner JA, Pignataro RM.
Comprehensive Wound Management, Third Edition (pp 365-385).
© 2024 Taylor and Francis Group.

information pertinent to the wound type. The information requested on the form is more likely to be relevant to the patient, and the clinician will not forget to ask certain questions or perform certain tests relevant to the etiology of the wound. For example, a pressure injury form may contain one of the risk assessment tools such as the Braden or Norton scale, and a form for neuropathic ulcers would contain the elements of foot screening. Another advantage of an etiology-specific form is that it can usually be printed on a single sheet. A single sheet is more likely to be read by other members of the wound management team and other parties who have an interest in the care provided. However, information should not be crammed into a single page such that the readability of the form is compromised. Etiology-specific forms become a problem when the clinician does not know the true cause of a wound. A clinician may not reach an accurate diagnosis even after the form has been completed, especially if a wound presents a difficult differential diagnosis. A compromise is the use of a generic wound care form supplemented with an etiology-specific form. An example of a generic integumentary documentation form is given in Figure 19-1. Supplemental forms specific to venous disease, pressure injuries, thermal injuries, and neuropathic injuries are provided in Figures 19-2, 19-3, 19-4, and 19-5, respectively. However, because electronic medical records (EMRs) are now commonplace, using one form and only documenting in the particular sections relevant to the patient can be simpler.

Proper documentation can be difficult if a logical sequence is not followed. In this chapter, the *Guide to Physical Therapist Practice* (*Guide*) concepts are used as a basis for documentation. This system is based on continuous development and testing of hypotheses of causal and contributing factors that have led to the patient's current state of health. The clinician must then select tests to confirm, refute, or modify hypotheses regarding these causal and contributing factors. As the clinician takes a verbal history or reads a history from another source, the process of developing hypotheses is already occurring. Frequently, a referring clinician has provided a diagnosis for the patient's condition. This referring diagnosis may be a good starting point but must not be the sole focus of the patient history or physical examination. On occasion, the referring diagnosis may be incomplete or inaccurate. In particular, the clinician must be wary of less common etiologies that may masquerade as common types of wounds.

To a great extent, the clinician must perform a complete physical examination and take a history as if none had already been done by another clinician. Failure to confirm data collected by another clinician produces the potential for casually accepting a referring diagnosis and missing a critical piece of information that either generates the diagnosis or contributes to the patient's condition. For example, a patient may be referred with a diagnosis

of cellulitis superior to the medial malleolus with wounds that have remained open for 2 years. Despite the referring diagnosis, the prudent clinician becomes suspicious of venous disease, so the questions and testing start down the road of confirming contributing factors for venous disease rather than accepting the diagnosis of an infection. If the patient reports a history of diabetes, the clinician will immediately begin asking questions related to both neuropathy and peripheral arterial disease. In both cases, the clinician will perform an examination of the peripheral circulation to rule out arterial disease, a contraindication for compression.

ELEMENTS OF THE HISTORY

For facilities other than acute care hospitals, a standardized history form becomes increasingly important. Hospital-based facilities will have a history and physical examination section in the patient's EMR that should contain all relevant information. However, information critical to the treatment plan for the wound should be kept in a specified wound section so an individual taking over care of the patient will not be required to read an entire chart. In addition, the hospital EMR provides lab values and lists medications. This information can supplement what is on the history. For example, a history of congestive heart failure or rheumatoid arthritis may not be explicitly documented in the history and physical. However, medications listed may cue the clinician to inquire about these conditions. In an outpatient facility, the standardized history form can be useful if done carefully. An example of an outpatient history form is given in Figure 19-6. Often, simply asking a patient to fill out the form is not sufficient. With an exhaustive listing of possible ailments, patients are likely to quickly run down the list of irrelevant items and miss an important problem that should have been identified. Key items should be confirmed verbally with the patient. If possible, this should be done with a family member or caregiver, and the patient should be asked directly whether they have any medical conditions that might be related to the wound.

Important questions are generated by both the wound's etiology and any additional diagnoses listed in the history. In particular, questions related to diabetes are critical. Anyone who reports a history of diabetes mellitus should be asked about glycemic control, including current blood glucose and hemoglobin A1c, to determine short- and long-term glycemic control. Questions about standing and walking are particularly important for lower extremity ulcers. A person with wounds consistent with venous disease needs to be asked about standing. A person with apparent neuropathic ulcers needs to be asked about walking, shoes, off-loading techniques used, and other items discussed in Chapter 11.

GENERIC INTEGUMENTARY DOCUMENTATION FORM

Patient_____ Age_____ M F   Clinician_____ Date_____

History
Chief complaint_____
Home arrangements_____
Support system_____
Occupation/education/hobbies/home activities_____
_____
Ambulation required for lifestyle_____
Standing required for lifestyle_____
Current lifestyle limitations_____
Medications_____
Past medical history _____
Previous treatment for condition_____

Review of Systems
Neuromuscular_____
Musculoskeletal_____
Cardiopulmonary_____
Integumentary_____

Physical Examination
Wound photo or drawing here:

Color_____ Odor_____ Drainage _____ Extent_____
Shape_____ Tissue in wound   Black_____ %   Yellow_____ %   Red_____ %

Surrounding Skin
Texture_____ Temperature_____ Swelling: -+   ++   +++   ++++
Color_____ Hair/nails_____ Ecchymosis_____ Hemosiderin_____
Demarcation_____ Maceration_____ Epiboly_____

Diagnosis Impaired integumentary integrity with:
_____Risk of injury   _____Superficial injury
_____Partial-thickness injury   _____Full-thickness injury
_____Full-thickness injury and subcutaneous involvement

Prognosis: Within_____days weeks months, and within_____visits, the patient is expected to:
_____

Plan of Care
Patient and family/caregiver education_____
Procedural interventions_____ frequency_____ duration_____
                                      _____ frequency_____ duration_____
Signature_____ Date_____

Figure 19-1. Generic integumentary documentation form contains a short section for history and physical examination items most directly related to the cause of the wound and several blanks to be filled with words, checks, or "+" signs. The use of this form does not presume any diagnosis or etiology. Instead, the form is a means of keeping the clinician "on track" using the *Guide*. The therapist collects data and performs special tests as needed to rule in or rule out the wound's cause. In the diagnosis section, the clinician chooses with a check mark one or more of the 5 listed diagnoses based on impairments and the *Guide*. The prognosis derives from the diagnosis and the special circumstances of the patient. The plan of care includes patient/family/caregiver education and procedural interventions. To an extent, "goals" are part of the prognosis section; specific documentation requirements may require goals related to functions necessary to the patient (eg, the patient will be able to stand for an 8-hour shift without complaining of pain; the patient will have sufficient range of motion for self-feeding). The final section is only present to allow individuals with a need to know what direct or "procedural" interventions are being performed for the patient, how frequently, and an expected time at which the intervention will no longer be needed. If documentation of functional outcomes is needed, a general initial evaluation form may also need to be used.

SUPPLEMENTAL DATA FOR DIAGNOSIS OF VENOUS ULCERS

Patient_____ Clinician_____ Date_____

Alternatives to standing _____

Location(s)_____

Status of surrounding skin_____

Size of wound(s)	Length_____cm	Width_____cm	Depth	Partial-thickness	Full-thickness
Ankle brachial index	Right_____	Left_____			
Temperature of right foot	normal	increased	decreased		
Temperature of left foot	normal	increased	decreased		
Capillary refill (right)	normal	sluggish	absent		
Capillary refill (left)	normal	sluggish	absent		
Foot volume	Right_____	Left_____			
Wound bed	% Red_____	% Yellow_____	% Black_____		
Color of granulation tissue	red	pink			
Drainage	minimal	moderate	copious		

Color of drainage _____

Compression therapy (specify)_____

Signature_____ Date_____

Figure 19-2. Supplemental data for diagnosis of venous ulcers is used for the patient who is determined by the clinician to have venous ulcers. This form is meant to supplement the generic integumentary documentation form. These items are more directly related to venous ulcer risk factors, prevention of recurrence, and appropriate treatment. Note in particular the items to rule out arterial insufficiency. These items include the ankle-brachial index, foot temperature, capillary refill, and color of granulation tissue. Items used to confirm the suspicion of venous ulcers are also listed and will be illustrated in Figure 19-8.

The patient should also be asked about any symptoms that accompany walking that may be suggestive of intermittent claudication. Questions about lifestyle, general health, vision, balance, and available care at home are important in developing a treatment plan that can be followed by the patient and any caregivers. Information to be documented was discussed thoroughly in Chapters 7 (history) and 8 (physical examination). Examples of completed documentation forms are given in Figures 19-7 through 19-11.

A list of prescription drugs, over-the-counter medications, and herbal remedies should be obtained. Often, patients will not remember all of the medications by name. Asking them to bring in and show all of their medications will improve the drug review's accuracy. Many patients are proactive and carry a list of their medications with them. Other patients are extremely careless with medications. An extreme example is a patient who kept all of their medications in a single bag and took pills of different shapes and colors as they saw fit.

ELEMENTS OF THE PHYSICAL EXAMINATION

The physical examination performed during the initial visit will be much more comprehensive than that of subsequent visits. In particular, general health and mobility and possible complicating factors that may influence the patient's ability to follow a treatment plan need to be explored. Subsequent visits must have some element of examination. However, they are focused more on whether the prognosis developed from the initial visit is still appropriate and gives the clinician the opportunity to explore complications not foreseen during the initial evaluation. General mobility should be evaluated and documented, even if the patient has no mobility. The lack of mobility weighs heavily in the prognosis of certain types of wounds, especially pressure injuries. The quality of gait is also important, particularly for the person with neuropathic feet. The loss of proprioception leads to unsteady gait, loss of heel-toe progression, and, in extreme cases, a wide-based gait with slapping of the foot onto the floor. The inability to control the foot and ankle during gait is a high-risk factor for the person with neuropathy due to increased shearing forces on the plantar surface.

Supplemental Data Form for Pressure Injuries

Patient_____ Clinician_____ Date_____

Stage of injury (identify location on figure at right with wound number)

1.	1	2	3	4	partially filled	filled	covered
2.	1	2	3	4	partially filled	filled	covered
3.	1	2	3	4	partially filled	filled	covered
4.	1	2	3	4	partially filled	filled	covered
5.	1	2	3	4	partially filled	filled	covered

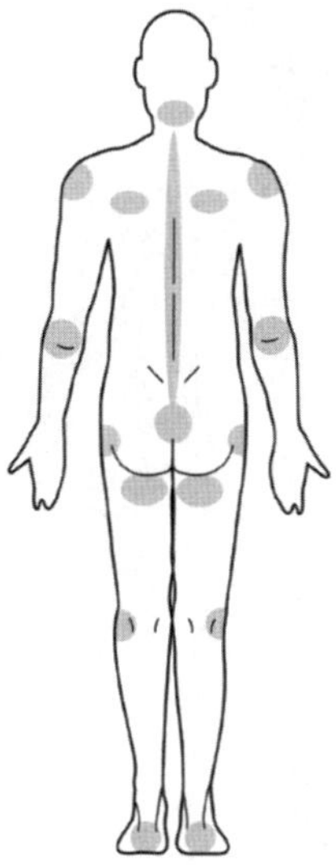

Size of injury (using identification key on right)

1. Length_____cm   Width_____cm   Depth_____cm
2. Length_____cm   Width_____cm   Depth_____cm
3. Length_____cm   Width_____cm   Depth_____cm
4. Length_____cm   Width_____cm   Depth_____cm
5. Length_____cm   Width_____cm   Depth_____cm

Tunneling, sinus tracts, undermining

1. Distance_____cm   Direction_____:00   Drainage_____
2. Distance_____cm   Direction_____:00   Drainage_____
3. Distance_____cm   Direction_____:00   Drainage_____
4. Distance_____cm   Direction_____:00   Drainage_____
5. Distance_____cm   Direction_____:00   Drainage_____

	1	2	3	4	5
Odor	_____	_____	_____	_____	_____
Drainage	_____	_____	_____	_____	_____
% R, Y, B	_____	_____	_____	_____	_____
Surrounding skin condition	_____	_____	_____	_____	_____

Signature_____ Date_____

Figure 19-3. Supplemental data form for pressure injuries is used for the patient with pressure injuries. The first area includes information on the depth and degree of healing of up to 5 injuries. Sadly, many patients will have more than 5 injuries, and a second or third supplemental data form for pressure injuries may be used. Depth of the injury is indicated by using numbers 1 through 4. As discussed in Chapter 10 and elsewhere in the text, many clinicians have difficulty handling documentation of a healing pressure injury. The last 3 columns of "Stage of injury" allow the clinician to document the progress of the wound in addition to the original depth of the injury by which the wound is meant to be staged. To the right, a figure used in Chapter 10 is placed on the form. Note that only a posterior view is used. In this view, wounds on the posterior side of the body and right and left sides can be circled, enumerated, and a line drawn to the circle or ellipse. This view covers a large fraction of pressure injuries, including the problem areas of the occiput, epicondyles of the elbow, sacrum, ischial tuberosities, and heels. If a wound is located on the anterior surface, a note can be written to indicate that the wound is not on the visible side and give a brief description (eg, chin and a line drawn to the figure to indicate the location on the anterior side). Due to the prevalence of tunneling, sinus tracts, and undermining with pressure injuries, a section has been devoted to describe them.

SUPPLEMENTAL FORM FOR THERMAL INJURY

Anterior
Adult head 4.5%   Child head 8.5%
Adult trunk 18%   Child trunk 18%
Adult upper extremity 4.5%   Child upper extremity 4.5%
Adult and Child 1%
Adult lower extremity 9%   Child lower extremity 6.5%

Posterior
Adult head 4.5%   Child head 8.5%
Adult trunk 18%   Child trunk 18%
Adult upper extremity 4.5%   Child upper extremity 4.5%
Adult lower extremity 9%   Child lower extremity 6.5%

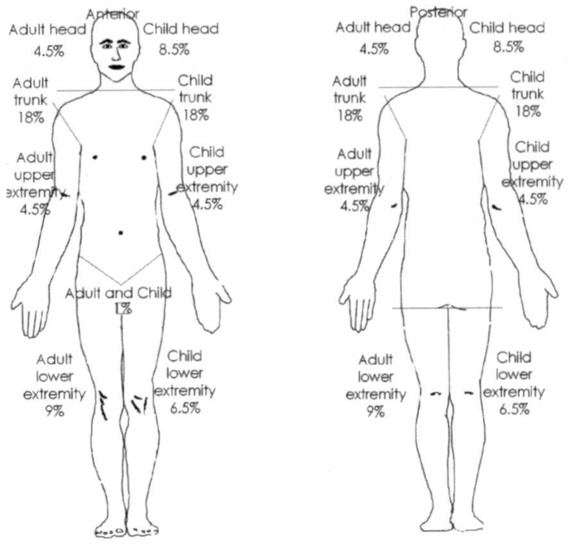

Indicate locations and depths of thermal injuries on the figure to the left.

- - Superficial thickness (1st degree)

//// Superficial partial thickness (2nd degree)

\\\ Deep partial thickness (deep dermal)

xxx Full thickness

	RUE	LUE	RLE	LLE	Anterior trunk	Posterior trunk
Deficits in range of motion	___	___	___	___	_____	_____
Deficits in strength	___	___	___	___	_____	_____
Active exercise	___	___	___	___	_____	_____
Active assisted exercise	___	___	___	___	_____	_____
Passive stretch	___	___	___	___	_____	_____
No movement allowed	___	___	___	___	_____	_____

Deficits in tolerance for bed mobility, bed exercise, position changes, ambulation (specify)_____

Indicate special positioning needs _____

Signature_____   Date_____

Figure 19-4. Supplemental form for thermal injury consists of figures to indicate the extent and depth of thermal injuries, including burns, scalds, and frostbite. This form may also be applicable to chemical and radiation injuries. Different patterns of shading are used to indicate the depth of injury. In some cases, the actual depth may not be certain, especially in the case of distinguishing a deep partial-thickness from a full-thickness wound. A key for the shading is given on the right. The next section is a table with a synopsis of neuromusculoskeletal impairments and appropriate types of movement for the 6 areas of the body, used as headings for the table. In many cases, thermal injuries are limited to 1 or 2 of the segments. For the deficits in range of motion and deficits in strength rows, the clinician may enter a ~ to indicate a deficit, a Ø to indicate no deficits in that body region, or may explicitly state a movement or muscle group affected. The next 4 rows of the table use the same 6 body regions, and a ~ is entered in 1 of the 4 rows under each column heading. At a glance, a clinician will know whether active range of motion, active-assisted, passive, or no movement is appropriate for the 6 regions. The clinician may make a note to indicate situations in which different types of movements are appropriate for different areas in 1 of the 6 categories given. For example, an injury may create a situation in which active range of motion is required for the hand, passive stretching is appropriate for the elbow, and active range of motion is appropriate for the shoulder. Moreover, certain directions of movement (eg, abduction or flexion) may need to be done in different ways. The next section addresses bed mobility, bed exercise, and ambulation.

SUPPLEMENTAL FORM FOR NEUROPATHIC ULCERS

Patient_____ Clinician_____ Date_____

Location(s): Indicate location of wounds on the diagram below and create a numeric key if there are multiple wounds.

Wound #	1	2	3	4	5
Wagner grade	_____	_____	_____	_____	_____
Size	_____	_____	_____	_____	_____
% Red	_____	_____	_____	_____	_____
% Yellow	_____	_____	_____	_____	_____
% Black	_____	_____	_____	_____	_____

Indicate location of callus on the diagram below with the symbol /////

Reflexes: AJ right   present   diminished   absent   AJ left   present   diminished   absent

Foot deformities (specify)_____

Gait deviations (specify)_____

Pulse (right)   4   3   2   1   0   (specify artery palpated)_____

Pulse (left)   4   3   2   1   0   (specify artery palpated)_____

Capillary refill (right)   normal   sluggish   absent

Capillary refill (left)   normal   sluggish   absent

Ankle brachial index   Right_____   Left_____

Right foot temperature   normal   decreased   increased (specify temperature)

Left foot temperature   normal   decreased   increased (specify temperature)

Sensory testing (indicate on the diagram below + for intact, +/- for diminished, - for absent

Left foot   Right foot

Dorsal   Plantar   Plantar   Dorsal

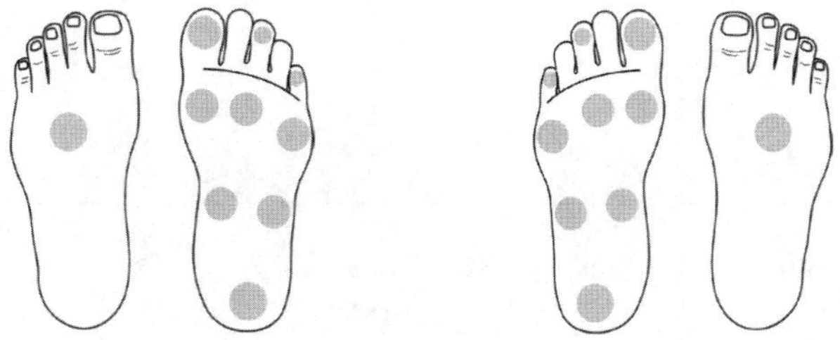

Signature_____   Date_____

Figure 19-5. Supplemental form for neuropathic ulcers. The term *diabetic foot ulcer* does not recognize that diabetes mellitus can cause both neuropathy and arterial insufficiency or that other diagnoses can cause neuropathy. The first item is the Wagner grade, in which 0 is an injury with intact skin; 1 is a shallow ulcer; 2 is a deep ulcer; 3 indicates infection of the wound or surrounding/underlying structures, especially osteomyelitis; 4 pertains to gangrene of the forefoot; and 5 indicates gangrene to most of the foot. The next section is used to document standard tests and measures for neuropathic ulcers and requires the filling of blanks or circling of items. The last item is a map of the feet. Four maps are given. On the left side are views of the plantar and dorsal left foot, and the right foot is on the right. The circles on the foot indicate the standard locations for sensory testing using a monofilament. The plantar foot has 9 locations, and the dorsal foot only one. In addition to the labels placed on the form, contours on the plantar figure and toenails on the dorsal figure are given to help identify the surface of the foot.

Sample History Form

List present conditions being managed by a licensed health care provider (physician, physical therapist, occupational therapist, speech therapist, audiologist, podiatrist, nurse, osteopath, psychologist, or other).

_____

_____

List current medications including prescriptions, over-the-counter medications, herbal or other self-administered remedies, and any dietary modifications. Obtain and review use of all of your medication bottles prior to filling out this part of the form.

_____

_____

List any surgical procedures and the condition for which they were performed.

_____

_____

List previous medical conditions, treatments received for them, and the outcomes of treatment.

_____

_____

Family History (circle all that apply):

Heart disease   Diseases of arteries or veins   Stroke   Diabetes   Respiratory disease

Have you been told that you have heart, lung, blood vessel, endocrine, digestive, kidney, skin, or any other disease?   yes   no

If so specify _____

Do you presently have any of the following symptoms (circle all that apply):

Chest pain	yes	no
Shortness of breath	yes	no
Dizziness or feeling faint	yes	no
Difficulty sleeping while lying flat in bed (need to raise head to breathe)	yes	no
Swelling of the legs, ankles, or feet	yes	no
Palpitations or abnormal heart rhythm	yes	no
Pain or cramping of legs with activity that is relieved by rest	yes	no

Loss of sensation of any part of the body	yes	no	specify_____
Coldness of any part of the body	yes	no	specify_____
Frequent urination	yes	no	
Getting up at night to urinate	yes	no	
Elevated blood sugar	yes	no	don't know
Night sweats	yes	no	
Change in appetite	yes	no	specify_____
Change in sleep pattern	yes	no	specify_____
Fever	yes	no	
Changes in pattern of bowel movement or urination	yes	no	

Specify the change _____

Unusual bleeding or discharges	yes	no	specify location _____
Pain resistant to over-the-counter medications	yes	no	
Pain that wakes you at night	yes	no	
Pain that does not change with activity or position	yes	no	

If yes to any of the last three questions above, specify the location of your pain _____

Red streaks	yes	no	specify location _____
Swollen lymph nodes/glands	yes	no	specify location _____
Changes in skin texture	yes	no	specify location _____
Loss of body hair	yes	no	specify location _____
Thickening of nails	yes	no	specify location _____

Figure 19-6. Sample history form. This form is made available to the patient before the first clinical visit to ensure accuracy, especially for list of medications. On clinic visit, review the form with the patient and assess their understanding of the items on the history form.

GENERIC INTEGUMENTARY DOCUMENTATION FORM

Patient___Stan Jones_____ Age _42_ (M)   F   Clinician _Linda Smith_   Date _7/19/23_

History

Chief complaint _Discomfort, weeping wound on leg, and discoloration around wound_

Home arrangements _Mobile home, 4 steps with single rail, step mother, 2 teenage brothers, 10-year-old sister live with pt_

Support system _Relatives living with pt, employer provides health insurance_

Occupation/education/hobbies/home activities _Cashier in convenience store, hunting, fishing, rebuilding autos_

Ambulation required for lifestyle _Primarily stands at cash register for 8-hour shift, sometimes with recreational activities_

Standing required for lifestyle _Stands almost entirety of waking hours_

Current lifestyle limitations _Discomfort to minor pain at work, has curtailed recreational activities_

Medications _Zoloft, Xanax, Prazosin_

Past Medical History _Recurrent leg ulcers, anxiety, HTN_

Previous treatment for condition _W/P, wet-to-dry dressings_

Review of Systems

    Neuromuscular   _WNL_

    Musculoskeletal   _WNL_

    Cardiopulmonary   _BP: 130/90, dilated, tortuous superficial leg veins in both legs_

    Integumentary   _Wound on medial, distal right leg, skin changes documented below_

Physical Examination

Wound photo or drawing here:

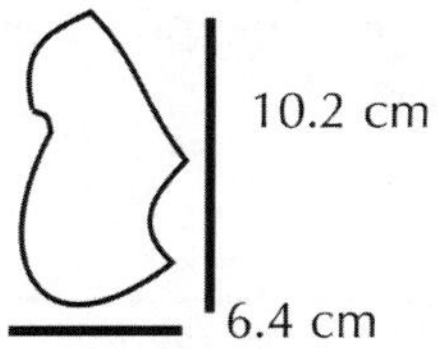

10.2 cm

6.4 cm

Color _red_____ Odor _Ø___ Drainage _copious serous___ Extent _see diagram, full-thickness____

Shape _irregular___ Tissue in wound: Black _0%_ Yellow _10%_ Red _90%_

Surrounding skin:

Texture _flaky__ Temperature _33.5°C_ Swelling: -   +   ++ (+++) ++++

Color _brown/yellow_ Hair/nails _WNL___ Ecchymosis _wound edges_ Hemosiderin _✓_

Demarcation _poor_____ Maceration _✓__ Epiboly _Ø_

Diagnosis   Impaired integumentary integrity with:

    _✓_ Risk of injury   __ Superficial injury

    __ Partial-thickness injury _✓_ Full-thickness injury

    __ Full-thickness injury and

        subcutaneous involvement

Prognosis   Within _3_ days weeks (months) and within _20_ visits, the patient is expected to:

Demonstrate preventive care, have full wound closure

Plan of Care

Patient and family/caregiver education _Causes and care for venous ulcers including self-performance of compression therapy_

Procedural interventions _debridement_____   frequency _3-5 days_ duration _3 weeks_

_____   _compression bandaging_   frequency _3-5 days_ duration _3 months_

Pt will be fit for custom stockings when leg volume normalizes   frequency _once____ duration _1 visit_

Signature _____*Linda Smith, PT*_____ Date_*7/19/23*_

Figure 19-7. Example of a generic integumentary documentation form. The forms have been designed to reduce redundancy as much as possible without sacrificing the "at a view" features of the forms.

SUPPLEMENTAL DATA FORM FOR DIAGNOSIS OF VENOUS ULCERS

Patient __Stan Jones_____   Clinician _Linda Smith_____   Date _7/19/23_____

Alternatives to standing _Store manager has agreed to allow pt to rotate between cashier work and stocking__

Location(s) _R medial leg, just proximal to medial malleolus_____

Status of surrounding skin _Hemosiderin staining, flaking, and weeping_____

Size of wound(s):   Length _10.2_ cm Width _6.4_ cm Depth partial-thickness ⟨full-thickness⟩

Ankle brachial index   Right __1.1__   Left __1.0__

Temperature of right foot   ⟨normal⟩   increased   decreased

Temperature of left foot   ⟨normal⟩   increased   decreased

Capillary refill (right)   ⟨normal⟩   sluggish   absent

Capillary refill (left)   ⟨normal⟩   sluggish   absent

Foot volume   right _1480_   left _1320_

Wound bed   % red _90_   % yellow _10_   % black _0_

Color of granulation tissue ⟨red⟩   pink

Drainage   minimal   moderate   ⟨copious⟩

Color of drainage   _clear_____

Compression therapy (specify) _4-layer compression bandaging prn, estimate 3 to 5 days between changes
initially; fit for custom stocking when volume normalizes_____

Signature_____Linda Smith, PT_____   Date ___7/19/23_____

Figure 19-8. Example of the venous ulcer form. This form is used if the patient is determined to have venous ulcerations. It is designed to eliminate lengthy descriptions and features components pertinent only to venous ulcers, including preventive measures and treatment specific to venous ulcers. In this example, the location of the wound proximal to the medial malleolus and condition of the surrounding skin are both consistent with venous ulcers. The next items are used to rule out arterial insufficiency. In this patient's case, we can see a normal ankle-brachial index, normal foot temperature, and normal capillary refill so we can assume that compression therapy is appropriate for this patient. Using a foot volumeter to quantify swelling of the lower extremities, clearly the right lower extremity is swollen. As detailed in the generic form, no edema has been observed in the left lower extremity but venous engorgement has been. This is a clear sign that the left lower extremity is at risk and the patient should be fitted with a custom stocking if feasible or use one of several alternatives discussed in Chapter 12 to reduce the risk of venous ulcers of the left leg. Note the blank for color of granulation tissue. This is another check for arterial insufficiency. Beefy, red granulation tissue, as in this example, indicates normal arterial inflow to the wound. Pink granulation tissue, on the other hand, is indicative of diminished arterial supply to the wound. Copious drainage is also consistent with uncontrolled venous pressure, although a recent dressing change could deceive the clinician. The clinician must ascertain when the current dressing was applied to estimate the degree of drainage. The last line is complementary to the treatment plan on the generic form. Because of the establishment of venous hypertension as the underlying cause of the wound, the specific form of compression therapy, rather than other forms of intervention described on the generic form, is specified on the supplemental venous ulcer form.

SUPPLEMENTAL DATA FORM FOR PRESSURE INJURIES

Patient __Tom Gray_____ Clinician __Jack Wilson_____ Date __9/30/23____

Stage of injury (identify location on figure at right with wound number)

1.	1	2	3	(4)	partially filled	filled	covered
2.	1	2	3	(4)	partially filled	filled	covered
3.	1	(2)	3	4	partially filled	filled	covered
4.	1	2	3	4	partially filled	filled	covered
5.	1	2	3	4	partially filled	filled	covered

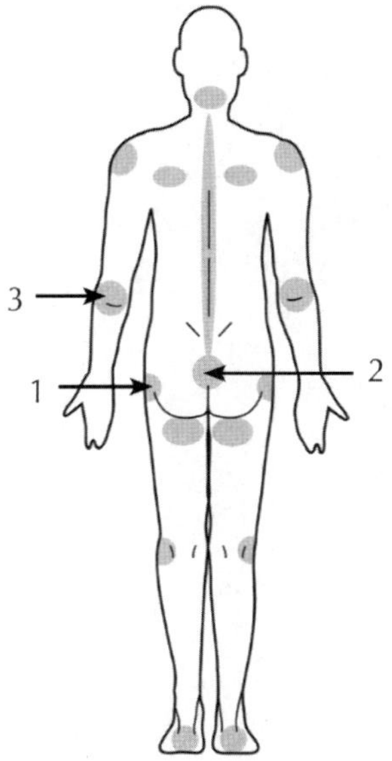

Size of injury (using identification key on right)

1.	Length _5.0_ cm	Width _3.5_ cm	Depth _6.2_ cm
2.	Length _4.6_ cm	Width _3.0_ cm	Depth _1.0_ cm
3.	Length _2.1_ cm	Width _1.7_ cm	Depth _N/A_ cm
4.	Length _____ cm	Width _____ cm	Depth _____ cm
5.	Length _____ cm	Width _____ cm	Depth _____ cm

Tunneling, sinus tracts, undermining

1.	Distance _2.0_ cm	Direction _12_ :00	Drainage _purulent_
2.	Distance _2.8_ cm	Direction _1__ :00	Drainage _gray_____
3.	Distance _____ cm	Direction ____ :00	Drainage _____
4.	Distance _____ cm	Direction ____ :00	Drainage _____
5.	Distance _____ cm	Direction ____ :00	Drainage _____

	1	2	3	4	5
Odor	foul	slight	N/A		
Drainage	purulent	min, serosang	N/A		
% R, Y, B	10, 50, 40	10, 80, 10	N/A		
Surrounding skin condition	inflamed	inflamed	WNL		

Signature_____ *Jack Wilson, RN, WOCN* _____ Date__9/30/23_____

Figure 19-9. Example of the pressure injury form. This is a relatively simple form that takes into account the frequent multiplicity of pressure injuries. Space for information for 5 injuries is available. In the first section, the stage of the injury as defined by the National Pressure Injury Advisory Panel (discussed in Chapter 10) and how much healing has occurred are documented.

SUPPLEMENTAL FORM FOR THERMAL INJURY

Patient _Ray Ator_ _____   Clinician _Lauren Greene_ _____   Date _5/5/23_ _____

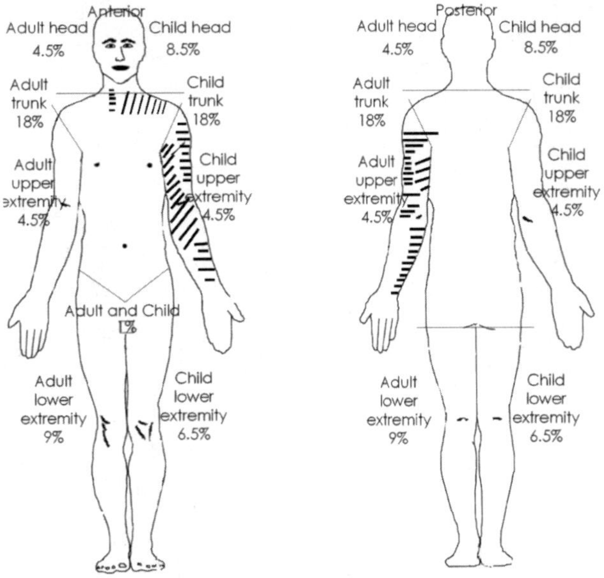

Indicate locations and depths of thermal injuries on figure to the left
- - Superficial thickness (1st degree)
//// Superficial partial thickness (2nd degree)
\\\ Deep partial thickness (deep dermal)
XXX Full thickness (3rd degree)

	RUE	LUE	RLE	LLE	Anterior trunk	Posterior trunk
Deficits in range of motion	Ø	✓ all	Ø	Ø	cerv ext	Ø
Deficits in strength	Ø	✓ all	Ø	Ø	Ø	Ø

Appropriate type of exercise

Active exercise	✓	✓	✓	✓	✓	✓
Active assisted exercise						
Passive stretch						
No movement allowed						

Deficits in tolerance for bed mobility, bed exercise, position changes, ambulation (specify) _Guarded, but functional secondary to left upper extremity and neck pain_

Indicate special positioning needs _Cervical extension, left shoulder abduction and extension_

Signature_____ _Lauren Greene, OT_ _____   Date_ _5/5/23_ _____

Figure 19-10. Example of the thermal injury form.

SUPPLEMENTAL FORM FOR NEUROPATHIC ULCERS

Patient___Brad Smith___ Clinician___Jim Brown___ Date___7/2/23___

Location(s): Indicate location of wounds on figure below and create numeric key if multiple wounds

Wound #	1	2	3	4	5
Wagner grade	3				
Size	5 cm x 3 cm				
% Red	90				
% Yellow	10				
% Black	0				

Indicate location of callus on the diagram below with the symbol /////

Reflexes: AJ right present diminished (absent) AJ left present diminished (absent)

Foot deformities (specify)___Hammer toes bilaterally___

Gait deviations (specify) ___Nonambulatory___

Pulse (right) 4 3 2 (1) 0 (specify artery palpated)___DP___
Pulse (left) 4 3 2 (1) 0 (specify artery palpated)___DP___

Capillary refill (right) normal (sluggish) absent
Capillary refill (left) normal (sluggish) absent
Ankle brachial index right___0.5___ left___0.6___
Right foot temperature normal (decreased) increased ___30.4°C___
Left foot temperature normal (decreased) increased ___30.2°C___

Sensory testing (indicate on the diagram below + for intact, +/- for diminished, - for absent

Left foot   Right foot

Dorsal   Plantar   Plantar   Dorsal

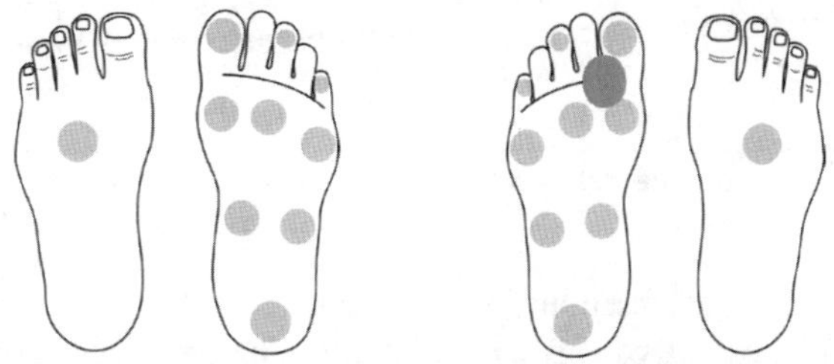

Signature___Jim Brown, DPT, CWS___ Date___7/2/23___

Figure 19-11. Example of the neuropathic ulcer form.

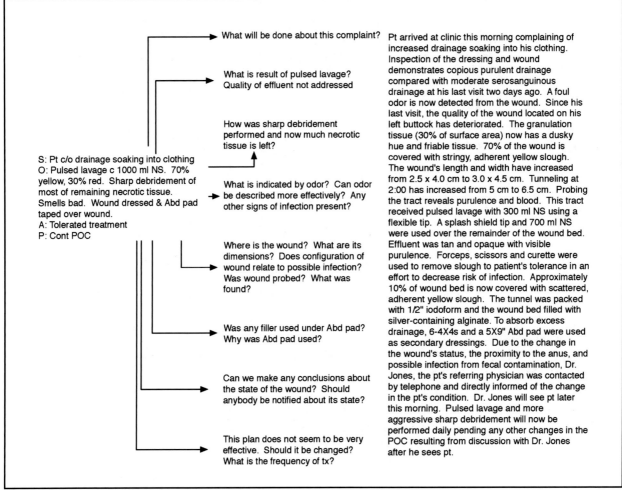

Figure 19-12. Example of poor documentation with demonstration of reworking into an effective progress note.

Strength, range of motion, sensation, and reflexes need to be addressed. The extent of this aspect of the evaluation needs to be ascertained at the time of the evaluation. Limited range of motion of the foot is also a major prognosticator of neuropathic ulcers. Sensory tests can be done quickly and can distinguish between small and large sensory neuron loss. Reflexes are particularly diagnostic of large neuron deficits in neuropathy but may also be informative for patients with other pathologies. Strength testing of the foot is similarly important, particularly for the individual with peripheral neuropathy. Loss of intrinsic foot muscle strength precedes critical foot deformities. The ankle-brachial index is considered to be a minimum standard for any patient with lower extremity ulcers. Suspected peripheral arterial disease should be quantified this way for possible referral to a vascular surgeon. A person with diabetes mellitus presenting with neuropathy of the lower extremities is at high risk for peripheral arterial disease and should be tested. Moreover, the person with venous ulcers needs to be tested to rule out arterial insufficiency before initiating compression therapy.

The wound itself and the surrounding skin need to be described thoroughly during the initial evaluation and each dressing change. For this reason, a section in the hospital EMR needs to be devoted to this aspect. Even if the dressing is not changed, the expectation is that the dressing at least be examined during each nursing shift for an inpatient. In settings outside a hospital, documentation of the wound and surrounding skin must be done for each visit. If the patient or a caregiver is tending to the wound between visits, the clinician needs to take a report from the patient or caregiver and document this report in the permanent record. The ability of the patient or caregiver to provide necessary care at home needs to be documented so the plan of care can be adjusted as needed.

Because a substantial amount of information is present on the initial evaluation, clinicians may be tempted to write excessively concise notes. An example of such a note is given in Figure 19-12. At a minimum, the location, color, odor, drainage, extent, and surrounding skin are documented. Anything that alters the diagnosis or prognosis must be stated explicitly, as diagrammed in

Figure 19-12. Any changes in the patient's other abilities from the initial evaluation should be examined regularly by physical examination or interview as set by facility procedures or as deemed necessary by the clinician. In addition to the physical examination of the wound, the patient should be interviewed, at least briefly during each visit, to determine whether changes have occurred since the initial evaluation and previous visits and whether any change is due to the etiology of the wound or related to work, home, recreation, or resources. When this information is documented appropriately, the need to modify the plan of care can be justified to all parties, including payers. If the patient or a caregiver is responsible for some aspects of wound management between visits, the adherence to the treatment plan should also be documented. The clinician needs to check for signs of nonadherence that might include the patient's knowledge of the details of the treatment plan, the condition of the wound, the condition of dressings, wear on shoes, changes in blood glucose, or other details relevant to the treatment plan. If the treatment plan outside the clinic is not being followed, modifications are likely to be needed. Careful documentation of nonadherence may be necessary to institute required changes in the treatment plan. If nonadherence is due to physical limitations, the patient may need to be seen more frequently in the outpatient or home health setting. A change from autolytic debridement to sharp debridement may be necessary if the patient is not willing or able to perform the necessary dressing changes or is unable to maintain the dressings' integrity. The patient may also need to be referred to a social worker or case manager to address deficits in social or financial support necessary to follow the treatment plan.

The treatment plan should be a logical extension of the history, physical examination, diagnosis, and prognosis. If these are documented carefully, the medical necessity and details of the treatment plan should be clear to third-party payers. In addition, other clinicians who may need to take over care of the patient will be better able to execute the plan. Bear in mind that due to the personal preferences of the patient, clinician, or caregiver, some details of how the plan is executed may vary from the initial plan. Documentation may be in either the well-established SOAP (Subjective, Objective, Assessment, and Plan) format or some other form, such as a narrative following the language developed in the *Guide*. The subjective portion corresponds roughly with the history taken from the patient. The objective section contains components of the history taken from medical records and the physical examination. The assessment section of a SOAP note will contain elements of diagnosis and sometimes elements of the prognosis. The plan section of a SOAP note contains the treatment plan, although some individuals will place functional objectives and goals with the "A" section. Comparing these 2 approaches, some aspects are common, but several items fall into different categories. For example, the information taken from the patient and that taken from medical records go into different parts of the SOAP note. In contrast, history is a complete section using the *Guide* approach. A comparison of documenting with these 2 approaches is given in Table 19-1.

PROGNOSIS

Prognosis is done fairly readily based on the *Guide* integumentary practice patterns B through E. Practice pattern A is related to preventing loss of integumentary integrity. Some of this pattern's elements may be important for a given patient who already has a wound to prevent recurrence of the wound or development of a wound in another location. A thorough history and physical examination will help determine whether any of the potential complications listed in the prognosis section of the preferred practice patterns might extend the time frame or lead to a new episode of care. The clinician needs to assess adherence constantly and, if necessary, modify the treatment plan to make adherence achievable so the prognosis can become achievable. The modifications may either increase or decrease the time frame and limit some of the expected outcomes. An example of a shortened time frame is when autolytic debridement was initially proposed, but sharp debridement was substituted in the treatment plan due to complications.

When developing the prognosis, one must be clear about the clinician's role in the episode of care. In many cases, the clinician in the acute care hospital is not expected to achieve complete healing of a wound but to achieve a clean and stable wound ready for some type of surgical repair such as grafting, or the goal is preparing the patient for discharge or transfer to the appropriate destination such as home with self-care or a caregiver or to a different type of facility. In other cases, typical of hospital- or resident-based facilities, one clinician may temporarily work with the patient, and another, who may be from a different discipline, takes over care once characteristics of the wound meet the established criteria. In an outpatient setting, the clinician will need to vary the frequency of visits and discharge the patient from the clinician's care as the characteristics of the wound change. Regardless of the setting, a time frame for complete healing or a prognosis for the wound's optimum condition should be developed. Variance from the final predicted outcome after discharge may be grounds for a new episode of care.

TABLE 19-1
Comparison of SOAP Note Documentation to Use of *Guide* Language

SOAP FORMAT	COMMON ELEMENTS	*GUIDE* LANGUAGE
Subjective	Chief complaint, history of the complaint, lifestyle, work, school, play	History
Objective	Review of systems, routine screening tests, tests specific to rule in/out suspected diagnosis	Physical examination
Assessment: Diagnosis or a description of the cluster of signs and symptoms; outcomes, functional goals, and time frames		Evaluation: Mental process, not written, in which information is analyzed critically Diagnosis: Identifying a cluster of signs and symptoms, often identified as a practice pattern Prognosis: Expected outcomes and time frame for achievement; discussion of complications
Plan	Specific interventions including patient education, behavior modification, direct interventions (eg, debridement and frequency and duration)	Plan of care

MEDICAL NECESSITY

A document giving the plan of care and showing medical necessity must be generated for Medicare and other reimbursement. To meet Medicare's criteria for medical necessity, documentation should support that (1) the treatment is necessary, (2) improvement of the condition is expected, (3) the proper clinician is providing the treatment, and (4) the condition will not improve or will become worse if treatment is not provided. Within the initial evaluation document, a succinct argument framed by medical necessity principles should be provided. A well-written plan of care describes the optimum combination of appropriate wound care and the reality of how the plan interacts with the patient. With sufficient experience, the plan of care will flow readily from the history and physical examination.

Given 2 patients with identical characteristics, 2 different plans of care are likely to be needed. Variance in the plan of care should be viewed as accommodations to the unique combinations of patient characteristics, including physical condition, resources, and lifestyle. Differences in the plan of care among patients with the same etiology should be supported explicitly by documentation. Although the accommodations may seem straightforward to the treating clinician, another person reading the documentation needs to read the explicit reasons to make appropriate decisions on reimbursement, the need for additional diagnostic testing, or the need for additional interventions such as surgery. These accommodations for individual differences need to be written with the concept of medical necessity in mind. Explicitly describe why each accommodation is necessary for the patient to benefit from the proposed plan of care. A well-documented initial evaluation that outlines the reasons for the choices made will generally meet all the documentation goals, including reimbursement, the ability of other clinicians to understand the treatment plan, and improved clinical decision making.

PHOTODOCUMENTATION

The phrase "a picture's worth a thousand words" is commonly used. This is frequently true in the case of open wounds. Words alone may fail to describe the appearance and the progression of healing adequately. In many cases, a hand-drawn diagram may be adequate, but in others the wound's quality needs to be captured more thoroughly. Photography is especially important for the wound containing vast amounts of necrotic tissue. In these cases, wounds frequently become much larger before they can heal. A good-quality photograph can show changes in the wound's quality and demonstrate complications that others may not have foreseen. This extra information can help the clinician explain the need for extended periods of care or re-evaluate the prognosis or plan of care. Some facilities also require pre- and postdebridement pictures to better support the coding submitted for reimbursement.

The first question that most clinicians have regarding photodocumentation of wounds is the most appropriate type of camera. At the last publication of this textbook, instant film (Polaroid) and 35-mm film cameras were still being utilized (Figure 19-13). However, since then, there has been a transition to digital photos and the use of tablets or cell phones as a way to obtain photos. Given the risk for violation of Health Insurance Portabiltiy and Accountability Act and patient privacy, the facility must have in place policies and procedures surrounding the use of such technology.

The standard for quality photographing of wounds is digital photography, whether via digital cameras or cell phones/tablets. Digital cameras combine the advantages of instant and 35-mm photographs. The clinician will know immediately whether the image is adequate. A wide range of price and resolution is available. Generally, higher-resolution digital cameras are more expensive. A balance needs to be struck between the required resolution and price. A camera with a zoom feature is desirable, especially for smaller wounds. In addition, one must decide on a medium for transferring the picture from the camera. Digital cameras now have the capacity to store hundreds of photographs at a time. Secure data cards and other memory devices holding several gigabytes are very affordable. Transferring the photographs may be done in several ways, including card readers, USB, and wireless connections. One must then consider how to store the digital pictures. At a minimum, photographs should be stored on a secure computer within the department. In addition, one may choose to print the picture or upload it to a computerized documentation system. Because the photographs do not require the purchase of film or the cost of film processing, digital photography is the most cost-effective means of photodocumentation. Another major advantage of digital photography is the ability to make as many copies of the picture as needed. One may track a wound's progress by arranging a series of digital photographs in either a video display or hard copy.

One area that seems like an advantage of digital photography is the availability of software to correct color problems and edit photos. However, this can be problematic for 2 reasons. Due to software correction availability, photographers may become complacent and not optimize setup for the photographs. In particular, the lack of adequate lighting and a tripod will lead to blurry pictures due to the combination of increased exposure time and camera movement. Another concern is the ability of those with the digital files to alter the photograph ("photoshopping") to promote their own agendas. Lawyers may claim that photos were altered to make a wound appear smaller or bigger than actual size. However, the presence of the ruler in the picture eliminates that concern.

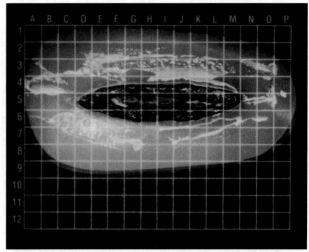

Figure 19-13. Example of Polaroid photo developed on grid film.

Use of Cell Phones or Tablets

Photographs obtained from cameras built into cellular phones are essentially cost free but historically provided relatively low resolution. As cell phones continue to advance with better cameras installed, this is no longer a major concern. Some facilities have policies against the use of personal cell phones or tablets for capturing photos, so these facilities will provide appropriate technology for staff to use.

General Photography Guidelines

Regardless of the type of camera used, several general rules need to be followed to optimize photodocumentation. The patient should always sign a photographic release form before photographs are taken. If the patient is a minor, a parent or guardian must sign the photographic release. An identification code for the patient, the date, and a measuring scale need to be present on each photograph; this usually depends on the facility's definition of patient identifiers. Patient identification should use a number, such as a medical record number or patient identification number, rather than the patient's name or initials. Disposable paper scales are commonly used within photographs. The patient's identifiers and the date are written on the scale; if possible, they can use patient ID stickers from EMRs. Ideally, the clinician will continue to use the camera at the same distance from the subject to better allow an eyeball comparison between photographs of the same wound. A digital camera must have a sufficient optical zoom range to achieve the same result. Digital zoom is not useful because it simply reduces the photograph's size with a corresponding decrease in resolution.

For at least the initial evaluation, a photograph needs to be taken that allows the wounded body part to be identified. Although one may be tempted to fill the entire photograph with the wound, the quality of the surrounding skin and other contributing factors in the diagnosis or prognosis should be captured in the photograph. In many cases, wounds are slow to heal due to the condition of the surrounding skin; therefore, sufficient surrounding skin needs to be in the photograph. Unless the wound is located on the face, the patient's face or anything else that could allow someone else to identify the patient should not be in the photograph. For wounds on the face, zoom enough to identify only what part of the face is involved and minimize the possibility of identifying the photograph's subject.

The background needs to be considered when taking any type of photograph. In many cases, the background will consist only of the patient's intact skin. If a background other than the patient's skin exists, avoid white or yellow. These colors reflect too much light and will distort the color of the wound. Use blue or green drapes in these cases. Also, avoid distracting objects within the photograph. Remove any equipment or personnel that might appear in the background. This problem is more likely to occur during the initial photograph showing the body part on which the wound is located. Carefully position the patient to allow the proper amount of light to strike the wound while optimizing patient comfort. Insufficient or excessive lighting will obscure the details of the wound, and colors will not be true. Avoid direct flash on the wound or flash too close to the wound. Excessive lighting or flash creates a bright picture with little contrast and inaccurate color. Be aware that direct flash will be reflected from moist surfaces. If flash is necessary, angle the camera so the flash is not reflected directly back toward the camera. Insufficient lighting will result in a dark picture with poor contrast and will distort the wound's color.

POTENTIAL PROBLEMS WITH DOCUMENTATION

Although seemingly trivial, elements of documentation have the potential to create problems at any time in the future. Other clinicians may not be able to decipher the plan of care, its rationale, or its details. For example, not documenting a tract's location and size may cause another clinician to miss it and fail to irrigate it during a subsequent visit adequately. A bad outcome such as sepsis or amputation, regardless of whether failure to adequately treat the wound contributed to the problem, could lead to a civil action seeking damages from the clinician or facility where the clinician practices. Inadequate documentation may lead to a lack of reimbursement from a third-party payer.

Each note must include the date and time of the visit. The lack of a date or time on each note can lead to the denial of payment. Inaccurate measurement of wound dimensions, particularly when multiple clinicians measure a wound, may give the impression of a wound that is fluctuating in size such that a trend toward healing or degeneration of the wound is obscured. The use of paper documentation requires handwriting. A hurried note often leads to illegibility that may lead to errors in treatment and may aid the plaintiff's case in a lawsuit. Abbreviations may not be understood. Facilities generally provide a list of acceptable abbreviations. Although some items in the list of unapproved abbreviations may seem absurd, facilities attempt to follow recommendations from agencies such as The Joint Commission. Most of the issues addressed by abbreviations are concerns about medication and surgical errors, but documentation rules must be applied equally to all clinicians, administrators, and technicians within the facility.

Although we would like to believe that our memories are flawless, as more time passes between a patient encounter and documentation, we become more likely to lose details. Ideally, documentation is done immediately following a patient encounter. Notes must be objective and accurate, containing sufficient detail for any other clinician or payer to understand the patient's condition. Exaggerating improvement in a wound's quality or size may lead a payer to conclude that subsequent visits were un-necessary and to deny payment. Stating that the wound is worse than it is to obtain greater payment is fraudulent. It could result in several severe penalties, including dismissal, loss of practice privileges, demand for repayment, and fines. Clinicians must focus the reader of notes on the problems that persist during an episode of care. If one states that the wound is decreasing in size and the wound bed is red, moist, and granulating but fails to mention that drainage is excessive, has a yellow/brown color, and the effluent from pulsed lavage within a tract is tan and opaque, payment requests are likely to be denied.

Another potential problem is the criticism of other clinicians. When writing a note, emphasize what needs to be done to resolve a problem that might have been caused by another clinician without explicitly stating that someone else did something wrong. For example, a scenario in which a referral with the diagnosis of cellulitis that is actually venous disease could be described simply in terms of the characteristics that led to the diagnosis of venous disease and not explicitly state that the referring diagnosis was wrong. Although what the patient states should be documented when it is pertinent, some patients will either deliberately or mistakenly provide incorrect information. If a patient is emphatic that another clinician did something wrong, remember that you were not present to confirm or deny what happened between them. A patient may be trying to get you to take sides in a dispute. If you take sides with the patient in such a situation, you may find yourself in an uncomfortable situation in the future as a witness in a lawsuit or having destroyed a relationship with another clinician un-necessarily. Keep your notations as objective as possible; do not blame another individual for a patient's condition. To ensure completeness of notations, facilities may adopt a chart review procedure. An example of a wound care chart review tool is shown in Figure 19-14.

LEGAL ISSUES

Our system of law allows 2 types of litigation: criminal and civil. Criminal litigation involves violating specific laws and prosecution by the local, state, or federal government. Criminal proceedings may result from fraudulent claims from third-party payers, assault, or battery. Although complaints of assault or battery against a patient are rare, excessive coercion perceived as a threat could be interpreted as assault, and performing a procedure on a patient without informed consent could be interpreted as battery.

Civil complaints are most likely to occur when a bad outcome follows an episode of care. In the context of wound care, the development of pressure injuries, sepsis, or amputation of an affected body part might become a focus of a civil complaint. Informed consent and a good relationship between the clinician and patient decrease the probability of a civil complaint. Winning a judgment in a civil action is dependent on 4 elements that can be related to documentation. The first element is the existence of a duty. If a clinician enters into an agreement to provide care to the patient, the first element is met. For example, a person who becomes a resident at a nursing home has entered into an agreement that the nursing home will provide an acceptable level of care. The nursing home now has a duty to that resident. The second element is breach of duty. Breach of duty could be either the omission of expected care or the commission of an act that harms a patient. Using the same example, failure to assess risk factors and provide interventions to prevent pressure injuries represents a breach of duty. The third element is injury caused by the breach of duty. Proximate cause between the breach of duty and harm to the patient must be proven. Proximate cause indicates a direct link between the breach of duty and injury. The plaintiff must show that the clinician's action or neglect was a substantial factor in the patient's injury and that the injury would not have occurred without the clinician's negligence. Pressure injuries caused by the lack of risk assessment and interventions to prevent them meet the third criterion. The fourth part is that actual damage occurred. Care given at a substandard level that does not harm the patient is not sufficient for winning a lawsuit. If the lack of turning or proper positioning does not lead to pressure injuries, no damages

may be awarded. The plaintiff's attorney must prove with the preponderance of evidence that the defendant is responsible for the plaintiff's damages. Damages may include lost wages, expenses (primarily but not exclusively medical) incurred by the plaintiff, and pain and suffering that resulted from the defendant's negligent care. Monetary loss resulting from pressure injuries and pain and suffering experienced by the nursing home resident represent damages sought by the plaintiff in this example.

The documentation of an initial evaluation establishes the duty of the clinician. Failure to provide informed consent and document the patient's condition and risk factors sets the stage for problems later. Any patient behaviors that might cause a bad outcome should be documented as they are discovered. This information could come from a verbal account or observation of the patient. For example, document any alternative treatments that the patient is performing (eg, having a dog lick the wound; soaking in Epsom salts; or the use of raw eggs, WD40 [WD-40 Company], or Windex [S.C. Johnson & Sons, Inc] on the wound). Also, document whether the patient is adherent in home care. Objective evidence of nonadherence, such as the condition of dressings and off-loading devices, should be documented. If a patient is apparently not performing regular dressing changes, cleansing the wound, or using off-loading devices, the clinician should document this nonadherence as soon as it is discovered. In addition to documenting problems caused by the patient, also explicitly document any intervention to correct the patient's behavior. Changes in the wound's characteristics such as worsening quantity or quality of drainage, odor, or deterioration of the wound bed must be documented as they occur along with interventions to address them, including any communication of the patient's condition with other clinicians. For example, if a wound is healing slowly, then grayish drainage and an odor become apparent, communication with the patient's referring physician should be performed and documented.

Teichman[1] has suggested a modification of the SOAP note as a means of clear documentation of informed consent. Teichman describes an acronym of SOOOAAP for Subjective, Objective, Opinion, Options, Advice, and Agreed Plan. Although subjective and objective are the same as the SOAP format, the assessment part is broken down into 3 parts that lend themselves directly to the concept of informed consent. Opinion emphasizes that the clinician is using the available information to reach a conclusion about the patient's condition while lowering the expectation that a firm diagnosis can be offered to every patient. The options section details possible courses of action. Rather than spelling out a treatment plan that necessarily follows from the clinical diagnosis, options implies that the patient has been given all possible information on which a course of action can be based. The advice section

Wound Care Chart Review Tool

Indicators: Clients with wounds will be appropriately cared for as evidenced by the following indicators:

Threshold: Goal is 85% on all indicators

Sample size: 100% or 10 charts for clients with a wound per quarter

Year: _____

Quarter: Jan to Mar   Apr to Jun   Jul to Sep   Oct to Dec

	Yes	No	N/A
1. Wound assessment done on admission			
A. Integumentary portion of Outcome and Assessment Information Set (OASIS) filled out	—	—	—
B. Wound assessment sheet initiated	—	—	—
C. Braden scale value computed	—	—	—
D. Integumentary area of point of contact (POC) filled out			
1. If Braden score <12 "Potential for impaired skin integrity demonstrated by" filled out	—	—	—
2. Wounds described in "Problem" section by location, type, stage or partial/full thickness, and size in centimeter	—	—	—
3. Steps of wound care included on "communication with MD" line of OASIS and "perform" section of plan of care. Wound care orders match treatment section of wound assessment sheet, including whether caregiver will be taught	—	—	—
E. Orders for wound care on 485 (plan of care form) includes technique; products, frequency, whether any caregiver will be taught	—	—	—
F. 485 includes "consult to be done by certified wound, ostomy, continence nurse (CWOCN) within 2 weeks"	—	—	—
2. Consistent and accurate wound assessments and wound related teaching documented on skilled nurse visit (SNV) notes			
A. Wound described with each dressing change			
1. Wound bed described	—	—	—
2. Drainage described	—	—	—
3. Surrounding tissue described	—	—	—
4. Signs or infection noted and MD notified or "No s/s infection noted" documented	—	—	—
5. Patient response to wound care noted	—	—	—
6. Wound care steps described	—	—	—
7. Wound location and type described	—	—	—
B. Accurate wound measurements done weekly			
1. L x W x D measured in centimeters to tenths	—	—	—
2. Includes measurement of deepest undermining and where undermining is located	—	—	—
3. Wound described as outlined above in 2A	—	—	—
4. Current wound care described	—	—	—
5. SNV notes evidence of teaching regarding wounds, wound care, products, pressure prevention, and/or skin care as appropriate	—	—	—
3. All changes in wound care and/or frequency done are accompanied by an MD order and Coordination of Care note	—	—	—
4. All MD orders are signed and returned	—	—	—

Figure 19-14. Tool used to ensure complete documentation for home health visits. (Developed by Megan Hughes, RN, CWOCN.)

describes what the clinician believes to be the optimal course of action. Finally, agreed plan emphasizes that the clinician and patient worked together to develop a plan of care. This subtle change in wording sends a strong message to any third parties that the patient was fully informed, options were discussed and based on the evidence available, and the patient chose to follow this plan of care. This flow of information in the SOOOAAP note may be contrasted to a typical SOAP note in which the clinician appears to have all of the power in the relationship. If a negative outcome occurs, the perception of the clinician holding all of the power leads easily to the conclusion by a third party that the patient was a victim, thereby increasing the likelihood of litigation. In contrast, a note written with the SOOOAAP format elements shows that the patient was not only informed of the evidence, options, and advice but was also a part of the decision process.

SUMMARY

Documentation is important for the obvious reason of maximizing reimbursement and avoiding civil judgments, but done well, it provides a road map for the episode of care. Information taken from the history section guides the physical examination, and the combined information is assessed by the clinician to develop a diagnosis and prognosis. The diagnosis and prognosis, in turn, guide the plan of care. The plan of care includes communication and coordination of care, patient education, and direct interventions. The patient's inability to adhere to the plan of care requires modification of patient education, changes in direct intervention, or the consultation of a social worker or other appropriate professionals to manage resources so that the patient becomes able to adhere to the plan of care. The patient's lifestyle, work, school, or play also need to be accommodated in the plan of care. Photography can be used to communicate visual aspects of the wound that words might not capture. Documentation of the patient's pertinent characteristics and the patient's wound decreases the likelihood of the denial of payment and civil litigation.

QUESTIONS

1. Why is documentation critical to a good outcome?
2. What is the role of documenting history?
3. How is this important with multiple clinicians working with the same patient?
4. How is physical examination related to history?
5. Explain how the physical examination might differ between a case with an obvious diagnosis and one without a clear diagnosis.
6. Contrast the subjective part of a SOAP note to the history and the physical examination's objective part.

REFERENCE

1. Teichman PG. Documentation tips for reducing malpractice risk. *Fam Pract Manag.* 2000;7(3):29-33.

BIBLIOGRAPHY

Brown G. Wound documentation: managing risk. *Adv Skin Wound Care.* 2006;19(3):155-167. doi:10.1097/00129334-200604000-00011

Centers for Medicare & Medicaid Services. Local coverage determination (LCD): wound care (L35125): general information. 2017. Accessed October 17, 2022. www.cms.gov/medicare-coverage-database/details/lcd-details.aspx?LCDId=35125

Classen NS. The basics of medical photography. *Acute Care Perspect.* 2000;8(2):7-11.

Hampton S. Accurate documentation and wound measurement. *Nurs Times.* 2015;111(48):16-19.

Hess CT. Understanding your documentation requirements. *Adv Skin Wound Care.* 2018;31(3):144. doi:10.1097/01.ASW.0000530374.61754.a3

Kinnunen UM, Saranto K, Ensio A, Iivanainen A, Dykes P. Developing the standardized wound care documentation model: a Delphi study to improve the quality of patient care documentation. *J Wound Ostomy Continence Nurs.* 2012;39(4):397-408. doi:10.1097/WON.0b013e318259c45b

Levine JM, Savino F, Peterson M, Wolf CR. Risk management for pressure ulcers: when the family shows up with a camera. *J Am Med Dir Assoc.* 2008;9(5):360-363.

20

Plan of Care

Irion GL, Gardner JA, Pignataro RM.
Comprehensive Wound Management, Third Edition (pp 387-401).
© 2024 Taylor and Francis Group.

TERMINOLOGY OF THE ICF MODEL

In years past, goals were set for a patient based on remediation of a documented impairment. For example, a deficit of range of motion would be remediated in terms of increased range of motion. Over time, however, the remediation of an impairment solely for the sake of remediation was questioned. Physical therapists were nudged in the direction of writing functional goals. As an example, shoulder range of motion would be improved to allow the patient to perform a task necessary to the individual's function in home, work, or community, such as dressing, operating machinery, and caring for children. Plans of care became hodgepodges of impairment and function-driven goals to be attained. Many clinicians either consciously or unconsciously began to incorporate the model of disablement into developing a plan of care. In November 1997, the American Physical Therapy Association published the *Guide to Physical Therapist Practice* (*Guide*). A second edition was published in January 2001. Guide 3.0 was updated in 2016 and was based on the *International Classification of Functioning, Disability and Health* (ICF), which is described later in this chapter. In April 2023, Guide 4.0 was released online. It focuses on more current issues in the physical therapy profession.

A given patient may be seen by a clinician at any point on the continuum from impairment, functional limitation, or disability. As defined in the *Guide*, impairment is a loss or abnormality of physiological, psychological, or anatomical structure or function; functional limitation is a restriction of the ability to perform at the level of the whole person, a physical action, activity or task in an efficient, typically expected, or competent manner; and disability is defined as the inability to engage in age-specific, gender-specific, or sex-specific roles in a particular context and physical environment. Placed in the context of the patient-clinician interaction, remediation of an impairment is not based on the impairment itself but to overcome functional limitations and prevent disability. Interaction may also occur to allow the patient to adapt to functional limitations to prevent or minimize disability or to retrain the patient for new roles following disability. In terms of wound management, the plan of care should not be focused on the "hole in the patient" but on the "whole patient." The outcome of the plan of care is ultimately to prevent or minimize functional limitations and disability secondary to integumentary impairments and to prevent secondary impairments. Secondary impairments result either directly or indirectly from another impairment. For example, the person placed on bed rest because of a neuropathic ulcer may develop cardiopulmonary complications caused by bed rest. Diminished cardiopulmonary function or cardiopulmonary disease would be a secondary impairment. Use of total contact casting or other

means of keeping the patient ambulatory is an example of preventing secondary impairments. This is an excellent example of how 2 interventions—bed rest and total contact casting—may address the same impairment, but one intervention is superior due to the prevention of a secondary impairment. Often, wounds represent secondary impairments. Cardiopulmonary, musculoskeletal, or neuromuscular impairments resulting in immobility may cause integumentary impairments (wounds). For example, an individual with a spinal cord injury is at high risk for the development of pressure injuries. An important role of the clinician is to prevent these secondary integumentary impairments by identifying how the skin is placed at risk due to cardiopulmonary, musculoskeletal, or neuromuscular impairments. The clinician then devises a plan of care to remediate the impairments that create the risk to the skin and prevent the secondary impairment manifesting itself as a wound.

INTERNATIONAL CLASSIFICATION OF FUNCTIONING, DISABILITY AND HEALTH

ICF is a worldwide collaborative effort of the World Health Organization (WHO) to facilitate multidisciplinary health care. This system is an effort to provide common language regarding health that is meant to be understandable across nations, languages, and disciplines and is built on the biopsychosocial model. The *Guide* is built on the disability model. The disability model was developed in an effort to encourage clinicians to consider more than a person's etiology in treatment planning. In contrast, the traditional medical model consists of obtaining a history and physical examination, performing a systems review, and conducting special tests to aid diagnosis. Following diagnosis, medicine or surgery is used to treat the diagnosed disease using standard care. The primary emphasis encouraged through the use of the disability model is preventing the progression of an impairment to a disability, a disability to a handicap, or an impairment directly to a handicap. The disability model incorporates elements of a person's situation that may cause impairment to become a disability or a handicap or cause a disability to become a handicap.

The disability model has several shortcomings. It does not explicitly direct clinicians to look at personal and environmental factors. It does not specify which activities are important to a given person. It does not specify how well a person participates in activities, and it lacks a means of quantifying a person's condition or comparing data across clinicians, facilities, settings, and nations. Although the disability model is an improvement over the traditional medical model, its greatest shortcoming remains the non-uniform language clinicians use, even when framing the person's problems within the disability model. Neither the traditional medical model nor the disability model has a standard for coding personal and environmental factors, and they have no explicit means of communicating activities and participation. Instead, clinicians tend to develop their own language. Language disparity tends to worsen as one compares language used within a given facility by members of the same discipline to different types of facilities and to members of different disciplines. Disparity in language is likely to result in difficulty interpreting others' documentation and time consumed seeking clarification from other clinicians.

The purpose of creating ICF is facilitating the communication of clinicians within and between disciplines. It is also designed to be a systematic language acting as a basis for analyzing health statistics. As opposed to International Classification of Diseases codes, ICF codes are meant to be independent of etiology or health care provider. Improvements of the ICF model over the disability model include a greater emphasis on a person's response to a given disease, a greater emphasis on patient-centered care, improved cross-discipline communication, and better integration with the biopsychosocial model. Within the framework of the ICF model, disability can mean physical, emotional, or social impairments manifesting themselves as limitations in activities and restrictions in participation. By its nature, the ICF model creates a patient-centered approach. The ICF model provides very specific definitions of terms commonly used in rehabilitation. The official WHO definitions of ICF terms are given in Table 20-1.

The ICF model operates under a small number of principles. Rather than drawing arbitrary distinctions between healthy and handicapped individuals, the model is based on the notion of a continuum of body structures, functions, activity limitations, and participation restrictions. For example, a person who cannot participate as a jockey in horse racing, as a professional basketball player, as a spelling bee competitor, or as an opera singer has some degree of impairment. A second major principle is that any specific impairment is equivalent without regard to its etiology (principle of equity/parity). A foot amputation, resulting from trauma, arterial disease, infection, or congenital anomaly, is treated identically within the model. In theory, the way a person receives a wound is not directly associated with the person's condition or problems. Etiology might, however, have an indirect effect through what are termed *contextual factors*. For example, depending on the wound's etiology, a person's psychological response may differ, which, in turn, may affect any activity limitations or participation restrictions related to the altered body structure or function.

TABLE 20-1
World Health Organization's Definitions of Terms Used With the ICF Model

Body Functions: Physiological functions of body systems (including psychological functions).

Body Structures: Anatomical parts of the body such as organs, limbs, and their components.

Impairments: Problems in body function or structure such as a significant deviation or loss.

Activity: Execution of a task or action by an individual.

Participation: Involvement in a life situation.

Activity Limitations: Difficulties an individual may have in executing activities.

Participation Restrictions: Problems an individual may experience in involvement in life situations.

Environmental Factors: Physical, social, and attitudinal environment in which people live and conduct their lives.

Data sources: Steiner et al, 2002; World Health Organization, 2002.

Contextual factors are divided into personal factors and environmental factors. Examples of personal factors given by the WHO include sex, age, other health conditions, coping style, social background, education, profession, past experience, and character style. According to the WHO, environmental factors include products and technology, natural environment and human-made changes to the environment, support and relationships, attitudes, services, systems, and policies. Using the ICF model places emphasis on relationships among the 3 core pieces of the model—body structure/function, activities, and participation—and the effects of the contextual factors on them. Activities and participation are placed in 9 specific categories: (1) learning and applying knowledge; (2) general tasks and demands; (3) communication; (4) movement; (5) self-care; (6) domestic life areas; (7) interpersonal interactions; (8) major life areas; and (9) community, social, and civic life.

Within the ICF model, impairments are given capacity qualifiers and performance qualifiers to aid in communicating the person's condition. The capacity qualifier refers to the person's ability to actually execute a task or action under ideal circumstances, whereas the performance qualifier communicates what the person actually does in their own environment. The use of personal assistance, assistive, or adaptive devices is not material in terms of capacity.

However, whether the person has access to assistance or equipment impacts performance. According to this model, performance of an activity may be restricted by alterations in body structure or function, activity limitations, personal factors, or environmental factors. Note, however, as depicted in Figure 20-1, that arrows are drawn in both directions among body structure/function, activity limitations, and participation restriction. Arrows are also drawn from contextual factors to these 3 core entities. For example, if a person is given an off-loading device, a walker, and personal assistance, they may be able to travel to health care providers, participate in activities related to wound care, and allow the neuropathic ulcer to heal.

USING THE ICF MODEL AS A FRAMEWORK FOR PLAN OF CARE

The person's needs and preferences are determined through a discussion of the person's problems and therapy goals and validated tools such as the SF-36 (Short-Form Health Survey). Components of the interview are open-ended questions with answers written in the person's own words. These questions are based directly on the ICF model (ie, which problems of the body functions are being experienced, which body structures are involved, what limitations of activities are being experienced, whether participation is being restricted in significant tasks or actions, and which environmental factors or personal factors are barriers or facilitators).

Following interviews and the collection of data from standardized written tools, guided physical examinations are performed by relevant members of the health care team. Impairments are then placed into the 3 categories of (1) body structures/functions, (2) activities, and (3) participation. A form has been developed by Steiner et al[1] specifically for the ICF model, which they termed the *Rehabilitation Problem-Solving Form* (RPS Form). Alternatively, a simple 3-row grid with 3 columns in the first 2 rows and 2 columns in the third row can be created (see Figure 20-1). The top row of the grid contains the interview and written data divided among the 3 core categories. The information obtained through physical examination is placed into the middle row within the appropriate 3 core categories. The third row consists of personal factors and environmental factors. The single clinician or preferably a health care team then looks for connections among the 8 blocks on the grid or the RPS-Form used. Circles and lines are drawn on the form to help visualize relationships among items in the 8 blocks. An assessment of any personal factors or environmental factors that might either cause or contribute to problems listed is made. Examining the completed form should cue clinicians to personal and environmental factors that

might impact connections among items on the form or grid. Clinicians may identify facilitators that could be exploited or barriers that could be overcome with the availability of specific environmental factors. Hypotheses related to cause and effect for the person's problems and factors contributing to, rather than causing, the effects are developed and analyzed critically. When factors directly or indirectly responsible for any structural or functional impairments, activity limitations, or participation restrictions are identified, a plan of care can be readily developed to address modifiable physical, personal, or environmental factors. The top section of the form or grid becomes useful in the reconciliation of differences between expectations of the patient and clinician(s). The patient may have expectations that are either too high or too low or misdirected in the opinion of the clinician. The patient and clinician must then find a suitable solution to any conflicts in expectations. Reviewing the relationships using a visual tool with the patient directly may expedite any conflict resolution.

COMPONENTS OF THE PLAN OF CARE

The plan of care is developed through the systematic process of examination, evaluation, diagnosis, and prognosis (Figure 20-2). Specific impairments are identified based on physical examination and risks of functional limitations and disability by evaluating the impact of the impairments on the patient's roles, lifestyle, home, resources, and available assistance. The clinician is responsible for taking a thorough history that may include general demographic information, social history, occupation/employment, growth and development, and living environment. In addition, the history of the current condition, current and prior functional status and activity level, current medications, past history of the current condition, past medical and surgical history, family history, health status, and social habits are considered in determining a diagnosis (Figure 20-3). Diagnosis is defined as a cluster of signs and symptoms, syndromes, or categories in the *Guide*. In contrast to the pathology-driven diagnostic categories used by physicians, the diagnoses described in the *Guide* are impairment driven. Based on the history and diagnosis, a prognosis is developed. Prognosis as defined in the *Guide* includes the predicted optimal level of improvement in function and the amount of time needed to reach that level. Prognosis may also include a prediction of the levels of improvement that may be reached at various intervals during the course of therapy. The plan of care describes the interventions to be used, goals, and outcomes of the interventions. In this model, *goals* refer specifically to remediation of impairments and outcomes related to

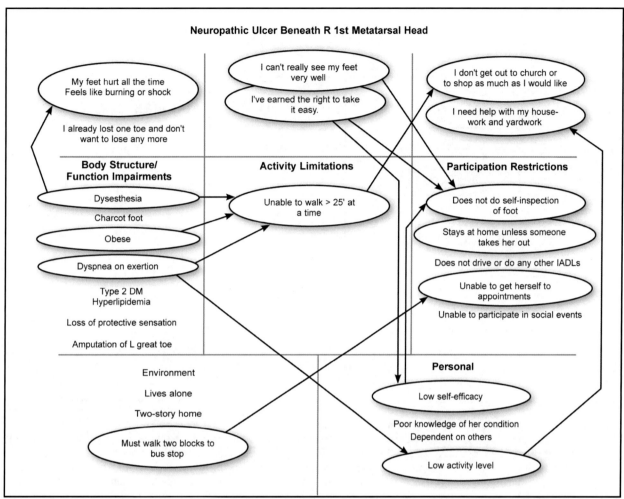

Figure 20-1. Using the ICF model to develop a plan of care. This tool is used to discover the patient's underlying problems so they can be addressed efficiently. The patient's participation restrictions were all traced to a small number of underlying problems (2 of them are not linked in this example to improve the clarity of this figure). She did not perform self-inspection of her feet because of diabetic retinopathy and low self-efficacy. She stayed at home unless someone transported her, which led to missing health care appointments. She was obese, unable to walk more than 25 feet, had dyspnea on exertion, and complained of foot pain. Because of these physical problems, she had a low activity level and was unable to perform any instrumental activities of daily living. Finally, her low self-efficacy was caused by the negative impact of physical deterioration and isolation on her self-esteem. These basic problems led to a downward spiral of inactivity and physical and emotional decline. Underlying problems uncovered by this approach included the need for greater social support to improve her self-efficacy and to take her to health care appointments. Treatment of her dysesthesia pharmacologically has increased her willingness to perform activities on her feet, including physical therapy. Physical therapy has increased her mobility and broken the cycle of inactivity and physical deterioration. As a result of addressing these 3 problems, the patient now has the ability to get out of her home, participate in social events, do light shopping, and take better control of her health problems. Now she is less reliant on home care and has a much brighter outlook. As a result of these changes in addition to wound care, her neuropathic ulcer has healed, and she is less likely to develop more ulcerations. As an exercise, finish connecting the remaining items on this figure. Then, think back to a current or past patient and populate another grid until you are ready to use this tool with new patients.

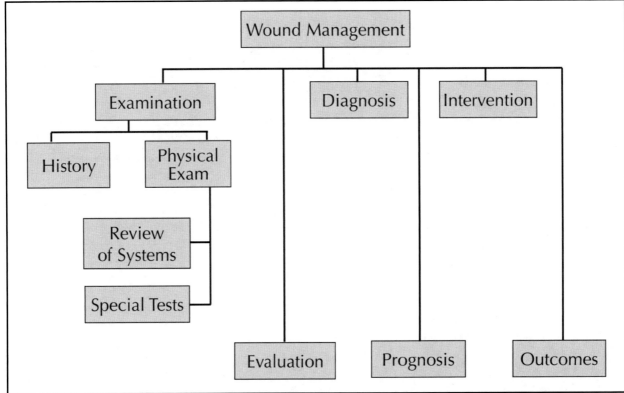

Figure 20-2. The plan of care begins with data gathering. The examination consists of a history and physical examination with a review of systems and special tests used to rule in or rule out suspected causes of the wound. Following data gathering, the clinician undergoes a mental processing of the data. This process is called the evaluation. Based on the data, the clinician develops the impairment-driven diagnosis according to the processes described in the *Guide*. Although not necessary for every patient, the clinician may also seek to confirm or refute a pathology-driven diagnosis. The prognosis is developed based on the diagnosis and unique combination of circumstances of the patient derived from the history and physical examination. Interventions are devised based on the examination, diagnosis, prognosis, and patient preferences and resources. Appropriate outcomes are derived in consultation with the patient, family, caregivers, and other involved clinicians.

minimizing functional limitations, optimizing health status, and preventing disability. The hope of clinicians is to prevent disability. Although not addressed specifically in the *Guide*, outcomes may be limited to minimizing disability, rather than preventing it. Common outcomes for wound management are shown in Figure 20-4. The plan of care may also include patient education, development of a maintenance program, and periodic reassessment of the maintenance program.

PROCEDURAL INTERVENTIONS

With respect to skin integrity, actions required of the clinician include identifying the cause of wounds and how to prevent recurrence, identifying factors that interfere with healing, appropriately selecting and applying wound care products, appropriate debridement (if required), and selection of adjunctive therapies as indicated. Categories of interventions are shown in Figure 20-5.

Fluid Balance

Healing is most effective if the wound microenvironment is optimized. This optimization includes maintaining an appropriate moisture level. A dry wound must be moistened, and a heavily draining wound needs to be managed either to absorb excessive moisture or to decrease the cause of the copious drainage. Macromolecules produced in the wound, including glycosaminoglycans, fibronectin, collagen, and growth factors, need to be retained in the wound while acceptable levels of nonpathogenic organisms and protection from pathogens in the environment are achieved. An appropriate microenvironment is usually accomplished through the use of occlusive dressings that retain fluid in the wound while either absorbing or allowing evaporation of excessive moisture. Maintaining wound temperature near core body temperature produces optimal fibroblast replication. Wound moisture is particularly critical to allow the migration of epithelial cells, movement of enzymes, growth factors, and structural molecules through

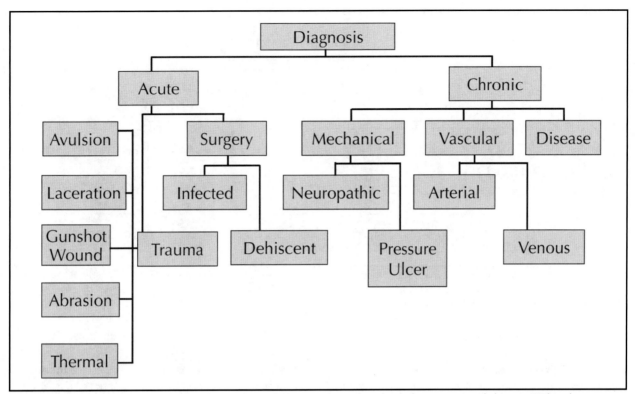

Figure 20-3. A flowchart to evaluate etiology of a wound. Wounds are first divided into acute and chronic. Within the category of acute wounds, causes are divided into traumatic and surgical wounds of the type most likely to be referred to a clinician other than a surgeon. Within the category of chronic wounds, the subcategories of mechanical, vascular, and disease are given. Although many other causes of wounds exist, for the purpose of this flowchart, only the most common are demonstrated.

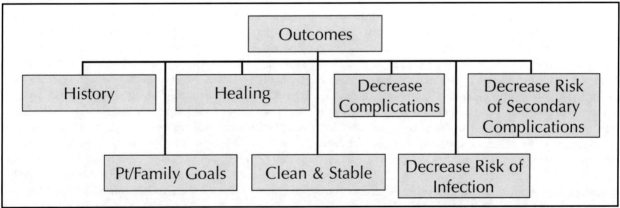

Figure 20-4. A flowchart for the development of outcomes and a select sample of them. Realistic outcomes are derived from understanding the patient's unique set of circumstances, such as resources, lifestyle, and physical condition, as well as the goals of the patient, family, and caregivers. Possible outcomes range from complete healing to reducing the risk of secondary complications that would likely exacerbate the condition of a patient with terminal disease.

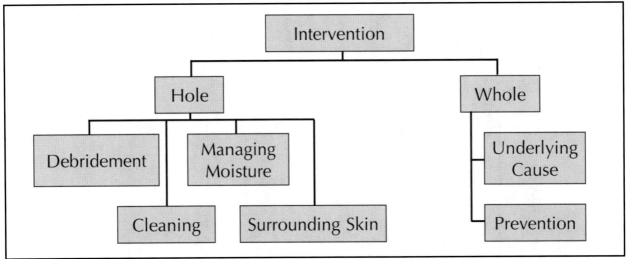

Figure 20-5. Interventions for wound management consist of treating the "hole in the patient" and the "whole of the patient." Interventions for addressing the wound itself include debridement, cleaning, managing drainage, and optimizing the health of the skin surrounding the wound. To benefit the patient as a whole, the underlying cause of the wound is addressed, and preventive measures are taken to prevent either recurrence of the wound or the development of new wounds elsewhere.

the wound. However, excessive moisture can cause maceration, injuring the source of epithelial cells needed to resurface the wound. Incontinence creates an even greater problem because of the acidity of urine and feces.

Allowing the wound to dry out was once encouraged as a means of preventing infection. However, this practice has been abandoned with research showing that dry wound beds impede wound healing. Although desiccated fibrin and blood act as a dressing to retain moisture below and keep out pathogens, scab formation slows epithelial cell migration as epithelial cells are forced to migrate deeply and through a dry environment. Scab formation is mainly an issue for wounds greater in diameter than a few millimeters. For narrow, especially linear wounds requiring minimal epithelial cell migration, scab formation is a minor issue. For superficial wounds, re-epithelialization can occur from appendages and wound edges, but for deep wounds involving the full thickness of dermis, epithelialization proceeds from the edges only, and full-thickness wounds greater than a few centimeters in diameter may require operative repair. Full-thickness or deeper wounds fill with granulation tissue before re-epithelialization. A moist wound bed assists in the migration and proliferation of fibroblasts as well as epithelialization.

Bacterial Balance

A second consideration is the issue of bacterial balance. Bacterial balance requires an understanding of infection, contamination, and colonization. All chronic open wounds are colonized by microbes, but clinicians should

not be careless in maintaining cleanliness of the wound. Contamination of a wound may increase the risk of infection. Although the immune system and the balance of microbes may keep a given pathogen from proliferating in the wound, the introduction of new bacteria or changing the environment of the wound may allow one bacterium to multiply rapidly and injure cells in the wound. Certain microbes may begin to digest the interstitial space, producing cellulitis, and spread subcutaneously, forming sinus tracts and additional abscesses. Although occlusion promotes the growth of cells needed for healing a wound, occlusion will also promote the growth of certain types of bacteria in the wound; therefore, infected wounds should not be occluded. Grossly contaminated wounds and wounds suspected to be infected should be allowed, at least initially, to heal by secondary intent until the wound is clean and stable. Any cavity in the tissue provides an environment conducive to bacterial overgrowth and prevents observation of the wound. Exposure to air and irrigation decrease the bacterial count but cause the wound to dry out, slowing healing. Therefore, the clinician must be ready to alter the treatment plan, depending on whether the goal is prevention/treatment of infection or promotion of granulation and epithelialization. Occlusive dressings are indicated when healing is to be promoted and the wound is not infected. Nonocclusive dressings are indicated in wounds that are infected or are at high risk for infection such as grossly contaminated wounds. Nonocclusive dressings should be used until the bacterial count is low enough to use occlusive dressings.

Drainage Management

The third consideration is the management of drainage. One aspect often neglected is the drainage caused by rough handling of wounds by the clinician or caregiver. By minimizing wound handling, inflammation is reduced. Inflammation caused by debridement, excessive irrigation, and frequent dressing changes leads to edema, serous drainage, and slowed healing. One means of reducing drainage is to debride necrotic tissue as rapidly as possible. Protracted debridement with daily or even twice daily rough handling of the wound and the persistence of necrotic tissue promote inflammation and lead to drainage. A number of dressings are available to absorb a wide range of drainage. Alginate/hydrofiber and foam dressings can absorb moderate to maximum drainage longer than other dressings, allowing for less frequent changes. When inflammation and drainage have decreased to suitable levels, hydrocolloid sheets and semipermeable films can be used to retain an appropriate level of moisture for several days. Purulent drainage, however, is a clear sign to stop occluding the wound. Purulence should be absorbed with either gauze or alginate. Although aggressive sharp debridement is preferred, wounds may be filled with antibiotic-soaked gauze if other factors indicate. Another problem caused by chronic inflammation due to rough handling is the leakage of fibrinogen into the wound bed. Fibrinogen may be converted to fibrin on the wound surface, causing a hard yellow material to form on the wound surface. This type of eschar is particularly difficult to debride. Curettage, ultrasonic debridement, or enzymatic debriders may be used to clear this material from the wound. In a dry wound, moisture can be both added and retained by using amorphous hydrogel on the wound bed and an occlusive dressing. When retaining moisture in a wound, some moisture may run over the surrounding skin, causing maceration. A moisture-barrier cream or skin sealant can be effective in preventing maceration.

FORMULATING THE PLAN OF CARE

The plan of care needs to flow from the items discussed previously. Given 2 patients with identical characteristics, 2 different plans of care are likely to be needed. Variances in the plan of care should be viewed as accommodations to the unique combinations of patient characteristics, including physical condition, cultural beliefs and behaviors, resources, and lifestyle. The plan of care needs to represent the optimum combination of appropriate wound care and the reality of how the plan interacts with the patient.

Treatment planning may follow 4 basic decision points in addition to accommodations for circumstances beyond the characteristics of the wound. The 4 basic decision points are (1) presence, suspicion, or reasonable assumption of impending infection; (2) type of debridement suited to the patient and the wound; (3) depth of tissue loss; and (4) management of drainage and the surrounding skin.

Presence, Suspicion, or Reasonable Assumption of Impending Infection

When infection is known to be present, it is suspected, or one may reasonably suspect that it will occur, treatment decisions are directed primarily toward managing infection. Interventions directed toward eliminating infection may, in fact, slow wound healing. However, infection is sufficiently serious to warrant precedence over other aspects of wound management. Other aspects are not ignored; rather, potential conflicts in management of the different aspects of the wound are resolved by allowing certain aspects to take precedence. Infection can be managed in a number of ways. Critically important to bear in mind is the relationship between the presence of necrotic tissue and infection. Necrotic tissue provides a foothold for pathogenic bacteria that otherwise would remain under control on a relatively clean wound surface. Based on this principle, infection can be managed by sharp debridement or other means of rapid debridement. The National Pressure Injury Advisory Panel recommends sharp debridement of pressure injuries with impending infection. The American Diabetes Association recommends aggressive sharp debridement of neuropathic ulcers. In addition to the use of sharp instruments, one may use pulsatile lavage, irrigation, or other forms of hydrotherapy to supplement the removal of necrotic tissue and bacteria. Application of antibiotics or surface antiseptics may be appropriate for a small number of days, particularly for acute wounds at risk of infection because of gross contamination from gunshot wounds, motor vehicle accidents, and agricultural and industrial accidents. Acute wounds, especially wounds that have not received care within several hours, will need aggressive lavage, debridement, and possibly treatment with antibiotics. The National Pressure Injury Advisory Panel recommends only a brief trial of surface treatment for pressure injuries that fail to respond to optimal care. The American Diabetes Association, on the other hand, does not recommend surface treatment at all, instead calling for sharp debridement and parenteral antibiotics specifically selected for the identified pathogen.

Type of Debridement Needed

The second point is the type of debridement utilized. Several factors come into play. Factors may include economics of the health care setting, patient satisfaction, patient/caregiver skill, and clinician skill. Debridement is necessary for any wound with necrotic tissue. The type of debridement, however, needs to be determined based on a number of institutional, personal, and wound characteristics. In the acute care setting in which discharge is dependent on the wound becoming clean and stable, rapid debridement is necessary. Some clinicians may choose to perform nonspecific mechanical types of debridement, often using hydrotherapy. Clinicians with the skill to perform sharp debridement can achieve a clean, stable wound much more rapidly than by using hydrotherapy alone. In many cases, especially with neuropathic ulcers, sharp debridement can be achieved in a single visit. The wound may need to be monitored, and some further minor debridement may be necessary if discharge is pending completion of a round of intravenous antibiotic treatment. In many cases, however, the patient is now discharged to home with home health visits to complete a course of intravenous antibiotics. If clinician skill or patient preference dictates against sharp debridement, pulsatile lavage with concurrent suction may be a reasonable alternative. Whirlpool therapy, however, is generally not a reasonable alternative. Whirlpool therapy may be preferred for wounds with a large surface area requiring low-level agitation and minor burns on extremities that require the cleansing of residues such as silver sulfadiazine. Soaking a wound to loosen necrotic tissue and pulling loose tissue with forceps once or twice a day is a common practice but offers no advantage over sharp debridement or pulsatile lavage with concurrent suction. Whirlpool agitation is generally ineffective at debriding areas of subcutaneous involvement with undermining, tunneling, and sinus tracts and risks contamination of wounds with flora from other submersed areas of the body. Within a limited depth of approximately 20 cm, flexible tips of pulsatile lavage units can readily reach these areas.

Whirlpool therapy should also be avoided for wounds due to venous disease. Edema is exacerbated by placing the limb in a dependent position with the thigh compressed against the edge of the tank and warm water increasing blood flow to the affected leg. In addition, the elevated temperature of typical whirlpool therapy increases the demand for blood flow in cases of peripheral arterial disease and increases the risk of further tissue injury in thermal injuries and skin with diminished sensation. Fragile skin, especially in an older patient, can be damaged by the agitation and maceration caused by soaking the extremity for 20 minutes.

When the time frame is not critical or the quality of life is not dependent on rapid debridement of the wound, autolytic and chemical debridement are reasonable. However, the patient or a caregiver must be able to determine if wound infection occurs. Infection demands immediate sharp debridement. In an outpatient or home health situation, a patient may express preference for autolytic or chemical debridement because of concern about pain or psychosocial factors. In a long-term care setting in which rapid debridement will not impact quality of life, the patient and clinician may agree to a more protracted but less invasive debridement procedure. For example, a bedfast individual with an open heel ulcer will not become ambulatory simply because of sharp debridement of the wound. On the other hand, a person who needs to be ambulatory and could be if not for a foot wound may decide on sharp debridement and total contact casting or one of its alternatives to become ambulatory sooner. A flowchart for debridement is shown in Figure 20-6.

Depth of Tissue Loss

The third decision point is the presence of subcutaneous tissue loss, including undermining, tunneling, and sinus tracts. When infection is present or debridement is ongoing, these tissue defects are often filled with gauze material. Dressings moistened with either normal saline or an antibiotic solution are typically used to fill these. Packing strip with or without iodine may be used for tunnels and sinus tracts. Packing strip comes in various widths and usually needs to be fanfolded as it is placed in a tunnel or sinus tract. Although the cotton material may promote inflammation of the tissue in the wound, absorption of infectious drainage and preventing occlusion that promotes growth of bacteria take precedence. Of particular importance is preventing wounds from closing over subcutaneous defects. Ideally, a wound fills completely with granulation and re-epithelializes. However, some patients may re-epithelialize too rapidly. Patients may be pleased that the wound has closed, but occlusion of necrotic tissue and purulence beneath the skin are likely to lead to a skin abscess in the near future. Such wounds must be kept open with packing strip and irrigated as much as possible to allow the wound to granulate fully before it closes. Larger undermined areas and simple areas of subcutaneous loss may be filled with moistened 4×4 or 2×2 gauze sponges or bandage rolls until the risk of infection is minimized. Note, however, that gauze sponges and bandage rolls are not designed for packing wounds. Packing strips are specifically manufactured to prevent the shedding of fibers that is likely to occur when gauze sponges and bandage rolls are used for packing wounds. Because of its design, 2-inch iodoform is less likely to cause inflammation than a 2-inch bandage roll.

Once the wound is stable, nonirritating filling materials should be substituted. Alginates, hydrofibers, and combinations with collagen are good choices for filling

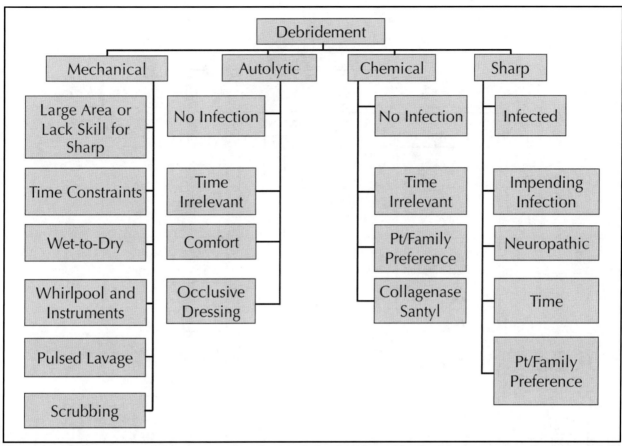

Figure 20-6. A flowchart outlining the reasons and methods for debridement by the 4 basic means: mechanical, autolytic, chemical, and sharp debridement.

these subcutaneous defects. Alginates and hydrofibers are available in both sheets and ribbons/ropes. These materials maintain their tensile strength while absorbing drainage and can be readily removed from the wound, even from tunnels and sinus tracts. Collagen present in the material is absorbed by the wound and may speed healing. A suitable secondary dressing needs to be placed over the wound based on the drainage and desired frequency of dressing change.

Management of Drainage

The fourth decision point is based on drainage and manipulation of the desired frequency of dressing change. With subcutaneous tissue loss, both a primary and secondary dressing are chosen. For a simpler full-thickness or partial-thickness wound, a primary dressing may be sufficient. The type of dressing chosen must be based on multiple factors, again based on the order of precedence discussed earlier—infection, debridement, subcutaneous involvement, and drainage. If a wound is infected and filled with gauze, a nonocclusive secondary dressing needs to be

used. Typical choices include bandage rolls, self-adherent gauze bandages, and abdominal pads taped over skin protectant. Bandage rolls may be used on any body part and can be fanfolded to increase absorption. Abdominal pads can be gently pulled back and retaped from one corner (or more if necessary) to inspect a wound. On occcasion, these absorbent materials may be used over materials such as alginates or hydrofibers to absorb copious drainage for a few days as inflammation resolves. An occlusive dressing is generally used over an occlusive type of wound filler (hydrogel, foam, or alginate/hydrofiber); however, initially the drainage may overwhelm most occlusive dressings, requiring the use of some combination of abdominal pads, multiple gauze sponges, and bandage rolls.

When occlusion of the wound is appropriate, the quantity of drainage and characteristics of the patient and dressings must be considered. A desiccated wound can be rehydrated with amorphous hydrogel covered with a simple dressing such as a semipermeable film. Light drainage from a partial-thickness or full-thickness wound without subcutaneous involvement may be managed with a semipermeable film. Hydrocolloids are the most occlusive wound dressing and are ideal for wounds that are clean and

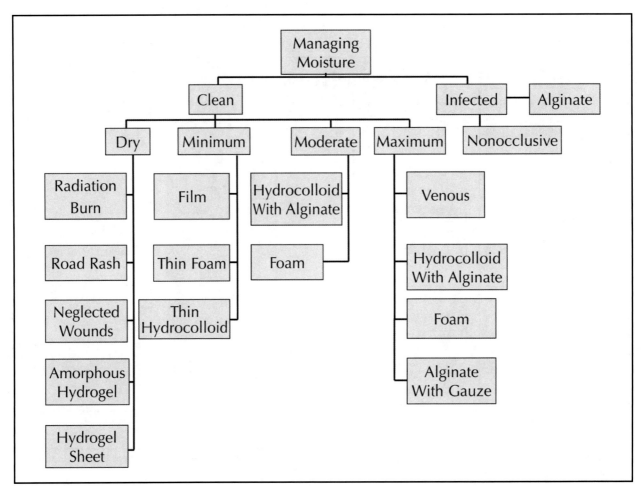

Figure 20-7. A flowchart for managing drainage. The first division is into clean wounds and infected wounds, with only non-occlusive dressings or alginates as options. Clean wounds are categorized by the quantity of drainage. Selected examples of wounds typically observed to have different levels of drainage and types of primary dressings appropriate for the drainage are listed.

stable and, therefore, only need to be protected. Ideally, the hydrocolloid dressing is left in place for 5 days or more. Depending on the drainage and extent of subcutaneous involvement, alginate, hydrofiber, or foam may be needed beneath the hydrocolloid sheet. The hydrocolloid dressing is changed at the desired interval of 5 to 7 days or earlier if the dressing becomes white and swollen. Leaving an over-hydrated occlusive dressing in place too long risks maceration of the surrounding tissue. Hydrogel sheets are popular dressings for abrasions as well as chemical and radiation burns due to their soothing effect. Water released from the hydrogel can macerate the surrounding skin, and evaporation of water from the hydrogel dressing can allow the wound bed to desiccate if it is left in place too long. Foam dressing materials are good choices when a wound is ready for occlusion, but drainage is too heavy for hydrocolloid sheets. For a heavily draining wound with subcutaneous involvement, foam sheets can be placed into a wound as a

primary dressing with a hydrocolloid secondary dressing. Composite dressings constructed of contact material surrounded with absorbent material and a waterproof exterior can also be used on this type of wound. Composite foam and film dressings may also be useful but may not last for the number of days desired by the clinician. In addition to the characteristics of the dressing materials, the patient characteristics and wound location must be considered. A bulky dressing should not be placed on an area where it will catch onto clothing and shoes or other items in the environment. If the person will be showering, a film, foam, or hydrogel dressing may not stay in place. Hydrocolloid sheets are waterproof on the outside and, if kept out of direct spray, can last several days even with showering. A flowchart for the management of moisture is shown in Figure 20-7 and one for managing the surrounding skin is shown in Figure 20-8.

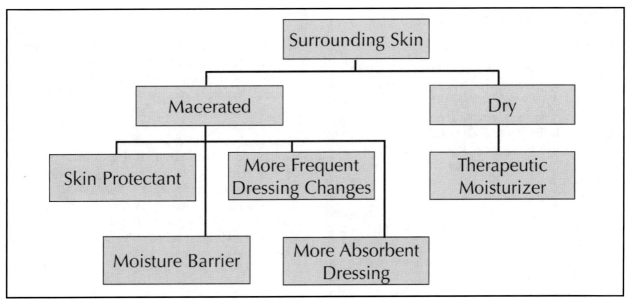

Figure 20-8. Care for the surrounding skin is divided into the categories of macerated and dry and possible solutions for optimizing the moisture of the surrounding skin.

Modifications for the Care of Aging Skin

Foremost, the choice of wound products to be used on the skin of older patients must take into account the fragile nature of their skin. Moreover, because of decreased inflammation and greater risk of malnutrition and dehydration, the clinician must assume a longer period for healing. Therefore, dressings that need to be changed frequently or have strong adhesive must be used with care or avoided. Tape of any kind must be used judiciously. In particular, silk and plastic tape should not be used. Nontape alternatives such as stretch netting should be considered. When occlusive dressings are chosen, hydrocolloids and semipermeable films should be used only if nonadherent foam or hydrogel sheets are not practical. If films or hydrocolloid sheets are to be used, skin protectant needs to be placed on the surrounding skin. In addition, the absorbency of the dressing needs to be optimized. Although thin hydrocolloid sheets permit better visualization of the wound, thicker hydrocolloid sheets may be necessary to prolong time between changes. Filling the wound with an absorbent material such as alginate or hydrofiber can also prolong the wearing time of hydrocolloid and semipermeable film dressings. When these dressings are removed, care must be taken to avoid injury to the skin. The skin should not be pulled with the dressing as it is removed. Gentle peeling of hydrocolloid sheets or stretching of a semipermeable film tangentially to the skin surface as the skin is held in place may reduce the risk of injury, as shown in Chapter 16. In addition

to selecting wound care products carefully, a number of other forms of skin protection should be considered. The skin of older adults tends to become dry and brittle and may fissure and tear with minor trauma. Therapeutic moisturizers may be necessary, especially during the winter or in low-humidity environments. Bed frames and rails should be inspected for sharp edges and padded as needed.

Cleansing of wounds of older adults needs to be done as gently as possible. Pulsatile lavage with suction may be done at a lower-impact pressure or replaced by gentle irrigation as necessary. Mechanical damage and maceration can result from vigorous whirlpool therapy for cleansing or nonselective debridement. For many older patients, the clinician must consider the risks and benefits of different types of debridement. Frequently, orders are received for whirlpool and wet-to-dry dressings on the wounds of older patients. Additives to the whirlpools or topical agents placed on the wound may cause severe injury to the wound or surrounding skin. Older patients in the terminal stage of an illness may not benefit from the full scale of options available from the clinician. The clinician must determine what benefits the patient will receive from any given intervention. Often, wound healing is not achievable due to the nutritional or cardiopulmonary status of the patient, and goals are limited to reducing the risk of infection and managing drainage and odor of the wound. If sharp debridement provides no benefit, a treatment plan optimizing autolytic debridement can be appropriate.

Optimizing Wound Healing in Children

Compared with adults, children have a better outcome from laceration repair. Children are less likely to have wound infections (2.1% vs 4.1%) and have a better cosmetic outcome than adults. Lacerations in children are irrigated less frequently than those of adults (53% vs 77%) and more frequently scrubbed (50% vs 45%). Comparing the characteristics of wounds of children and adults, wounds in children are much more likely to occur on the head (86% vs 38%), to be linear and shorter, less likely to be contaminated, and more commonly caused by blunt trauma compared with adults. The greater prevalence of children's wounds on the highly vascular head may be responsible for the lower infection rate, rather than some intrinsic difference in wound healing between children and adults. Although children are believed to have a greater ability to heal than adults, several factors relevant to children may slow healing. Children, especially neonates, have a greater surface area to body mass ratio and more difficulty in regulating body temperature than adults, which may impair healing. Young children, like older adults, are at greater risk of malnutrition, especially in the presence of digestive disease or prematurity. Premature neonates have more fragile skin than full-term infants and, as such, are more susceptible to wounds due to weaker intracellular attachments. Due to the tremendous instrumentation required in the neonatal intensive care unit, premature infants are at great risk for cutaneous injury during handling. Moreover, multiple lines and equipment in conjunction with a lack of voluntary movement may place the neonate at risk of pressure injuries from this instrumentation. In particular, infants are susceptible to occipital pressure injuries due to the disproportionate head size. Risk factors for children in intensive care include age less than 36 months, ventricular septal defect (study involved children receiving open heart surgery), intubation longer than 7 days, and being in intensive care longer than 8 days. Infants are also at risk of skin injury secondary to persistent contact with urine and feces on the perineal skin.

PATIENT EDUCATION

The *Guide* specifically addresses patient education as one of the components of the therapist's interaction with a patient/client, in addition to procedural interventions, documentation, communication, and coordination of patient care. Each patient has a unique educational and lifetime learning background and level of self-efficacy. Some individuals are in a position of directly supervising and performing the bulk of their care, whereas others are completely dependent on others in developing and carrying out a plan of care. Therefore, the clinician must interview the patient, family, and caregivers to ascertain their levels of understanding of the process by which the wound developed and how to facilitate its healing. Topics for discussion include the etiology of the wound, rudimentary principles of wound healing, the purposes and mechanisms of action of any interventions, and expected outcomes. Most individuals will not be able to process all of this information at once and will need periodic reinforcement, including opportunities for the patient to discuss progress during each visit and to ask questions. The clinician should also periodically assess the patient's or caregiver's cognitive (knowledge), psychomotor (ability to apply the knowledge), and affective (attitudes toward the process) learning.

COORDINATION AND COMMUNICATION

Each clinician has an ethical obligation to provide optimum care within their range of knowledge, skills, and abilities. As part of this, the clinician is obligated ethically to refer a patient to a clinician with the appropriate knowledge, skills, and abilities to provide optimal benefit for the patient. In the case of peripheral arterial disease, the patient obviously needs the services of a vascular surgeon. If a wound becomes infected or infection cannot be controlled by sharp debridement, referral to an infectious disease specialist or surgeon becomes necessary. If a wound requires more extensive debridement than can be managed without an operating room, requires general anesthesia, or if the patient has tunneling or sinus tracts that will need to be opened, referral to a surgeon is needed. If a clinician lacks skill at sharp debridement, this aspect of care needs to be turned over to a person who is skilled. If the clinician wishes to continue to see patients likely to need sharp debridement, the clinician should undergo appropriate training and ensure that this intervention is supported by legal regulations and guidelines within their practice environment. Other potential situations requiring referrals include complicated cases of nutritional risk, management of incontinence, need for splints, adaptive or assistive devices, orthoses, prostheses, mobility or activity of daily living training, psychological counseling, assistance in obtaining financial resources and caregivers, vocational training, or creating a plan of care within constraints imposed by payers.

SUMMARY

The plan of care is a blueprint for interventions provided based on the history and physical examination of the patient, a diagnosis of the cause of the wound healing, and the prognosis for healing. It is modified based on a unique set of circumstances related to the patient's ability to follow through with the plan. Decision points include the need to treat infection, the type of debridement needed, filling subcutaneous defects, and managing drainage to optimize wound moisture while simultaneously maintaining the integrity of the surrounding skin. The skin of older adults and neonates is at greater risk of injury due to anatomical and physiologic differences. Older skin has less contact area, has decreased thickness and blood flow, and is vulnerable to tearing and bleeding. A number of risk factors for injury are present in neonates, especially premature infants. Decreased ability to regulate heat, potential for malnourishment, inability to reposition, and the presence of multiple lines and devices increase the risk of injury and slow healing. Both infants and older adults need to be handled gently to avoid skin injury. The ICF model is described as a tool for treatment planning by identifying the relationships among physical impairments, activity limitations, participation restrictions, and personal and environmental factors.

QUESTIONS

1. How does the care setting affect the plan of care?

2. How might an immobile terminally ill patient's plan of care differ from an ambulatory person's plan of care for a foot wound?

3. What 2 critical functions do dressings perform in managing wound drainage?

4. What are critical reasons for performing sharp debridement?

5. Under what circumstances would sharp debridement not be performed?

6. What characteristics need to be considered in choosing a dressing that patients will need to change at home?

7. Explain the greater risk of tearing and bleeding that occur in the skin of older people.

8. Describe steps that can be taken to minimize damage to the skin of the infant and older patient.

9. List risk factors for skin injury and slow wound healing commonly present in premature infants.

REFERENCE

1. Steiner WA, Ryser L, Huber E, Uebelhart D, Aeschlimann A, Stucki G. Use of the ICF model as a clinical problem-solving tool in physical therapy and rehabilitation medicine. *Phys Ther.* 2002;82(11):1098-1107.

BIBLIOGRAPHY

American Physical Therapy Association. *Guide to Physical Therapist Practice.* Accessed October 17, 2022. http://guidetoptpractice.apta.org/

Dijkers MP, Hart T, Whyte J, Zanca JM, Packel A, Tsaousides T. Rehabilitation treatment taxonomy: implications and continuations. *Arch Phys Med Rehabil.* 2014;95(1 Suppl):S45-54.e2. doi:10.1016/j.apmr.2013.05.033

Gordon A, Kozin ED, Keswani SG, et al. Permissive environment in postnatal wounds induced by adenoviral-mediated overexpression of the anti-inflammatory cytokine interleukin-10 prevents scar formation. *Wound Repair Regen.* 2008;16(1):70-79.

Helgeson K, Smith AR. Process for applying the international classification of functioning, disability and health model to a patient with patellar dislocation. *Phys Ther.* 2008;88(8):956-964.

Hollander JE, Singer AJ, Valentine S. Comparison of wound care practices in pediatric and adult lacerations repaired in the emergency department. *Pediatr Emerg Care.* 1998;14(1):15-18.

Jette AM. Toward a common language for function, disability and health. *Phys Ther.* 2006;86(5):726-734.

Johnson AM, Woltenberg LN, Heinss SH, Carper R, Taylor S, Kuperstein J. Whole person health: using experiential learning and the ICF model as a tool for introductory interprofessional collaborative practice. *J Allied Health.* 2020;49(2):86-91.

Malloy-McDonald MB. Skin care for high-risk neonates. *J Wound Ostomy Continence Nurs.* 1995;22(4):177-182.

Neidig JRE, Kleiber C, Oppliger RA. Risk factors associated with pressure ulcers in the pediatric patient following open-heart surgery. *Prog Cardiovasc Nurs.* 1989;4(3):99-106.

Pieper B, Templin T, Dobal M, Jacox A. Prevalence and types of wounds among children receiving care in the home. *Ostomy Wound Manage.* 2000;46(4):36-42.

Roaldsen KS, Rollman O, Torebjörk E, Olsson E, Stanghelle JK. Functional ability in female leg ulcer patients—a challenge for physiotherapy. *Physiother Res Int.* 2006;11(4):191-203.

Verbrugge LM, Jette AM. The disablement process. *Soc Sci Med.* 1994;38(1):1-14.

World Health Organization. *Towards a common language for functioning, disability and health.* 2002; Author.

21

Regulations and Reimbursement

OBJECTIVES

- Discuss Medicare and typical state licensing regulations relevant to wound management.
- Discuss issues related to reimbursement for wound management services.
- Describe how to build a wound management team to optimize wound management.

However contentious and subject to rapid and dramatic change, the issues discussed in this chapter are important for a healthy practice that allows our patients/clients to benefit from our services. Unfortunately, a detailed description of what is optimal or even allowable in terms of reimbursement is likely to be outdated before many readers use this text. Changes occur due to federal legislation and rules dictated by government agencies such as the Centers for Medicare & Medicaid Services (CMS). Prudence dictates that each facility has an individual responsible for analysis of the multitude of health care rules and regulations that may impact reimbursement. Depending on the case mix of individual facilities, these issues may require adjustments to staffing. An attempt will be made to discuss general principles that are unlikely to change in the near future.

REGULATIONS

Issues concerning both regulation and reimbursement are often related. With Medicare as the largest third-party payer and other payers generally following CMS's policies, regulations developed for CMS affect reimbursement profoundly. Pro bono cases are an important part of our social responsibility; however, when developing a plan of care, both wound care products and services rendered will need to be reimbursable in the vast majority of cases for the facility's fiscal health. CMS expended over $1.6 trillion in 2021 for Medicare and Medicaid recipients. With such a large amount of money, volumes of regulations are written in an attempt to use the available money most efficiently. CMS regulations do not vary across states or among carriers or fiscal intermediaries (companies contracted to manage Medicare Parts A and B). However, the implementation of regulations may vary substantially, such that another may not cover services covered in one state or by a certain CMS contractor. Although only a small number of insurance companies serve as Medicare contractors, staff in different states may have different interpretations of a given Medicare rule. Within a given contractor, different personnel are likely to have different interpretations of the same rule. This situation is exacerbated by job turnover within these companies. Individuals working for CMS contractors can be educated to understand the role of different interventions for a patient's various characteristics. However, the loss of that employee forces the clinician to educate another. CMS attempts to improve uniformity by periodically distributing explicit instructions to its contractors on certain issues. Although the regulations often appear arbitrary and more favorable to specific settings and providers than others, we must learn to work within these regulations while providing appropriate and fiscally responsible care and advocating for policy changes when needed.

Medicare requires the evaluation and interventions involved in wound management to be performed by appropriately trained and licensed individuals. In some cases, state laws may permit tremendous latitude in assigning personnel to direct patient care. Regardless of the letter of the law, ethical, moral, and risk management principles must be applied to staffing decisions. The potential risk of harming a patient can never be justified by assigning direct patient care to individuals lacking appropriate training or licensing regardless of what individual state practice acts may allow. Moreover, fee schedules are based on the use of appropriate personnel; billing for direct patient care provided by an individual lacking the training specified by Medicare requirements could be ruled Medicare fraud and lead to severe consequences.

State licensing requirements generally become an issue on 2 points. First, does the patient have direct access to your services or must they be referred, usually through a family practitioner or other medical specialist? The second concern is how the state practice acts for the different providers are written in terms of debridement. Individuals in each state need to determine current regulations for referral and sharp debridement. In general, physicians (including podiatrists), physician assistants, and physical therapists are permitted to perform sharp debridement. Advanced practice nurses and other health care providers may be allowed within given states.

REIMBURSEMENT ISSUES

Charges for direct interventions generally eligible for reimbursement by CMS include those for evaluation, debridement, wound stimulation by high-volt pulsed current or pulsed electromagnetic field, and negative pressure wound therapy, in addition to those traditionally used beyond treatment of the wound itself. Only specific types of wounds are eligible for payment under debridement codes. These wound types are surgical wounds that must be left open to heal by secondary intention; infected open wounds; wounds caused by trauma or surgery; or wounds related to "complicating metabolic, vascular, or pressure factors." This list covers the most common wounds discussed in Chapters 11 to 14 and nearly all of those produced by unusual causes, as described in Chapter 18. Uncomplicated abrasions and lacerations are specifically excluded. CMS does not consider the use of treatments other than debridement, negative pressure wound therapy, hyperbaric oxygen, and high-volt pulsed current and pulsed electromagnetic field stimulation as medically necessary.

The American Medical Association (AMA), working with CMS, has developed a coding system for billing for services termed *Common Procedural Terminology* (CPT). The term CPT is a registered trademark of the AMA, which reserves all rights to the term CPT and the individual descriptions of each code. Because CPT is copyrighted material, only short descriptors of each code are allowed in publications other than the AMA's official annual publication, *CPT Current Procedural Terminology*, and a monthly publication called *CPT Assistant*. Descriptions of individual CPT codes discussed in this text are not the complete official description, but the AMA's shortened version is deemed acceptable. Codes may be added, deleted, or descriptions modified on an annual basis by the AMA. Reimbursement amounts and requirements are also subject to change following notice by CMS. More complete descriptions and requirements for the use of any given CPT code can be obtained from official AMA sources or the websites of CMS contractors. CMS establishes Healthcare Common Procedure Coding System (HCPCS) codes for supplies, equipment, and temporary or unusual situations. Three levels of HCPCS codes are in existence at the time of this writing. Level I includes the CPT codes, written by an AMA committee to aid in Medicare administration. Level II represents codes developed by CMS either temporarily or to handle durable medical equipment (eg, specialty beds and surgical supplies such as wound dressings and compression bandages). Level III is developed to handle unique situations.

The original philosophy for CPT codes was that payment would be based on the service provided rather than the provider. However, this philosophy has changed first with the codes for evaluation, which are now provider dependent. Until 2000, debridement codes existed only under the surgical section of the codes. Sharp debridement had been paid to nonphysician providers under one of the surgical codes 11040 to 11044 by some CMS contractors. However, other contractors would not provide payment despite the ruling that Medicare payment for sharp debridement is allowed for physical therapists, podiatrists, physicians, and advanced practice nurses with specialized training. Payment under other plans or as part of a diagnosis-related group (DRG) may allow others to perform sharp debridement. The major problem with reimbursement under the surgical codes was the cost determined for reimbursing debridement as a surgical procedure and the absence of a code that reflected the lower cost of providing sharp debridement in a nonsurgical environment. In the revisions for 2001, CPT code 97601 for the removal of devitalized tissue from wounds by selective debridement without anesthesia was implemented. Within the description for this code, examples of allowable means of debridement included both selective and nonselective means of debridement. Whirlpool, pulsatile lavage, and selective sharp debridement with scissors, scalpel, and forceps were given as examples. Reimbursement under this code bundled any topical application(s), wound assessment, and instruction(s) for ongoing care per session, not the time spent performing the service. Moreover, for reimbursement, an evaluative component is expected with each session. The CPT code 97602 was created at the same time to designate nonselective debridement using procedures not requiring skilled services. As of 2019, this code is not separately payable under Medicare because it is considered a nonskilled service. The application of wet-to-dry dressings, enzymatic debriders, and scrubbing are included under this code. Some CMS contractors may consider whirlpool therapy to belong to this category and deny payment if a whirlpool bill is submitted under codes 97597 or 97598.

New codes were implemented in 2005 for "active wound care management" with a description implying selective debridement. The 2 codes 97597 and 97598 cover the same service, differing only in the size of the wound, and are limited to removing necrotic tissue with the expectation that the procedure can be done selectively (selective debridement). Selective debridement of wounds with a 20 cm^2 or smaller surface area is coded 97597; the same procedure for a wound with a surface area greater than 20 cm^2 is coded 97598. The payment for 97598 has been greater than for 97597, but both were increased to the same amount for 2019. When a wound greater than 20 cm^2 is debrided, both 97597 and 97598 are billed. None of the debridement codes are time based. Payment is the same regardless of time spent, cost of dressings and other supplies applied, or the amount of assistance required to perform the service. However, ambulatory care patients seen in a physician-based clinic can be billed through office visit codes 99201 to 99215. The CPT codes 99201 to 99205 pertain to 5 levels of care for new patients with the

descriptors problem focused, expanded, detailed, comprehensive, and high complexity assigned to these 5 codes, respectively. Codes 99211 to 99215 are used for outpatient visits by established patients using the same 5 descriptors. Based on the time and other resources used for the office visit, 1 of the 5 levels for either a new or established patient is chosen. For example, a simple follow-up examination of a patient would be billed as 99211. Extensive, time-consuming debridement and use of expensive dressings could be billed as 99215. Other CPT codes that might be utilized in wound care are 16020, 16025, and 16030, which are for debridement of partial-thickness burn injuries (small, medium, large), and codes 97605 and 97606 for negative pressure wound therapy.

When billing for debridement, codes for excisional debridement (11040 series) and selective debridement (97597 and 97598) cannot be used on the same day for the same wound. Appropriate use of both sets of codes would be excisional debridement by a surgeon on one day, followed by selective debridement no sooner than the next day by a physical therapist, advanced practice nurse, or physician assistant. For 2008, a category III CPT was developed for "low frequency, non-contact, non-thermal ultrasound," code 0183T. T codes are essentially temporary tracking codes; CMS "tracks" these codes for a period of time to see how often they are used and determine whether a category I CPT code should be assigned. In 2014, the 0183T code was replaced with the 97610 code. CPT code 97610 can be used as a stand-alone code; however, it is not separately payable when done in conjunction with debridement.

Codes in the 11040 series pertain to surgical excision of tissue as a means of debridement and may require anesthesia. The codes for selective debridement, 97597/8, are to be used by physicians when the service performed is the same as that provided by a physical therapist or nurse. However, when viable tissue, such as subcutaneous tissue, muscle, or bone, is involved (incisional debridement), the surgeon must use the 11040 series.

Codes are available for foot care (CPT codes 11055 to 11057) and nail care (CPT codes 11720 and 11721), but foot care is generally considered a maintenance service. Medicare will not cover it except under specific circumstances elaborated by CMS under its Routine Foot Care policy (ARA-02-043). This policy lists many appropriate conditions that might become foot threatening without appropriate foot care. Conditions include diabetes mellitus and a large number of other neuropathic and metabolic diseases. Routine foot care includes nail debridement, but nail debridement is included in the Routine Foot Care policy exceptions for systemic conditions.

CMS defines nail debridement as a "significant reduction in the thickness and length of the nail to the tolerance of the patient with the aim of allowing the patient to ambulate without pain." This definition is then further qualified by stating that simple trimming by cutting or grinding is not considered debridement. Superficial fungal infections that do not cause significant symptoms are not covered. If the patient is nonambulatory, CMS will only cover nail debridement of mycotic nails resulting in pain or secondary infection that results from dystrophic nails.

Medicare covers foot exams, including associated treatment once every 6 months for eligible individuals with a documented loss of protective sensation if the patient has not been seen by a "foot care specialist" within this 6-month period. CMS requires a diagnosis of loss of protective sensation to be established by standardized testing with the 5.07 monofilament, including 5 sites on each foot's plantar surface. The full 10-point exam endorsed by the American Diabetes Association is not required. The criterion of the American Podiatric Medicine Association is considered acceptable. This criterion requires failure to detect the 5.07 Semmes-Weinstein monofilament at 2 or more sites out of 5 tested on either foot. Examination required by CMS includes patient history and a minimum of visual inspection of the feet, monofilament testing, an examination of foot structure, biomechanics, vascular status, and need for special footwear. Patient education, local care of superficial wounds, debridement of callus, and trimming and debridement of nails are included in the payment for the semiannual visit. A large number of qualifiers are included in the policies covering foot care and nail debridement. The reader is directed to the CMS website to view these details.

If callus removal is performed during a selective debridement procedure, payment is only provided through 97597 or 97598. An additional submission for payment under 11055 to 11057 will be denied. Similarly, if only callus removal is performed, a claim for selective debridement will be denied. Therefore, the additional resources needed for callus removal are absorbed by the clinic performing the selective debridement. Due to the restrictive nature of CPT codes available, a clinic visit for a 10-cm^2 neuropathic ulcer that includes 45 to 60 minutes of wound and callus debridement will be reimbursed at a lower rate than a 15-minute procedure on a 22-cm^2 wound. Specific indications and limitations of coverage and medical necessity in general and guidelines specific to debridement CPT codes are listed verbatim in Table 21-1.

Medicare regulations related to electrical stimulation and pulsed electromagnetic field (see Table 21-1) require that a period of "appropriate standard wound care has been tried for at least 30 days and there are no measurable signs of healing." The phrase "appropriate standard wound care" is vague but implies that CMS has the right to deny coverage if the documentation does not support the expected level of care. Similarly, the phrase "no measurable signs of healing" is vague. Failure of wound dimensions to decrease is unlikely to satisfy requirements. The quality of the wound must also be considered. Documented evidence

of decreased bioburden, improved quality of surrounding skin, and wound bed within 30 days prior to initiation of electrical stimulation for wound healing is likely to lead to payment denial. Additionally, CMS will deny any claims for electrical stimulation once the wound bed is 100% re-epithelialized. Also, note that CMS will only cover electrical stimulation for chronic wounds, specified as "stage 3 and 4 pressure injuries, arterial ulcers, diabetic ulcers and venous stasis ulcers." Table 21-2 provides guidelines for documentation from CMS.

A list of CPT codes considered to be wound management is given in Table 21-3. New devices and technology are introduced every year that will claim to be the ultimate in wound healing. Clinicians must do their due diligence in understanding the technology and any research or evidence that supports it. Additionally, CMS may not cover many of these new technologies or may only cover them for very specific diagnoses, so again the clinician must investigate and understand the technology thoroughly before using it.

A large number of CPT codes are now available for cellular and/or tissue-based products. This number reflects the increasing technologic advancements and types of skin replacements. Different ranges of CPT codes are available for different combinations of living, nonliving, allografts, xenografts, and acellular matrix products. The use of these codes requires a physician to harvest the graft (as appropriate) and care for the donor site. The skin replacement/substitute application requires "surgical" fixation, which means a surgeon must do it. This fixation may include staples, sutures, or adhesives. The use of a wound dressing to hold the material in place does not meet the requirements for using the CPT codes. A range of CPT codes for each type of material is used to delineate the site and the skin substitute's size. When billing for application of these materials, concurrent billing for surgical debridement (11040-11042) or creation of a recipient site (15000) is not allowed because it is expected that wound bed preparation is done prior to placement of the skin substitute.

A trend for CMS is incorporating supplies necessary for performing a task into the payment for a given CPT code. This is termed *bundling*. When billing, one must be aware of what supplies are bundled. Billing for both the task and the supplies or individual tasks covered by a code is termed *unbundling*. The use of a code that pays a higher rate than the code that CMS considers appropriate for the level of care provided is termed *upcoding*. Both unbundling and upcoding are considered forms of fraud by CMS.

CMS requires a discount on procedures that are bilateral in nature. Specifically noted by CMS is the application of an Unna's boot (29580). Instead of paying double for an application of 2 Unna's boots (one on each leg), CMS pays 50% for the second procedure, and the modifier -50 is used to indicate bilateral application. Substantial documentation

TABLE 21-1
CMS Coverage Indications, Limitations, and/or Medical Necessity

This Local Coverage Determination (LCD) offers coverage indications and guidelines for wound care involving debridement; electrical stimulation and electromagnetic therapy; negative pressure wound therapy; low-frequency, noncontact, nonthermal ultrasound (MIST Therapy); and topical oxygen therapy (TOT).

For the purposes of this LCD, wound care is defined as care of wounds that are refractory to healing or have complicated healing cycles either because of the nature of the wound itself or because of complicating metabolic and/or physiological factors.

Active wound care procedures are performed to remove necrotic tissue and/or devitalized tissue to promote healing. Providers are responsible to determine medical necessity and use the appropriate current CPT/HCPCS code for service provided. Please consult the current AMA CPT book for the complete code description of the procedures being performed to submit claims.

This LCD supplements but does not replace, modify, or supersede existing Medicare-applicable National Coverage Determinations (NCDs) or payment policy rules and regulations for additional wound care. Federal statute and subsequent Medicare regulations regarding provision and payment for medical services are lengthy. They are not repeated in this LCD. Neither Medicare payment policy rules nor this LCD replace, modify, or supersede applicable state statutes regarding medical practice or other health practice professions acts, definitions, and/or scopes of practice. All providers who report services for Medicare payment must fully understand and follow all existing laws, regulations, and rules for Medicare payment for additional wound care sessions and must properly submit only valid claims for them. Please review and understand them and apply the medical necessity provisions in the policy within the context of the manual rules. Relevant CMS manual instructions and policies are provided in the CMS National Coverage Policy section.

This policy *does not* address metabolically active human skin equivalent/substitute dressings, burns, skin cancer or hyperbaric oxygen therapy.

DEBRIDEMENT

Debridement is defined as the removal of foreign material and/or devitalized or contaminated tissue from or adjacent to a traumatic or infected wound until surrounding healthy tissue is exposed. This LCD applies to debridement of localized areas such as wounds and ulcers. The mere removal of secretions, cleansing of a wound, does not represent a debridement service.

At least one of the following conditions must be present and documented:

- Pressure injury, stage 2, 3 or 4
- Venous or arterial insufficiency ulcers
- Dehiscenced wounds
- Wounds with exposed hardware or bone
- Neuropathic ulcers
- Neuroischemic ulcers
- Diabetic foot ulcer(s)
- Complications of surgically created or traumatic wound where accelerated granulation therapy is necessary that cannot be achieved by other available topical wound treatment.

Should deep tissue pressure injury or stage 2 injury progress to unstageable, stage 3, or stage 4 requiring debridement, then documentation supporting this must be included in the medical record.

(*continued*)

TABLE 21-1 (CONTINUED)

CMS Coverage Indications, Limitations, and/or Medical Necessity

GOALS OF DEBRIDEMENT
Remove devitalized tissue
Decrease risk of infection
Promote wound healing
Prevent further complications

DEBRIDEMENT MAY BE CATEGORIZED AS SELECTIVE OR NONSELECTIVE
Selective debridement refers to the removal of specific, targeted areas of devitalized or necrotic tissue from a wound along the margin of viable tissue. Occasional bleeding and pain may occur. The routine application of a topical or local anesthetic does not elevate active wound care management to surgical debridement. Selective debridement includes selective removal of necrotic tissue by sharp dissection including with scissors, scalpel, and forceps; and selective removal of necrotic tissue by high-pressure water jet. Selective debridement should only be done under the specific order of a physician.

Wound Care Nonselective Debridement Includes the Following:
• Surgical debridement is excision or wide resection of all necrotic or devitalized tissue, possibly including excision of the viable wound margin. This is usually carried out in the operating room by a surgeon. Anesthesia is usually required. It is frequently used for deep tissue infection, drainage of abscess or involved tendon sheath, or debridement of bone.
• Sharp debridement is the removal of necrotic or foreign material just above the level of viable tissue and is performed in an office setting or at the patient's bedside with or without the use of local anesthesia. Sharp debridement is less aggressive than surgical debridement but has the advantage of rapidly improving the healing conditions in the ulcer. These typically are the services of recurrent, superficial, or repeated wound care.
• Enzymatic debridement is debridement with topical enzymes used when the necrotic substances to be removed from a wound are protein, fiber, and collagen. The manufacturer's product insert contains indications, contraindications, precautions, dosage, and administration guidelines.
• Wet-to-moist dressing is used to keep the wound moist. This type of dressing is used to remove drainage and necrotic tissue from wounds.

Debridement of the wound(s), if indicated, must be performed judiciously and at appropriate intervals. Medicare expects that with appropriate care and no extenuating medical or surgical complications or setbacks, wound volume or surface dimensions should decrease over time or wounds optimally will demonstrate granulation tissue. Wounds that fail to demonstrate measurable reduction in size at 2 to 4 weeks despite appropriate therapy are unlikely to heal. There is also literature to support that a reduction of less than 40% for venous and less than 50% for diabetic ulcers at 4 weeks is an overall predictor of outcome for healing.
Medicare expects the wound care treatment plan to be modified in the event that appropriate healing is not achieved. Debridement should be performed by a health care professional acting within the scope of their legal authority.

Evidence of Improvement Includes Measurable Changes (Decreases) of Some of the Following:
Drainage (color, amount, consistency)
Inflammation
Swelling
Pain
Wound dimensions (diameter, depth, tunneling)
Necrotic tissue/slough

(continued)

TABLE 21-1 (CONTINUED)
CMS Coverage Indications, Limitations, and/or Medical Necessity

USE OF EVALUATION AND MANAGEMENT (E/M) CODES IN CONJUNCTION WITH DEBRIDEMENT(S)

Patients who have chronic wounds may frequently have underlying medical problems that require concomitant management in order to bring about wound closure. In addition, patients may require education, other services, and coordination of care both in the preoperative and postoperative phases of the debridement procedure. An E/M service provided and documented on the same day as a debridement service may be covered by Medicare only when the documentation clearly establishes the service as a "separately identifiable service" that was reasonable and necessary, as well as distinct, from the debridement service(s) provided.

BIOPHYSICAL AGENTS

Biophysical agents or modalities such as electrical stimulation; induced electrical stimulation; negative pressure wound therapy; hyperbaric oxygen; and noncontact, nonthermal ultrasound all add some form of energy to the wound bed to help drive the healing process forward, especially in the compromised tissues of patients who tend to get pressure injuries.

ELECTRICAL STIMULATION AND ELECTROMAGNETIC THERAPY

Please refer to CMS Publication 100-03, *Medicare National Coverage Determination Manual*, Chapter 1-Part 4, § 270.1 *Electrical Stimulation (ES) and Electromagnetic Therapy for the Treatment of Wounds*.

NEGATIVE PRESSURE WOUND THERAPY

Negative pressure wound therapy (NPWT), utilizing either durable or disposable medical equipment, involves the application of controlled or intermittent negative pressure to a properly dressed wound cavity. Suction (negative pressure) is applied under airtight wound dressings to promote the healing of open wounds *resistant to prior treatments*. Coverage of traditional NPWT (tNPWT) device/unit/type or supplies is under DME, and providers should consult their DME LCD for specific coverage, parameters, and guidelines.

LOW-FREQUENCY, NONCONTACT, NONTHERMAL ULTRASOUND (MIST THERAPY)

Low frequency, noncontact, nonthermal ultrasound is a system that uses continuous low-frequency ultrasonic energy to atomize a liquid and deliver continuous low-frequency ultrasound to the wound bed. This modality is often referred to as "MIST Therapy."

There should be documented improvements in the wound(s) evident after 6 MIST treatments.

Improvements include documented reduction in pain, necrotic tissue, or wound size or improved granulation tissue. Continuing MIST treatments for wounds demonstrating no improvement after 6 treatments is considered not reasonable and not necessary. No more than 18 services of MIST Therapy within a 6-week period will be considered reasonable and necessary. Also, MIST Therapy treatments would be separately billable if other active wound management and/or wound debridement is not performed.

TOPICAL OXYGEN THERAPY

Refer to Change Request (CR) 10220, *Hyperbaric Oxygen (HBO) Therapy, Section C, Topical Application of Oxygen*.

Reproduced from Centers for Medicare & Medicaid Services. Local Coverage Determination (LCD): Wound Care (L35125): General information. 2017. Accessed October 19, 2022. www.cms.gov/medicare-coverage-database/details/lcd-details.aspx?LCDId=35125

TABLE 21-2
CMS Documentation Guidelines

DOCUMENTATION

The medical record must clearly show that the criteria under Coverage Indications, Limitations, and/or Medical Necessity have been met. The medical record must include a certified plan of care containing a treatment plan with goals, physician follow-up, the expected frequency and duration of the skilled treatment, and the potential to heal. With continuation of a treatment plan, there needs to be ongoing evidence of the effectiveness of the plan, including diminishing area and depth of the ulceration, resolution of surrounding erythema and/or wound exudates, decreasing symptomatology, and overall assessment of wound status (such as stable, improved, worsening, etc) documented. Appropriate modification of treatment plan, when necessitated by failure of wounds to improve, must be demonstrated. The record must document complicating factors for wound healing as well as measures taken to control complicating factors when debridement is part of the plan. Medical records must be made available to Medicare on request.

The patient's medical record must contain clearly documented evidence of the progress of the wound's response to treatment at each visit. This documentation must include, at a minimum:

Current wound volume (surface dimensions and depth).

- Presence (and extent of) or absence of obvious signs of infection.
- Presence (and extent of) or absence of necrotic, devitalized, or nonviable tissue or other material in the wound that is expected to inhibit healing or promote adjacent tissue breakdown.

When debridement is reported, the debridement procedure notes should demonstrate tissue removal (ie, skin, full or partial thickness; subcutaneous tissue; muscle and/or bone), the method used to debride (eg, hydrostatic, sharp, abrasion, etc), and the character of the wound (including dimensions, description of necrotic material present, before and after debridement; and after debridement the description of tissue removed including amount in cm^2, degree of epithelialization, etc). Procedure notes should also include the severity of tissue destruction, undermining or tunneling, necrosis, infection, or evidence of reduced circulation.

When performing debridement of a single wound, report depth using the deepest level of tissue removed. In multiple wounds, sum the surface area of those wounds that are at the same depth, but do not combine sums from different depths. See current CPT book for coding guidance.

Active debridement must be performed under a treatment plan as any other therapy service, outlining specific goals, duration, frequency, modalities, an anticipated endpoint, and other pertinent factors as they may apply. Departure from this plan must be documented.

Documentation for debridement exceeding utilization guidelines must include a complete description of the wound, progress toward healing, complications that have delayed healing, and a projected number of additional treatments necessary.

Appropriate evaluation and management of contributory medical conditions or other factors affecting the course of wound healing (such as nutritional status or other predisposing conditions) should be addressed in the record at intervals consistent with the nature of the condition or factor.

Photographic documentation of wounds immediately before and after debridement is recommended for prolonged or repetitive debridement services and may be requested by this contractor for payment of claims.

When wound care is provided by the therapist, for both in- and outpatient wound care, the medical record is required to have the following documentation:

- Physician order(s) for therapy/wound care services and signed plan of treatment (also known as a *plan of care*) detailing treatment modalities for therapy/wound care services must be established as soon as possible or within 30 days.
- Initial evaluation of therapy/wound care services.
- Wound characteristics such as diameter, depth, color, presence of exudates, or necrotic.

(continued)

TABLE 21-2 (CONTINUED)
CMS Documentation Guidelines

- Previous wound care services administered including date and modalities of treatment.
- Every 10 days, progress notes to include current wound status, measurements (including size and depth), and the treatment provided.
- Description of instrument used for selective or sharp debridement (eg, forceps, scalpel, scissors, tweezers, high-pressure water jet, etc).
- Certification/recertification for therapy/wound care services.
- Actual minutes provided to support each timed service/HCPCS provided.

UTILIZATION GUIDELINES

Prolonged, repetitive debridement services require adequate documentation of complicating circumstances that reasonably necessitated additional services. The record must clearly document the failure of wounds to improve to support the medical necessity for removal of muscle and/or bone for complicated management of wounds.

Coverage of traditional negative pressure wound therapy (tNPWT) device/unit/type, or supplies is covered under the Durable Medical Equipment benefit (Social Security Act §1861(s)(6)), and providers should consult their DME LCD for specific coverage, parameters, and guidelines.

Negative pressure wound therapy only receives coverage when medical necessity continues to be met and there is documented evidence of clear benefit from the NPWT treatment already provided.

The number of debridements and NPWT for a wound within the context of a palliative treatment plan (ie, when wounds are not expected to heal or when patients are in an end-of-life situation) would be expected to be of a limited frequency and duration consistent with that of palliative care.

The extent and number of services provided should be medically necessary and reasonable based on the documented medical evaluation of the patient's condition, diagnosis, and plan.

Only when medical necessity continues to be met and there is documented evidence of clear benefit from the services provided should services be continued. When services are performed in excess of anticipated peer norms based on data analysis, the services may be subject to medical review.

SUMMARY OF EVIDENCE FROM COMMENT PERIOD (09/26/2019-11/10/2019)

Overall conclusions:

Included in this LCD are the revisions to add debridement for stage 2 pressure injuries, diabetic foot ulcers (DFU), and chronic nonpressure ulcers with severity limited to breakdown of the skin when biofilm or devitalization is present. It is clear, and never under reconsideration, that a standard treatment of wounds includes debridement of devitalized tissue including necrotic, infected, slough, debris, and tissue with abnormal granulation. Prior to the reconsideration, debridement was limited to stage 3 and 4 pressure injuries. The reconsideration requested the addition of stage 2, DFU (listed in addition to neuroischemic ulceration), and nonpressure wounds with limited skin breakdown.

Although literature directly discussing stage 2 pressure injury and the value of debridement may be limited, we accept the premise of the National Pressure Ulcer Advisory Panel stating "there is strong informed clinical consensus to support the role of debridement in wound bed preparation, despite the ethically understandable lack of randomized controlled trials directly comparing debridement to no debridement in human subjects." There is ample evidence demonstrating debridement of ulcers with biofilm or devitalized tissue, regardless of the stage. It is therefore reasonable and medically necessary, and considered the medically accepted standard of care, to treat with debridement. Biofilms and devitalized tissue can be found both on the surface and in deeper wounds. Accepting the premise that wounds with biofilms and devitalized tissue require debridement, it is then accepted that stage 2 pressure injury and nonpressure wounds with limited skin breakdown may require debridement for proper wound healing.

(continued)

TABLE 21-2 (CONTINUED)
CMS Documentation Guidelines

It has been and continues to be accepted that DFU require debridement as part of standard wound healing practices. Prior to this reconsideration request, DFU were categorized as part of neuroischemic ulcerations, understanding the mechanism of most diabetic wounds arise from a vascular or neurologic etiology. The request in the reconsideration was to specifically add DFU for coverage. The reviewed literature and comments support evidence for diabetic foot wounds with an etiology other than neurological or ischemic injury. Such other causes include deformity, limited ankle range of motion, high plantar foot pressures, minor trauma, previous ulceration or amputation, and visual impairment. Evidence has shown that debridement of diabetic foot ulcers enhances the healing process when combined with standard wound care for a diabetic foot ulcer. Accepting that not all DFU are neuroischemic and continuing to accept that debridement is an important part of the wound treatment, the LCD has been changed to specifically identify DFU for coverage independent of neurological and ischemic injuries.

Reproduced from Centers for Medicare & Medicaid Services. Local Coverage Determination (LCD): Wound Care (L35125): General information. 2017. Accessed October 19, 2022. www.cms.gov/medicare-coverage-database/details/lcd-details.aspx?LCDId=35125

TABLE 21-3
CPT Codes Relevant to Wound Management

29445	Application of a cast
29581	Multilayer compression below knee
29582	Multilayer compression above knee
97610	Low-frequency, noncontact ultrasound
97597	Pertains to excisional debridement using either high-pressure water jet with or without suction or sharp instruments. This includes topical applications, wound assessment, instructions for ongoing care (patient education). Any use of whirlpool is bundled in the charge. This provides payment for the first 20 cm^2.
97598	Code added to receive payment for each additional 20 cm^2
97602	Code used for nonselective debridement without anesthesia. Examples provided include wet-to-moist dressings, enzymatic debridement, abrasion, and larva therapy. This also includes any topical applications and instructions for ongoing care.
97605	Code used for negative pressure of wound therapy wounds < 50 cm^2 of using reusable equipment. It also includes patient education and topical applications.
97606	Code used in place of 97605 for wounds > 50 cm^2
97607	Code used for wounds ≤ 50 cm^2 using disposable, nondurable equipment
97608	Code used in place of 97607 for wounds > 50 cm^2
G0239	Electromagnetic therapy for pressure, diabetic, venous, and arterial ulcers
G0281	Unattended electrical stimulation for pressure, diabetic, venous, and arterial ulcers
G0282	Unattended electrical stimulation for wounds other than listed above

Codes 11042 to 11047 are used for surgical debridement (incisional debridement). 11042 applies to subcutaneous tissue, 11043 refers to muscle and/or fascia, and 11044 refers to bone, all for the first 20 cm^2. 11045 is used with additional increments of 20 cm^2.

CPT® is a trademark of the American Medical Association. Current Procedural Terminology © 2017 American Medical Association. All rights reserved. The descriptions appearing in this publication are the acceptable short versions. Please consult an official CPT publication for complete descriptions.

of the need for 2 separate applications on different days might be acceptable once (eg, a venous disease diagnosis on the second leg was made later). Subsequent visits would require bilateral application whenever medically feasible.

Outpatient or home services performed under a physician's supervision fall under the "incident-to" rule. The incident-to rule applies to Part B of Medicare and is paid to the physician as if the physician were performing the care. This rule does not apply to inpatient hospitals, skilled nursing facilities, and hospital outpatient departments. The incident-to rule requires that the services rendered are "integral" parts of the physician's professional service, a normal part of the patient's plan of care, the physician performs the initial service, and the physician remains actively involved in the patient's care. These requirements imply that the incident-to services are rendered on an established patient with an established plan of care in place. Services provided by nonphysicians under this rule must be those that either are commonly not billed individually or are billed under the physician's charges, such as dressing changes and application of enzymatic debriders that would otherwise be performed by the physician as part of the charge. Those allowed to perform "incident-to" services must be considered the physician's employees, whether directly employed or contracting with the physician. The relationship between the person rendering the incident-to services and the physician must be part of the documentation. The physician must be nearby (eg, in the same office suite) but does not need to be present in the room where treatment is being provided. In addition, individual nonphysicians working for physicians may bill under their own National Provider Identifier (NPI) for services within their scopes of practice under specific circumstances. These services must be those that would be payable to a physician for the same service, the provider must have their own NPI, and state laws/regulations must be met. If these conditions are met, the physician is not required to be present. However, CMS pays at a lower rate if the nonphysician's NPI is used for billing.

Although Medicare covers a large portion of expensive technology and supplies to facilitate wound healing, copayments for office visits, procedures, and supplies obtained from DME suppliers are required. Copayments for expensive dressings and procedures may discourage the patient or clinician from using them. Not collecting the copayment as an incentive for the patient to utilize services is not allowable; both clinics and DME suppliers are required to "make every effort" to collect copayments. Failure to do so can result in punitive action from CMS, which could include decreased payments, suspension from participating in CMS programs, or even exclusion. Higher copayments must be considered during treatment planning. Patients may be willing to incur costlier copayments per visit if they

can heal more rapidly and save money compared with a more protracted course of treatment. Clinicians may also suggest that patients obtain secondary insurance to cover the 20% Medicare does not pay. In addition to copayments, clinicians must consider the possibility of capped benefits. Patients will be required to pay for services that exceed capped amounts. Congress has required CMS to cap therapy services, but this was removed in 2018. Although caps on services by CMS have been removed, clinicians must be mindful of caps imposed by private insurers for patients with coverage other than Medicare or Medicaid.

ICD-10 CODES

A limited number of *International Classification of Diseases, 10th Revision, Clinical Modification* (ICD-10-CM) codes may be used for the patient's diagnosis to receive reimbursement under debridement codes. New 2019 ICD-10 codes for wound care came into effect on October 1, 2018. Software is used to determine whether the CPT codes used for billing are appropriate given the ICD-10 code used for a patient's diagnosis. If an appropriate ICD-10 code is not present, automatic denial of claims will occur for CPT codes 11042, 11043, 11044, 16020, 16025, 16030, 97597, 97598, 97605, and 97606. With the development of ICD-10, many new codes were added for wounds, which allows for a more specific description of wounds. For example, ICD-9 code 891.0, Open wound of knee, leg [except thigh], and ankle, without mention of complication is now much more detailed in ICD-10, breaking it down into S81.009A, Unspecified open wound, unspecified knee, initial encounter; S81.809A, Unspecified open wound, unspecified lower leg, initial encounter; or S91.0091, Unspecified open wound, unspecified ankle, initial encounter. To be even more correct, one should specify left vs right to decrease the risk of denial. Also, one should specify initial encounter with an A, subsequent encounter with a D, or sequela encounter with an S. Sequela is "used for complications or conditions that arise as a result of a condition, such as scar formation after a burn."

Other allowable diagnoses for payment under CPT codes related to wound management are gas gangrene, atherosclerosis of the "native arteries of the extremities," lower extremity venous disease, skin infection, necrotizing fasciitis, and gangrene. More restrictive codes must accompany claims for physical therapy evaluation. Acceptable ICD-10 codes for reimbursement of the physical therapy evaluation to occur along with payment for selective debridement include burns (second or third degree), pressure injuries, and chronic ulcers of the lower extremities.

MEETING MEDICARE DOCUMENTATION REQUIREMENTS FOR REIMBURSEMENT

Based on current regulations, 3 key items are needed to satisfy Medicare requirements for documentation: medical necessity, progress, and progress relative to the resources used. The first item to document is whether the patient's condition justifies the level of care given. The patient's condition(s), including any complicating factors that weigh in intervention choice, should be included. In addition to documenting the need, the documentation should support the intervention(s) based on what is likely to occur if the intervention is not done, that the appropriate person is carrying out the intervention, and the likelihood of the intervention being successful. For example, a necrotic wound that is either infected or at risk for infection justifies the intervention of sharp debridement by a physical therapist, advanced practice nurse, podiatrist, or physician. The risks of spreading infection, failure to heal, and possible amputation should also be discussed. Moreover, suppose more frequent outpatient visits are needed due to the patient's or patient's caregivers limited ability to care for the wound. In that case, documentation should be provided to support the greater number of visits. The addition of electrical stimulation needs to be supported by documented lack of healing despite appropriate wound management for a minimum of 30 days.

The second item to document is how well the patient is responding to the intervention. Patient response to treatment needs to be described in progress reports. A brief mention that the patient is responding well to treatment is not sufficient. The documented progress should be related directly to the desired outcomes or goals listed on the initial evaluation. The documentation should indicate objective measures of improvement, including removing necrotic tissue, wound bed appearance, drainage, and wound dimensions. Descriptions indicating improved healing or potential for healing, such as improving the surrounding skin, may be necessary. Simple wound measurements may not be sufficient to capture the true improvement in a wound's condition, especially early in the treatment plan, because wounds may actually increase in size with debridement.

The third item to document is whether the resources used are appropriate for the progress observed. If the treatment plan fails to produce progress, explaining why this happened and steps to overcome impediments, including a change in the treatment plan, need to be documented. For example, if the patient is unable or unwilling to perform required dressing changes or compression therapy, a brief narrative explaining complications and defining a new course needs to be written. All 3 of these issues will be supported more readily by photographic documentation. Exact wording for Medicare documentation requirements is given in Table 21-2.

By today's standards, the ability to bill CMS for services requires a computerized billing system and individuals trained in using the software. For example, billing regulations from an outpatient clinic require the entry of several codes to describe the service performed. Other codes used for billing when services are provided in a hospital outpatient setting under the outpatient prospective payment system include therapy revenue codes to receive payment under the Medicare Physician Fee Schedule. Software termed the Integrated Outpatient Code Editor, regulated by CMS, then determines the appropriate Ambulatory Payment Classification.

Dressings and Topical Medications

Under Ambulatory Payment Classification rules, the cost of any dressings or topical agents used is bundled into the payment for the procedure performed. If the patient has received any dressings or medications for home use, these are not to be used for outpatient therapy. Additionally, the use of free samples distributed to a clinic is not allowed.

Although dressing changes themselves are not billable because this is not a skilled service, dressing materials, as well as chemical debriders for patients to use at home, are billed under the appropriate HCPCS code. Under Medicare Part B, surgical/wound dressings (primary and secondary) are covered under specific criteria—the dressings are medically necessary for treating a wound caused by or treated by a surgical procedure or when debridement of a wound is medically necessary. Dressings are not covered for stage 1 pressure injuries or first-degree (superficial) burns. No payment is given for skin sealants or barriers, skin cleansers, or irrigating solutions or solutions used to moisten gauze, topical antiseptics and topical antibiotics, or enzymatic debriding agents. Orders must be signed by a health care practitioner (see previous discussion) with the type of dressing, size, the number used each time, frequency of dressing change, and expected duration. New orders are required if a new dressing is added and if the quantity increases. A new order is also required every 3 months for each dressing used. DMERC (durable medical equipment regional carrier) regulations provide utilization guides; therefore, dressing change frequency should match these guidelines when ordered. The guidelines are listed in Chapter 16. You should consult your DMERC for current DMERC guidelines.

An issue determined by CMS relates to the use of silver or honey dressings. CMS has ruled that coding for silver or honey dressings will be based on the dressing materials and features as they would be for any other dressing regardless of the presence of silver or honey. Therefore, dressings must be billed to the DMERC based on the existing HCPCS code definitions. More expensive dressings with other components may not be cost-effective because CMS will not pay for them. However, if they accelerate healing, it is prudent and ethical to use the more expensive dressings.

"PRESENT ON ADMISSION" AND TAG F-314

New regulations have been developed to motivate health care facilities to reduce costs. In 2007, CMS determined that they would no longer pay for any additional costs due to specific complications occurring during hospitalization. These include infections associated with bladder catheterization, vascular access, and median sternotomy. Other problems included in this directive are blood incompatibility, air embolism, falls, pressure injuries, and objects left in a patient's body after surgery. Of particular interest is the need to document any pressure injuries present within 48 hours of admission to a facility. CMS will not pay costs associated with the development of pressure injuries not documented as present within this 48-hour time span. The regulation specific to pressure injuries is labeled F-314 by CMS for long-term care facilities. Specifically, it states, "Based on the Comprehensive Assessment of a resident, the facility must: a) ensure that a resident that enters the facility without pressure sores does not develop pressure sores unless the individual's clinical condition demonstrates that they were unavoidable; b) promote the prevention of pressure ulcer development; c) promote the healing of pressure ulcers that are present (including prevention of infection to the extent possible); and d) prevent the development of additional pressure ulcers."

COST-EFFECTIVENESS

This topic is often uncomfortable for clinicians and a seemingly endless battleground between clinicians and administrators. However, several studies have indicated that optimal wound care is often more cost-effective than lower cost-per-visit alternatives.[1] For example, Bolton et al[1] showed a range of 53% to 615% greater care costs to use gauze dressings on various types of ulcers compared with clinically more prudent choices of hydrocolloid dressings (see Table 4 in Bolton et al article). Frequently, the argument for a given type of intervention is based on the cost of materials and not the cost of labor or the likelihood of attaining goals set for the intervention. The cost of a single

application of gauze is much less than a hydrocolloid sheet, but the cost of applying gauze to a wound 3 to 4 times daily for 5 days is much greater than the single application of a hydrocolloid sheet. Even the cost of materials thought to be cheaper can become much greater depending on the frequency of dressing changes and the quantity of gauze used for each dressing change. Second, the larger picture of direct and indirect costs of wound care needs to be analyzed for the different options. Direct costs include the materials for primary and secondary dressings; materials used for wound cleansing, debridement, and dressing change such as bottles of saline, additional gauze, gloves, gowns, masks, shoe covers, and tape; and labor involved in these activities, including the cost of setting up and cleaning, especially when considering whirlpool therapy. Large quantities of water, the cost of filling tanks, disinfecting tanks, and quality checks on infection control can become very high relative to other wound management aspects. Other equipment may include pressure relief/reducing devices, operating room time, surgical procedures, and pharmacy. Potential indirect costs include prolonged treatment (increased inpatient days and increased home health or outpatient visits), loss of days of work by the patient, treatment of complications of slower healing, costs of waste disposal driven higher by more frequent dressing changes, and the potential for litigation if a suboptimal plan is followed. One common example is the comparison of whirlpool therapy with pulsed lavage. Although the cost for materials for pulsatile lavage is greater than whirlpool, the much greater cost in clinician's time and possibly slower achievement of the same outcome can make whirlpool therapy much more expensive.

Another example is the provision of sharp debridement. One visit for sharp debridement may be more expensive than a single visit for hydrotherapy for debridement, but the faster outcome from sharp debridement can make the cost per outcome achieved much lower for selective sharp debridement compared with using hydrotherapy and disposable or sterilizable instruments to remove small amounts of necrotic tissue over several days. Although each clinical unit must make its own decisions regarding the cost-effectiveness of treatments, the issue of quality of life must be considered along with the more typical issues of decreased wound size, pain relief, debridement, and risk frequency of infection.

WOUND MANAGEMENT TEAMS

Successful management of patients with wounds, especially those managed under DRGs, requires coordination, communication, and cooperation. Teams in an acute care facility typically consist of a physician, physical therapist, clinical dietitian, and wound ostomy continence nurse. Some facilities may include occupational therapists and other personnel, such as nursing aides or patient care assistants. These individuals are integral to the team because they tend to see the patient most frequently and assist with toileting, personal hygiene, and repositioning. Each individual on the team plays an important role due to the individual's unique training within their discipline and the individual's experience. The key to success is to determine ahead of time what responsibilities each member of the team will have. Waiting until the program is under way to assign responsibilities is likely to create hard feelings within the group, perhaps creating a siege mentality and dividing the group. Members need to clearly elaborate what their individual skills are and the patient populations with which the individual clinician is familiar. Flowcharts designed from this information allow each clinician to determine the next step in the sequence and refer, when necessary, to a different discipline.

A common pitfall is the assumption of hierarchical knowledge within the team. One individual is unlikely to have all of the knowledge and skills of the other clinicians. Optimal staffing would include a sufficient number of clinicians of different disciplines and specialization, so any given patient could be seen by a member or combination of members of the wound care team with the appropriate knowledge and skills for each situation. Therefore, any patient would receive all of the necessary evaluations, education, and direct interventions leading to optimal care. A team is likely to have several members who have substantially overlapping knowledge or abilities, along with a smaller number with highly specialized skills.

Every team requires a leader to be functional. The team leader is not necessarily a physician but should be a person with the vision, passion, commitment, and interpersonal skills necessary for the team to be functional. In many clinics, the team leader is a physical therapist, nurse, or dietitian who has the respect of the other team members and other key leaders of the facility. This person is most likely the one who recognizes how to weed out inefficiency and improve patient satisfaction without creating a stressful environment. A preliminary team representing typical disciplines needs to be assembled, and the perceived roles of members of each discipline need to be shared with the other members. Often members of one discipline understand very little of the training and experience of other members. Preliminary flowcharts identifying each member of the wound care team's roles should be designed by a small number of members of the team and submitted for approval by the team as a whole. Attempts to design flowcharts by the entire team are unlikely to be fruitful. A subgroup of more than 4 to 5 individuals is likely to bog down on details, whereas a group smaller than 3 is likely to miss details. Sharing the work of the subgroup with the entire development team is used to improve the product.

Turf battles may still arise; therefore, one of the first agenda items on such committees is a series of team-building exercises and establishment of rules of conduct for the meetings. Agreeing to a consensus process as opposed to a majority process may improve the group's workings as well. When a flowchart is developed, a review of previous cases or hypothetical ("paper") patients can be used to identify any modifications needed. Several rounds of this exercise may be necessary to fine-tune the processes of the team.

In putting the actual team together, team leaders must recognize that the presence of too many or too few members from a given discipline can create an unhealthy environment and the destructive nature of the development of cliques. Any perception of a subgroup of the team "ganging up" will quickly destroy objectivity and undermine any trust built within the group. Meetings of the development committee need to be scheduled regularly with an optimal interval. Often weekly meetings are used. This time allows individual work to be accomplished between meetings and meaningful reflection to occur. Longer intervals cause members to lose focus and for other events to take precedence over the committee's work. In any environment, but especially in a DRG environment such as acute care hospitals in which the team's effectiveness may determine the length of stay, the team's cost-effectiveness is important. Generally, the DRG environment encourages facilities to discharge patients as rapidly as possible, which may require continued care following discharge. Lack of coordination of patient care and waiting for orders to be written may delay discharge or result in premature patient discharge. Often continued care is necessary in the form of home health, outpatient physical therapy, or inpatient rehabilitation.

For this reason, case managers should be members of the team. Having a wound care team in place with autonomy is more likely to result in a timely and appropriate care level. In facilities without well-defined teams, conflicts are common. Individual physicians may write orders for outdated, inappropriate, or inefficient treatment plans. When approached about revising their orders, some physicians may become defensive or hostile. Conflicts may also arise from the multiplicity of physicians involved with individual patients. A primary care physician, general surgeon, orthopedic surgeon, endocrinologist, infectious disease specialist, internal medicine specialist, and others may be involved in the care of a patient with a wound. Without the wound care team's authority to manage the patient's wounds, different physicians may write conflicting plans, or none of the physicians may actually take responsibility for the wounds. Therefore, all physicians involved with patients with wounds must be willing to refer patients to the team without any micromanagement. The referring physician's input is important to the team's ability to develop and execute a plan of care. However, they must be free of constraints placed on them by individual physicians.

SUMMARY

The execution of a plan of care must consider several nonpatient issues including legal limits on personnel performing services, CMS regulations, and the payment provided by CMS and other payers for services. CMS rules are tremendously complex with a seemingly endless list of acronyms applied to different types of facilities and providers. Billing CMS for services requires a working knowledge of the most current ICD and CPT codes, dedicated software, and personnel. One must learn what is included in CPT codes and whether CMS considers the service provided under the CPT code as medically necessary for a given ICD code. Failure to utilize codes correctly could result in unbundling and upcoding, which can then lead to punitive action by CMS. CMS services are contracted to several private companies with employees who may interpret CMS regulations differently. A good working relationship with the contractor can greatly reduce the possibility of denial of payments. CMS contractors and health care service providers can work together to ensure that patients receive the most appropriate care and that fair reimbursement is paid. Cost-effectiveness of care and development of wound care teams are necessary to optimize care and fiscal responsibility. Cultures of individual facilities can undermine wound care teams' autonomy and disrupt morale to the point of the team disbanding. Overcoming a facility's culture can become an overwhelming task, requiring a strong leader with support from the facility's highest administration levels for patients to receive optimum care.

QUESTIONS

1. Who determines which interventions a physical therapist is permitted to perform?

2. In most states, which professionals are allowed to perform sharp debridement based on their licenses alone?

3. Does a physical therapy license allow sharp debridement in your state or other states where you might practice?

4. What is the implication of the American Physical Therapy Association's position statement regarding physical therapy assistants performing sharp debridement?

5. Who may provide a referral for wound management by a physical therapist?

6. In acute care, what is the basis for payment in general?

7. In acute care, how is payment for wound management provided?

8. What is the implication of using more expensive interventions in acute care?

9. In an outpatient setting, what aspects of wound management will be paid?

10. What is the basis for payment in outpatient care?

11. In outpatient physical therapy, what is the implication of using more expensive interventions?

12. In which setting can more expensive interventions be paid at a greater rate?

13. Under what circumstances can a physical therapist be paid for wound interventions beyond debridement and modalities?

14. Under what circumstances are dressing changes billable?

15. What types of payments are available to physicians in a freestanding clinic?

16. Under what circumstance are these payments available to physical therapists?

REFERENCE

1. Bolton LL, van Rijswijk L, Shaffer FA. Quality wound care equals cost-effective wound care: a clinical model. *Adv Wound Care.* 1997;10(4):33-38.

BIBLIOGRAPHY

Centers for Medicare & Medicaid Services. Local Coverage Determination (LCD): Wound Care (L35125): General information. 2017. Accessed October 19, 2022. www.cms.gov/medicare-coverage-database/details/lcd-details.aspx?LCDId=35125

de Leon J, Bohn GA, DiDomenico L, et al. Wound care centers: critical thinking and treatment strategies for wounds. *Wounds.* 2016;28(10):S1-S23.

Demiralp B, Soltoff S, Koenig L. Hospital patients with severe wounds: early evidence on the impact of Medicare payment changes on treatment patterns and outcomes. *J Med Econ.* 2019;22(3):266-272. doi:10.1080/13696998.2018.1559599

Fife CE, Walker D, Farrow W, Otto G. Wound center facility billing: a retrospective analysis of time, wound size, and acuity scoring for determining facility level of service. *Ostomy Wound Manage.* 2007;53(1):34-44.

Nussbaum SR, Carter MJ, Fife CE, et al. An economic evaluation of the impact, cost, and Medicare policy implications of chronic nonhealing wounds. *Value Health.* 2018;21(1):27-32. doi:10.1016/j.jval.2017.07.007

WOUND CARE RESOURCES

Organizations

- Alliance of Wound Care Stakeholders: https://www.woundcarestakeholders.org/
- APTA Section on Clinical Electrophysiology and Wound Management: http://www.aptasce-wm.org/
- American Professional Wound Care Association (APWCA): http://www.apwca.org/
- Amputee Coalition of America: http://www.amputee-coalition.org/
- Association for the Advancement of Wound Care (AAWC): https://aawconline.memberclicks.net/
- National Pressure Injury Advisory Panel (NPIAP): http://www.npiap.com
- Undersea & Hyperbaric Medical Society (UHMS): http://uhms.org/
- Wound, Ostomy and Continence Nurses Society: http://www.wocn.org/
- Wound Healing Society: http://woundheal.org/

Certifications

- American Board of Physical Therapy Specialties: https://specialization.apta.org/become-a-specialist/wound-management
- American Board of Wound Management: https://abwmcertified.org (multidisciplinary accreditation in wound management)
- National Alliance of Wound Care (NAWC): http://www.nawccb.org/ (national wound care credentialing).
- Wound Care Plus: https://mywoundcareplus.com/ (education and certification in wound care).
- Wound Ostomy Continence Nursing Certification Board (WOCNCB): http://www.wocncb.org/

Educational Meetings

- Symposium for Advanced Wound Care: http://www.sawc.net/ (official meeting site for the AAWC)
- European Wound Management Association: https://ewma.org

Journals

- *Advances in Skin & Wound Care* (Lippincott Williams & Wilkins): http://www.woundcarejournal.com/
- *American Journal of Infection Control*: www.apic.org
- *Journal of the American Podiatric Medical Association*: http://www.japmaonline.org
- *Journal of Wound Care*: http://www.journalofwound-care.com/
- *Journal of WOCN*: www.jwocnonline.com
- *Open Access Journal of Plastic Surgery*: http://www.eplasty.com/
- *Podiatry Today*: www.podiatrytoday.com
- *Wound Repair and Regeneration*: https://onlinelibrary.wiley.com/journal/1524475x
- *Wounds*: www.woundsresearch.com

Educational Websites

- APTA Evidence-Based Resources: https://www.apta.org/patient-care/evidence-based-practice-resources
- Lab Tests Online: http://www.labtestsonline.org/ (information on interpretation of lab test results and listing of lab tests appropriate for given conditions)
- National Guideline Clearinghouse: http://www.guide-lines.gov/ (searchable database of clinical guidelines, including those related to skin and wound care)
- RxList. The Internet Drug Index: https://www.rxlist.com
- Worldwide Wounds: http://www.worldwidewounds.com/
- Wound Care Education Institute: https://www.wcei.net/
- Wound Care Learning Network: https://www.hmpgloballearningnetwork.com/site/woundcare
- Wound Management & Prevention: https://www.hmpgloballearningnetwork.com/site/wmp

INDEX